T0261539

INTERNATIONAL REVIEW OF CHILD NEUROLOGY SERIES

NEURODEVELOPMENTAL DISABILITIES: CLINICAL AND SCIENTIFIC FOUNDATIONS

Edited by

Michael Shevell

Editor: Hilary M. Hart
Managing Director, Mac Keith Press: Caroline Black
Project Manager: Mirjana Misina
Indexer: Susan Boobis

First published in this edition 2009 by
Mac Keith Press, 6 Market Road, London N7 9PW, UK
British Library Cataloguing-in-Publication data

A catalogue record of this book is available from the British Library

ISBN: 978-1-898683-70-4 (hardback)
ISBN: 978-1-898683-67-4 (paperback)

Typeset by Graphicraft Limited, Hong Kong
Printed by The Lavenham Press Ltd., Water Street, Lavenham, Suffolk, UK

Cover image: Axial T2-weighted image of an infant at 26 weeks gestational age. Superimposed on the image are lines representing the direction of greatest water diffusion for each voxel (orientation of the principal eigenvector). See Chapter 9, Figure 3.

INTERNATIONAL REVIEW OF CHILD NEUROLOGY SERIES

NEURODEVELOPMENTAL DISABILITIES: CLINICAL AND SCIENTIFIC FOUNDATIONS

Edited by

MICHAEL SHEVELL

Montreal Children's Hospital, Quebec, Canada

2009
MAC KEITH PRESS
for the
INTERNATIONAL CHILD NEUROLOGY ASSOCIATION

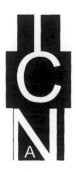

INTERNATIONAL REVIEW OF CHILD NEUROLOGY SERIES

CONTENTS

AUTHORS' APPOINTMENTS

Stephen Ashwal — Distinguished Professor of Pediatrics, Chair, Division of Pediatric Neurology, Department of Pediatrics, Loma Linda University School of Medicine, Loma Linda, California

François Bolduc — Assistant Professor, Department of Pediatrics, University of Alberta, Stollery Children's Hospital, Edmonton, Canada

Sara S Cathey — Clinical Geneticist, Greenwood Genetic Center, North Charleston, South Carolina

Brian R Christie — Michael Smith Senior Scholar, Division of Medical Sciences and The Island Medical Program, University of Victoria, Victoria, Canada, Cellular and Physiological Sciences, University of British Columbia, Vancouver Canada

David L Coulter — Associate Professor of Neurology, Harvard Medical School, Department of Neurology, Children's Hospital Boston, Boston, Massachusetts

Johanna Darrah — Professor, Faculty of Rehabilitation Medicine, University of Alberta, Edmonton, Alberta

Carolyn Drews-Botsch — Emory University School of Public Health, Atlanta, Georgia

Adré du Plessis — Fetal Neonatal Neurology Program, Department of Neurology, Harvard Medical School, Boston, Massachusetts

Brennan D Eadie — Division of Medical Sciences and The Island Medical Program, University of Victoria, Victoria, Canada, Cellular and Physiological Sciences, Faculty of Medicine, University of British Columbia, Vancouver, Canada

Carl Ernst — Department of Psychology, University of British Columbia, Vancouver, BC

Frances Page Glascoe — Adjunct Professor of Pediatrics, Vanderbilt University, Nashville, Tennessee

Pierre Gressens — Director, Inserm, Hopital Robert Debre, Paris, France

Sally Hartley — Professor of Communication and Health, University of East Anglia, Norwich, United Kingdom

Kenton R Holden   Professor, Departments of Neurosciences and Pediatrics, Medical University of South Carolina, Charleston, South Carolina, Greenwood Genetic Center, North Charleston, South Carolina

Terrie Inder   Associate Professor, Departments of Pediatrics, Neurology & Radiology, Washington University, St Louis Children's Hospital, St Louis, Missouri

Michael V Johnston   Kennedy Krieger Institute and Departments of Neurology, Pediatrics and Physical Medicine and Rehabilitation, Johns Hopkins University School of Medicine, Baltimore, Maryland

David A Kube   Associate Professor of Pediatrics, University of Tennessee Health Science Center, UT Boling Center for Developmental Disabilities, Memphis, Tennessee

Catherine Limperopoulos   School of Physical & Occupational Therapy, Departments of Neurology/Neurosurgery and Pediatrics, McGill University, Montreal Children's Hospital-McGill University Health Centre, Montreal, Canada

Annette Majnemer   Professor, School of Physical & Occupational Therapy, McGill University, Montreal, Canada

Elysa J Marco   Assistant Professor, Department of Neurology, University of California San Francisco, San Francisco, California

Kevin P. Marks   General Practitioner and Clinical Assistant Professor, Peace Health Medical Group, Eugene, Oregon and Oregon Health and Science University School of Medicine, Department of General Pediatrics, Portland, Oregon

Barbara Mazer   Assistant Professor, School of Physical & Occupational Therapy, McGill University, Montreal, Canada

David J Michelson   Assistant Professor of Pediatrics, Division of Pediatric Neurology, Department of Pediatrics, Loma Linda University School of Medicine, Loma Linda, California

Michael E Msall   Professor of Pediatrics, University of Chicago Pritzker School of Medicine, Kennedy Research Center on Intellectual and Developmental Disabilities, Section of Development and Behavioral Pediatrics, Comer and LaRabida Children's Hospitals, Chicago, Illinois

Jeff Neil   Green Professor of Neurology, Pediatrics and Radiology, Washington University, St. Louis, Missouri

Charles RJC Newton   Professor of Tropical Neurosciences and Paediatrics, Institute of Child Health, University College London, London, United Kingdom

Frederick B Palmer	Shainberg Professor of Pediatrics, University of Tennessee Health Science Center, Director-UT Boling Center for Developmental Disabilities, Memphis, Tennessee
Jennifer J Park	University of Chicago Pritzker School of Medicine, Kennedy Research Center on Intellectual and Developmental Disabilities, Section of Developmental and Behavioral Pediatrics, Comer and LaRabida Children's Hospitals, Chicago, Illinois
Sheryl L Rimrodt	Department of Developmental Cognitive Neurology, Kennedy Krieger Institute and Department of Pediatrics, Johns Hopkins University School of Medicine, Baltimore, Maryland
Elliott H Sherr	Director, Brain Development Research Program, Department of Neurology, University of California, San Francisco, San Francisco, California
Michael Shevell	Professor, Departments of Neurology/Neurosurgery & Pediatrics, McGill University, Division of Pediatric Neurology, Montreal Children's Hospital-McGill University Health Centre, Montreal, Canada
Myriam Srour	Fellow in Neurogenetics, Hôpital Notre-Dame, Université de Montréal, Montreal, Canada
Andrea K Titterness	Division of Medical Sciences and The Island Medical Program, University of Victoria, Victoria, Canada, Neuroscience Program, University of British Columbia, Vancouver, Canada
Tim Tully	Cold Spring Harbor Laboratory, Cold Spring Harbor, New York
Cristina O Vasuta	Department of Psychiatry, Faculty of Medicine, University of British Columbia, Vancouver, Canada
Alina J Webber	Cellular and Physiological Sciences, Faculty of Medicine, University of British Columbia, Vancouver, Canada
Richard I Webster	TY Nelson Departments of Neurology and Neurosurgery, Children's Hospital at Westmead, Sydney University, Sydney NSW, Australia
Jerome Y Yager	Professor and Head, Section of Pediatric Neurosciences, Stollery Children's Hospital, University of Alberta, Edmonton, Alberta
Marshalyn Yeargin-Allsopp	National Center on Birth Defects and Developmental Disabilities, Centers for Disease Control and Prevention, Atlanta, Georgia

PREFACE

A common problem in child health, neurodevelopmental disabilities are a core and essential feature in the practice of the clinical pediatric neurosciences. Despite these disorders being common and challenging, it is rare to encounter a book that comprehensively deals with the various aspects of these particular clinical problems. Substantial recent advances in genetics, molecular biology and imaging, as well as in the rehabilitation sciences, have added much in recent years to our understanding and treatment of these particular disorders.

I am particularly pleased that the International Child Neurology Association and Mac Keith Press have chosen to devote this year's book of the International Review of Child Neurology Series to this particular topic. The responsibility for co-ordinating this multi-author effort was taken seriously by myself and I am grateful for the confidence shown in me in undertaking this matter by the International Child Neurology Association.

I owe thanks to a number of individuals for this effort and I would be remiss if these were not mentioned at the very onset.

All of the contributing authors were a pleasure to work with and each brought their own personal perspective and high level of accomplishment in their particular field to addressing varying aspects of neurodevelopmental disabilities. I have very much appreciated the ongoing support during the preparation of this particular book of the supervising editor of the International Review of Child Neurology Series, Dr Charles Newton.

I owe individual thanks to my teachers in child neurology and genetics who have inspired me to achieve in this most interesting and challenging of subspecialties. These teachers have included Drs Gordon Watters, Bernard Rosenblatt, Kenneth Silver, Frederick Andermann and David Rosenblatt. Over the years, I have been blessed by a number of terrific pediatric neurology residents and fellows who, through my teaching of neurology, have also inspired me to continue to ask questions and to learn. My current colleagues at the Montreal Children's Hospital-McGill University Health Centre (Drs Bernard Rosenblatt, Chantal Poulin, Marie-Emmanuelle Dilenge and Alison Moore) have provided me with a warm and nurturing work environment that enables me to undertake much in the way of extra-curricular efforts.

Much of the administrative and secretarial work pertaining to this particular book has been undertaken by Alba Rinaldi, and to her unflagging efforts great thanks are due by myself.

I would also like to single out my daughters, Allison and Meaghan, who have been and continue to be the best course in normal child and adolescent development that any father could ask for.

Finally and most importantly, I must give thanks to Annette Majnemer, my partner in so many things in life, who has taught me and inspired me throughout her own career that there are many questions to be asked and many answers to be aspired to. Without her, I would not have accomplished what I have.

Michael Shevell, MD, CM, FRCPC
Professor (with Tenure)
Departments of Neurology/Neurosurgery & Pediatrics
McGill University
Division of Pediatric Neurology
Montreal Children's Hospital

1
CONCEPTS AND DEFINITIONS IN NEURODEVELOPMENTAL DISABILITY

Michael Shevell

Definitions provide the mechanism to limit and demarcate the outlines of 'something' clearly, by explicitly providing its distinctive core features and immutable 'essence' or 'quality.' Definitions are declarative statements of meaning which are a dynamic product of usage and consensus which may change over time as our understanding of a concept changes. The objective of a definition is to provide for clarity and agreement in both verbal and written communication (Webster's Encyclopedic Dictionary 1988).

Broadly speaking, 'neurodevelopmental disability' as a concept brings together under one rubric a group of related, but clinically distinct, chronic disorders whose essential and unifying feature is a documented disturbance in developmental progress, either quantitative or qualitative, or both, compared with established norms in one or more recognized developmental domains (American Psychiatric Association 1994). These domains traditionally include: motor (gross or fine), speech/language, cognition, personal/social, and activities of daily living. These domains are in themselves not mutually exclusive or independent. Collectively, these disorders are a common problem in child health which challenges practitioners at varying levels, including, but not limited to, accurate timely recognition, diagnosis, causation, intervention, resource allocation, and outcomes (First and Palfrey 1994).

Individual subtypes of neurodevelopmental disability defined below are essentially 'symptom complexes,' rather than specific disorders or diseases (Sherr and Shevell 2006). Etiologically heterogeneous, neurodevelopmental disability subtypes are diagnosed not by objective laboratory testing, but rather by observed clinical features. These subtypes can be conceptualized as 'terms of convenience' that encapsulate a number of commonly encountered children sharing impairments, which mandates a common diagnostic evaluation and approach, and broadly share medical requirements and therapeutic needs and individual/family challenges to participation and integration. In effect, they provide a shorthand way of communication between health professionals. Their conceptualization and recognition, in both a timely and accurate manner, are challenged by the awareness that the development of the child is an ongoing dynamic process involving the complex interplay of intrinsic (i.e. child) and extrinsic (i.e. families, environmental) factors, whose individual trajectories need not be smooth or consistent across time (Darrah et al.

2003). There is also a wide variation of 'normal' to be accepted, and drawing a clear boundary line between normal and abnormal is often problematic when going from the general concept to the specific child. Ideally, the diagnosis of the subtypes outlined below should occur *over* time, rather than at a single point of clinical convenience (i.e. snapshot).

GLOBAL DEVELOPMENTAL DELAY

For the young child (i.e. less than 5 years of age), objective measurement of intelligence and cognition requires a consistent, standardized, and reliable measure of what is in essence an inferred concept. It also requires a universally agreed upon and widely applicable definition of intelligence itself. Both achieving this definition and an agreed upon measure of cognition have proved problematic, indeed elusive, to date in this age group (Gould 1981). Thus, the neurodevelopmental disability subtype of 'global developmental delay' has emerged to describe the child with limitations and delay in the widespread acquisition of skills that are directly observable and measurable in the context of the natural progression of all children (Simeonsson and Sharp 1992, Simeonsson and Simeonsson 2001). These skills are both developmental and functional in conceptualization and can be tracked systematically across time. Global developmental delay refers to a disturbance across a variety of developmental domains, which is defined operationally as a significant delay in two or more developmental domains (Shevell et al. 2003). From a practical standpoint, delay in two domains usually, but not invariably or necessarily, implies delay that is observable in all domains.

MENTAL RETARDATION/INTELLECTUAL DISABILITY

Global developmental delay may be an early marker of what is termed mental retardation,[1] which is typically diagnosable in the child older than 5 years of age. The present consensus definition of 'mental retardation,' put forward by the American Association on Mental Retardation (now the American Association on Intellectual and Developmental Disabilities) in 2002, describes this entity as 'a disability characterized by significant limitation both in intellectual functioning and adaptive behaviour as expressed in conceptual, social and practical adaptive skills' (American Association on Mental Retardation 2002). Thus, the definition of mental retardation goes beyond a significant limitation in intelligence or cognition conceptualized as general mental capabilities, which is best objectively captured through an 'intelligence quotient' (IQ) score (subject to its own potential intrinsic errors in measurement) to include limitations in adaptive behavior (Spreat 1999). Adaptive

---

[1] UK usage: learning disability.

behavior is conceptualized as skills that an individual learns in order to function in the context of his/her everyday life. These skills include those that are conceptual, practical, and social in orientation. Limitations in these skills impair performance and substantially dampen the ability to anticipate correctly and respond to the changes and demands encountered in daily life. Standards with respect to personal independence and social responsibility are not met. Intellectual disability is the currently preferred term for mental retardation (Schalock et al. 2007).

Clearly, global developmental delay and mental retardation are complementary, but non-synonymous, terms that share common features yet have distinctive characteristics (Sherr and Shevell 2006). At their core, they both represent a defect or disorder in learning. Though standardized testing solidifies their accurate diagnosis, the reality is that in practice experienced clinical judgment is typically substituted for such detailed intensive standardized testing (Sherr and Shevell 2006). Still to be determined through longitudinal studies is the precise relationship between these two related entities (Peterson et al. 1998).

DEVELOPMENTAL LANGUAGE IMPAIRMENT

'Developmental language impairment' is characterized by a predominant, almost exclusive, delay in the speech/language domain (Webster and Shevell 2004). Developmental language impairment features either an expressive or receptive deficit in the absence of any observed cognitive limitations, significant hearing loss or co-existing autistic features (Nass and Trauner 2006). A multitude of synonymous terms have been utilized including (but not limited to) specific language impairment, developmental language disorders, and developmental dysphasia. Various elements of language may be affected including articulation, phonologic decoding and programing, oral motor planning (dyspraxia), semantics, syntax, lexicon, and pragmatics. Though various classification schemes for developmental language impairment have been put forward, consensus agreement on the precise subcategorization for this neurodevelopmental disability subtype remains elusive thus far.

Longitudinal studies have emphasized that the delay in language skills initially observed in the child is not merely one of maturational delay (Shevell et al. 2005). Indeed, the documented delay may over time not be solely restricted to the language domain, with early language delay perhaps functioning as a harbinger of later observed and more early recognized cognitive difficulties. Careful studies at the time of diagnosis have suggested that these children may often have overlooked, indeed subtle, neurologic and motor difficulties that may impact on overall developmental trajectory and thus have therapeutic implications (Webster et al. 2008). Thus, labeling a child originally with a developmental language impairment may be a matter of the language domain's degree and predominance of impairment, rather than the apparent exclusivity of this domain's deficit.

AUTISTIC SPECTRUM DISORDERS

'Autistic spectrum disorders' have also been known by various terms including autism syndrome and pervasive developmental disorders. First described in the 1940s, diagnostic criteria for this neurobehavioral syndrome have been extended over time, resulting in more children with milder and varying degrees of deficits meriting the 'autistic' diagnostic label (Hirtz et al. 2006). This broadening clinical phenotype accounts for much of the recent observed 'autism epidemic.'

Present criteria encapsulated in the Diagnostic and Statistical Manual of Mental Disorders, 4th edition revised (DSM-IVR) define a range of deficits that reflects a quantitative *and* qualitative impairment in both reciprocal social interactions and language skills, combined with a restrictive repertoire and stereotyped patterns of behavior, interest, and activities (American Psychiatric Association 1994). The qualitative impairment in social interaction is signaled by abnormalities in non-verbal behavior, peer relationships, sharing with others, and demonstrated reciprocity. Language impairment is signaled by actual delay, repetitive idiosyncratic or non-varied language use, and conversational limitations with respect to initiating and sustaining a conversation. Motor mannerisms, adherence to routine, and observed restricted patterns of interests or bizarre preoccupations frequently characterize behavior in the autistic child. Among children with autistic spectrum disorders, there is marked variability in the precise distribution and actual severity of symptoms. Cognitive function also can be highly variable between affected individuals.

Diagnosis of an autistic spectrum disorder requires an application of a DSM-IVR diagnostic checklist or standardized interview (e.g. Autism Diagnostic Interview (ADI), Autism Diagnostic Observaton Schedule (ADOS)) or the application of a widely accepted autism rating scale (e.g. Childhood Autism Rating Scale (CARS)) (Hirtz et al. 2006). Some children may not reach the threshold for formal diagnosis of an autistic spectrum disorder; thus the label of a 'pervasive developmental delay – not otherwise specified' or a 'global developmental delay with autistic features' may be warranted (Shevell et al. 2001). The distinction between these two entities is not clear at this time and they may be synonymous with widely overlapping terms or diagnostic formulations.

CEREBRAL PALSY

The concept of 'cerebral palsy' dates from the latter part of the 19th century (Ingram 1994) and the penultimate consensus definition states that cerebral palsy is 'an umbrella term covering a group of non-progressive, but often changing, motor impairments syndromes secondary to lesions or anomalies of the brain arising in the early stages of its development' (Mutch et al. 1992). Cerebral palsy is clearly conceptualized as a symptom complex featuring heterogeneous etiology, pathologies, and clinical manifestations (Shevell and Bodensteiner 2004) and the most recent consensus definition highlights a disorder of movement and posture with activity limitations and a varying range of associated sensory, behavioral, cognitive, perceptual, language, medical, and musculo-skeletal difficulties (Rosenbaum et al. 2007).

The non-progressive nature of cerebral palsy refers to the underlying pathologic lesions that neither progress nor resolve once they occur. Neurodegenerative, neurometabolic, and neoplastic processes do not underlie cerebral palsy; however, some controversy exists regarding the inclusion of potentially progressive vascular (i.e. moyamoya) or traumatic (i.e. shaken baby syndrome) etiologies under this term. While the pathologic lesion may not change, clearly the clinical manifestations of a child's cerebral palsy may evolve over time, reflecting the interplay of the lesion with a dynamic maturing nervous system (Badawi et al. 1998).

Motor impairment is at the core of cerebral palsy (Minear 1956) and is manifested by motor delay, gait disturbance, and objective neurologic findings involving changes in tone (typically increased), passive resistance to stretch, the quality of possible limb movements (i.e. dyskinesias), the presence of primitive reflexes, and the exaggeration of stretch reflexes. The combination and severity of observed features and the resulting impairments are highly variable. Furthermore, the observed motor difficulties may co-exist with developmental impairments in other domains (e.g. global developmental), cognitive and/or adaptive limitations (e.g. mental retardation), primary sensory impairments (e.g. hearing or visual loss), learning disorders (e.g. learning disability or attention-deficit–hyperactivity disorder), or a seizure disorder (e.g. epilepsy) (von Wendt et al. 1985).

By definition, only lesions affecting the brain can result in cerebral palsy and only those occurring in the early stages of brain development prior to its complete maturation (Mutch et al. 1992). The precise timeframe corresponding to this early stage has not been consistently and universally agreed upon (Stanley et al. 2000). This has led to local geographic variation in etiologic patterns for cerebral palsy reported depending on the precise local 'early' timeframe employed.

GROSS MOTOR DELAY

Like developmental language impairment, 'gross motor delay' is delay affecting exclusively or predominantly a single developmental domain, in this instance motor skills (either gross or fine in character). It is a single domain developmental delay (Shevell et al. 2000). Children with isolated cerebral palsy and no other impairments have gross motor delay, but not all children with gross motor delay have cerebral palsy. This is so because some children with gross motor delay will either not have objective neurologic findings, aside from the motor delay itself, or they may indeed manifest an etiology arising not from the brain but rather from the spinal cord or peripheral nervous system (i.e. lower motor unit).

OTHER NEURODEVELOPMENTAL DISABILITIES

While primary sensory impairments occur at increased frequency in the setting of the neurodevelopmental disabilities, occasionally they occur in isolation, manifesting as either hearing loss (i.e. 'deafness') or visual impairment (i.e. 'blindness'), which brings forth unique and particular challenges to the affected child, family, and those involved in primary care, especially from a rehabilitative perspective. Previously intact school age children may manifest, in the context of school attendance, either a 'specific learning disability' or an 'attention-deficit–hyperactivity disorder,' both of which can be considered as a neurodevelopmental disability subtype. Developmental co-ordination disorder is a recently parsed and defined neurodevelopmental disability that provides a diagnostic label to children previously considered as 'clumsy' or 'maladroit.' Diagnosis of this particular neurodevelopmental disability is based on currently formulated DSM-IVR criteria.

INTERNATIONAL CLASSIFICATION OF FUNCTIONING, DISABILITY AND HEALTH

The above definitions reflect a pronounced and somewhat narrowly configured biomedical approach which may be overtly limiting or narrow when considering chronic health conditions such as the neurodevelopmental disabilities. While not altering the basic unifying definitions in any way, a complementary framework is offered by consideration of the International Classification of Functioning, Disability and Health (ICF) (World Health Organization 2001). The product of a decade of effort by the World Health Organization (WHO), the ICF offers a different model for disability and functioning which is more holistic and robustly biopsychosocial in orientation (Fig. 1.1).

This model emphasizes the continual bi-directional dynamic interaction between contextual factors and health conditions (Rosenbaum and Stewart 2004). Contextual factors may be personal (i.e. age, gender, education, lifestyle) or environmental (i.e. social, cultural, institutional, financial). Disability is envisioned as a social construct, reflecting the unique product of the interactions between the individual and the broader family, community, and society in which the individual resides. In this schema, activity and participation are important potentially modifiable determinants of health that could – and should – be addressed through intervention (i.e. therapy). By being a social construct, the range of modifications that may affect disability is broadened considerably. Indeed, desired modifications are individualized to fit the particular needs of the individual family unit. Furthermore, by expanding outcomes beyond that of the modification of body structures or function alone, the potential for therapeutic change and benefit is also considerably expanded.

The ICF model can be applied in a unique and particular way to each child with a neurodevelopmental disability. Within this framework, properly speaking

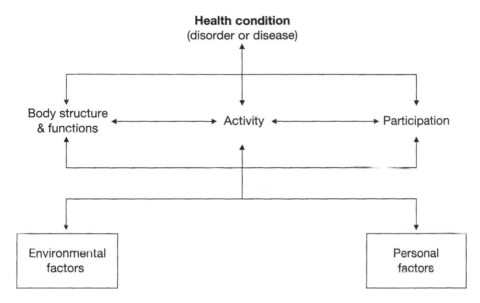

Fig. 1.1. World Health Organization model for health and functioning.

the disability does not rest with the child. This has led to the emergence of a 'family centered care' approach to intervention (Rosenbaum et al. 1998). Rather than fixing the deficit, however physiologically defined, therapeutic efforts are directed at resolving difficulties and barriers to participation and activity that are identified by the child and family as subjectively desired goals. Together with our emerging scientific understanding of childhood neurodevelopmental disability, this offers the hope of improving overall outcomes for these children.

ACKNOWLEDGMENTS
MS is grateful for the support of the MCH Foundation and YCC during the writing of this manuscript. Alba Rinaldi provided the necessary secretarial assistance.

REFERENCES
American Association on Mental Retardation (AAMR) (2002) *Mental Retardation: Definition, Classification and Systems of Support.* Washington, DC: American Association on Mental Retardation.
American Psychiatric Association (1994) *Diagnostic and Statistical Manual of Mental Disorders,* 4th edn. Washington, DC: American Psychiatric Association.
Badawi N, Watson L, Petterson B, Blair E, Slee J, Haan E, et al. (1998) What constitutes cerebral palsy? *Dev Med Child Neurol* 40: 520–527.
Darrah J, Hodge M, Magall-Evans J, Kembhavi G (2003) Stability of serial assessments of motor and communication abilities in typically developing infants: implications for screening. *Early Hum Dev* 72: 97–110.

First LR, Palfrey JS (1994) The infant or young child with developmental delay. *N Engl J Med* 330: 478–483.

Gould SJ (1981) *The Mismeasure of Man.* New York: WW Norton.

Hirtz DG, Wagner A, Filipek PA (2006) Autistic spectrum disorders. In: Swaiman KF, Ashwal S, Ferreiro DF (eds) *Pediatric Neurology: Principles & Practice, 4th edn.* Philadelphia: Mosby Elsevier, pp 905–936.

Ingram TTS (1994) A historical view of the definition and classification of the cerebral palsies. In: Stanley F, Alberman E (eds) *The Epidemiology of the Cerebral Palsies.* London: Spastics International Medical Publications, pp 1–11.

Minear WL (1956) A classification of cerebral palsy. *Pediatrics* 18: 841–852.

Mutch L, Alberman E, Hagberg B, Kodama K, Perat MV (1992) Cerebral palsy epidemiology: where are we now and where are we going? *Dev Med Child Neurol* 34: 547–551.

Nass R, Trauner DA (2006) Developmental language disorders. In: Swaiman KF, Ashwal S, Ferreiro DF (eds) *Pediatric Neurology: Principles & Practice, 4th edn.* Philadelphia: Mosby Elsevier, pp 845–854.

Petersen MC, Kube DA, Palmer FB (1998) Classification of developmental delays. *Semin Pediatr Neurol* 5: 2–14.

Rosenbaum P, King S, Law M, et al. (1998) Family-centred services: a conceptual framework and research review. *Phys Occup Ther Pediatr* 18: 1–20.

Rosenbaum P, Paneth N, Leviton A, Goldstein M, Bax M, Damiano D, et al. (2007) A report: the definition and classification of cerebral palsy. *Dev Med Child Neurol* 49: 8–14.

Rosenbaum P, Stewart D (2004) The World Health Organization International Classification of Functioning, Disability and Health: a model to guide clinical thinking, practice and research in the field of cerebral palsy. *Semin Pediatr Neurol* 11: 5–10.

Schalock RL, Luckasson RA, Shogren KA, Borthwick-Duffy S, Bradley V, Buntinx WH, et al. (2007) The remaining of mental retardation: understanding the change to the term intellectual disability. *Intellect Dev Disabil* 45: 116–124.

Sherr EH, Shevell MI (2006) Mental retardation and global developmental delay. In: KF, Ashwal S, Ferreiro DF (eds) *Pediatric Neurology: Principles & Practice, 4th edn.* Swaiman, Philadelphia: Mosby Elsevier, pp 799–820.

Shevell M, Ashwal S, Donley D, Flint J, Gingold M, Hirtz D, et al. (2003) Practice parameter: evaluation of the child with global developmental delay. Report of the Quality Standards Subcommittee of the American Academy of Neurology and the Practice Committee of the Child Neurology Society. *Neurology* 60: 367–380.

Shevell MI, Bodensteiner JB (2004) Cerebral palsy: defining the problem. *Semin Pediatr Neurol* 11: 2–4.

Shevell MI, Majnemer A, Rosenbaum P, Abrahamowicz M (2000) Etiologic yield in single domain developmental delay: a prospective study. *J Pediatr* 37: 633–637.

Shevell MI, Majnemer A, Rosenbaum P, Abrahamowicz M (2001) Etiologic yield of autistic spectrum disorders: a prospective study. *J Child Neurol* 16: 509–512.

Shevell MI, Majnemer A, Webster R, Platt R, Birnbaum R (2005) Outcomes at school age of preschool children diagnosed with developmental language impairment. *Pediatr Neurol* 32: 264–269.

Simeonsson RJ, Sharp MC (1992) Developmental delays. In: Hoekelman RA, Friedman SB, Nelson NM, et al. (eds) *Primary Pediatric Care.* St Louis: CV Mosby, pp 867–870.

Simeonsson RJ, Simeonsson NW (2001) Developmental surveillance and intervention. In: Hoekelman RA, Adam HM, Nelson NM, et al. (eds) *Primary Pediatric Care, 4th edn.* St Louis: CV Mosby, pp 274–280.

Spreat S (1999) Psychometric standards for adaptive behavior assessment. In: Schalock RL (ed) *Adaptive Behavior and its Measurement: Implications for the Field of Mental Retardation.* Washington, DC: American Association on Mental Retardation.

Stanley F, Blair D, Alberman E (2000) What are the cerebral palsies? In: *Cerebral Palsies: Epidemiology & Causal Pathways.* London: Mac Keith Press, pp 8–13.

von Wendt L, Rantakallio P, Saukkonen AL, Tuisku M, Mäkinen H (1985) Cerebral palsy and additional handicaps in a 1-year birth cohort from northern Finland: a prospective follow-up study to the age of 14 years. *Ann Clin Res* 17: 156–161.

Webster's Encyclopedic Dictionary (1988) New York: Lexicon Publications.

Webster R, Shevell MI (2004) The neurobiology of specific language impairment. *J Child Neurol* 19: 471–481.

Webster RI, Erdos C, Evans K, Majnemer A, Saigal G, Kehayia E, et al. (2008) Neurological and magnetic resonance imaging findings in children with developmental language impairment. *J Child Neurol* 23: 870–877.

World Health Organization (2001) *International Classification of Functioning, Disability and Health (ICF).* Geneva, Switzerland: World Health Organization.

2

THE EPIDEMIOLOGY OF SELECTED NEURODEVELOPMENTAL DISABILITIES – AN OVERVIEW

Marshalyn Yeargin-Allsopp and Carolyn Drews-Botsch[1]

Developmental disabilities are an important public health issue. Overall, an estimated 17% of children in the United States have a disability, and about 2% of all children will require lifelong care for their disability (Boyle and Cordero 2005). Boyle and Cordero estimated that the economic costs of four major disabilities (mental retardation/intellectual disability, cerebral palsy, hearing loss, and vision impairment) exceeded $50 billion based on 2003 dollars (Boyle and Cordero 2005). The epidemiology of neurodevelopmental disabilities is a rapidly evolving field that is an important complement to clinical investigation and practice. Epidemiologic data can inform the development of prevention programs and the identification of the clinical and educational needs of children with neurodevelopmental disabilities (Paneth 2005). This chapter discusses basic epidemiologic concepts and their application to better our understanding of the selected neurodevelopmental disabilities that will be the focus of this book (i.e. mental retardation/intellectual disability, developmental language disorders).

EPIDEMIOLOGIC METHODS

Epidemiology is the study of the distribution of diseases in populations (Last 2000). The underlying assumption is that diseases are not randomly distributed throughout the population, but are concentrated within specific segments of the population because of environmental and intrinsic host characteristics. In other words, 'disease' is caused by factors that can be identified through an understanding of who gets the 'disease.' Therefore, the goals of epidemiology are to determine the extent of disease in various segments of the population, to understand the natural history of the disease, and to identify possible risk factors and definite causes (Paneth 2005).

---

[1] The findings and conclusions in this report are those of the authors and do not necessarily represent the views of the Centers for Disease Control and Prevention.

Epidemiologic studies are dichotomized into two main types: (1) descriptive studies, and (2) analytic studies. Descriptive studies evaluate the distribution of disease in a population, while analytic studies focus on comparing the distribution of disease in more than one population with the purpose of identifying those factors that are associated with differential probabilities of disease occurrence.

MEASURES OF DISEASE OCCURRENCE

The occurrence of disease in a population is generally measured as some type of ratio to avoid differences related to the absolute size of the underlying population. The numerator is a count of the number of cases of disease within a population and the denominator is a standardized measure or unit of population size. Counting the number of cases requires operationally precisely defining the condition and then counting all the individuals within a defined population that meet that particular definition. Given a specific condition, two basic types of numerators are available: cases that are newly developing (i.e. incident cases) or cases of disease present in a population at a given point in time (i.e. prevalent cases).

Different types of denominators create different measures of disease occurrence. A risk or cumulative incidence defines the proportion of new cases in a population at risk. Thus, the population at-risk is the denominator, and the numerator is the number of newly developing cases within that particular at risk population. The cumulative incidence is reported as cases per unit of population during a specific time interval. There are a variety of key features of the cumulative incidence. First, it is a true proportion, that is the numerator is part of the denominator. Thus, the cumulative incidence represents the proportion of the population that will develop the disease in a particular time period. However, it should be noted that the cumulative incidence varies by the length of the follow-up period. For example, among infants born in the United States in 2001, newborns have a 0.45% risk of dying within the first 28 days of life, a 0.68% risk of dying within the first year of life and a 100% risk of dying within 200 years (National Center for Health Statistics 2005).

New cases of disease can also be described as an incidence rate, also known as the incidence density. The numerator for the incidence rate is defined as the number of new cases of disease developing in a population divided by the amount of person-time spent at-risk. In theory, this is an instantaneous measure, known as the 'force of morbidity.' In practice, it is measured as an average incidence rate over a defined period.

However, the utility of incidence measures is limited in studies of developmental delay and neurodevelopmental disabilities (Durkin 2002). It may be impossible to identify incident cases because their onset is unknown, and it may be impossible to identify individuals who are truly free from disease and are at risk of developing such impairments, particularly because such conditions may often develop *in utero* or shortly after birth. As a result, prevalence measures are more common than incidence measures in epidemiologic studies of developmental delay and neuro-developmental disabilities. The prevalence of a condition, like the cumulative incidence, is a true proportion, varies between 0 and 1, and is calculated as the number of cases present in a population at a single point in time divided by the total number of individuals in the population at that point in time.

Incidence and prevalence are numerically related. The prevalent pool of subjects is the rate of subjects flowing into the diseased proportion (incidence rate) minus the rate of subjects flowing out of the diseased population, either by being cured or by death. Numerically, this is represented by *Prevalence odds = Incidence density × Average duration of disease* when the risk is stable and in- and out-migration of subjects are balanced (Rothman and Greenland 1998, Morabia 2005). Thus, factors that influence the incidence density, the cure rate, or case fatality rate, can all affect the prevalence of disease in a population. From a causal perspective, associations between suspected etiologic factors and a neurodevelopmental condition must be assessed cautiously and the likelihood that the observed association results from a relationship with the duration of disease, rather than with incidence, must be carefully considered.

MEASURES OF ASSOCIATION

Analytic epidemiologic studies assess the relationship between an exposure and an outcome by comparing statistically the occurrence of disease in an exposed population with the occurrence in an unexposed population. Just as there are varying methods of assessing disease occurrence, there are a variety of methods of assessing the association between exposure and disease. In its simplest formulation, the incidence of disease among exposed individuals is compared with the incidence among unexposed individuals. This is the basic cohort study in which the incidence of disease, either cumulative incidence or incidence density, is assessed in a group of exposed individuals and compared with the incidence among a known unexposed group of individuals.

There are two ways to compare the incidence in two populations: (1) as a difference, or (2) as a ratio. Taking a ratio of the incidence measures indicates the proportional change in incidence related to exposure. This measure is termed the risk ratio, or the cumulative incidence ratio when comparing cumulative incidences. The term rate ratio, or incidence density ratio, is used when the ratio of incidence rates is calculated. One can also calculate analogous difference measures. That is, the risk difference and the rate difference by subtracting the incidence among unexposed individuals from the incidence among exposed individuals.

For cohort studies, the choice between difference and ratio measures is often up to the discretion of the investigator. However, case–control studies commonly estimate odds ratios. Case–control studies start with a sample of individuals with disease and a sample of similar individuals who did not develop disease. The odds of exposure (i.e. Proportion exposed ÷ Proportion unexposed) among individuals with the disease are compared with the odds among those who do not have the condition. Assuming that the baseline risk for controls is similar to that of the cases, this exposure odds ratio will estimate the rate ratio when the controls are selected to represent person-time at risk and will estimate the prevalence odds ratio when prevalent cases are selected. The exposure odds ratio will estimate the cumulative incidence ratio when controls are sampled at the beginning of follow-up (i.e. in a case–cohort study) or when the controls are sampled from the non-cases at the end of follow-up and the condition is a relatively rare occurrence.

BIAS

These measures of association and the statistical tests that accompany them are merely that – measures of association. They do not tell the investigator anything about actual causation. The first question that should arise is whether or not the observed association is valid. In other words, on average does the observed associ-ation represent the true relationship between exposure and outcome? There are three main types of bias that arise in epidemiologic studies: (1) information bias, (2) selection bias and (3) confounding.

Information bias occurs because the variables in the study are not measured accurately. The errors may be in assessing the outcome, the exposure, and/or co-variates that are included in the study. Mismeasurement is extremely common in epidemiology. Etiologic heterogeneity is another common cause of information bias. We know relatively little about the causes of, and differences between, some con-ditions so they often get lumped together even if they are actually distinct entities. To the extent that we understand the differences between conditions with similar developmental phenotypes, we should separate these conditions. However, because we often know relatively little about the pathogenesis of neurodevelopmental conditions, it is difficult to make appropriate separations, which results in possi-ble misclassification of some cases.

In general, errors in the exposure and outcome information bias the observed association towards the null, creating a conservative bias in studies in which an association has been observed (Hofler 2005). However, if the diagnosis or the report-ing of exposure differs by the other variable (exposure or outcome), the direction of bias is unpredictable. This is of particular concern for associations that are highly visible to the community, such as the alleged association between autism and child-hood vaccinations (Andrews et al. 2002) or for information reported by parents who are grieving because of a condition and/or disability in their child. Further, because many neurodevelopmental outcomes have subtle signs early in life, the diag-nosis may depend on a variety of factors such as socioeconomic status, parental education level, access to health care, an index of suspicion among health care workers, and referral for testing by teachers and other educators. Any of these factors could create differences in the magnitude of errors in the direction of either diagnosis and/or exposure.

Selection bias occurs because of differences in who is selected for evaluation. In a cohort study, such bias would occur if there were differences in loss to follow-up by exposure status and/or the risk of outcome. For example, if high social class individuals whose children have a disability migrate from an area in search of better services, this could create a selection bias. In case–control studies this occurs if disease and exposure interact to affect the actual selection for inclusion in the study.

Confounding occurs when the effect of the exposure of interest on the outcome is mixed with the effect of an extraneous variable because a third variable, the co-variate, is an independent risk factor for the outcome and is also associated with the exposure of interest. Because social class is a strong risk factor for cognitive development (Drews et al. 1995) and is also associated with preterm birth (Foster et al. 2000), social class will be a confounder of a study assessing the impact of preterm birth on later cognitive development. However, unlike the bias resulting from misclassification and selection bias, the investigator can eliminate the bias resulting from confounding by carefully controlling for the co-variate in statistical analysis.

ASSESSING CAUSATION IN EPIDEMIOLOGY

Ultimately, one is usually interested in making causal statements about associations between disease and exposure. However, epidemiology is only good at assessing associations. Further, epidemiologic arguments are inductive, rather than deductive. In other words, we can only disprove hypotheses formally or inclusively, not prove them (Buck 1975). For example, statistical tests can disprove the null hypothesis that no association exists between an exposure and an outcome. More precisely, we can make a statistical argument that it is unlikely that the occurrence of disease is the same in exposed and unexposed populations, but we can never prove conclusively that there is no association in some segment of the population.

Disproving the null hypothesis of no association between an exposure and an outcome is not the same as actually proving causality. There are a number of reasons that disease occurrence could differ between exposed and unexposed populations. How then does one determine that an exposure is causally related to a disease? In 1965, Sir Bradford Hill developed a set of criteria that he claimed could be used to argue that an observed association between an exposure and a disease represented a true causal relationship (Hill 1965). First, the temporal sequence had to be correct. For an exposure to cause an outcome, it had to precede the development of the condition. This, in fact, is part of the definition of causation and, unlike the rest of Hill's criteria, is required for the observed association to be causal. However, in some respects this is difficult to assess for developmental exposures because the onset of a neurodevelopmental outcome is often difficult to determine, and it usually precedes the diagnosis by a substantial period of time. Thus, this criterion must be carefully determined for neurodevelopmental outcomes.

Hill's other criteria are meant to argue that bias or sampling differences are unlikely to explain the observed association. For example, he argued that an association in which there is a specific exposure–disease relationship and an observed dose–response curve is more likely to be causal than an association without these characteristics. However, there are difficulties in applying these criteria to neurodevelopmental conditions. Dose–response curves may not be observed for neurodevelopmental conditions because an exposure resulting in cell death, for example, may result in spontaneous miscarriage and/or stillbirth at high levels, but result in developmental delay at lower exposure levels. Additionally, developmental events are highly sequential and timed. Therefore, an exposure may result in a specific congenital malformation at one point in development, a different malformation at a different point in time, and developmental delay when exposure occurs during a third developmental period. So, when assessing causality of neurodevelopmental outcomes, one should consider how the developmental sequence is likely to impact the observed associations and outcomes. Thus, the nature of neurodevelopmental conditions affects significantly our ability to conduct confident epidemiologic studies.

MENTAL RETARDATION/INTELLECTUAL DISABILITY

DISEASE DESCRIPTION AND CLASSIFICATION

Although there are a variety of definitions of mental retardation/intellectual disability (MR/ID) in current use (Table 2.1), the core feature of MR/ID is significantly subaverage general intellectual functioning accompanied by significant limitations in adaptive functioning. MR/ID has traditionally been divided into levels of severity based on the statistical distribution of a measured intelligence quotient (IQ) with cutoff points based on the number of standard deviations (1 SD = 15 points) below the accepted statistical population mean IQ of 100 (Table 2.2). The American Association on Mental Retardation (AAMR) (Luckasson et al. 2002) uses a three-step approach to defining the severity of mental retardation (Luckasson et al. 1992). This change is believed to be more relevant to the provision of actual needed services (Luckasson et al. 1992, Leonard and Wen 2002). Similarly, in the tenth revision of the International Classification of Diseases (ICD-10), the need for varying supports is also included as one of the indicators differentiating mild from severe mental retardation (Table 2.2).

PREVALENCE

The prevalence of MR/ID has rarely been assessed through clinical examination of an entire population. Therefore, an 'administrative' prevalence is often employed. The administrative prevalence is defined as the proportion of individuals who have been defined, for administrative purposes such as education, as having MR/ID.

TABLE 2.1
Definitions of mental retardation

American Psychiatric Association Diagnostic and Statistical Manual of Mental Disorder, Fourth Edition (DSM-IV)[a]
Significantly subaverage general intellectual functioning (Criterion A) that is accompanied by significant limitations in adaptive functioning in at least at two of the following skill areas: communication, self-care, home living, social/interpersonal skills, use of community resources, self-direction, functional academic skills, work, leisure, health, and safety (Criterion B). The onset must occur before 18 years (Criterion C)

American Association on Mental Retardation (AAMR)[b]
A disability characterized by significant limitations both in intellectual functioning and adaptive behavior as expressed in conceptual, social, and practical adaptive skills. The disability originates before age 18

World Health Organization (WHO)
International Classification of Diseases, Ninth Revision, Clinical Modification (ICD-9)[c]
Subnormal intellectual functioning which originates during the developmental period

International Classification of Diseases, Tenth Revision (ICD-10)[d]
A condition of arrested or incomplete development of the mind, which is especially characterized by impairment of skills manifested during the developmental period, skills which contribute to the overall level of intelligence, i.e. cognitive, language, motor, and social abilities

International Classification of Impairments, Disabilities, and Handicaps (ICIDH)[e]
Intellectual impairments include those of intelligence, memory, and thought. Includes disturbances of the rate and degree of development of cognitive functions, such as perception, attention, memory, and thinking and their deterioration as a result of pathologic process

International Classification of Functioning, Disability, and Health (ICF)[f]
Classified with intellectual growth, intellectual retardation, and dementia under Intellectual Functions: 'General mental functions, required to understand and constructively integrate the various mental functions, including all cognitive functions and their development over the life span'

[a] American Psychiatric Association (1994) *Diagnostic and Statistical Manual of Mental Disorders, Fourth Edition* (DSM-IV). Washington DC: American Psychiatric Association.
[b] Luckasson R, Coulter DL, Polloway EA, Reiss S, Schalock R, Snell ME, et al. (2002) *Mental Retardation: Definition, Classification and Level of Supports.* Washington DC: American Association on Mental Retardation.
[c] *International Classification of Diseases,* Ninth Revision (1988) Clinical Modification (ICD-9CM). Washington, DC: Public Health Service, US Department of Health and Human Service.
[d] World Health Organization (WHO) (1992) *International Classification of Diseases, Tenth Revision* (ICD-10). Geneva, Switzerland: World Health Organization.
[e] World Health Organization (WHO) (1980) *International Classification of Impairments, Disability, and Handicaps.* Geneva, Switzerland: World Health Organization.
[f] World Health Organization (WHO) (2001) *International Classification of Functioning, Disability, and Health.* Geneva, Switzerland: World Health Organization.

TABLE 2.2
Subclassification of mental retardation by IQ

Level of retardation	DSM-IV[a]	AAMR[b] Intensity of support	ICD-9CM[c]	ICD-10[d]	ICIDH[e] Impairments of intelligence	ICF[f,g]
			IQ range			
Mild	50–55 to 70	Intermittent	50–70	50–69	Mild IQ (50–70) Individuals who can acquire practical skills and functional reading and arithmetic abilities with special education, and can be guided towards social conformity	Mild problem (slight, low: 5–24%)
Moderate	35–40 to 50–55	Limited	35–49	35–49	Moderate IQ (35–49) Individuals can learn simple communication, elementary health and safety habits, and simple manual skills, but do not progress in functional reading or arithmetic	Moderate problem (medium, fair: 25–49%)
Severe	20–25 to 35–40	Extensive	20–34	20–34	Severe IQ (20–34) Individuals can profit from systematic habit training	Severe problem (high, extreme: 50–95%)
Profound	Below 20–25	Pervasive	0–20	0–20	Profound IQ (Under 20; Individuals might respond to skill training in the use of legs, hands, and jaws	Complete problem (total: 96–100%)

[a] American Psychiatric Association (1994) *Diagnostic and Statistical Manual of Mental Disorders, Fourth Edition* (DSM-IV). Washington DC: American Psychiatric Association.
[b] Luckasson R, Coulter DL, Polloway EA, Reiss S, Schalock R, Snell ME, et al. (2002) *Mental Retardation: Definition, Classification and Level of Supports*. Washington DC: American Association on Mental Retardation.
[c] *International Classification of Diseases*, Ninth Revision (1988) Clinical Modification (ICD-9CM). Washington, DC: Public Health Service, US Department of Health and Human Service.
[d] World Health Organization (WHO) (1992) *International Classification of Diseases, Tenth Revision* (ICD-10). Geneva, Switzerland: World Health Organization.
[e] World Health Organization (WHO) (1980) *International Classification of Impairments, Disability, and Handicap*. Geneva, Switzerland: World Health Organization.
[f] World Health Organization (WHO) (2001) *International Classification of Functioning, Disability, and Health*. Geneva, Switzerland: World Health Organization.
[g] IQ is not a construct in ICF. All three components classifed in ICF: (1) body functions and structures; (2) activities and participation; and (3) environmental factors, are quantified using the same generic scale, from 'no problem' to 'complete problem'.

Further, most epidemiologic studies of MR/ID have estimated the administrative prevalence using a case definition that relies exclusively on the results of IQ testing. Incorporating adaptive functioning into case definitions for epidemiologic studies has been difficult because of the lack of standardization regarding administration of these tests (Schumpert, personal communication).

Assuming a normal distribution of intelligence, with a mean of 100 and a standard deviation of 15, the prevalence of MR would be *expected* to be 23 per 1000 (Larson et al. 2001). However, in a recent review of 43 studies, the observed prevalence of mental retardation in children 5–19 years of age ranged from 2 to 85 per 1000 (Roeleveld et al. 1997), with 10 per 1000 being considered to be the most likely 'true' estimate (Mercer 1973b, Jacobson and Janicki 1983, Munro 1986, Lipkin 1991, Yeargin-Allsopp and Murphy 1992, Yeargin-Allsopp et al. 1992, Murphy et al. 1995).

Most epidemiologic studies have defined mild MR/ID (MMR/ID) as an IQ 50–55 to 70–75, and severe MR/ID (SMR/ID) as an IQ <50 (Kiely 1987, Roeleveld et al. 1997). Three-quarters (75–80%) of individuals with MR are usually reported to have MMR/ID (Murphy et al. 1998). Many reviews of international epidemiologic studies have suggested that the prevalence of SMR/ID is approximately 2–4 per 1000 in children (Fryers 1984, Kiely 1987, Starza-Smith 1989, Roeleveld et al. 1997) and adults (Reschly 1992). This range has been reported for both developed and developing countries (Kiely 1987, Roeleveld et al. 1997, Leonard and Wen 2002), with 3.8 per 1000 considered being a reliable estimate (Roeleveld et al. 1997). The reported prevalence of MMR/ID has been much more variable than for SMR/ID. It is not known whether this represented true differences in the rate in different populations or methodologic differences in the studies. However, Roeleveld et al. (1997) concluded that 29.8 per 1000 is a reasonable estimate of the prevalence of MMR.

Social and Demographic Characteristics

The observed prevalence of MR/ID varies by a number of population characteristics including age, gender, and socioeconomic status. The observed prevalence of MR/ID usually peaks at 10–14 years of age (Kiely 1987, McLaren and Bryson 1987). Murphy et al. (1995) reported that the prevalence of mental retardation varied from 1 per 1000 in children under the age of 5, to 97 per 1000 in children 10–14 years of age. This is probably due to diagnosis of children, particularly those with MMR/ID, within educational settings, rather than incident cases occurring during the school years. Thus, in considering the prevalence of MR/ID, the age of population captured in the denominator must be carefully considered (Murphy et al. 1998).

MR/ID is found more commonly in males than in females, with an observed male:female ratio of approximately 1.5:1 (Leonard and Wen 2002). Roeleveld found that the excess of males was higher for MMR/ID, with ratios ranging from 1.4:1 in the Netherlands to 1.8:1 in Sweden (Kiely 1987, Murphy et al. 1995, Roeleveld et al. 1997). The male:female ratio for SMR/ID has been reported to be 1.2:1 (Roeleveld et al. 1997). Biologic factors, such as X-linked conditions (Tariverdian and Vogel 2000, Chelly and Mandel 2001), could result in a greater occurrence of MR/ID among boys than girls (Partington et al. 2000). Social factors, such as behaviors that might cause boys to receive greater attention and thus be tested, are believed to be responsible for at least some of the male preponderance in MMR/ID.

The inverse relationship between socioeconomic status and prevalence of MR/ID has been well documented (Stein and Susser 1960, Birch et al. 1970, Rutter et al. 1970, Mercer 1973a, Broman et al. 1987, Decouflé and Boyle 1995, Yeargin-Allsopp et al. 1995). Studies have consistently shown that MMR/ID is largely of unknown etiology and is highly correlated with lower socioeconomic status (Munro 1986, Kiely 1987, Drews et al. 1995, Yeargin-Allsopp et al. 1995). Drews et al. (1995) examined MR/ID associated *with* neurologic conditions (non-isolated MR/ID) and *without* neurologic conditions (isolated MR/ID). The findings from that study support the idea that there are two distinct types of MR/ID: isolated MR/ID, which is mainly influenced by social and demographic factors, and MR/ID with other neurologic condition, which is more likely to be severe and is largely affected by biologic or pathologic factors (Decouflé and Boyle 1995, Drews et al. 1995, Croen et al. 2001).

Racial and ethnic differences in the prevalence of MR/ID have also been reported. In the United States, African-American children and children born to Hispanic and Asian mothers have higher rates of MR/ID than do Caucasian children (Murphy et al. 1995, Yeargin-Allsopp et al. 1995, Croen et al. 2001). Similarly, a higher rate of MR/ID has been reported among Australian indigenous (i.e. Aboriginal) children than among Caucasians (Leonard and Wen 2002). Confounding by socioeconomic factors is assumed to contribute to these differences. However, an excess of MR/ID among African-American children compared with Caucasian children in metropolitan Atlanta remained after controlling for sociodemographic factors (Yeargin-Allsopp et al. 1995).

Maternal age at delivery is another risk factor for MR/ID (Broman et al. 1987, Drews et al. 1995). This association varies with the level of MR/ID. Children whose mothers were teenagers (ages 15–19) at the time of delivery had a slightly increased risk for *mild MR/ID* than did children of older mothers. However, children whose mothers were older (i.e. 40–44 years) had a greater risk for *moderate to severe MR/ID* than did children whose mothers were in their twenties at the time of delivery (Chapman et al. 2002). The latter finding may be related to the increased risk of various chromosomal disorders with increased maternal age.

ETIOLOGY AND RISK FACTORS

A recent review by Leonard and Wen (2002) found that the proportion of MR/ID cases with a known etiology varied from 22% in metropolitan Atlanta to 77% in

Sweden. The proportion with a known etiology varies with the intensity of the diagnostic work-up and the definition of a known cause. Stringent criteria for what constitutes a 'cause' leads to a larger proportion of undetermined etiology (McLaren and Bryson 1987, Yeargin-Allsopp et al. 1997). The causes of MR/ID also differ by level of severity of MR/ID. Three-quarters (75–80%) of children with SMR/ID have an identified cause of their disability (McLaren and Bryson 1987, Yeargin-Allsopp et al. 1997, Leonard and Wen 2002). In contrast, most studies have reported a recognized etiology for fewer than half (25–40%) of children with MMR/ID (McLaren and Bryson 1987). However, the low proportion of children with mild MR with a recognized etiology has been challenged as a result of improved diagnostic capabilities (Shevell et al. 2003) and the scrutiny into the contribution of environmental factors, such as lead and mercury exposure (Mendola et al. 2002).

More than 500 genetic diseases are known to cause MR/ID. However, most are rare and do not contribute substantially to the overall prevalence of MR/ID (Flint and Wilkie 1996, Murphy et al. 1998). Chromosomal disorders are the most common known cause of mental retardation, accounting for 5–19% of all cases of MR/ID (Czeizel et al. 1990, Schaefer and Bodensteiner 1992, Yeargin-Allsopp et al. 1997, Hou et al. 1998, Murphy et al. 1998), and a higher proportion of cases of SMR/ID. Down syndrome (1 per 800 live births) (National Center on Birth Defects and Developmental Disabilities, 2004) accounts for 10–15% of all MR/ID cases (Leonard and Wen 2002), and at least two-thirds of all genetic causes of mental retardation (Yeargin-Allsopp et al. 1997, Fernell 1998, Hou et al. 1998, Cans et al. 1999, Stromme and Hagberg 2000). Other prominent causes of MR/ID include fragile X syndrome (1 per 4000 males and 1 per 8000 females) (Turner et al. 1996); and Prader–Willi syndrome (Leonard and Wen 2002).

Prenatal events are believed to contribute to the majority of causes of MR/ID (Yeargin-Allsopp et al. 1997, Fernell 1998). Fetal alcohol syndrome accounted for about 8% of the cases of MR/ID in Norway and metropolitan Atlanta (Leonard and Wen 2002). Other prenatal exposures that have been associated with MR/ID include: maternal smoking (Rantakallio and Koiranen 1987, Roeleveld et al. 1992, Drews et al. 1996); maternal prescribed medications during pregnancy such as hydantoins (Hanson 1986, Adams et al. 1990, Scolnik et al. 1994, Holmes et al. 2005); maternal medical conditions, particularly thyroid disease (Haddow et al. 1999, Qian et al. 2000); urinary tract infections (McDermott et al. 2001); maternal phenylketonuria (Lenke and Levy 1980, Waisbren et al. 1997); and intrauterine infections (Murphy et al. 1998). Birth defects are more common in children with MR/ID. However, this association may result from shared etiology. Low birth weight (<2500g), pre-term delivery (<37 weeks' gestation), and intrauterine growth restriction have been associated with MR/ID. Twins and other multiples are at increased risk for MR/ID (Boyle et al. 1997), probably because of the effect of multiple gestation on fetal growth and gestational age.

Perinatal asphyxia was once thought to be a major contributor to MR/ID and other developmental disabilities. However, one study found asphyxia recorded in the medical records of only about 5% of children with MR/ID (Yeargin-Allsopp et al. 1997). Additionally, relatively few cases of MR/ID are caused by perinatal infections, including group B streptococcus (CDC 1997) and herpes simplex virus (AAP 2003). Neonatal screening has been shown to be effective in preventing MR/ID resulting from most metabolic and endocrine disorders. In metropolitan Atlanta between 1981 and 1991, only 2 of 148 cases of MR/ID were related to phenyl-ketonuria, homocystinuria, maple syrup urine disease, tyrosinemia, hypothyroidism or classic galactosemia (CDC 1999).

Postnatal causes account for 3–15% of the cases of MR/ID (McLaren and Bryson 1987, Yeargin-Allsopp et al. 1997, Murphy et al. 1998). Further, MR/ID attributed to postnatal events such as lead exposure (Needleman 1992a, 1992b, Mendola et al. 2002); methylmercury exposure (Harada 1968, Marsh et al. 1987, Mendola et al. 2002, Davidson et al. 2004); traumatic brain injuries (CDC 1996, Yeargin-Allsopp et al. 1997); and postnatally acquired infections (CDC 1996, Yeargin-Allsopp et al. 1997) are frequently preventable causes.

COMMUNICATION DISORDERS

Speech and language disorders, which include developmental language disorders or specific language impairment, refer to problems in communication and related areas such as oral motor function. The disorders range from sound substitutions to an inability to understand or use either language or an oral motor mechanism for functional speech and/or feeding. The cause is often unknown, but known causes include hearing loss, neurologic disorders, brain injury, mental retardation, drug abuse, and physical impairments such as cleft lip or palate (National Information Center for Children and Youth with Disabilities 2000). Some communication disorders of childhood are developmental, hence they might be transient, while others are more serious with lifelong consequences that affect learning, socialization, and employment.

Chronic speech disorders are defined as difficulty producing speech sounds or problems with voice quality. The prevalence of such disorders is 16 per 1000 children under the age of 18 years of age (American Speech-Language-Hearing Association 2004). In the 2000–2001 school year, 18.9% of school age children received services for speech or language disorders under the Individuals with Disabilities Education Act (IDEA) Part B. This figure does not include children who had speech or language problems that were secondary to another associated condition (US Department of Education 2002).

Specific language impairment refers to a significant deficit in linguistic functioning that does not result from deficits in hearing, intelligence, or motor functioning (Shamas et al. 1998). Estimates of the prevalence of specific language impairment during preschool and early years range from 2% to 8%, with an overall median prevalence of 5.9% (8% for boys and 6% for girls) (Tomblin et al. 1997). Further, over the 10-year period from the 1991–1992 to the 2000–2001 school years, there was a 10% increase in the number of children receiving services for speech or language impairment (US Department of Education 2002). In 2003, 1 129 260 American children received special services for speech or language impairments under IDEA Part B. After specific learning disabilities, it is the second most common disability classification (US Department of Education 2004). Currently, relatively little is known about definite risk factors underlying etiologic conditions.

CONCLUSIONS
The epidemiology of neurodevelopmental disabilities is a rapidly evolving field that is an important complement to clinical investigation and practice. Epidemiologic data can assist in developing prevention programs and in identifying the clinical and educational burden of providing services to children with developmental disabilities. However, the nature of developmental disabilities makes such investigations methodogically difficult. Therefore, in developing and using this knowledge, clinicians, educators, and researchers need to define these conditions clearly and precisely, understand their developmental timing, subdivide these conditions into etiologic and diagnostic homogeneous subgroups and constructs, identify the population to which the measure of occurrence applies, and recognize the possible sources of error and bias that may result from the methods used. As the field of neurodevelopmental disabilities epidemiology evolves, the information available to clinicians and parents will improve, allowing for better decisions for the families, the children, and the communities affected by these unfortunately relatively prevalent conditions.

REFERENCES
Adams J, Voorhees CV, Middaugh LD (1990) Developmental neurotoxicity of anticonvulsants: human and animal evidence on phenytoin. *Neurotoxicol Teratol* 12: 203–214.
American Academy of Pediatrics (AAP) (2003) Group B streptococcal infections. In: Pickering LK (ed) *Redbook: 2003 Report of the Committee on Infectious Diseases, 26th edn.* Elk Grove Village, IL: American Academy of Pediatrics. p 584.
American Speech-Language-Hearing Association (2004) Communication facts: incidence and prevalence of communication disorders and hearing loss in children. Retrieved November 11, 2005, from http://www.asja.org.
Andrews N, Miller E, Taylor B, Lingam R, Simmons A, Stowe J, et al. (2002) Recall bias, MMR, and autism. *Arch Dis Child* 87: 493–494.
Birch HG, Richardson SA, Baird D, Horobin G (1970) *Mental Subnormality in the Community.* Baltimore: Williams & Wilkins.
Boyle CA, Cordero JF (2005) Birth defects and disabilities: a public health issue for the 21st century. *Am J Public Health* 95: 1884–1886.
Boyle CA, Keddie A, Holmgreen P (1997) The risk of mental retardation in twins. *Soc Pediatr Epidemiol Res* 11: A10.

Broman S, Nichols Pl, Shaughnessy P, Kennedy W (1987) *Retardation in Young Children: A Developmental Study of Cognitive Development*. Hillsdale, NJ: Lawrence Erlbaum Associates.

Buck C (1975) Popper's philosophy for epidemiologists. *Int J Epidemiol* 4: 159–167.

Cans C, Wilhelm L, Baille MF, du Mazaubrun C, Grandjean H, Rumeau-Rouquette C (1999) Aetiological findings and associated factors in children with severe mental retardation. *Dev Med Child Neurol* 41: 233–239.

Centers for Disease Control and Prevention (CDC) (1996) Postnatal causes of developmental disabilities in children aged 3–10 years – Atlanta, Georgia, 1991. *MMWR* 45: 130–134.

Centers for Disease Control and Prevention (CDC) (1997) Decreasing incidence of perinatal Group B streptococcal disease. United States, 1993–1995. *MMWR* 46: 473–477.

Centers for Disease Control and Prevention (CDC) (1999) Mental retardation following diagnosis of a metabolic disorder in children aged 3–10 years – metropolitan Atlanta, Georgia, 1991–1994. *MMWR* 48: 353–356.

Chapman DA, Scott K, Mason C (2002) Early risk factors for mental retardation: role of maternal age and maternal education. *Am J Ment Retard* 1: 46–59.

Chelly J, Mandel JL (2001) Monogenic causes of X-linked mental retardation. *Nat Rev Genet* 2: 669 680.

Croen LA, Grether JK, Selvin S (2001) The epidemiology of mental retardation of unknown cause. *Pediatrics* 107(6): E86. Retrieved January 23, 2006, from http://pediatrics.aappublications. org/cgi/content/full/107/6/e86.

Czeizel A, Sankaranarayanan K, Szondy M (1990) The load of genetic and partially genetic diseases in man. *Mutat Res* 232: 291.

Davidson PW, Myers J, Weiss B (2004) Mercury exposure and child development outcomes. *Pediatrics* 113: 1023–1027.

Decouflé P, Boyle CA (1995) The relationship between maternal education and mental retardation in 10-year-old children. *Ann Epidemiol* 5: 347–353.

Drews CD, Murphy CC, Yeargin-Allsopp M, Decouflé P (1996) The relationship between idiopathic mental retardation and maternal smoking during pregnancy. *Pediatrics* 97: 547–553.

Drews CD, Yeargin-Allsopp M, Decoufle P, Murphy CC (1995) Variation in the influence of selected sociodemographic risk factors for mental retardation. *Am J Public Health* 85: 329–334.

Durkin M (2002) The epidemiology of developmental disabilities in low-income countries. *Ment Retard Dev Disabil Res Rev* 8: 206–211.

Fernell E (1998) Aetiological factors and prevalence of severe mental retardation in children in a Swedish municipality: the possible role of consanguinity. *Dev Med Child Neurol* 40: 608–611.

Flint J, Wilkie AOM (1996) The genetics of mental retardation. *Br Med Bull* 52: 453–464.

Foster HW, Wu L, Bracken MB, Semenya K, Thomas J, Thomas J (2000) Intergenerational effects of high socioeconomic status on low birthweight and preterm birth in African Americans. *J Natl Med Assoc* 92: 213–21.

Fryers T (1984) *The Epidemiology of Severed Intellectual Impairment: The Dynamics of Prevalence*. London: Academic Press.

Haddow JE, Palomaki GE, Allan WC, Williams JR, Knight GJ, Gagnon J, et al. (1999) Maternal thyroid deficiency during pregnancy and subsequent neuropsychological development of the child. *N Engl J Med* 341: 549–555.

Hanson JW (1986) Teratogen update: fetal hydantoin effects. *Teratology* 33: 349–353.

Harada Y (1968) Congenital (or fetal) Minamata disease. Study Group of Minimata Disease. Kumamoto, Japan: Kumamoto University: pp 93–117.

Hill AB (1965) The environment and disease: association or causation? *Proc R Soc Med* 58: 295–300.

Hofler M (2005) The effect of misclassification on the estimation of association: a review. *Int J Methods Psychiatr Res* 14: 92–101.

Holmes LB, Coull BA, Dorfman J, Rosenberger P (2005) The correlation of deficits in IQ with midface and digit hypoplasia in children exposed in utero to anticonvulsant drugs. *J Pediatr* 146: 118–122.

Hou JW, Wang TR, Chuang SM (1998) An epidemiological and aetiological study of children with intellectual disability in Taiwan. *J Intellect Disabil Res* 42: 137–143.

Jacobson JW, Janicki MP (1983) Observed prevalence of multiple developmental disabilities. *Ment Retard* 21: 87–94.

Kiely M (1987) The prevalence of mental retardation. *Epidemiol Rev* 9: 194–218.

Larson SA, Lakin KC, Anderson L, Kwak N, Lee JH, Anderson D (2001) Prevalence of mental retardation and developmental disabilities: estimates from the 1994/1995 National Health Interview Survey Disability Supplements. *Am J Ment Retard* 106: 231–252.

Last JM (2000) *A Dictionary of Epidemiology, 4th ed.* New York: Oxford University Press.

Lenke RR, Levy HL (1980) Maternal phenylketonuria and hyperphenylalaninemia: an international survey of the outcome of untreated and treated pregnancies. *N Engl J Med* 303: 1202–1208.

Leonard H, Wen X (2002) The epidemiology of mental retardation: challenges and opportunities in the new millennium. *Ment Retard Dev Disabil Res Rev* 8: 117–134.

Lipkin P (1991) Epidemiology of the developmental disabilities. In: Capute AJ, Accardo PJ (eds) *Developmental Disabilities in Infancy and Childhood.* Baltimore, MD: Paul H. Brookes Publishing Co, pp 43–67.

Luckasson R, Coulter DL, Polloway EA, Reiss S, Schalock RL, Snell ME, et al. (2002) *Mental Retardation: Definition, Classification and Systems of Supports.* Washington, DC: American Association on Mental Retardation.

Luckasson R, Schalock RL, Snell ME, Spitalnik DM (1992) The 1992 AAMR definition and preschool children: response from the Committee on Terminology and Classification. *Ment Retard* 34: 247–253.

Marsh DO, Clarkson TW, Cox C, Myers GJ, Amin-Zaki L, Al-Tikriti S (1987) Fetal methylmercury poisoning: relationship between concentration in single strands of maternal hair and child effects. *Arch Neurol* 44: 1017–1022.

McDermott S, Daguise V, Mann H, Szwejbka L, Callaghan W (2001) Perinatal risk for mortality and mental retardation associated with maternal urinary tract infections. *J Fam Pract* 50: 433–437.

McLaren J, Bryson SE (1987) Review of recent epidemiological studies of mental retardation: prevalence, associated disorders, and etiology. *Am J Ment Retard* 92: 243–254.

Mendola P, Selevan S, Gutter S, Rice D (2002) Environmental factors associated with a spectrum of neurodevelopmental deficits. *Ment Retard Dev Disabil Res Rev* 8: 188–197.

Mercer JR (1973a) *Labeling the Mentally Retarded.* Berkeley: University of California Press.

Mercer J (1973b) The myth of 3% prevalence. *Monogr Am Assoc Ment Defic* 1: 1–18.

Morabia A (ed) (2005) A history of epidemiologic methods and concepts. *Am J Epidemiol* 161: 604–605.

Munro JD (1986) Epidemiology and the extent of mental retardation. *Psychiatr Clin North Am* 9: 591–624.

Murphy CC, Boyle C, Schendel D, Decouflé P, Yeargin-Allsopp M (1998) Epidemiology of mental retardation in children. *Ment Retard Dev Disabil Res Rev* 4: 6–13.

Murphy CC, Yeargin-Allsopp M, Decouflé P, Drews C (1995) The administrative prevalence of mental retardation in 10-year-old children in metropolitan Atlanta, 1985 through 1987. *Am J Public Health* 85: 319–323.

National Center on Birth Defects and Developmental Disabilities (2004) Risk factors for Down Syndrome. Atlanta, GA: Centers for Disease Control and Prevention. Retrieved December 28, 2005, from http://www.cdc.gov/ncbddd/bd/ds.htm.

National Center for Health Statistics (2005) Final nation data. Retrieved December 28, 2005, from http://www.marchofdimes.com/peristats.

National Information Center for Children and Youth with Disabilities (2000) NICHCY – Info about speech and language disorders. Fact sheet number 11 (FS11). Retrieved December 28, 2005, from http://www.kidsource.com/NICHCY/speech.html.

Needleman H (ed) (1992a) *Low Level Lead Exposure: The clinical implications of current research.* New York: Raven Press.

Needleman H (1992b) *Human Lead Exposure.* Boca Raton: CRC Press.

Paneth N (2005) Nature and uses of epidemiology. Retrieved January 23, 2006, from http://www.pitt.edu/-super1/lecture/lec8011/index.htm.

Partington M, Mowat D, Einfeld S, Tonge B, Turner G (2000) Genes on the X chromosome are important in undiagnosed mental retardation. *Am J Med Genet* 92: 57–61.

Qian M, Wang D, Chen Z (2000) A preliminary meta-analysis of 36 studies on impairment of intelligence development induced by iodine deficiency. *Am J Prev Med* 24: 75–77.

Rantakallio P, Korainen M (1987) Neurologic handicaps among children whose mothers smoked during pregnancy. *Prev Med* 16: 597–606.

Reschly D (1992) Mental retardation: conceptual foundations, definitional criteria, and diagnostic operations. In: Hooper S, Hynd G, Mattison R (eds) *Developmental Disorders: Diagnostic criteria and clinical assessment.* Hillsdale: Lawrence Erlbaum Associates.

Roeleveld N, Vingerhoets E, Zielhius GA, Gabreëls F (1992) Mental retardation associated with parental smoking and alcohol consumption before, during, and after pregnancy. *Prev Med* 21: 110–119.

Roeleveld N, Zielhuis GA, Gabreels F (1997) The prevalence of mental retardation: a critical review of recent literature. *Dev Med Child Neurol* 39: 125–132.

Rothman KJ, Greenland S, eds. (1998) *Modern Epidemiology, 2nd edn.* Philadelphia, PA: Lippicott-Raven.

Rutter M, Tizard J, Whitmore K (1970) *Education, Health and Behavior: Psychological and medical study of childhood development.* New York: John Wiley.

Schaefer GB, Bodensteiner JB (1992) Evaluation of the child with idiopathic mental retardation. *Pediatr Clin North Am* 39: 929–943.

Scolnik D, Nulman I, Rover J, Gladstone D, Czuchta D, Gardner HA, et al. (1994) Neurodevelopment of children exposed in utero to phenytoin and carbamazepine monotherapy. *JAMA* 271: 767–770.

Shamas GH, Wiig EH, Secord WA (1998) *Human Communication Disorders: An Introduction, 5th edn.* Boston: Allyn & Bacon.

Shevell M, Ashwal S, Donley D, Flint J, Gingold M, Hirtz D, et al. (2003) Practice parameter: evaluation of the child with global developmental delay. *Neurology* 60: 367–380.

Starza-Smith A (1989) Recent trends in prevalence studies of children with severe mental retardation. *Disabil Soc* 4: 177–195.

Stein Z, Susser M (1960) The families of dull children and classification for predicting careers. *Br J Prev Soc Med* 14: 83–88.

Stromme P, Hagberg G (2000) Aetiology in severe and mild mental retardation: a population-based study of Norwegian children. *Dev Med Child Neurol* 42: 76–86.

Tariverdian G, Vogel F (2000) Some problems in the genetics of X-linked mental retardation. *Cytogenet Cell Genet* 91: 278–284.

Tomblin JB, Smith E, Zhang X (1997) Epidemiology of specific language impairment: prenatal and perinatal risk factors. *J Commun Disord* 30: 325–344.

Turner G, Webb T, Wake S, Robinson H (1996) Prevalence of fragile X syndrome. *Am J Med Genet* 64: 196–197.

US Department of Education (2002) 24th Annual Report to Congress on the Implementation of the Individuals with Disabilities Education Act, Section 618. Jessup, MD: Ed Pubs, Education Publication Center, US Department of Education.

US Department of Education (2004) Individual with Disabilities Education Act (IDEA) Data. Number of Children Served Under IDEA by Disability and Age Group, 1994–2003. Retrieved January 21, 2005, from http://www.ideadata.org/tables27th/ar_aa9.xls.

Waisbren SE, Rokni H, Bailey I, Rohr F, Brown T, Warner-Rogers J (1997) Social factors and the meaning of food in adherence to medical diets: results of a maternal phenylketonuria summer camp. *J Inherit Metab Dis* 20: 21–27.

Yeargin-Allsopp M, Drews CD, Decouflé P, Murphy CC (1995) Mild mental retardation in black and white children in metropolitan Atlanta: a case–control study. *Am J Public Health* 85: 324–328.

Yeargin-Allsopp M, Murphy CC (1992) Response to Letter to the Editor: Underestimation of the incidence of mental retardation. *Pediatrics* 90: 653–654.

Yeargin-Allsopp M, Murphy CC, Cordero JF, Decouflé P, Hollowell J (1997) Reported biomedical causes and associated medical conditions for mental retardation among 10-year-old children, metropolitan Atlanta, 1985 to 1987. *Dev Med Child Neurol* 39: 142–149.

Yeargin-Allsopp M, Murphy CC, Oakley GP, Sikes K (1992) A multiple-source method for studying the prevalence of developmental disabilities in children: the Metropolitan Atlanta Developmental Disabilities Study. *Pediatrics* 89: 624–630.

3

THE CHANGING PANORAMA OF PRESCHOOL DISABILITY: BIOMEDICAL AND SOCIAL RISKS

Michael E Msall and Jennifer J Park

Approximately 37 million people were living in poverty in the United States in 2005, which represented 12.6% of the population. That figure was 17.6% for children under 18 years, suggesting that children were disproportionately exposed to the adverse affects of poverty (US Census Bureau 2006). Although the rate of poverty among children with disability is not available for 2005, recent studies and reports suggest the figure is higher than that of children without disabilities (Fujiura and Yamaki 2000, US Census Bureau 2005). In 2000, it was estimated that 28% of children with disability lived in households below the federal poverty level, while the figure was 16% for children without disability (Fujiura and Yamaki 2000). The US Census Bureau has stated that in 1999 the poverty rate for families raising children with disability was 21.8%, compared to 12.6% for families with children without disability (US Census Bureau 2005).

These data indicate that children with disability are more likely to live in impoverished situations than their peers without disability and only describe a portion of families with limited resources. Many economists and child developmental specialists consider incomes of 2–3 times above the official federal poverty level as the minimum requirements for a 'living' wage. While these data show that child disability and poverty are related, they do not tell us if one causes the other; that is, if family poverty is the outcome of child disability or if child disability is the result of family poverty. The data also fail to illustrate the delicate interplay of both disability and poverty on the cognitive, health, and social outcomes of children exposed to both elements.

This chapter reviews the influence of biomedical and social risks on preschool children (birth to age 5 years) and how with current knowledge the risks and suboptimal outcomes can be reduced or minimized. This chapter focuses on the US experience which reflects that of an economically wealthy nation with an advanced health care network yet with an intrinsically unequal distribution of wealth and accessibility to educational, social, medical, and rehabilitation resources.

TABLE 3.1
Prevalence of neurodevelopmental and genetic disorders in US children 0–5 years (population: 20 million)

	Rates per 1000	Children (N)
Neurodevelopmental disorders		
Cerebral palsy	2.5	50 000
ID-MR (IQ 50–55)	5	100 000
Autistic spectrum disorder	2	40 000
Hearing loss (>50db)	2	40 000
Visual loss (<20/200)	0.5	10 000
Technology dependent	1	20 000
Any neurodevelopmental disorder	20	400 000
Neurologic and genetic disorders		
Down syndrome	1	20 000
Fragile X	1	20 000
Fetal alcohol	1	20 000
Neonatal encephalopathy	7.5	150 000
Epilepsy	5	100 000
Spina bifida	0.5	10 000
Muscular dystrophy	0.5	5000
Congenital heart disease	7	140 000
Any congenital disease	30	600 000

ID-MR, intellectual disability–mental retardation.

BIOMEDICAL AND SOCIAL RISK FACTORS AND DISABILITY

The two most important categorical determinants of disability and developmental delay are biomedical and social risk factors. Biomedical risk factors are related to biologic elements such as genetic, chromosomal, or neurologic disorders. These are illustrated in Table 3.1.

Social risk factors denote suboptimal home and community environment such as domestic violence, child abuse, drug addiction, crime, and gang activity (Holzmann and Jorgensen 2000). In many cases, social risks are closely tied to a family's wealth and socioeconomic status (SES). Disabilities that render adverse outcomes in preschool children independent of their parents' SES include fragile X syndrome, Down syndrome, autism spectrum disorder, cerebral palsy, spina bifida, Rett syndrome, and Prader–Willi syndrome. Disabilities that are highly related to poverty and low SES are fetal alcohol spectrum disorder, preterm birth (i.e. prior to 37 weeks' gestation), low birth weight (less than 2500g), and mild intellectual disability (i.e. IQ scores more than 2 standard deviation below the mean with adaptive difficulties). Of these, low birth weight and mild intellectual disability affects 7% of newborns and 1 out of 7 preschoolers, respectively (Table 3.2).

TABLE 3.2
Epidemiology of preschool psychologic risks in US children (2000)

Risk factors	Percentage
Children under 6 years in poverty	
African-Americans	48
Hispanics	43
Caucasians	15
In deep poverty[a]	13
African-Americans in deep poverty[a]	33
Psychosocial risks	
Parents with < high school education	25
Single mothers	37
Teenaged mothers	38
Maternal mental health disorder	5
Children in foster care	2
Children who are homeless	1
Biomedical risks	
Low birth weight (<2500g)	7
Very low birth weight	1–2
Child abuse and neglect	10
Illicit substance exposure[b]	10
No prenatal care	5
Prenatal exposure to tobacco	20
Prenatal exposure to alcohol	10
Childhood failure to thrive	5
Childhood lead level	5
Developmental risks	
Motor delay[c]	5
Speech language[c]	20
Global developmental delay[c]	10
Suboptimal cognitive development	15

[a] Deep poverty = 50% below poverty line.
[b] Includes cocaine, heroin, and marijuana.
[c] Standard scores of more than 1.5 SD below the mean for age.

COST OF DISABILITY IN CHILDREN
Children with disability live in households where there are less financial resources. These families are more likely to live in poverty than those children without disabilities. Children with special care needs account for 13% of the child population in the United States (Palfrey 2006), and 1 in every 26 families in the United States reported raising children whose special needs result in sufficient challenges

to limit academic or community participation (US Census Bureau 2005). This means approximately 2.8 million families in the United States were raising at least one child with disability between the ages of 5 and 17. That figure accounts for 9.2% of the 30.7 million families raising children in the United States at the time. It was also noted that families with members who had disability were more likely than other families to receive social security and public assistance, and were less likely to be employed or to own their own residence. In 2000, the rates of families without members with disability receiving Supplemental Security Income and any public assistance or welfare were 0.9% and 2.7%, respectively, but the figures for families with children with disability were 9.1% and 11.4%. While the median income of families raising children without disability was $50 098, the same figure for families raising children with disability was $38 332 (US Census Bureau 2005).

The cost of caring for children with disabilities brought on by biologic and/or social risk factors can either push families into poverty or, in the case of families with pre-existing low income, into deeper poverty. This exposes the already vulnerable children to the additional adverse health and developmental effects of poverty such as poor nutrition, inadequate housing and medical care, and a lack of access to quality child care and schools. Some of the most common assistance associated with caring for children with disabilities includes rehabilitation therapies (e.g. physical therapy, occupational, and speech therapy), medication, counseling and educational services, adaptive equipment, primary and specialty medical care, and family supports (Perrin 2002, Parish and Cloud 2006). It is estimated that the cost associated with special education is generally 2.3 times higher than the cost of a student with no special needs (Roth et al. 2004), while health care costs of children with special care needs were over 3 times more than the cost of children without special care needs (Newacheck and Kim 2005). Since private insurance, Medicaid, and the State Children's Health Insurance Program do not meet all financial burdens, the cost of medical and educational assistance as well as special equipment for disabled children largely rests on the family (Parish and Cloud 2006). This is especially trying for families that are already in poverty or low SES. Children with special care needs in low income families (<200% of federal poverty level) are over 10 times more likely to have financially burdensome expenses (i.e. out-of-pocket expenditure that is over 5% of the family income) than higher income families (≥400% of federal poverty level) (Newacheck and Kim 2005).

PRENATAL EFFECTS OF POVERTY: PRETERM BIRTH AND LOW BIRTH WEIGHT STATUS
Advances in pediatric medicine have increased the survival of infants with adverse health risks such as preterm birth, very low birth weight, and extremely low birth weight status (Msall and Tremont 2002). However, the number of children born preterm and/or with low birth weight status have actually increased in recent years

(March of Dimes 2005). The adverse environmental and social conditions that are associated with increased risks for children to be born preterm and/or with low birth weight status extends well beyond their childhood. The number of children living in low income families has increased since 2000 (National Center for Children in Poverty 2006). In addition, certain high risk behaviors have also increased, such as the rate of binge drinking among childbearing-age US women (ages 18–44) which rose from 12% in 2001 to 13.1% in 2003 (March of Dimes 2005).

Several biomedical and social risk factors are associated with preterm birth and low birth weight. Infants from multiple births (twins, triplets, or more), infants born to mothers with chronic health conditions (e.g. diabetes, high blood pressure, and heart problems), and infants born to mothers who engaged in 'risky' behaviors prior to the child's birth (e.g. tobacco and alcohol use, narcotic and opiate exposure) are more likely to have offspring who are born preterm and with low birth weight (Bishai and Koren 1999, Weitzman et al. 2002, March of Dimes 2005).

Although preterm birth and low birth weight can occur in pregnancies across all socioeconomic and racial backgrounds, poverty and low SES are strongly related to preterm birth and low birth weight (Huston 1991). African-American infants are more than 1.5 times more likely than Caucasian infants to be born preterm (<37 weeks' gestation). Infants born to African-American mothers were also 2.5 times more likely to be born very preterm (<32 weeks' gestation) than their white peers (March of Dimes 2005). This racial discrepancy in preterm birth and low birth weight parallels the national discrepancy in wealth distribution. African-Americans have the lowest 3-year average median income (2003–2005) among racial groups in the United States (US Census Bureau 2006), and while only 10% of white children are poor, 34% of African-American children and 30% of Hispanic children are from families below the official poverty level (annual income below $19 307 for a family of four) (Palfrey 2006). Poverty and low SES increase the risks of substance use among pregnant and childbearing-age women. Rates of marijuana, cocaine, tobacco, and alcohol use are higher for women who are unmarried, unemployed, and have less than a college education (Huston 1991, Hans 1999). It has been suggested that the prevalence of substance abuse, illicit drug use, and smoking among women from impoverished or low SES background is largely due to the pervasive sense of helplessness, low self-esteem, difficulties coping with repetitive stress, and pressure from coping with difficult financial situations in everyday living (Huston 1991, Weitzman et al. 2002).

Lack of prenatal care also puts infants born to women from impoverished or low SES background at risk for preterm birth and low birth weight. Women who receive prenatal care are more likely to detect and identify prenatal complications or health problems early and are more likely to have access to educational and support services (e.g. counseling) and referrals to reduce risky behaviors such as substance use and poor nutrition (March of Dimes 2005). Approximately 3.5% of pregnant

TABLE 3.3
Impact of birth weight on school-age outcomes

Birth weight (g)	Very good/excellent health (%)	Poor/fair health (%)	Functional limitation (%)[a]	No limitation (%)
<1500	69	6	20	79
1501–2499	78	3	10.3	88
2500–2999	80	2.4	8	91
≥3000	84	1.5	6.7	93

Source: National Health Interview Survey 1997–2000.
[a] In age-appropriate motor, self-care, communication/sensory, or learning skills.

women in 2003 either began prenatal care late (i.e. in the third trimester) or received no prenatal care at all, with Native American and African-American mothers at least twice as likely as white mothers to receive late prenatal care or no prenatal care (7.6% and 6%, respectively, compared to 2.1% of white mothers) (March of Dimes 2005). Women living below poverty level who are unmarried, are under the age 20 and over 35 years with fewer years of overall education are more likely to receive less prenatal care (Huston 1991). It should be pointed out that even with standardized prenatal care, the complex causal pathways that can lead to dramatic decreases (or increases) in preterm birth are not known. The adverse effects of preterm birth and low birth weight include a spectrum of health, developmental, and behavioral outcomes (Msall et al. 1998, Thompson et al. 2003, March of Dimes 2005). Table 3.3 summarizes the impact of birth weight on school age outcomes using data from the National Health Interview Survey (NHIS) for the 1997–2000 cohorts (Msall et al. 2003a).

In this particular cohort, 408 children (1.2%) were born with very low birth weight status (<1500g); 2185 children (6.2%) were born with low birth weight status (1500–2499g); 6289 children (17.8%) were born with birth weights of 2500–2999g; and 26 404 children were born with a birth weight of over 3000g. There were significantly lower ratings of very good and excellent health, as well as disproportionately high rates of functional limitations in mobility, communication, sensory, and learning skills amongst children with indicators of poverty. In addition, indicators of child well-being and disability were worse for children with higher indicators of poverty (such as Medicaid health insurance) (Msall et al. 2003a). Among school children on Medicaid (an indicator of poverty and social disadvantage), functional disability occurred in 35% of children who weighed less than 1500g at birth, 15% of children who weighed 1500–2499g at birth, and 13% of children who weighted over 2500g at birth. Poor health was present in 14%, 7%, and 5% of these groups, respectively (Msall et al. 2003b).

Low birth weight infants are also more likely to have emotional and behavioral problems, learning disorders and lower cognitive abilities, than infants born with normal birth weight (Weitzman et al. 2002). However, with adequate management and supports, these conditions do not preclude a child born with low birth weight completing high school and achieving eventual successes in adulthood (Hack 2006; Saigal et al. 2007).

POVERTY: SUBOPTIMAL PRESCHOOL ENVIRONMENTS AND CHILD OUTCOMES

In addition to the aforementioned risks, poverty and low SES can have other detrimental consequences to a child's cognitive, health, and behavioral development. The adverse effect of poverty and low SES seems to have the most impact during early childhood, especially in the preschool years (Brooks-Gunn and Duncan 1997, Bradley and Corwyn 2002). In many cases, the effects of poverty and low SES on cognitive, health, and behavioral outcomes of children not only feed off of each other, but they can be combined with pre-existing biomedical risk factors, thus increasing the suboptimal outcomes of economically disadvantaged children. For example, a child born with very low birth weight and hearing loss who does not receive proper audiologic attention and care because of the complexity of factors facing the parents in accessing pediatric subspecialists has a higher chance of experiencing additional later learning, behavior, and communicative challenges.

COGNITIVE DEVELOPMENT

Although it is not certain to what extent the adverse outcomes of poverty and low SES in childhood influence adolescence and adulthood, it appears that cognitive development especially is most affected by poverty during the early stages of childhood (Brooks-Gunn and Duncan 1997). Several researchers indicate that poverty and low SES are strong predictors of school attendance, high school drop-out, and college enrollment, with a particularly strong relationship between SES and verbal skills and SES and developmental learning experiences (Brooks-Gunn and Duncan, 1997, Battin-Pearson et al. 2000). The lack of educational attainment among the impoverished and low SES populations limits developmental learning experiences (Brooks-Gunn and Duncan 1997, Battin-Pearson et al. 2000). This lack of educational attainment among the impoverished and low SES population could be related to the fact that children from low SES backgrounds disproportionately lack access to cognitively stimulating resources and activities such as books, cassette tapes, educational toys, visits to the museum, and related parent–child learning activities (Huston 1991, Bradley et al. 2001, Bradley and Corwyn 2002).

The lack of parent–child interaction may also have a role in the suboptimal cognitive development of children from poor families. In a study by Hart and Risley (1980), children from middle class families received verbal input of over 30 000 000 words by age 3, with 83% of these verbal interactions being educational and positive in content and 17% being negative and disciplinary in content. However, children from poor African-American families received inputs of 10 000 000 words by age 3 with 29% of these verbal interactions being educational and positive in content while 21% were negative and disciplinary. Such differences resulted in less verbal abilities, lower IQ, and poorer educational achievement throughout childhood (Hart and Risley 1980). In another study (Bradley et al. 2001), non-poor mothers were shown to be twice as likely as poor mothers to read to their children three or more times a week during infancy and early childhood. It was also noted that more well-to-do mothers were more likely than their poor counterparts to speak to their children or respond to their children verbally (Bradley et al. 2001).

HEALTH

Children from impoverished and low SES backgrounds are more likely to suffer setbacks in physical health because of poor nutrition, lack of medical care, lack of transportation to medical facilities, and hazardous living conditions. Studies have shown that children from impoverished backgrounds are less likely to receive regular physical check-ups or visits to the doctor's office, be immunized, receive dental care, receive proper nourishment, and have health insurance (Huston 1991, Hertzman and Wiens 1996, Duncan and Brooks-Gunn 2000). Factors that contribute to these outcomes are low parent income or unemployment, a shortage of community health professionals, problems with accessing transportation, available child care, and time management (Huston 1991). Children from impoverished backgrounds are also more likely to experience adverse environments such as lead poisoning, asthma, and injuries as a result of living in overcrowded older buildings and neighborhoods with limited safety precautions in place for young children (Huston 1991, Brooks-Gunn and Duncan 1997, Palfrey 2006).

Adverse health outcomes due to social risk factors in children living in poverty and low SES can result in mild to severe child disability in cognition, communication, and sensory skills. Children from poor backgrounds are more likely to be affected with mild intellectual disability, visual and hearing impairment, and disabilities related to accidental injuries (Huston 1991, Reading 1997).

Exposure to violence also results in health problems for children from an early age. Children who are exposed to domestic violence, abuse, and community violence are more likely to have asthma, gastrointestinal problems, and school absences (Graham-Bermann and Seng 2005). Abusive and/or negligent parents are more likely to either ignore or undermine child health conditions that need medical treatment (Flaherty et al. 2006).

EMOTIONAL, BEHAVIORAL, AND MENTAL HEALTH

Poverty and low SES affects emotional and behavioral development of children through experiences of hunger, abuse, parental neglect, social isolation, and directly witnessing various acts of violence within the community. Children exposed to such adverse outcomes are more likely to suffer from emotional and behavioral problems including attention-deficit–hyperactivity disorder (ADHD), depression, anxiety, sexual promiscuity, teenage pregnancy, and substance abuse (Huston 1991, Brooks-Gunn and Duncan 1997, Reading 1997, Tenney-Soeiro and Wilson 2004). It is also noted that children with developmental delays have a higher risk for behavioral problems (Committee on Children with Disabilities 2001).

Hunger, one of the many byproducts of poverty and low SES, can affect a child's mental health. According to national research, approximately 12.4 million children in the United States experienced food insecurity in 2005 (US Department of Agriculture 2005). Hungry children are more likely to experience anxiety and depressive symptoms, probably due to stress caused by unpredictable and irregular eating patterns and food resources. The high stress level of mothers who are under pressure or struggling to provide for their children's most basic needs can also affect their children's emotional well-being (Weinreb et al. 2002).

PREVENTIVE INTERVENTIONS

Although the effects of biomedical and social risk factors of poverty and low SES can have devastating outcomes on child development, these effects can be reduced or minimized with early preventive educational and social interventions. These interventions are especially important, considering that in many cases biomedical risks caused by the prenatal effects of poverty and low SES (such as preterm birth and low birth weight) can be worsened by conditions of suboptimal postnatal social and familial environments. Children at highest risk for mild intellectual disability in elementary school years who receive educational intervention during the preschool interval are more likely to show appropriate average intellectual performance than those who have not received such direct intervention (Ramey et al. 1978, Campbell et al. 2001). Some analyses have even demonstrated that the severity of the postnatal effects of low SES (such as maternal education level) are a more significant predictor of eventual child language and cognitive performance than actual prenatal exposure to substances such as tobacco, cocaine, marijuana, and alcohol (Hurt et al. 1997, Arendt et al. 2004). Frank et al. (2005), in addition to finding 'no negative effect of prenatal cocaine exposure on WPPSI-R IQ scores identified at 4 years,' noted that children with a history of prenatal cocaine exposure can benefit from early intervention and preschool enrichment programs that enhance outcomes for low income students. Considering that many studies have demonstrated that 'the socio-cultural environment not only has a direct influence on children's intellectual competence, but acts in conjunction with biological factors to magnify or dampen their potentially adverse effects on mental and physical development,' the importance of intervention programs to help prevent the negative outcomes of biologic and social risk factors due to low SES cannot be overemphasized (Camp et al. 1998).

IDENTIFYING THE 'AT-RISK' POPULATION
In order for children to receive the benefits of early intervention, they must either have obvious developmental delays or be 'at-risk' for subsequent delay and disability. The latter, although more challenging to identify, is nevertheless a very important criteria because 'some conditions associated with developmental delay may not produce observable impairment until the affected children are older and then possibly untreatable' (Camp et al. 1998). Several studies have suggested using certain maternal, perinatal, neonatal, and demographic characteristics available at birth to identify children at later risk for mild intellectual disability, developmental delay, and educational difficulties. These characteristics include: (1) low SES of the family, (2) low maternal education, (3) low levels of maternal cognitive performance, (4) minority status, (5) single parenthood, and (6) third or later born child (Ramey et al. 1978, Finkelstein and Ramey 1980, Camp et al. 1998).

Successful early intervention programs not only enhance behavioral and cognitive development of 'at-risk' children, but they also offer family supports by promoting parent–child interaction and parenting skills. Bailey et al. (1999) observed that 'early intervention is not a discrete event but rather a complex series of interactions and transactions centered around the accomplishment of two basic tasks: nurturing and enhancing the development and behavior of the infant or toddler with a disability, and sustaining their families.'

THREE LESSONS FROM PREVIOUS STUDIES
THE INFANT HEALTH AND DEVELOPMENT PROGRAM: COMPREHENSIVE INTERVENTIONS FOR CHILDREN WHO WERE BORN PRETERM
The Infant Health and Development Program (IHDP) was a multicenter study designed to evaluate the effects of early intervention on health and developmental outcomes of low birth weight survivors. Nine hundred and eighty five (N = 985) preterm, low birth weight infants from Boston, Dallas, Little Rock, Miami, New Haven, New York, Philadelphia, and Seattle were recruited in 1985–86 (37% of the recruits weighed 2001–2500g, 37% weighed 1501–2000g, and 26% weighed less than 1501g at birth). Of those, 377 were randomly assigned to the intervention group while the remaining 608 were assigned to the follow-up only group (i.e. comparison group). During the study, children from both groups were both given medical care and received a series of developmental and social assessments. The IHDP standard of care for all comparison group children included developmental and rehabilitation referrals to early intervention and community providers when delays were detected (Gross et al. 1997).

Children in the IHDP intervention group and their families experienced quality home visits and center-based early childhood full-day education utilizing a validated developmental curriculum (Gross et al. 1997, Bradley and Corwyn 2002). The home visits began at neonatal discharge and the center-based early childhood educational experience began when the infants were 1 year of age. Both home visits and early educational interventions lasted until the children were 3 years of age.

The home visits were conducted on a weekly basis during the first year and bi-weekly in years 2 and 3. The home visiting lessons consisted of relationship-based learning with a focus on enhancing communication skills and facilitating parent problem solving for child behavior stressors and family challenges. The center-based interventions operated 7–9 hours a day, 5 days a week, with children encouraged to attend a minimum of 4 hours per day. Staff to children ratio was 1:3 between 12 and 23 months, and 1:4 for ages 24–36 months. The curriculum was centered on games and activities that addressed cognitive, fine motor, language, gross motor, social, and self-help skills.

Three-year follow-up of both intervention and comparison groups revealed substantial differentials in the percentage of children with borderline (IQ 71–84) and impaired (IQ ≤70) intellectual performance. Among children with the highest participation rates, 1 in 13 had cognitive impairments. In contrast, 2 in 5 children with the lowest participation rates had cognitive impairments. In addition, the program's greatest impact occurred among children whose mothers had low IQs. Approximately 40% of children from the comparison group had intellectual disability at age 3 if their mothers had cognitive disabilities, compared with 15% of intervention children whose mothers also had a cognitive disability.

The assessment of cognitive, behavioral, and health outcomes of the participants at 3 years of age showed that children in the intervention group had significantly higher scores on the cognitive tests and receptive vocabulary tests than did the comparison group (Gross et al. 1997). The intervention group also scored lower on reported behavior problems than the comparison group. Among children who survived birth weights of less than 1500g, the mean Stanford Binet IQ of the intervention group was 88 compared with 80 in the comparison group. These scores increased to 92 and 82, respectively, among the very low birth weight survivors if the children with cerebral palsy (presumably acquired prior to neonatal discharge) were excluded from the cognitive testing data. Among children who survived birth weights of less than 1000g, the scores were 87 and 80, respectively, with scores of 93 and 85 when extremely low birth weight survivors without cerebral palsy were not included for their cognitive scores. Overall, the evident short-term benefit of the IHDP intervention was that intellectual disability suggest mental retardation could be prevented among children at dual jeopardy because of preterm birth and parents with cognitive disability.

THE HARDY STUDY: ADVERSE EARLY CHILD ENVIRONMENTS AND ADULT OUTCOMES IN BALTIMORE

Hardy and colleagues examined the impact of early childhood adversity in inner city mothers and the outcomes for their children when adult (Hardy and Shapiro

1999). The offspring were examined at ages 27–33 years old. These children had been born between 1959 and 1966 in Baltimore and their mothers were living in poverty at the time of the children's birth. Of the 1758 adults, 68% had completed high school, and 76% were living independently without public support. Seventy-five percent had deferred having their first child until age 20 years or older. However, there were both sex and racial differentials for adult outcomes of children who had experienced adversity. Seventy-three percent of girls graduated from high school compared with only 64% of the boys. Seventy-three percent of whites completed high school compared with only 48% of African-American children in the study.

Further analysis of this cohort examined the impact of educational achievement on adult success. The factors most predictive of high school completion were average or better reading skills at age 8 years, not repeating a grade in school, and not becoming a teen parent. Thus, even among those children at highest social risk, positive outcomes can be obtained or enhanced if there is early educational success (Hardy and Shapiro 1999).

BROOKLINE PRESCHOOL PROJECT: QUALITY EARLY CHILDHOOD EDUCATION

Palfrey et al. (2005) examined 120 adults at age 25 who had participated in comprehensive preschool services in Brookline, Massachusetts involving both inner city Boston and suburban preschoolers. In this cohort, one-third of the families were African-American, Latino, or Asian. Outcomes included physical and mental health, education, independent living, and risk-taking behaviors.

Of the inner-city participants followed at age 25, 84% were employed, 28% had incomes below the poverty level (<$20 000 per year), 8% had been suspended from high school, and mean education level was 2.3 years beyond high school. Sixty-four percent of the participants rated their current health as very good or excellent.

In the inner-city group that did not receive comprehensive preschool interventions, outcomes at age 25 were less than optimal. There was 71% employment and 72% poverty. In addition, 20% had been suspended from high school, most had not completed college, and they averaged 1.2 years of education after high school. Only 42% rated their health status as very good or excellent. Overall, inner city adults who had received comprehensive preschool services had increased access to medical care, higher levels of health efficacy, more positive health behaviors, and less depression compared with adult inner city peers who had not received comprehensive preschool services. Lastly, young adults who had participated in this program had more educational attainment, higher income levels, more responsible health care behaviors, and a positive sense of well-being (Palfrey et al. 2005).

CONCLUSIONS

The IHDP, Baltimore, and Brookline projects collectively demonstrate that groups with biologic and social disadvantages or social disadvantages alone benefit from quality comprehensive early childhood health development and family supports. Outcomes were modified by targeted intervention although the intervention was by no means a 'magic bullet' which fixed all problems. It is the complex interplay of risk, developmental impacts, and missed opportunities once targeted that are critical to successful eventual outcomes.

This reinforces the importance of a biopsychosocial model when we examine the complex trajectories of children at risk and their access to developmentally promoting preschool services. In addition, health professionals must not assume that comprehensive preschool supports are followed by access to quality elementary and high schools. About 50 years ago, Drillien and associates demonstrated that preterm children who escaped severe neurologic impairments and who were born into educated and middle class families had academic achievement scores similar to their term siblings. In contrast, preterm children who escaped severe neurologic impairment but grew up in social disadvantage had significantly worse academic and cognitive outcomes than their siblings (Drillien 1967).

Most recently, Heckman (2006) examined the importance of investing in skill formation and preschool child development prevention services for children in poverty. The analysis emphasizes the difficulties that later interventionist programs (special education, behavioral health, juvenile justice) have in remediating earlier deficits. Investments in prevention and early childhood appeared to substantially increase the chances of having sufficient cognitive and non-cognitive skills essential for later adult success. Among the latter skills are motivation, perseverance, and tenacity. The analysis reveals that it is more cost-effective to proactively invest in skill formation in the preschool years, than remediate later skill deficits in middle childhood and adolescence. This is because later attainment builds on early cognitive, communicative, social, and emotional competencies. In addition, compensatory interventions in middle childhood and adolescence are far from 100% effective. In addition, there are serious gaps in community-wide access to fully meet vulnerable children's needs.

Our challenge in the developmental neurosciences continues to be how to best understand the complex interplay of brain structure and function with respect to biologic and social vulnerability. By taking a biopsychosocial framework to these complex challenges, we can promote a proactive habilitative and educational approach for children who are at highest biologic and social risk. For children with severe challenges, our efforts require understanding markers and mechanisms that disrupt cognitive, communicative, and adaptive pathways that underlie successful learning and development.

ACKNOWLEDGMENTS
Supported in part by 1U01HD37614 entitled 'NICHD Family and Child Well Being Network: Child Disability,' the Children's Guild of Buffalo, and the Grant

Healthcare Foundation of Chicago. Larry Gray, Peter Smith, Tom Blondis, Ron Espinal, Lainie Ross, Lyn Kahana, Mike Schreiber, Bree Andrews, Dilek Bishku, Jill Glick, Diana Ryan, A Timosciek and the University of Chicago Early Intervention outreach team provided valuable feedback.

REFERENCES

Arendt RE, Short EJ, Singer LT, Minnes S, Hewitt J, Flynn S, et al. (2004) Children prenatally exposed to cocaine: developmental outcomes and environmental risks at seven years of age. *J Dev Behav Pediatr* 25: 83–90.

Bailey DB Jr, Aytch LS, Odom SL, Symons F, Wolery M (1999) Early intervention as we know it. *Ment Retard Dev Disabil Res Rev* 5: 11–20.

Battin-Pearson S, Abbott RD, Hill KG, Catalano RF, Hawkins JD (2000) Predictors of early high school dropout: a test of five theories. *J Educat Psychol* 92: 568–582.

Bishai R, Koren G (1999) Maternal and obstetric effects of prenatal drug exposure. *Clin Perinatol* 26: 75–86.

Bradley RH, Corwyn RF (2002) Socioeconomic status and child development. *Annu Rev Psychol* 53: 371–99.

Bradley RH, Corwyn RF, McAdoo HP, Coll CG (2001) The home environments of children in the United States part I: variations by age, ethnicity, and poverty status. *Child Dev* 72: 1844–1867.

Brooks-Gunn J, Duncan GJ (1997) The effects of poverty on children. *Future Child* 7: 55–71.

Camp BW, Broman SH, Nichols PL, Leff M (1998) Maternal and neonatal risk factors for mental retardation: defining the 'at-risk' child. *Early Hum Dev* 50: 159–173.

Campbell FA, Pungello EP, Miller-Johnson S, Burchinal M, Ramey CT (2001) The development of cognitive and academic abilities: growth curves from an early childhood educational experiment. *Dev Psychol* 37: 231–242.

Committee on Children with Disabilities (2001) American Academy of Pediatrics: Developmental surveillance and screening of infants and young children. *Pediatics* 108: 192–196.

Drillien CM (1967) The incidence of mental and physical handicaps in school age children of very low birth weight. *Pediatrics* 39: 238–247.

Duncan GJ, Brooks-Gunn J (2000) Family poverty, welfare reform, and child development. *Child Dev* 71: 188–196.

Finkelstein NW, Ramey CT (1980) Information from birth certificates as a risk index for educational handicap. *Am J Ment Defic* 84: 546–52.

Flaherty EG, Thompson R, Litrownik AJ, Theodore A, English DJ, Black MM, et al. (2006) Effect of early childhood adversity on child health. *Arch Pediatr Adolesc Med* 160: 1232–1238.

Frank DA, Rose-Jacobs R, Beeghly M, Wilbur M, Bellinger D, Cabral H (2005) Level of prenatal cocaine exposure and 48-month IQ: importance of preschool enrichment. *Neurotoxicol Teratol* 27: 15–28.

Fujiura GT, Yamaki K (2000) Trends in demography of childhood poverty and disability. *Except Child* 66: 187–199.

Graham-Bermann SA, Seng J (2005) Violence exposure and traumatic stress symptoms as additional predictors of health problems in high-risk children. *J Pediatr* 146: 349–354.

Gross T, Spiker D, Haynes C (eds) (1997) *Helping Low Birth Weight, Premature Babies. The Infant Health and Development Program.* Stanford, California: Stanford University Press.

Hack M (2006) Young adult outcomes of very-low-birth-weight children. *Semin Fetal Neonatal Med* 11: 127–137.

Hans SL (1999) Demographic and psychosocial characteristics of substance-abusing pregnant women. *Clin Perinatol* 26(1): 55–74.

Hardy JB, Shapiro S. (1999) Pathways to Adulthood: A Three-Generation Urban Study, 1960–1994. http://dir.niehs.nih.gov/direb/studies/cpp/pathway/cb2420fg.pdf

Hart B, Risley TR (1980) In vivo language intervention: unanticipated general effects. *J Appl Behav Anal* 13: 407–432.

Heckman JJ (2006) Skill formation and the economics of investing in disadvantaged children. *Science* 312: 1900–1902.

Hertzman C, Wiens M (1996) Child development and long-term outcomes: a population health perspective and summary of successful interventions. *Soc Sci Med* 43: 1083–1095.

Holzmann R, Jorgensen S (2000) *Social Risk Management: A new conceptual framework for Social Protection, and beyond.* Washington, DC: World Bank.

Hurt H, Malmud E, Betancourt L, Brodsky NL, Giannetta J (1997) A prospective evaluation of early language development in children with in utero cocaine exposure and in control subjects. *J Pediatr* 130: 310–312.

Huston AC (ed) (1991) *Children in Poverty: Child Development and Public Policy.* Cambridge, UK: Cambridge University Press.

March of Dimes (2005) March of Dimes Data Book for Policy Makers. Maternal, Infant, and Child Health in the United States. Office of Government Affairs, March of Dimes.

Msall ME, Tremont MR (2002) Measuring functional outcomes after prematurity: developmental impact of very low birth weight and extremely low birth weight status on childhood disability. *Ment Retard Dev Disabil Res Rev* 8: 258–272.

Msall ME, Bier JA, LaGasse L, Tremont M, Lester B (1998) The vulnerable preschool child: the impact of biomedical and social risks on neurodevelopmental function. *Semin Pediatr Neurol* 5: 52–61.

Msall ME, Rogers ML, Avery RC, Hogan DP (2003a) Impact of birthweight status on school age outcomes in the 1997–2000 National Health Interview Surveys. *Dev Med Child Neurol* 45 (Suppl 96): 38, SP 13.

Msall ME, Rogers ML, Avery RC, Hogan DP (2003b) Effect of health insurance coverage on school age outcomes for low and very low birthweight children in the 1997–2000 National Health Interview Surveys. *Dev Med Child Neurol* 45 (Suppl 96): 40, SP 18.

National Center for Children in Poverty (2006) Low-Income Children in the United States, National and State Trend Data, 1995–2005. http://www.nccp.org/media/nst06a_text.pdf.

Newacheck PW, Kim SE (2005) A national profile of health care utilization and expenditures for children with special health care needs. *Arch Pediatr Adolesc Med* 159: 10–17.

Palfrey JS (2006) *Child Health in America: Making a Difference Through Advocacy.* Baltimore, MS: Johns Hopkins University Press.

Palfrey JS, Hauser-Cram P, Bronson MB, Warfield ME, Sirin S, Chan E (2005) The Brookline Early Education Project: a 25-year follow-up study of a family-centered early health and development intervention. *Pediatrics* 116: 144–152.

Parish SL, Cloud JM (2006) Financial well-being of young children with disabilities and their families. *Soc Work* 51: 223–232.

Perrin JM (2002) Health services research for children with disabilities. *Milbank Q* 80: 303–324.

Ramey CT, Stedman DJ, Borders-Patterson A, Mengel W (1978) Predicting school failure from information available at birth. *Am J Ment Defic* 82: 525–534.

Reading R (1997) Poverty and the health of children and adolescents. *Arch Dis Child* 76: 463–467.

Roth J, Figlio DN, Chen Y, Ariet M, Carter RL, Resnick MB, et al. (2004) Maternal and infant factors associated with excess kindergarten costs. *Pediatrics* 114: 720–728.

Saigal S, Stoskopf B, Boyle M, Paneth N, Pinelli J, Streiner D, et al. (2007) Comparison of current health, functional limitations, and health care use of young adults who were born with extremely low birth weight and normal birth weight. *Pediatrics* 119: e562–73.

Tenney-Soeiro R, Wilson C (2004) An update on child abuse and neglect. *Curr Opin Pediatr* 16: 233–237.

Thompson JR, Carter RL, Edwards AR, Roth J, Ariet M, Ross NL, et al. (2003) A population-based study of the effects of birth weight on early developmental delay or disability in children. *Am J Perinatol* 20: 321–332.

US Census Bureau (2005) Disability and American Families: 2000. http://www.census.gov/prod/2005pubs/censr-23.pdf.

US Census Bureau (2006) Income, Poverty, and Health Insurance Coverage in the United States: 2005. http://www.census.gov/prod/2006pubs/p60-231.pdf.

US Department of Agriculture (2005) Measuring Food Security in the United States: Household Food Security in the United States, 2005. http://www.ers.usda.gov/Publications/ERR29/ERR29.pdf.

Weinreb L, Wehler C, Perloff J, Scott R, Hosmer D, Sagor L, Gundersen C (2002) Hunger: its impact on children's health and mental health. *Pediatrics* 110: e41.

Weitzman M, Byrd RS, Aligne CA, Moss M (2002) The effects of tobacco exposure on children's behavioral and cognitive functioning: implications for clinical and public health policy and future research. *Neurotoxicol Teratol* 24: 397–406.

4

ETHICS AND COMMON MORALITY IN NEURODEVELOPMENTAL DISABILITIES

Michael Shevell

Children with neurodevelopmental disabilities represent a 'doubly vulnerable' population that is the by-product of both age and impairment who ultimately depend on the protection of others for their ethical treatment (Shevell 1998). Unfortunately, recent history is replete with examples from a variety of geographic locales and sociopolitical cultures, where such protection was sadly lacking leading to what frankly must be termed a egregious abuse and neglect of this population (Sherr and Shevell 2006). The result of such abuse and neglect were grievous harms to these individuals, sometimes beyond our human capacity to fully comprehend and understand as caring persons.

Ethics is the branch of philosophy that seeks to identify the principles that should underlie 'ideal' human behavior (Cooke 1996). It is rationally based, utilizing reason and logic applied rigorously to formulate what should be the basis for correct decisions and actions (Jonsen et al. 1986). It goes beyond the situational to elaborate unifying themes that cross all aspects of human endeavor and behavior. These unifying themes are truly beyond the restraints of either time or place.

Morality concerns itself with actual conduct in society. It defines, through consensually derived rules and guidelines, conduct that is deemed by society to be acceptable which is typically expressed as codes of behavior (e.g. legal) (Coulter 2006). Derived from the universal themes of ethics, morality is shaped by the realities of the societal situation that are created and encountered in human evolution. Individuals in a society, for the sake of harmony, seek to conduct themselves in accordance with this morality or they risk exclusion, marginalization, opprobrium, or punishment by the collective group.

Thus, what we encounter in our everyday practice is not ethics per se, although it permeates the substrata, but rather a 'common morality.' This common morality can be conceptualized as the common sense, generally accepted understanding of socially approved norms of human conduct. In the Western world, these norms tend to be derived from a 'deontologic' perspective which emphasizes the primacy of recognized duties and obligations in which ethical behavior is driven and evaluated by the actual intention(s) that underlie actions (Solomon and Higgins 1996). Careful study has consensually elaborated four specific, but non-absolute, duties that are transformed into the rules that shape the common morality as applied to the medical sphere of decisions, behavior and interactions. These four duties shaping our medically targeted common morality are autonomy, beneficence, non-maleficence, and justice (Bernat 1994a).

The principle of autonomy and its explicit recognition have shaped much of the change in clinical ethics and medical practice over the past century (Bernat 2002). Autonomy recognizes a respect for others in conferring the locus and power of personal choices and decisions on the individual. It reflects individual uniqueness and empowerment. Autonomy encapsulates 'self-rule,' in that it is the individual who can best determine most responsibly and accurately what is best for that particular individual. Such decisions must be free of the constraints of controlling influences and any duress, however defined. However, autonomy does not intrinsically exist for all persons. To be truly autonomous, the individual must have the capacity to understand the choices available and the specific consequences of these choices. This implies a cognitive capability that is acquired over time which is lacking in the young child and/or the cognitively impaired. Autonomy is the bedrock and essence of informed consent.

Beneficence refers to the principle of undertaking actions that do or promote good (Culver and Gert 1984). Medically, this refers to the prevention and treatment of illness, the alleviation of pain, suffering, and disability, and the facilitation of health in its broadest sense. At the individual level, this implies that actions undertaken should be in the best interests of the patient. This leads to consideration of issues pertaining to 'quality of life,' which raises questions regarding possible subjectivity and perspective. This is especially problematic when the individual does not have the acquired capacity to articulate what is in his/her best interests and burdens are perceived to accrue to others (i.e. family, society).

Related to beneficence is the principle of non-maleficence, essentially articulated as 'primum non nocere' – first do no harm (Culver and Gert 1984). Actions should be undertaken to deliberately avoid and, if unavoidable, minimize the infliction of any evident harms. When both harms and benefits may occur, the balance of benefits versus harms as the result of an action should be demonstrably in favor of desirable beneficial effects. Difficulties arise when trying to establish a priori a hierarchy of desirable benefits and harms anticipated. This may not always be self-evident and benefits and harms may occur possibly (i.e. less than 50% chance) or probably (i.e. greater than 50% chance) rather than inevitably. A doctrine of minimizing risks in direct proportion to the benefits anticipated has evolved, as well as the practice of accepting greater risks if so chosen directly by the autonomous affected individual (Beauchamp and Childrens 1989).

Justice refers to the principle of fairness that mandates the equal treatment of equals (Rawls 1971). However, limitations in resources may challenge our capacity to be fair to all. Defining and recognizing equals (i.e. persons) may also be compromised in situations of perceived limited resources. Perspectives of fairness may also change depending on whether standards of need, merit, potential contribution, or effort should achieve primacy. Factors both within and beyond the control of the affected individual may be taken into account. Fairness applied across society may limit the practitioner's effort to provide optimal care to an individual patient. Finally, who should be empowered to decide what is fair? From a historical perspective, justice has been the moral principle most often compromised with respect to children with a neurodevelopmental disability and the results of such compromise have often been grievous harms to these children.

PERSONHOOD

The above duties and obligations are owed by mutual consent to those who are persons. Personhood is the attribute or quality that confers moral status (Field and Behrman 2004). Since we (i.e. sentient individuals capable of reading this sentence) perceive ourselves as persons, we treat other persons as we wish ourselves to be treated. This rule (labeled the 'Golden Rule' in some traditions) transcends religious beliefs and cultural affinities and can be considered universal in its applicability. Thus, an essential issue is what defines personhood? The key question then becomes: Are all humans persons? If not, which humans are persons with moral status and which are not? A knowledge of history reveals that an invariable precondition of all systematic historic harms directed at particular individuals or groups is initially considering them as non-persons or less than full persons.

Religious viewpoints often consider the presence of a soul or spirit which in some way captures an aspect of the divine as the marker of personhood (Berrigan 2000). Western rationalist traditions emphasize the presence of reason (Fletcher 1979). This includes the capacity to reflect, to be aware of oneself and one's individual uniqueness, and the ability to relate in a meaningful way to others who are also persons. This implies developmental and cognitive skills which may be lacking in a disabled child. This raises the challenge of establishing objective fair criteria for determining personhood. Is personhood and its attached moral status an 'all or none' or varying phenomenon, one that can be acquired and lost over time, which is then reflected in variations in the moral obligation(s) owed to others? Or are limitations in personhood not a modifier of what are essentially human rights to the equal application and availability of the duties of beneficence, maleficence, and justice? Easy answers to these questions and challenges do not exist and cannot be foreseen to be universally achieved in a manner that will be satisfactory to the wide variety of existing viewpoints conferred by religion, culture, and tradition. To maximally avoid potential harms, a conservative approach in defining personhood may be the most conciliatory if we value harmony in our societal relations.

CONSENT

Respect for autonomy mandates that every medical act is predicated on an informed, valid, and voluntary consent (Shevell 1998). In order to provide consent, an individual must be competent, that is capable of fully comprehending the details of the situation, the options available (if any), and the specific consequences of selecting each of these options (Bernat 2002). Competence is not yet present in the young child, especially one who is also cognitively disabled. Competence need not be an 'all or none' phenomenon (Bernat 1994b, 2002).

Thus, in the situation of incompetence, or less than full competence, one must rely on proxy decision-making which logically must be rendered in the disabled child from a 'best interest' rather than a 'substituted judgment' perspective (Shevell 1998). This involves an objective detailed analysis of actual or anticipated burdens and benefits that may result from a particular action that is independent of any values that may have been expressed by the incompetent individual. This often, especially in the context of a difficult decision, is made with reference to the 'quality of life' of the affected individual. Quality of life has both subjective and objective elements (Martyn 1994). Those that are objective tend to be historically emphasized since they are discrete and measurable, frequently against an implied standard of individual worth established by society (i.e. productivity, intelligence). Subjective elements are more elusive and difficult to capture, but may be more meaningful to the individual. Furthermore, it must always be remembered that the 'value of a life' and its actual 'quality' are not synonymous terms.

The need for proxy decision-making also mandates careful consideration of who makes the decision. Clearly, the preference lies with the immediate family who typically provide the locale of day-to-day supportive care (Bernat 1994c). However, this imparts a burden of care to the family that may affect and bias an independent 'best interest' analysis. In addition, in the setting of family disruption (i.e. divorce), there may be conflicts between potential proxy decision-makers. Furthermore, the vulnerability of disabled children mandates that they be protected from proxies who may in themselves be unreasonable, irrational, or punitive. Thus, a degree of medical paternalism in this situation can be justified to some extent (Cooke 1994). It has also been noted that rarely is cognitive or physical disability in and of itself in isolation sufficient moral grounds for special selective treatment or the denial of potentially beneficial treatment.

CLINICAL RESEARCH
Initial formulation of a code of clinical research ethics was prompted by the Nuremberg war crime trials of physicians involved in harmful human experimentation during the regime of the Third Reich (Grodin 1992). The Nuremberg Code incorporated the need for voluntary informed consent, knowing avoidance of harms, and the scientific integrity of both the investigator and the experimental protocol (Judgement 1992). Subsequent clinical research ethic guidelines have built upon these tenets. Surprisingly, the Nuremberg Code in its final formulation was silent on the issue of research involving incompetent individuals such as children

with neurodevelopmental disabilities. Subsequent guidelines have focused on the need for proxy consent and the minimization of potential risk exposure as a result of research participation (Shevell 2002). This is an explicit recognition of the vulnerability of this particular population (Shevell 2002).

It is generally accepted that the cognitively or physically disabled should not be used as 'samples of convenience' for research that could just as well be carried out utilizing competent adults or less vulnerable, that is non-disabled, children (Task Force 1982). Indeed, the participation of the disabled in research projects should be largely limited to investigating those issues directly related to their specific disability (Shevell 2002). The research should in some way benefit either the subjects themselves or the disability-specific peer group of which they are a member.

Controversy has existed regarding the acceptable risk exposure for vulnerable children, especially in the context of research that is not directly beneficial and is either therapeutic or diagnostic in orientation. The standard usually applied regarding acceptable risks in such a situation is 'slightly more than minimal'; however, the precise meaning of this term is still open to debate (US Dept HHS 1991). Most would agree that caution in the context of risk exposure is warranted given the absence of the ability to directly provide consent for participation and it is incumbent upon investigators, institutions, institutional review boards, and granting/funding agencies that sponsor research to exercise responsibility at a variety of levels regarding acting as a protector of the welfare of vulnerable subjects. While challenges exist in the moral conduct of research involving children with a neurodevelopmental disability, it is important that these challenges not result in research in this population being avoided as too difficult to undertake, which would lead to the entirely undesired effect of creating a class of 'therapeutic orphans' who as a group do not participate in, and therefore may not benefit from, medical advances (Levine 1989).

JUSTICE

While consensus exists that justice is a desired ethical principle that should underlie our common morality, achieving justice has challenged all societies at a practical level. A conflict exists between our desire for fairness and fair treatment, especially for ourselves and those we care about, and our recognition that there are inevitably finite limits to resources. In particular, an intrinsic conflict exists between society's attempt to distribute resources and the health practitioner's obligation to provide optimal care for the individual patient. Furthermore, the pretext of limited available resources has often been utilized as the rationale to justify unethical behaviors towards the disabled (Parent and Shevell 1998).

The debate on this topic focuses on establishing an appropriate standard of fairness that is objectively and equally applied both within the context of finite resources and the valuation of individual worth (Outka 1974). Equal access appears preferential to utilitarian or libertarian approaches. The former is difficult, if not impossible, to measure objectively and the latter eventually inevitably attaches the prospect of economic wealth as a lever to access. Limited resources will temper equal access and thus the emphasis on the utilization of public resources is to provide access to services of proven value that positively impact on broadly defined health and welfare measures of those affected. It can be foreseen that this will often lead to confrontation between different groups as they assert their competing claim to scarce resources. Thus, better-organized groups, both politically and financially, may triumph in the public arena. An option exists to minimize this potential conflict by collectively advocating for more health care resources on a societal level.

CONCLUSIONS
Much progress has clearly been made on establishing a common morality in health care for children with neurodevelopmental disabilities. Basic principles of autonomy, beneficence, non-maleficence, and justice have been incorporated into everyday medical practice. This has brought changes in how we view and treat such children, imparting greater dignity and intrinsic value, and enhancing awareness of our collective and individual moral obligations. Challenges remain, especially in achieving true justice, yet if the recent past is prologue to the future, we can anticipate further progress, which, when combined with our scientific advances, can only improve the health and welfare of these children.

ACKNOWLEDGMENTS
MS is grateful for the support of the MCH Foundation and YCC during the writing of this manuscript. Alba Rinaldi provided the necessary secretarial assistance.

REFERENCES
Beauchamp TL, Childrens JF (1989) *Principles of Biomedical Ethics (3rd edn)*. New York: Oxford University Press.
Bernat JL (1994a) Ethical theory. In: Bernat JL (ed) *Ethical Issues in Neurology*. Boston: Butterworth-Heinemann, pp. 3–22.
Bernat JL (1994b) Mental retardation. In: Bernat JL (ed) *Ethical Issues in Neurology*. Boston: Butterworth-Heinemann, pp 245–264.
Bernat JL (1994c) Clinical ethics and the law. In: Bernat JL (ed) *Ethical Issues in Neurology*. Boston: Butterworth-Heinemann, pp 65–88.
Bernat JL (2002) Informed consent in pediatric neurology. *Semin Pediatr Neurol* 9: 10–18.
Berrigan D (2000) God is love. *Noah Homes Newsl* Spring issue: 2.
Cooke RE (1994) Vulnerable children. In: Grodin MA, Glantz LH (eds) *Children as Research Subjects: Science, Ethics and Law*. New York: Oxford University Press, pp 193–214.
Cooke RE (1996) Ethics, law, and developmental disabilities. In: Capute AJ, Accardo PJ (eds) *Developmental Disabilities in Infancy and Childhood (2nd edn)*. Baltimore: Paul H Brookes, pp 609–618.
Coulter DL (2006) Ethical issues in child neurology. In: Swaiman KF, Ashwal S, Ferreiro M (eds) *Pediatric Neurology Principle & Practice (4th edn)*. Philadelphia: Mosby Elsevier, pp 2587–2398.

Culver GM, Gert B (1984) Basic ethical concepts in neurological practice. *Semin Neurol* 4: 1–8.

Field MJ, Behrman RE (eds) (2004) *Ethical Conduct of Clinical Research Involving Children.* Washington DC: National Academy Press.

Fletcher J (1979) *Humanhood: Essays in Biomedical Ethics.* Buffalo, NY: Prometheus Books.

Grodin MA (1992) Historical origins of the Nuremberg Code. In: Annas GJ, Grodin MA (eds) *The Nazi Doctors and the Nuremberg Code. Human Rights in Human Experimentation.* Oxford: Oxford University Press, pp 121–144.

Jonsen AR, Siegler M, Winslade WJ (1986) *Clinical Ethics* (2nd edn). New York: Macmillan, p 3.95.

Judgement. In: Annas GJ, Grodin MA (eds) (1992) *The Nazi doctors and the Nuremberg Code: Human Rights in Human Experimentation.* Oxford: Oxford University Press, pp 94–107.

Levine RJ (1989) Children as research subjects. In: Kopelman LM, Moskop JC (eds) *Children and Health Care: Moral and Social Issues.* Kluwer Academic Publishers, pp 73–87.

Martyn SR (1994) Substituted judgement, best interests, and the need for best respect. *Camb Q Health Ethics* 3: 195–208.

Outka G (1974) Social justice and equal access to health care. *J Relig Ethics* 2: 11–32.

Parent S, Shevell MI (1998) The 'first to perish': child euthanasia in the Third Reich. *Arch Pediatr Adolsec Med* 152: 79–86.

Rawls JA (1971) *A Theory of Justice.* Cambridge: Harvard University Press.

Sherr EH, Shevell MI (2006) Mental retardation and global developmental delay. In: Swaiman KF, Ashwal S, Ferreiro M (eds) *Pediatric Neurology; Principle & Practice* (4th edn). Philadelphia: Mosby Elsevier, pp 799–820.

Shevell MI (1998) Clinical ethics and developmental delay. *Semin Pediatr Neurol* 5: 70–75.

Shevell MI (2002) Ethics of clinical research in children. *Semin Pediatr Neurol* 9: 46–52.

Solomon RC, Higgins KM (1996) *A Short History of Philosophy.* New York: Oxford University Press, pp 210–214.

Task Force on Legal and Ethical Issues (1982) Experimentation with mentally handicapped subjects. In: Edwards RB (ed) *Psychiatry and Ethics: Insanity, Rational Autonomy, and Mental Health Care.* Buffalo: Prometheus Books, pp 224–229.

US Department of Health and Human Services (1991) Protections of human subjects. Title 45 *Code of Federal Regulations* Part 46.

5

POLICY AND GOALS FOR THE FUTURE FOR INDIVIDUALS WITH NEURODEVELOPMENTAL DISABILITIES

David L Coulter

Disability policy is a shifting and constantly changing set of strategies developed by advocates, researchers, and professionals, and implemented by both public and private organizations. It exists inevitably in the gap between what should be and what is. Current policy represents a moving snapshot of this gap, as governments and organizations seek to maximize outcomes within the reality of what are often limited and at times scarce resources. The gap varies tremendously between and within countries, based on the worldwide variability in research knowledge, public attitudes, and available financial resources. This discussion emphasizes policy goals as an approximation of what should be, using present best available research and expert consensus. Current policy is described as a reflection of what is, at least at the time of this review. The discussion reviews primarily American and Western European policies, where the gap between what should be and what is appears to be is narrower than in developing nations where resources are more limited. Because disability policy by its nature changes over time, a brief review of historical trends is needed to understand how we arrived at where we are today. This will also help explain and provide a conceptualization of how to get to where we should go in the future.

HISTORICAL OVERVIEW

Disability policy has evolved over the centuries and will undoubtedly continue change in response to new research and public attitudes. Analysis of the early history of disability is complicated by the evolving relatively recent understanding of disability. This means that one must be cautious when attempting to apply current concepts to an analysis of these early sources. For example, numerous references to disability are found in the Bible, but rarely identified as such. Did Moses have a speech impediment (such as stuttering) or was he just a poor public speaker? Jesus cast out demons from people with a variety of what we would call disabilities (i.e. epilepsy), but does that mean Jesus considered such people to be sinful? Muhammad specifically called upon his followers to take care of people with disabilities, which was a fairly new concept at the time. The idea of demonic possession as a cause for mental illness and disability was common in Christian Europe throughout the

Middle Ages, but other sources suggest that disability was also sometimes considered a natural part of the human condition. Thus, it is hard to gain a coherent understanding of disability policy during these early pre-modern eras (Scheerenberger 1983, Braddock and Parish 2002).

By the 17th century, society was beginning to understand the difference between mental illness and intellectual disability; 'madmen' put wrong ideas together, while 'idiots' have very few ideas at all and cannot reason from them. Since both groups often committed crimes or were unable to support themselves, institutional facilities such as almshouses and prisons often grouped together individuals with mental illness and intellectual disability as well as common criminals. Public policy did not really begin to provide for people with disabilities as a distinct group until fairly modern times. Schools for the deaf and the blind began to emerge in Europe by the 18th century and somewhat later in the United States. Society recognized an obligation to pay for the support of people with intellectual disability, which was sometimes done by 'auctioning off' the person to a bidding family that was willing to provide care (Scheerenberger 1983).

In the 19th century, schools for children with intellectual disability were established in Europe and America, under the influence of reformers such as Jean Itard, Edouard Seguin, Samuel Gridley Howe, and Hervey Wilbur. The goal of these schools (sometimes referred to as training schools) was to educate the student so that he/she could re-enter society as a productive adult. As the number of children with intellectual disability began to overwhelm the capacity of these initially small private schools, reformers sought to gain public support for opening larger publicly funded institutions. Public policy supported the establishment of many such institutions during 1850–1900, with the initial goal of educating and training residents to return to public life. When economic conditions deteriorated and residents could not find work, the emphasis gradually changed to focus primarily on permanent custodial care. By 1900, there were 171 institutions for persons with intellectual disability in 21 countries, including 25 in the United States (Barr 1904).

This emphasis on physical separation from society received strong support from the eugenics movement of the early 20th century. 'Mental defectives' were seen as threats to society because of their ability to reproduce and 'pass on' their intellectual disability to their children. Prohibition of marriage and involuntary sterilization were widespread public policy responses to this perceived threat (Trent 1994). Even after the rejection of eugenics and recognition of the murderous euthanasia program directed specifically at disabled children and adults in Nazi Germany, public policy continued to support the segregation of people with intellectual disabilities in custodial institutions throughout the middle of the 20th century. Indeed, the number of residents with intellectual disability living in public institutions peaked in 1967 in the United States, when there were almost 200 000 such persons living in these facilities (Braddock and Parish 2002).

To an extent, the institutional approach to public services was driven by a medicalized model of disability focused on medical diagnosis and treatment. Institutions were usually run by physicians and staffed by nurses. It was also supported by a social construction of disability that viewed disability as a threat to society (Trent 1994). The past 50 years have seen a gradual shift in thinking about disability to emphasize self-determination and the value of social roles played by individuals with disabilities. Political advocacy by and for people with disabilities has led to most of the public policy changes in recent times (Noll and Trent 2004). Supported by federal laws and Supreme Court decisions in the United States, public policy began to focus on discharging people from institutions and providing community-based services instead. Passage of the Americans with Disabilities Act in 1990 provided key legal support for these policies. However, the most recent data show that 41 000 persons are still living in public institutions (Braddock et al. 2005). The United Nations has also passed important declarations on human rights for persons with disabilities that provide international policy guidance in this area.

Thus, current disability policy reflects this long history as well as modern thinking about the role of people with disabilities in society. Vestiges of outdated approaches still persist despite ongoing efforts to change them.

DISABILITY POLICY GOALS

In 2003 an invitational conference was held in Washington, DC, to identify research and policy goals for people with developmental disabilities. The purpose of the conference was to survey and analyze existing research and policy in order to develop comprehensive goals that would serve as guides for future work. The project received funding from 10 federal agencies, as well as support from a number of professional societies and academic institutions. Over 200 national experts participated in 12 work groups, which were designed to cover all aspects of the field across the lifespan. These work groups focused on:

1 Young children with, or at risk for, developmental disabilities
2 Effective education in the least restrictive setting
3 Transitions from home and school to the roles and supports of adulthood
4 Positive supports for behavioral, mental health, communication, and crisis needs
5 Comprehensive health supports and health promotion
6 Biomedical research for primary and secondary prevention
7 Employment and productive life roles
8 Access and support for community lives, homes, and social roles
9 Support of families and family life across the lifespan
10 Self-advocacy, self-determination, and social freedom and opportunity
11 Emerging technologies
12 Healthy aging and community participation

The proceedings of the conference, including the reviews and recommendations of the 12 work groups, were published by the American Association on Mental Retardation (Lakin and Turnbull 2005) to serve as a benchmark and guide for shaping future research efforts and policy discussion. These results are summarized in the discussion that follows. The specific policy goals recommended and endorsed by the work groups are listed in the Appendix.

YOUNG CHILDREN AT RISK

Federal US policy has supported special education for children with disabilities for many years. A number of laws, including the Head Start Act, the Education for All Handicapped Children Act, and the Individuals with Disabilities Education Act, have provided guidance and support for programs serving young children at risk. More recently, the National Research Council of the National Academy of Sciences published reviews and recommendations in this area (National Research Council and Institute of Medicine 2000, National Research Council 2001). Several professional groups have also published policy recommendations for practice (Bredekamp and Copple 1997, Sandall et al. 2005).

Identification of young children at risk varies greatly from one location to another. This is partly related to differences in eligibility criteria, the use of different instruments and measures for screening and referral, and the need to understand cultural and linguistic diversity in child development. Some have raised questions regarding early identification of young children at risk (Wolery and Bailey 2002):

1 What factors cause some children to be identified earlier than others?
2 What are the earliest symptoms and signs of an emerging disability?
3 What are the best strategies for identification?
4 How can the process of identification be culturally sensitive and fair to all?

Programs and interventions for young children at risk also vary greatly from one location to another. Research supports specific strategies, but resources are not always sufficient to replicate these idealized programs in community settings. Clearly, more research is needed to define what interventions are most effective in producing the desired outcomes at a cost that can be sustained by local resources (Wolery and Bailey 2002). Since young children at risk depend primarily on their families for developmental support, and many intervention programs rely extensively on family participation, families need to be able to make good choices and to become effective educators for their children. Intervention strategies thus need to be sensitive to cultural differences in how families support their child's development. Professionals (including therapists and educators) need to be well-trained in child development, effective intervention techniques, and family support.

Effective Education

Education has been the cornerstone of intervention for children and adolescents with disabilities for more than a century. Educational policy has varied greatly over the years, moving broadly from an emphasis in the past on removal and segregation in separate and often isolated facilities, to the current emphasis on inclusion (e.g. mainstreaming) as much as possible in the same programs and facilities used by all students. The idea that all children with disabilities are entitled to education is relatively new, having been established in the United States only in the last 50 years. In many countries, this idea is still an unfulfilled dream. Current educational policy in the United States is defined by federal laws that mandates a free and appropriate public education for all children, including children with even the most severe disabilities. In general, education is to occur in the 'least restrictive setting,' that is most similar to the regular classroom, taking into account the special needs of the child with disabilities. In practice, this means that children with disabilities are included in the regular classroom for some programs but also removed from the classroom for special educational programs that are tailored to their individual needs. Considerable research has documented the value of inclusive education for children with disabilities, and for those without, as well as identifying effective educational strategies for achieving good outcomes (McLaughlin et al. 2005).

Transition to Adulthood

The transition to adulthood is typically marked by the end of special education, which usually occurs around age 18–22 years depending on local educational policy. What happens next is not always clear. Young adults with disabilities may continue into post-secondary education, enter vocational training, participate in the adult work force, or enroll in adult day programs and sheltered workshops. Many will continue to live with their natural family, but others will move out to live in various community-based settings including group homes and supported living environments. One of the major challenges during this transition to adulthood is learning how to participate in community-based social, leisure, and recreational opportunities in order to have a personally satisfying and fulfilling life as an adult. Federal policy concerning transitioning to adulthood is contained in the Rehabilitation Act, the Americans with Disabilities Act, the Individuals with Disabilities Education Act, and the No Child Left Behind Act. Transition services are defined as a coordinated set of activities designed on an individual basis that help the student move from school to post-school activities. In general, current policy requires identification of individually determined transition service needs starting at age 14.

Transition services may include functional vocational assessment, pre-vocational and vocational training, and instruction in adult living skills including community participation skills. Policy also focuses on achieving educational outcomes, including school graduation. An increasing emphasis is being placed on post-secondary education as opportunities develop for young people with disabilities to attend college, supported by policies than ensure appropriate accommodations for people with disabilities. More work, however, is needed to develop lifelong learning opportunities for adults with disabilities, but little actual policy guidance is currently available in this area.

POSITIVE BEHAVIORAL SUPPORTS

Positive behavioral supports are broadly recognized as the optimal response to challenging behaviors in persons with developmental disabilities (Carr et al. 2002). Current federal policy expressed in the Individuals with Disabilities Education Act requires schools to use positive behavioral support techniques. Major American professional associations, including the American Association on Intellectual and Developmental Disabilities (formerly the American Association on Mental Retardation), the Arc of the United States, the Council on Exceptional Children, TASH (formerly the Association for Persons with Severe Handicaps), the American Psychological Association, and the National Association of School Psychologists, have clear policy statements endorsing positive behavioral supports as the standard of practice for their field. Most also have clear policy statements opposing aversive, negative, or punishment-based behavioral intervention strategies. Positive behavioral supports are consistent with, and indeed derived partly from, the science of applied behavioral analysis, which is the current standard of practice for treating persons with autism (Tuchman and Rapin 2006).

Positive behavioral support emphasizes the use of functional behavioral analysis and individual behavioral support plans. Functional behavioral analysis identifies the target behavior, examines the antecedent situations and conditions in which the behavior occurs, and considers the typical consequences of the behavior. These data are then analyzed to discover potential instigating factors that may have initiated the behavior and maintaining factors that cause the individual to continue behaving in such a manner. Hypotheses are generated to explain the functional significance or purpose of the behavior, such as avoidance, escape from undesired situations, communication of feelings (such as pain, anxiety, or discomfort), or gaining access to desired objects, activities, or social situations. Results of the functional behavioral analysis are then used to generate an individualized behavioral support plan, which may involve treatment of causative physical and mental health conditions, environmental changes that encourage positive behavior which includes the development of new, desirable behavioral skills, the cessation of unintentional rewards for problem behaviors, and the provision of new rewards for desirable behaviors. Research has confirmed the relative effectiveness of these techniques (Repp and Horner 1999). Current and future policy should address the development, dissemination, and application of programs to provide positive behavioral supports and the training of teachers, therapists, and other professionals in the use of these methods.

Health Supports and Health Promotion

Health policy goals for persons with developmental disabilities are based on several national consensus documents, most prominently the report of the Surgeon General of the United States (US Public Health Service 2002) and a related report on mental health policy goals (National Institutes of Health 2001). Additional guidance is provided in the general policy goals outlined in *Healthy People 2010* (US Public Health Service 2000). International support for many of these policy goals was documented.

The Community Health Supports Model was developed to replace the Medical Model as a way to conceptualize and plan health supports for persons with developmental disabilities (Coulter 2004). This model is described in Fig. 5.1. Health conditions, together with biomedical, social, behavioral, and educational risk factors, lead to problems in functioning, which can be considered as potential opportunities for interventions to improve functioning. Support needs reflect physical, mental, behavioral, emotional, social, and environmental health problems, and specific support activities and interventions are designed to address each of these problems. Health support activities must be reassessed continually and revised as needed to improve their ability to produce the desired outcomes, taking into account the individual's changing preferences, personal growth, life situation, and health status. Health promotion is an important aspect of support for which there is an emerging body of research evidence in persons with intellectual disability (Nehring 2005).

Comprehensive reviews of the health status of persons with developmental disabilities document the gaps in care that currently exist (Horowitz et al. 2000). These gaps are related to limited access to care, variable and often insufficient health care financing, and inadequate training of health care professionals in the treatment of persons with disabilities. Medicaid remains the most important source of health care financing for persons with developmental disabilities in the United States, but coverage varies widely from one state to another. Some countries offer systematic, universal, and consistent access to health care for all citizens, but other countries (particularly those with limited public financial resources) provide little or no access for persons with disabilities (Zinkin and McConachie 1995). Training varies widely, but the recent development of training programs such as that for neurodevelopmental disabilities in the United States should improve the situation in the future. Health care policy should encourage better training in this area for general practitioners as well as for neurologists and other specialists (e.g. pediatricians, psyciatrists) involved in caring for persons with developmental disabilities.

Primary and Secondary Prevention

Primary prevention involves prevention of the actual underlying condition causing disability, while secondary prevention involves treatment that prevents an existing

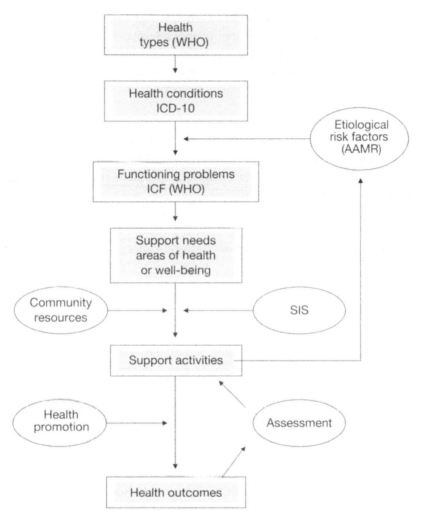

Fig. 5.1. Community health supports model.

condition from resulting in additional disability. Prenatal care that prevents preterm birth is an example of primary prevention, while dietary treatment of infants born with phenylketonuria is an example of secondary prevention. When the etiology of developmental disability is reconceptualized as a set of biomedical, social, behavioral, and education risk factors that interact across the individual's lifespan, then strategies that specifically address these individualized risk factors can be seen as methods for primary and secondary prevention. In this way, personal wellness (or individual well-being) becomes the individual's unique experience of prevention (Coulter 1996).

Opportunities for prevention derive from new and ongoing research describing the genetic, neurologic, and environmental influences on child development. The pace of this research is such that any attempt to review it is immediately out of date, but Smith (2005) provides a useful current synthesis. Current policy related to prevention focuses on a number of proven strategies that address known genetic and environmental factors:

1 Federal, state and locally funded programs to provide prenatal care and nutritional support for mothers and infants
2 Universal newborn screening for recognized inherited, treatable disorders of metabolism (e.g. phenylketonuria)
3 Mandated screening for lead poisoning in young children
4 Required immunization schedules to prevent communicable diseases that can cause acquired disability (e.g. measles, bacterial meningitis).

Each of these areas could be expanded through new policy initiatives, after research has demonstrated the cost-effectiveness of such approaches. For example, pre-conception testing to identify genetic risks in potential parents could lead to pre-implantation *in vitro* diagnosis of embryos at risk and selection of those that do not have the genetic condition leading to disability. Universal newborn screening could ideally be expanded to include more treatable metabolic disorders, such as mitochondrial diseases and fatty acid oxidation disorders. Environmental testing of young children could also be expanded, given the large number of potential toxins present in the environment, but the current state of research in this area is inadequate to support such widespread and diverse testing at this time. Ongoing research on immunization has led to rapid expansion of available prevention, but the widespread availability of these immunization schedules is limited, especially in developing countries where the need is greatest. Research policy also needs to address the continued development of potential curative treatments, such as molecular or stem cell based interventions, that could reverse potentially disabling conditions.

EMPLOYMENT

The capacity of individuals with intellectual disability to work productively is well-known historically. The initial development of 'training schools' was to train people with intellectual disability to become productive contributing members of society. The rapid growth of residential institutions during the 19th century was made possible by the productive labor of those who lived there. This labor, largely unpaid, provided the material and financial resources that kept the institution viable on an ongoing basis. Many institutions raised or grew their own food on the institutional farm, using resident labor to do the farm work. Other residents were involved in workshops located on the institutional property, producing goods and services used internally as well as externally. Many institutions were thus 'self-sufficient' because they relied on the unpaid labor of those who lived there. As institutions declined in the 20th century and individuals with intellectual disability remained in the community, usually living at home, opportunities to work were often limited. Sheltered workshops were developed as a place where people could work and be paid at a very low rate (i.e. sub-minimum wage). During the past 40 years, however, additional work options have been developed and supported by a variety of federal laws and directed policies.

Research has shown that people with intellectual disability vary in their ability to work. Some are capable of independent employment in the regular workforce, while others require supports to become productive. These supports often include 'job coaches' who assist the individual to perform the required tasks, ideally 'fading' their involvement as the individual acquires the required skills needed to become more independent. Others with more significant disabilities may need to work in a special environment where ongoing support is present. Wages vary but typically remain low. Current policy is intended to assist individuals to work in the most independent and productive setting possible, taking into account their personal needs and skills. Ideally, competitive employment opportunities for people with intellectual disabilities are characterized by:

1 An informed choice and decision-making regarding where to work and what to do
2 Inclusion of the individual in the regular workforce to the maximum extent feasible
3 Development of a career path with opportunities for potential advancement
4 Parity in wages, hours of employment, and benefits for equal work
5 Parity in possible work options
6 The opportunity to be employed promptly and efficiently (Wehman et al. 2003).

The reality is that most individuals with intellectual disability remain unemployed or underemployed. Although the number of such persons involved in competitive and supported work has increased gradually during the past few decades, the absolute numbers remain low. Many, if not most, are still working in sheltered workshops. Those who do work competitively are often stuck in low-wage, dead-end jobs with little capacity for possible advancement. Many inspirational stories of people with disabilities who have become exemplary workers in the competitive workforce document the largely untapped resource represented by this pool of individuals who are ready, able, and often willing to work. Potential competition with non-disabled workers is a major perceived barrier to the development of policy to address this issue fully. In a society where many people are unemployed or more typically underemployed, people with disabilities will be the least likely to find work. Achieving the ideals described above continues to be a major policy challenge.

COMMUNITY LIFE

The majority of adults with intellectual disability live at home with their families. Others live in community-based settings such as group homes, usually with 3–6 residents, and a few live independently or in supported living environments. Current policy strongly supports the expansion and improvement of community-based services, including the recruitment, training, and retention of high-quality direct support professionals to work with persons living in these settings (Lakin et al. 2005). Living in the community does not always guarantee effective participation or social inclusion in the life of the community, but it does clearly facilitate it and renders it a possibility. Public policy may encourage social inclusion but simply cannot force it. Nonetheless, many parents whose adult children have moved out of the family home and into a supported living setting such as a group home have observed that their child now has a much better social life and greater community participation than they could provide in the family home. This depends to a large extent on the skills, interests, and intrinsic humanity of the direct support workers involved in a particular individual's life. Policy influences this indirectly when it encourages and rewards these workers who do their job well. Unfortunately, many direct support workers are grossly underpaid and do not stay long in these particular jobs.

Policy can encourage the expression of personal autonomy by allowing individuals more choice and control over the funding that is available to support them, allowing them to select community-based settings and activities that meet their personal goals. Support for self-determination and person-centered planning are key elements of this approach to funding policy.

Abuse of persons with intellectual disability is common, affecting 25–50% of such persons according to various surveys (Lakin et al. 2005). Such abuse can occur in family homes, institutions, schools, group homes, and in the community at large. The judicial system often fails to report and investigate such abuses adequately. Legal policy needs to improve in order to protect persons with disabilities.

FAMILY SUPPORT

The overarching goal of family support is to improve and enhance the quality of life of the entire family, because the quality of life of the individual with intellectual and developmental disabilities often depends largely on the quality of life of the immediate family. Turnbull et al. (2005) provide a comprehensive review of the literature on family support, noting the various laws and cases that provide policy direction in this area. Family support means that families are provided with the required resources and means needed and have sufficient personal choice and control to select the supports that are most appropriate for them. Such supports need to be sensitive to cultural diversity. Policy is somewhat varied in this area, often with good intentions that are insufficiently funded because of trends in local economies. Issues affecting families often cut across a broad variety of challenges, including health, education, work, community living, and aging. Thus, policy needs to provide much better collaboration and cooperation between all of the various bureaucratic and non-governmental agencies involved.

SELF-DETERMINATION AND SELF-ADVOCACY

Self-determination means that the individual has the power to determine and control key aspects of his/her life. One needs to have the freedom and opportunity to choose, the knowledge and experience to make good choices, and the authority to make choices and accept responsibility for them. As a general principle, self-determination is the cornerstone of much international policy regarding human rights and has been endorsed by the United Nations in several documents on civil and political rights. However, it has not always been extended to people with intellectual and developmental disabilities. Self-advocacy refers to the ability of people with disabilities to speak up and to assert their own right to self-determination. At one level, a person with even profound disability who communicates a choice or preference is advocating for himself/herself. At a more systematic level, self-advocates have organized into many local and national groups and have had important influences on legislation and national policy related to disability. They are often included as advisors and consultants when policy is being evaluated.

In a general sense, the principal policy goal related to self-determination is to provide the resources and opportunities for individuals with disabilities to obtain and exert control over important aspects of their lives. This is expressed in the self-advocacy slogan, 'Nothing about us without us.' It can be understood also from a social power perspective as a nascent political movement to obtain power for those who do not have it (Whitehead and Hughey 2004). In the future, merely listening to people with disabilities will not be enough. Policy-makers and society at large will have to actually give them the proportionate power they need to achieve true self-determination.

EMERGING TECHNOLOGIES

Technologic support for persons with disabilities is a fairly recent phenomenon which has resulted in improved functioning and participation for many persons who have obtained access to these supports. Several federal laws, most prominently the Americans with Disabilities Act, have expanded access to a wide range of assistive technology. Promoting access to this technology is an important policy goal. Achievement of this goal is influenced by several related factors:

1 Development of effective technologies to assist individuals without unreasonable difficulty
2 Refinement of existing technologies to improve their accessibility for those in need
3 Research to add new technologic capacity, based on advances in science and engineering
4 Dissemination of information about existing technology to potential consumers
5 Training of providers in making assistive technology available to those in need
6 Funding to provide often-expensive technology supports to all individuals with disabilities who could benefit from them

For fairly obvious reasons, policy to accomplish these goals is more feasible in countries with sophisticated and extensive financial and technologic resources than in countries where such resources are limited. International efforts are needed to redress this disparity and make the benefits of assistive technology more available worldwide. Access to emerging Internet-based and informatic driven technologies could be useful in these international efforts.

AGING

Many of the issues for people with intellectual and developmental disabilities who are aging are similar to those of the general population. The need for comprehensive residential, health, financial, and social supports is common to all. Nonetheless, there are also specific issues for people with lifelong disabilities that are unique to their situation. These include issues related to the underlying condition which may be progressive, such as the dementia that often occurs in persons with Down syndrome. Research on healthy aging in persons with neurodevelopmental disabilities is fairly limited, and research policy should support expanded work in this area (Davidson et al. 2003). Health promotion is as important for aging individuals with developmental disabilities as for anyone else, including careful attention to diet, nutrition, activity, and exercise (Nehring 2005). With these commonalities of need, public policy should foster interdisciplinary cooperation between systems serving people with neurodevelopmental disabilities (i.e. state disability agencies) and systems serving people who are aging (i.e. state agencies for seniors).

APPENDIX: POLICY GOALS
YOUNG CHILDREN AT RISK

1 Children with or at risk for developmental disabilities will be identified as early as possible so that they can access quality services.
2 Measurable, cost-effective, and sound intervention strategies will be available to support the health and well-being of all children and to strengthen their ability to participate fully in family and community life.

3 Families will be able to make informed decisions and partner effectively with professionals to achieve positive outcomes.

4 All children and families will have access to community-based, coordinated systems of effective services from supportive and skilled personnel who value individual and cultural differences, provide continuity of supports, and promote community inclusion.

EFFECTIVE EDUCATION

1 All children and youth with intellectual and developmental disabilities will receive an individually referenced, culturally relevant, effective education leading to valued post-school outcomes and provided in the least restrictive setting, such as education in the general education school and classroom.

2 Parents and families and youth with intellectual and developmental disabilities will be full partners in determining what constitutes an effective education as well as the least restrictive setting.

3 Accountability standards and procedures will be sufficient to ensure that each child or youth with intellectual and developmental disabilities receives an effective education within the least restrictive setting.

4 Children and youth with intellectual and developmental disabilities will have access to sufficient human and fiscal resources, supports and services required for them to be effectively educated in the least restrictive setting.

TRANSITION TO ADULTHOOD

1 Efforts will increase to promote self-determination and self-advocacy by students.

2 Students with intellectual and developmental disabilities will have access to the general standards-based curriculum.

3 Graduation rates of students with intellectual and developmental disabilities will increase.

4 Schools will work with other appropriate agencies to ensure that students have access to, and fully participate in, supports for post-secondary education and community living opportunities.

5 Families will have informed participation in education and life planning, decision-making, and promotion of self-advocacy for their transition-aged children.

6 Collaboration and cross-systems links will be created at all levels to support student self-determination, self-advocacy, and achievement of meaningful school, post-school, and adult role outcomes.

7 A qualified workforce will be available to address the needs of youth with intellectual and developmental disabilities.

8 All students with intellectual and developmental disabilities will have full, active participation in all aspects of social, recreational, and leisure community life.

POSITIVE BEHAVIORAL SUPPORTS

1 Individuals with intellectual and developmental disabilities and problem behavior and/or mental health disorders will have ongoing access to appropriate assessment that guides support practices, including person-centered planning, mental health and medical evaluation, and functional behavioral assessment.
2 Individuals with intellectual and developmental disabilities will have access to effective, positive, and evidence-based behavioral, mental health, medical, and social supports needed to: (a) prevent and reduce problem behaviors or mental disorders; (b) support social resilience; and (c) promote desired lifestyle outcomes.
3 Individuals with intellectual and developmental disabilities and problem behavior will have access to ongoing monitoring of the extent to which behavioral support plans are implemented and are effective.
4 Systems of care, including policy, organizational, and quality assurance variables, will be established across the lifespan to enable the effective and sustained implementation of positive behavioral and mental health supports.
5 Comprehensive systems of care will be developed that include crisis prevention, intervention, and follow-up services.
6 A sufficient number of leadership, direct support, and support coordination personnel who are trained in the theory and practice of positive behavioral support will be available to individuals, families, schools, workplaces, and local communities.

HEALTH SUPPORTS AND HEALTH PROMOTION

1 People with intellectual and developmental disabilities will have access to high quality health care that is appropriate, affordable, timely, comprehensive, and provided in their communities without regard to their ability to pay.
2 The health care system for people with intellectual and developmental disabilities will promote their inclusion in the community.
3 People with intellectual and developmental disabilities and their families will partner with health care providers to access and use health information to make choices and decisions about their own health care.
4 People with intellectual and developmental disabilities will be treated with respect by health care providers who are well trained to respond to their general and specific health needs.
5 People with intellectual and developmental disabilities will have the opportunity to participate in the full range of health promotion and wellness activities available to other children and adults.

6 People with intellectual and developmental disabilities will have access to comprehensive mental health, behavioral, and other allied services and supports to meet their needs within the community.

7 Knowledge about the health status and needs of people with intellectual and developmental disabilities will be identified, evaluated, and expanded across the lifespan.

PRIMARY AND SECONDARY PREVENTION

1 New scientific techniques emerging from genetics, neurobiology, molecular biology, imaging, toxicology, behavioral/cognitive sciences, and related fields will be applied to specific mechanisms that interfere with development throughout the lifespan to reduce primary and secondary disability.

2 Screening and diagnosis of conditions associated with intellectual and developmental disabilities will be employed to maximize opportunities for effective prevention or early intervention.

3 Genetic, pharmacologic, metabolic, and bioengineering advances will be employed to understand, treat, or cure intellectual and developmental disabilities across the lifespan.

4 Access to screening, diagnosis, and treatment approaches will be provided without disparities in the availability or quality of such services.

EMPLOYMENT

1 Access to adequately supported competitive employment, customized employment, self-employment, or other integrated work will be available to people with intellectual and developmental disabilities to promote their inclusion and productivity.

2 Students will be involved in multiple paid integrated work experiences prior to leaving school and will leave school with a job or other work-related vocational plans.

3 Federal and state funding programs will support integrated employment and full-day support in the community.

4 Policy and funding emphasizing personal control of employment support resources will grow and be available to all people with intellectual and developmental disabilities.

5 Employers will be partners and customers of vocational support programs in order to increase employment and career opportunities.

6 Individual with intellectual and developmental disabilities will have full and equal access to specialized and generic resources that provide job training and job placement support as needed to secure desired employment outcomes.

7 Business ownership by people with intellectual and developmental disabilities will be supported as a viable employment option by relevant public agencies.

COMMUNITY LIFE

1 People with intellectual and developmental disabilities will live in and participate fully in their communities.
2 People will choose the community supports they need and want, and exercise control in the selection of how these supports are provided.
3 People will have access to stable, skilled, community-based support providers when and to the extent they are needed.
4 People will have personally satisfying lives and valued social roles.
5 People will be safe, have the assistance they need to manage life's risks, and be free from exploitation by others.

FAMILY LIFE

1 Family–professional partnerships will be used in research, policy-making, and the planning and delivery of supports and services, so that families will control their own destinies, with due regard for the autonomy of adult family members with disabilities to control their own lives.
2 Families will participate fully in communities of their choice to obtain comprehensive, inclusive, locally based, and culturally responsive services.
3 Services and supports for all families of people with disabilities will be readily available, accessible, appropriate, affordable, and accountable to them.
4 Families will participate in directing the use of public and private funding authorized and appropriated to benefit them and their family members with intellectual and developmental disabilities.
5 Families and professionals will have access to state of the art knowledge and best practices regarding supports for people with intellectual and developmental disabilities and will collaborate in applying this knowledge.
6 Research and policy initiatives will include and respect the perspective of siblings of people with intellectual and developmental disabilities.

SELF-DETERMINATION AND SELF-ADVOCACY

1 People with intellectual and developmental disabilities will be equal partners in research about them.
2 People with intellectual and developmental disabilities will make informed decisions about all aspects of their lives.

3 People with intellectual and developmental disabilities will have the opportunity to build their capacity, including their knowledge, skill, and resources, in order to control their own lives and contribute to their communities.
4 People with intellectual and developmental disabilities will have control over their resources, including funding and supports.
5 People with intellectual and developmental disabilities will have meaningful opportunities and supports to enable them to advocate for themselves and to demonstrate leadership.
6 People with intellectual and developmental disabilities will have the freedom and opportunity to participate in social activities and have the social relationships that they desire.

TECHNOLOGY

1 Research will be promoted and expanded on the application of current and emerging technologies for people with intellectual and developmental disabilities.
2 A national network of research centers will be developed to focus on the application of technology to people with cognitive and other disabilities.
3 Undergraduate and graduate training programs will be established to promote fundamental competencies and skills needed to provide education about the use of technology for people with intellectual and developmental disabilities.
4 Information regarding technology will be available and accessible to individuals with disabilities, their families, and their support networks.

AGING

1 Communities will utilize universal design, environmental modifications, and technologies that provide full accessibility for people with disabilities as they age.
2 Families and other caregivers of older adults with intellectual and developmental disabilities will receive sufficient economic, social, and emotional supports to enable them to provide care as both parents and family members with disabilities age.
3 Older adults with intellectual and developmental disabilities will live in community settings of their choice, with sufficient supports to maximize their independence, transportation, safety, personal assistance, and economic security.
4 Older adults with intellectual and developmental disabilities will have opportunities for valued social participation in community life, including friendships and strong social networks.
5 Adults with intellectual and developmental disabilities will enjoy more healthy aging with increased longevity and better physical and behavioral health as they age.

ADDENDUM

Updated information may be found in the special issue of *Mental Retardation and Developmental Disabilities Research Reviews* on Public Policy Aspects of Developmental Disabilities, edited by Susan Parish and Glen Fujiura.

REFERENCES

Barr MW (1904) *Mental Defectives.* Philadelphia: Blakiston's.

Braddock D, Hemp R, Rizzolo MC (2005) *The State of the States in Developmental Disabilities.* Washington DC: American Association on Mental Retardation.

Braddock D, Parish SL (2002) An institutional history of disability. In: Braddock D (ed) *Disability at the Dawn of the 21st Century.* Washington, DC: American Association on Mental Retardation.

Bredekamp S, Copple C (1997) *Developmentally Appropriate Practice in Early Childhood Programs.* Washington, DC: National Association for the Education of Young Children.

Carr EG, Dunlap G, Horner RH, et al. (2002) Positive behavioral support: evolution of an applied science. *J Positive Behav Intervent* 4: 4–16.

Coulter DL (1996) Prevention as a form of support. *Ment Retard* 34: 108–116.

Coulter DL (2004) *Health for People with Intellectual Disabilities in the 21st Century: the Community Health Supports Model.* Keynote paper presented at the Annual Meeting of the American Association on Mental Retardation, Philadelphia, May 2004.

Davidson PW, Heller T, Janicki MP, Hyer K (2003) *The Tampa Scientific Conference on Intellectual Disability, Aging and Health.* Chicago: University of Chicago Press.

Horowitz SM, Kerker BD, Owens PL, Zigler E (2000) *The Health Status of Persons with Mental Retardation.* New Haven, CT: Yale University Press.

Lakin KC, Gardner J, Larson S, Wheeler B (2005) Access and support for community lives, homes and social roles. In: Lakin KC, Turnbull AP (eds) *National Goals and Research for People with Intellectual and Developmental Disabilities.* Washington, DC: American Association on Mental Retardation, pp 179–215.

Lakin KC, Turnbull AP (2005) *National Goals and Research for People with Intellectual and Developmental Disabilities.* Washington, DC: American Association on Mental Retardation.

McLaughlin M, Blacher J, Duffy, S, et al. (2005) Effective education in the least restrictive setting. In: Lakin KC, Turnbull AP (eds) *National Goals and Research for People with Intellectual and Developmental Disabilities.* Washington, DC: American Association on Mental Retardation, pp 39–63.

National Institutes of Health (2001) *Emotional and Behavioral Health in Persons with Mental Retardation and Developmental Disabilities.* Bethesda, MD.

National Research Council (2001) *Eager to Learn: Educating our Preschoolers.* Washington, DC: National Academy Press.

National Research Council and Institute of Medicine (2000) *From Neurons to Neighborhoods: The Science of Early Child Development.* Washington, DC: National Academy Press.

Nehring W (ed) (2005) *Health Promotion for Persons with Intellectual and Developmental Disabilities.* Washington, DC: American Association on Mental Retardation.

Noll S, Trent JW (2004) *Mental Retardation in America.* New York: New York University Press.

Parish SL, Fijiura G (2007) Public policy aspects of the developmental disabilities (eds). *Mental Retardation* and *Developmental Disabilities Research Reviews,* 13: 107–194.

Repp AC, Horner RH (1999) *Functional Analysis of Problem Behavior: From Effective Assessment to Effective Support.* Belmont, CA: Wadsworth.

Sandall S, Hemmeter ML, Smith BJ, McLean ME (eds) (2005) *DEC Recommended Practices: A Comprehensive Guide for Practical Application in Early Intervention and Early Childhood Special Education.* Longmont, CO: Sopris West.

Scheerenberger RC (1983) *A History of Mental Retardation.* Baltimore: Brookes.

Smith M (2005) *Mental Retardation and Developmental Delay: Genetic and Epigenetic Factors.* Oxford: Oxford University Press.

Trent JW (1994) *Inventing the Feeble Mind: A History of Mental Retardation in the United States.* Berkeley, CA: University of California Press.

Tuchman R, Rapin I (eds) (2006) *Autism: A Neurological Disorder of Early Brain Development.* London: Mac Keith Press.

Turnbull AP, Turnbull R, Agosta J, et al. (2005) Support of families and family life across the lifespan. In: Lakin KC, Turnbull AP (eds) *National Goals and Research for People with Intellectual and Developmental Disabilities.* Washington, DC: American Association on Mental Retardation, pp 217–256.

US Public Health Service (2000) *Healthy People 2010.* Washington, DC: US Public Health Service.

US Public Health Service (2002) *Closing the Gap: A National Blueprint for Improving the Health of Individuals with Mental Retardation.* Washington, DC: US Public Health Service.

Wehman P, Revell WG, Brooke V (2003) Competitive employment: has it become the 'first choice' yet? *J Disabil Policy Studies* 14: 163–173.

Whitehead TD, Hughey JB (2004) *Exploring Self-Advocacy from a Social Power Perspective.* New York: Nova.

Wolery M, Bailey DB (2002) Early childhood special education research. *J Early Intervent* 25: 88–99.

Zinkin P, McConachie H (eds) (1995) *Disabled Children and Developing Countries.* London: Mac Keith Press.

6

CHILDREN WITH DEVELOPMENTAL DISABILITIES IN THE MAJORITY OF THE WORLD

Sally Hartley and Charles RJC Newton

INTRODUCTION AND OVERVIEW

The majority of children with neurodevelopmental disabilities are thought to live in 'developing countries' (Helander 2000), more recently called majority world countries (MWC). These countries are those where economic growth, modernization, political freedom, social justice, and the general quality of people's lives are considered to be inadequate by people from more developed countries (Stone 1999). The causes and outcome of children with neurodevelopmental disabilities in these countries appear to be different from more developed countries. In these countries, access to medical and rehabilitative services for children with neurodevelopmental disabilities is mainly confined to urban centers (Helander 1993).

The identification of children with disabilities in MWC is problematic, making estimates of the total burden of disability difficult. Disability depends upon cultural and social perceptions, with identification based upon causality, valued and devalued attributes, and often anticipated adult status (Groce 1999). Attributes determine the detection of disability within society; thus, those societies that value physical strength will identify children with physical impairment more readily. Causality often dictates the manner in which children with disabilities are treated within society, and can include 'evil' spirits, 'witchcraft,' as well as more recognizable biomedical causes. However, for the purposes of estimating the burden, and comparing the prevalence between regions, definitions that can be used across cultures have been developed.

INTERNATIONAL CLASSIFICATION OF DISABILITY

In 1980, the World Health Organization (WHO) set out definitions for impairment, disability, and handicap in the manual of International Classification of Impairment, Disability and Handicap. This classification was revised in 1997 to focus on components of health rather than on the consequences of diseases, thus offering a broader biopsychosocial perspective with a functional view of health-related conditions. Under the auspices of the WHO, International Classification of Impairment, Disability and Handicap developed into the International Classification of Function

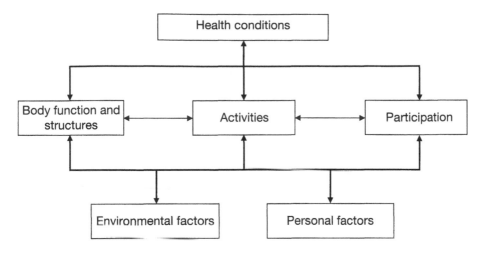

Fig. 6.1. The International Classification of Function (ICF) model of functioning and disability.

(ICF) in 2001 (Fig. 6.1). The ICF provides a common worldwide language and framework for the description of human functioning and disability as an important component of health and social care. This standardization of language resulted in the establishment of a culturally neutral applicable tool covering the whole lifespan which could be used in survey questionnaires. It also can be used to facilitate the comparison of data nationally and internationally.

ICF IN RELATION TO THESE PROBLEMS AND SOLUTIONS

The ICF is a classification scheme produced through an extensive consultation process. This process included representatives of all stakeholder parties (disabled people themselves, medical, education, and rehabilitative experts from developed countries and MWC). The consultation process took place over a 10-year period and the outcome offers an alternative conceptual basis for developing services to meet the needs of children with neurodevelopmental disabilities in the majority of the world. The classification defines disablement as a dynamic interaction between the child (i.e. their personality and intrinsic qualities), any impairment to their body structure and function, the people who relate to them, and the environmental context in which they live (WHO 2001). The needs generated by this complex interactive and constantly changing situation cannot be met by a rigid and focused service delivery system. A flexible and holistic approach is required. The classification scheme makes clear that disablement is a multidimensional dynamic and indeed largely a social phenomenon. For example, the examination of the dimensions of disablement show that impairment is not the only component of disability and this implies that 'treatment' needs to tackle all potentially modifiable, both intrinsic and extrinsic to the individual, components to be effective.

At the same time as developing the ICF, the WHO aimed to determine the 'global burden of disease' by calculating the disability-adjusted life years (DALYs) attributed to each individual person with a disability. The DALY is a statistical measurement for the value of lives lived with a disability. This is defined as the sum of two components: years of healthy life lost due to preterm mortality and the years lived with disability, the latter taking into account the burden of chronic conditions rather than focusing only on mortality. Thus, disability starting in childhood, particularly if associated with preterm mortality, will contribute significantly to the global burden of disease as measured by the DALY.

The DALY assumes a 'reduced value' of lives lived with a disability. This was conceptualized by economists and is not in line with the current thinking about disability and what such individuals might be able to contribute to society. Recent debate has reframed disability as a social issue relating to human rights and integration. The strong link made by DALY between disability and disease pushes the debate back into the medical model and away from the biopsychosocial dimensions represented in the ICF. Furthermore, the values assigned to various impairments are often based on the impact of impairment in adults living in developed countries and may not reflect what actually happens to children in MWC. There are few data on disabilities in children to calculate the various DALYs accurately.

BURDEN OF DISABILITY

In developed countries, people with impairment or disability are identified from computerized administrative data available from service records and registries, or from organized studies that follow a birth cohort of children (Mung'Ala-Odera and Newton 2007). However, in MWC, these sources of data are either not available or of such poor quality that any estimate based upon them is unreliable. The addition of questions to national censuses have not been found to be reliable (Chen and Simeonsson 1993) and studies and key informants tend to underestimate the true prevalence (Thorburn et al. 1991). Thus, in these areas, population censuses and sample surveys using questionnaires have been used to screen for children with impairments (Mung'Ala-Odera and Newton 2007), but these approaches vary in terms of execution, cost, and accuracy. Recently, another approach has been adopted in which stunting and poverty as potential markers of developmental impairment were used (Grantham-McGregor et al. 2007). With this approach, it has been estimated that at least 200 million children aged under 5 years in the world fail to reach their potential in cognitive and socioemotional development (Grantham-McGregor et al. 2007), but this staggering figure itself is likely to be an underestimate.

The Ten Questions Questionnaire (TQQ) was developed to screen for disability in children (Zaman et al. 1990). It has 10 questions designed for administration to parents of children aged 2–9 years, as a screening tool. It has been shown to be a valid instrument to detect moderate or severe neurologic impairment and disability

(Durkin et al. 1995, Mung'Ala-Odera et al. 2004), but it is not sensitive in the detection of mild impairments. It is expensive to administer and is more of a research tool than a means for rapidly identifying children for the provision of needed services. However, it has provided a tool that can be used in many parts of the world and thus allows comparison of the prevalence of impairments between different world regions.

The problem in identifying and characterizing disabilities in children living in MWC is the multidimensional nature of disablement and the lack of cultural and language-specific tools for assessment. The adaptation of assessments developed for Western populations is problematic on two counts. First, because the process is often extensive, the parameters often change so that they do not assess the skills tested in the original tests. Secondly, tools tend to concentrate on assessing impairment and do not adequately address limitations of activity, participation restrictions, and environmental (i.e. barrier or facilitator) factors. Furthermore, there is a severe shortage of skilled people who can administer these tests in the MWC, particularly therapists and psychologists.

The WHO has begun to address some of these issues and has recently published revised charts for growth and motor development based upon five sites (Ghana, India, Norway, Oman and the USA) scattered throughout the world (de Onis et al. 2006). There were no significant consistent differences in milestone achievement ages detected between boys and girls. The contribution of intersite heterogeneity to the total variance was only 5% for the achievement of some motor skills such as hands-and-knees crawling, standing alone, and walking alone, but nearly 15% for other skills such as sitting without support, standing with assistance, and walking with assistance. It was thought that intersite differences were due to culture-specific parental care behaviors, but the analyses support the appropriateness of pooling data from all sites and for both sexes for the purpose of developing an international standard for gross motor development.

There is considerable variation in the prevalence of disability and impairment measured by the TQQ in different regions of the developing world (Table 6.1). The highest prevalences were reported from South (Couper 2002) and East Africa (Mung'Ala-Odera et al. 2006), although the domains most affected varied considerably. The prevalence within a region appears to be greater in rural than urban areas. This may be caused by the lack of antenatal and perinatal care in these areas, because two of these studies identified these factors as independent risk factors for developing eventual neurologic impairment. The lower prevalence recorded in the younger age group may be due to difficulties in assessing this age group, especially for cognition and the differences in the varied assessment procedures. There are also marked differences in the prevalence of the documented motor impairments, which may be caused by methodologic differences or the fact that many children with motor deficits die within the first few years after the etiologic insult (Carter

TABLE 6.1
A comparison of prevalence rates (per 1000) of severe and moderate impairment in eight studies that used the Ten Questions Questionnaire (TQQ) across the world

Place	Year of study	Author	Age	Type of population	Population	Any NI	Cognitive	Motor	Epilepsy	Hearing	Vision
Bangladesh	1987–1988	(Zaman et al. 1992)	6–9	Rural and urban	5352	19	7	1	0.2	9	2
Ghana	2000	(Biritwum et al. 2001)	6–9	Rural and urban	594	17	–	–	–	–	–
Jamaica	1987–1988	(Paul et al. 1992)	2–9	Urban	5468	25	19	2	0.4	4	0.8
Kenya	2001–2002	(Mung'Ala-Odera et al. 2006)	6–9	Rural	10 218	61	31	5	41	14	2
Pakistan	1987–1988	(Durkin et al. 1998)	2–9	Rural and urban	6365	44	19	20	15.5	5	15
Saudi Arabia	1999	(Milaat et al. 2001)	6–12	Urban	1550	37	–	–	–	–	–
South Africa	2001	(Couper 2002)	6–9	Rural	*	63	67	30	13	36	25
South Africa	2001	(Christianson et al. 2002)	2–9	Rural	6692	–	36	–	–	–	–

NI, Neurologic Impairment.
* population not known

et al. 2005a). This may explain the relatively low prevalence of cerebral palsy seen in some regions, particularly in rural areas.

There are no comparable studies of disability or impairment in the West. However, for specific impairment domains, for example intellectual disability, the prevalence in MWC appears at least twice that noted in countries such as Australia (1.4/1000) (Leonard et al. 2003), Finland (11.9/1000) (Rantakallio and von Wendt 1986), and for severe intellectual disability in Sweden (4.5/1000) (Fernell 1998).

CAUSES OF IMPAIRMENT IN MWC

The causes of neurological impairment in children living in MWC are often undetermined, because there is a lack of documentation during the antenatal and perinatal periods, and lack of investigative facilities. Many conditions (Fig. 6.2) that affect child development are more common in MWC, while others such as preterm birth are associated with early mortality. In the recent global estimate (Grantham McGregor et al. 2007), four factors were identified from the review of literature

Causes of impairment that may be more common in developing countries
- Genetic diseases
  - areas of consanguity
- Prenatal exposure
  - alcohol
- Intrauterine growth retardation
  - low birth weight
- Birth asphyxia
- Malnutrition
  - iron deficiency
  - micronutrient deficiencies
- Metabolic
  - thyroid disorders
- Infectious diseases
  - malaria
  - bacterial meningitis
  - encephalitis
  - helminth infections
  - HIV
  - otitis media
- Toxins
  - lead poisoning
- Trauma

Aggravating situations
- Poverty
- Lack of health care
- Famine
- Natural disasters
- Maternal ill-health
  - depression
- Child labour
- Orphanhood
- Neglect and abuse
- War

These aggravating situations are all related to environmental factors of the ICF and are major determinants of disability

Fig. 6.2. Causes and aggravating factors of impaired neurodevelopment in majority world countries.

in which the evidence was compelling: (1) poor nutrition leading to stunting, (2) iodine deficiency, (3) iron deficient anaemia, and (4) inadequate cognitive stimulation (i.e. psychosocial deprivation) (Walker et al. 2007). There is also evidence to suggest that intrauterine growth restriction, malaria, maternal depression, exposure to violence, and exposure to heavy metals are associated with poor development in children in MWC.

POOR NUTRITION

It is estimated that, in MWC, one-third of children less than 5 years old are stunted (defined as height-for-age below 2 standard deviations of reference values). Stunting is caused by poor nutrition and aggravated by frequent infections. It is associated with poor childhood development and performance at school. Food supplements can improve motor and cognitive development (Walker et al. 2007).

IODINE DEFICIENCY

In 2004, the WHO estimated that one-third of the world's population have insufficient iodine intake (WHO 2004). This can lead to congenital hypothyroidism, making it the most commonly preventable cause of cognitive impairment worldwide. In two meta-analyses, iodine deficiency decreases IQ scores by more than 10 points (Walker et al. 2007). The timing of supplementation to prevent cognitive impairment is crucial, because evidence from China suggests that supplementation should occur in the first two trimesters of pregnancy to prevent moderate and severe neurologic impairment and improve later eventual child development (Cao et al. 1994).

IRON DEFICIENCY ANAEMIA

It is estimated that over one-quarter of children living in MWC have iron deficiency anaemia, and this may impair child development, particularly motor, cognitive, and emotional development. There have been many studies in MWC that demonstrate the improvement in child development within months following the administration of iron (Grantham-McGregor and Ani 2001). More recently, there have been longer follow-up studies demonstrating the long-term effects of iron deficiency in terms of lower IQ and motor scores, poor school performance, and behavioral problems (Walker et al. 2007).

INFECTIOUS DISEASES

Infectious diseases involving the central nervous system are much more common in MWC than in developed countries. Bacterial meningitis, viral encephalitis, and malaria are major causes. When these disorders occur, they appear to be more severe and associated with a greater degree of neurologic impairment than in the West. For example, nearly half of the children who survived pneumococcal or haemophilus meningitis in Africa have neurologic sequelae (Peltola 2001). Over 2 billion people are exposed to falciparum malaria in the world, with children in sub-Saharan Africa accounting for over 80% of those infected. Severe malaria is associated with neurologic and cognitive sequelae (Kihara et al. 2006), and it is estimated that over 250 000 child have an impairment caused by malaria each year (Carter et al. 2005b). Other infections that lead to impaired child development include HIV and diarrheal disease. Lastly, intestinal helminths, a major cause of iron deficiency anaemia, may impair child development by this and other mechanisms.

Environmental Toxins

Children in MWC are often exposed to harmful substances, either *in utero* or environmental toxins. Fetal alcohol syndrome is common in many regions, particularly those that are associated with manufacture of alcohol (May et al. 2000). Other drugs that affect the fetus are not that common in the MWC. The WHO estimated that 40% of children have elevated lead levels, which lead to cognitive and motor impairment. Arsenic contamination of drinking water is particularly common in South-East Asia, and this is associated with impaired cognition. Other toxins, such as manganese and pesticides, have been associated with impaired neurodevelopment (Walker et al. 2007).

Psychosocial Factors

Child development is dependent on many psychosocial factors, many of which are profoundly perturbed in children in MWC. Three aspects of parenting have been consistently related to children's overall cognitive and emotional well-being (1) cognitive stimulation, (2) caregiver sensitivity and responsiveness to the child, and (3) caregiver affect (Walker et al. 2007). Caregivers of children in MWC often have chronic ill health, live in poverty with overcrowding, and sometimes under extreme conditions such as famine or war. These factors will impair the ability of these caregivers to provide basic care and stimulation for their children in these circumstances. Furthermore, their sensitivity and response are poorer than in developed countries. Studies from MWC suggest that early cognitive stimulation improves cognitive abilities (Walker et al. 2007). Other factors such maternal depression and exposure to violence are also more common in MWC and can have profound effects on the child's development.

Case–control studies have identified the following risk factors of neurologic impairment (1) lack of prenatal care, (2) birth difficulties, (3) home births, (4) lack of maternal education, and (5) maternal age >30 years at the time of birth of the child. In a large study of risk factors in Bangladesh (Durkin et al. 2000), multivariate analyses identified maternal goiter, postnatal brain infections, consanguinity, and landless agriculture work as independently associated with the prevalence of severe cognitive impairment, while maternal illiteracy, landlessness, maternal history of pregnancy loss, and small for gestational age at birth were independent risk factors for mild cognitive disabilities. Studies in Nepal and Kenya found that neonatal encephalopathy (Ellis et al. 2000), neonatal tetanus (Barlow et al. 2001), neonatal jaundice and sepsis (Gordon et al. 2005) were important causes of neurodevelopmental delay in these areas.

NEURODEVELOPMENTAL IMPAIRMENTS

Of the domains of neurodevelopmental impairments in children, global developmental delay, mental retardation/intellectual disability, language impairment, and motor impairment are the most conspicuous.

GLOBAL DEVELOPMENTAL DELAY

There are few studies that address global delay in MWC, partly because of the lack of culturally appropriate tools and trained staff. A study in Saudi Arabia, in which 3-year-old children were screened with the Denver Developmental Scale, estimated the prevalence to be 24/1000 (Eapen et al. 2006).

There are limited data on the causes of global delay because most countries lack facilities for thorough investigation. In 247 Turkish children with developmental delay in whom chromosomal analysis and neuroimaging could be performed, perinatal complications (21%), cerebral dysgenesis (18%), chromosomal abnormalities (9%), genetic/dysmorphic syndromes (3%), metabolic disorders (4%), hypothyroidism (4%), neurocutaneous syndromes (3%), and intrauterine infection (2%) were identified in 64% of the children (Ozmen et al. 2005). This study and other studies from MWC highlight the importance of hypothyroidism and infections as common causes of global developmental delay in these regions.

MENTAL RETARDATION/INTELLECTUAL DISABILITY

It is thought that 2/1000 children will have conditions that will lead to severe mental retardation/intellectual disability, often in conjunction with other disabilities. These may result from a number of genetic conditions or diseases such as meningitis. Down syndrome is the single most important condition leading to severe mental retardation/intellectual disability (Sunders 1984, Baldwin et al. 1990). However, the survival rates in MWC differ according to available medical facilities and other factors such as employment, war, and natural disasters *inter alia*.

The conditions that lead to mild to moderate mental retardation/intellectual disability in the MWC are not usually medical. They are more likely to be a result of a combination of poor nutrition and understimulation. Within the population, the prevalence of such impairments can be estimated statistically using measures of intelligence. This has little functional value as the tests of intelligence are culturally bound and the results highly skewed in favor of developed countries. In surveys, prevalence estimates vary widely depending upon the method of measurement employed. By definition, an IQ screening method will lead to relatively high numbers of children being identified. If parental anxiety over educational progress is used as a means of identifying mental retardation/intellectual disability, this will lead to variable results, depending on the value placed on the educational system. Measures of social and functional attainment will probably result in relatively low numbers because children with mild mental retardation/intellectual disability are usually able to function very well in family life, and are therefore not noticeably different from their peers (Sunders 1984, Baldwin et al. 1990).

LANGUAGE IMPAIRMENT

People communicate in many different ways, mainly through using language, which may be spoken, written, or signed. However, there are several ways to communicate without using verbal language. These include gestures, pictures, body language, facial expression, and actions such as walking away or always being present. Some experts believe that the majority (60–90%) of communication is in fact non-verbal (Knapp and Hall 2002). Although the words 'language' and 'communication' are used interchangeably, the two concepts are different. Language 'is a body of words and the systems for their use common to a people who are of the same community or nation, the same geographical area, or the same cultural tradition' (http://www.infoplease. com). Language can be spoken, written, or signed. Communication can be defined as 'imparting or interchange of thoughts, opinions, or information by speech, writing, or signs.' Non-linguistic ways of communicating include gestures, pictures, body language, and facial expression.

Impaired language ability is therefore quite specific to the skill of using a system of symbols. At a simple level, key aspects of language are recognized as semantics (study of meaning), syntax (study of grammar), phonology (study of sounds), and morphology (study of form or structure). These symbols, which can be written or spoken, are used to communicate thoughts, ideas, and feelings. The processes in which language are used involve two processes: expression and reception.

Language impairment can occur when any of these areas are affected. Limited language functioning is associated with developmental delay and sometimes associated cognitive and underlying hearing impairments. The prevalence of language impairment in developed countries is estimated to be about 2% (Enderby and Philipp 1986), but the prevalence in MWC remains unknown. Some conditions that are common in MWC cause specific language impairments. For example, exposure to severe falciparum malaria is associated with difficulties in phonology, pragmatics, receptive vocabulary, and lexical semantics (Carter et al. 2006). As the burden of malaria is large, it is potentially one of the most common causes of language impairment in MWC.

Studies conducted in Uganda (Hartley 1998) and Zimbabwe (WHO 1997) have shown that about half of children with disabilities have communication difficulties.

Much can be done to improve communication, with relatively simple means and using non-professionals.

MOTOR IMPAIRMENT

Cerebral palsy and polio are major causes of motor impairment in MWC. The incidence of cerebral palsy is likely to be high, but surveys conducted in older children find the prevalence is low because few children survive given limited health care services especially in rural areas. With the improvement of medical services in MWC, the chances of survival for children with cerebral palsy has also improved. It is noticeable that as the incidence of polio decreases, with improved vaccination coverage and health education, cerebral palsy has become a more prominent condition in many MWC.

INTERVENTIONS

Many of the causes of developmental delay in MWC are preventable, although the logistics of providing appropriate interventions can be problematic within these regions. The four leading causes of poor performance in MWC (i.e. stunting, iodine deficiency, iron deficiency anaemia, and inadequate cognitive stimulation) can be addressed, but often require sustained commitment from governments and non-governmental organizations to implement. Alleviation of poverty, specifically the systematic prevention of food and medical shortages, are likely to make a significant impact on the prevention of neurodevelopmental impairment. Besides the treatment of nutrient deficiencies, much can be done to promote child development in MWC. Effective programs that provide direct learning experiences to children and families have been tested in these countries (Engle et al. 2007). They need to be targeted towards the younger and most disadvantaged children and integrated with family support, and health, nutritional, or educational systems.

SERVICES AVAILABLE

Services for disabled persons in MWC are usually technically limited in comparison with their more developed counterparts in other parts of the world. The United Nations estimates that only 3% of people with disabilities in the world who require rehabilitative care actually receive it (Groce 1999). There is a lack appropriate equipment and trained staff. Rehabilitation services tend to serve a very small percentage of the population, because of their location and financial restrictions. In particular, services available in the MWC are concentrated in urban areas. Finally, the relevance of available services in terms of meeting the needs of the children and their families is sometimes questioned. This centrally located, low coverage service also means that there is very little knowledge about the size and nature of this population group in these countries as a whole. Generally, the problems faced by these children and their families remain unknown, with policies and plans developed from estimates and experiences in more developed parts of the world that may not be analogous.

COMMUNITY-BASED REHABILITATION PROGRAMS

Community-based rehabilitation is 'a strategy within community development for the rehabilitation, equalization of opportunities and social integration of all people with disabilities. It is implemented through the combined efforts of disabled people themselves, their families and communities and the appropriate health, education and vocational and social services' (ILO et al. 2004). As such it is the rehabilitation strategy promoted by the WHO and it maps closely onto the dimensions of dis-ablement outlined in the ICF. Community-based rehabilitation programs therefore do not only target the medical determinants of disablement, but also the relevant social and environmental factors limiting activity and participation. In this way, it is thought to be a more effective strategy for improving the quality of the lives of disabled people and their families. However, it remains rigorously unevaluated in scientific terms as, like other complex health interventions, it presents some con-siderable challenges to research design and interpretation, especially in the context of MWC.

CONCLUSIONS

Developmental disabilities are more common in children living in MWC, but the causes are often different and can vary considerably from one region to another. Accurate estimation of the actual burden is hampered by a lack of cultural specific tools for assessing children, trained personnel to administer screening and diag-nostic tests, and lack of investigative facilities to determine the underlying cause. Prevention of the major causes of poor development is possible, but requires a con-certed effort from a number of different organizations. Services for children with disability are inadequate and hospital-based services are often not used by children with disabilities. Community-based rehabilitation programs offer a solution, but have not yet been properly evaluated for effectiveness.

REFERENCES

Baldwin S, Asindua S, Stanfield P (1990) Survey of childhood disabilities within a community-based programme for the rehabilitation of the disabled in Kibwezi division, Kenya. AMREF report, pp 1–45.

Barlow JL, Mung'Ala-Odera V, Gona J, Newton CR (2001) Brain damage after neonatal tetanus in a rural Kenyan hospital. *Trop Med Int Health* 6: 305–308.

Biritwum RB, Devres JP, Ofosu-Amaah S, Marfo C, Essah ER (2001) Prevalence of children with disabilities in central region, Ghana. *West Afr J Med* 20: 249–255.

Cao XY, Jiang XM, Dou ZH, Rakeman MA, Zhang ML, O'Donnell K, et al. (1994) Timing of vulnerability of the brain to iodine deficiency in endemic cretinism. *N Engl J Med* 331: 1739–1744.

Carter JA, Lees JA, Gona JK, Murira G, Rimba K, Neville BG, et al. (2006) Severe falciparum malaria and acquired childhood language disorder. *Dev Med Child Neurol* 48: 51–57.

Carter JA, Mung'Ala-Odera V, Neville BG, Murira G, Mturi N, Musumba C, et al. (2005a) Persistent neurocognitive impairments associated with severe falciparum malaria in Kenyan children. *J Neurol Neurosurg Psychiatry* 76: 476–481.

Carter JA, Ross AJ, Neville BG, Obiero E, Katana K, Mung'Ala-Odera V, et al. (2005b) Developmental impairments following severe falciparum malaria in children. *Trop Med Int Health* 10: 3–10.

Chen J, Simeonsson RJ (1993) Prevention of childhood disability in the People's Republic of China. *Child Care Health Dev* 19: 71–88.

Christianson AL, Zwane ME, Manga P, Rosen E, Venter A, Downs D, et al. (2002) Children with intellectual disability in rural South Africa: prevalence and associated disability. *J Intellect Disabil Res* 46: 179–186.

Couper J (2002) Prevalence of childhood disability in rural KwaZulu-Natal. *S Afr Med J* 92: 549–552.

de Onis M, Garza C, Onyango AW, Martorell R (2006) WHO Child Growth Charts. *Acta Paediatr Scand* 95: 1–106.

Durkin MS, Hasan ZM, Hasan KZ (1998) Prevalence and correlates of mental retardation among children in Karachi, Pakistan. *Am J Epidemiol* 147: 281–288.

Durkin MS, Khan NZ, Davidson LL, Huq S, Munir S, Rasul E, et al. (2000) Prenatal and postnatal risk factors for mental retardation among children in Bangladesh. *Am J Epidemiol* 152: 1024–1033.

Durkin MS, Wang W, Shrout PE, Zaman SS, Hasan ZM, Desai P, et al. (1995) Evaluating a ten questions screen for childhood disability: reliability and internal structure in different cultures. *J Clin Epidemiol* 48: 657–666.

Eapen V, Zoubeidi T, Yunis F, Gururaj AK, Sabri S, Ghubash R (2006) Prevalence and psychosocial correlates of global developmental delay in 3-year-old children in the United Arab Emirates. *J Psychosom Res* 61: 321–326.

Ellis M, Manndhar N, Manandhar DS, Costello AM (2000) Risk factors for neonatal encephalopathy in Kathmandu, Nepal, a developing country: unmatched case–control study. *BMJ* 320: 1229–1236.

Enderby P, Philipp R (1986) Speech and language handicap: towards knowing the size of the problem. *Br J Disord Commun* 21: 151–165.

Engle PL, Black MM, Behrman JR, Cabral de MM, Gertler PJ, Kapiriri L, et al. (2007) Strategies to avoid the loss of developmental potential in more than 200 million children in the developing world. *Lancet* 369: 229–242.

Fernell E (1998) Aetiological factors and prevalence of severe mental retardation in children in a Swedish municipality: the possible role of consanguinity. *Dev Med Child Neurol* 40: 608–611.

Gordon AL, English M, Tumaini DJ, Karisa M, Newton CR (2005) Neurological and developmental outcome of neonatal jaundice and sepsis in rural Kenya. *Trop Med Int Health* 10: 1114–1120.

Grantham-McGregor S, Ani C (2001) A review of studies on the effect of iron deficiency on cognitive development in children. *J Nutr* 131: 649S–666S.

Grantham-McGregor S, Cheung YB, Cueto S, Glewwe P, Richter L, Strupp B (2007) Developmental potential in the first 5 years for children in developing countries. *Lancet* 369: 60–70.

Groce NE (1999) Disability in cross-cultural perspective: rethinking disability. *Lancet* 354: 756–757.

Hartley S (1998) Service development to meet the needs of 'people with communication disabilities' in developing countries. *Disabil Rehabil* 20: 277–284.

Helander E (1993) *Prejudice and Dignity: an introduction to community based rehabilitation.* New York: United Nations Development Programme.

Helander E (2000) 25 years of community-based rehabilitation. *Asia Pacific Disability Rehabilitation Journal* 11: 4–9.

ILO, UNESCO, and WHO. (2004) CBR: a strategy for rehabiliation, equalization of opportunities poverty reduction and social inclusion of people with disabilities. Joint Position Paper.

Kihara M, Carter JA, Newton CR (2006) The effect of *Plasmodium falciparum* on cognition: a systematic review. *Trop Med Int Health* 11: 386–397.

Knapp ML, Hall JA (2002) *Nonverbal Communication in Human Interaction.* Belmont, CA: Wadsworth.

Leonard H, Petterson B, Bower C, Sanders R (2003) Prevalence of intellectual disability in Western Australia. *Paediatr Perinat Epidemiol* 17: 58–67.

May PA, Brooke L, Gossage JP, Croxford J, Adnams C, Jones KL, et al. (2000) Epidemiology of fetal alcohol syndrome in a South African community in the Western Cape Province. *Am J Public Health* 90: 1905–1912.

Milaat WA, Ghabrah TM, Al Bar HM, Abalkhail BA, Kordy MN (2001) Population-based survey of childhood disability in eastern Jeddah using the ten questions tool. *Disabil Rehabil* 23: 199–203.

Mung'Ala-Odera, Meehan R, Njuguna P, Mturi N, Alcock K, Carter JA, et al. (2004) Validity and reliability of the 'Ten Questions' questionnaire for detecting moderate to severe neurological impairment in children aged 6–9 years in rural Kenya. *Neuroepidemiology* 23: 67–72.

Mung'Ala-Odera V, Meehan R, Njuguna P, Mturi N, Alcock K, Carter JA, et al. (2006) Prevalence and risk factors of neurological disability and impairment in children living in rural Kenya. *Int J Epidemiol* 35: 683–688.

Mung'Ala-Odera V, Newton CRJC (2007) Identifying children with neurological impairment and disability in resource-poor countries. *Child Care Health Dev* 33: 249–256.

Ozmen M, Tatli B, Aydinli N, Caliskan M, Demirkol M, Kayserili H (2005) Etiologic evaluation in 247 children with global developmental delay at Istanbul, Turkey. *J Trop Pediatr* 51: 310–313.

Paul TJ, Desai P, Thorburn MJ (1992) The prevalence of childhood disability and related medical diagnoses in Clarendon, Jamaica. *West Indian Med J* 41: 8–11.

Peltola H (2001) Burden of meningitis and other severe bacterial infections of children in Africa: implications for prevention. *Clin Infect Dis* 32: 64–75.

Rantakallio P, von Wendt L (1986) Mental retardation and subnormality in a birth cohort of 12,000 children in Northern Finland. *Am J Ment Defic* 90: 380–387.

Stone E (1999) *Disability and Development.* Leeds: Disability Press.

Sunders CA (ed) (1984) *Handicapped Children: an epidemiological study in Nigerian children. Developmental perspectives.* London: Mac Keith Press.

Thorburn MJ, Desai P, Durkin M (1991) A comparison of efficacy of the key informant and community survey methods in the identification of childhood disability in Jamaica. *Ann Epidemiol* 1: 255–261.

Walker SP, Wachs TD, Gardner JM, Lozoff B, Wasserman GA, Pollitt E, et al. (2007) Child development: risk factors for adverse outcomes in developing countries. *Lancet* 369: 145–157.

WHO (2001) *International Classifications of Functioning, Disability and Health* (IFC) Geneva: World Health Organization.

World Health Organization (WHO) (1997) *Let's Communicate: A Handbook for People Working with Children with Communication Difficulties.* Geneva: World Health Organization.

World Health Organization (WHO) (2004) *Global Database on Iodine Deficiency: Iodine Status Worldwide.* Geneva: World Health Organization.

Zaman SS, Khan NZ, Islam S, Banu S, Dixit S, Shrout P, et al. (1990) Validity of the 'Ten Questions' for screening serious childhood disability: results from urban Bangladesh. *Int J Epidemiol* 19: 613–620.

Zaman SS, Khan NZ, Islam S, Durkin M (1992) *Childhood Disabilities in Bangladash.* Bangladesh Protibondhi Foundation.

7

SCREENING FOR DEVELOPMENTAL AND BEHAVIORAL PROBLEMS

Frances Page Glascoe and Kevin P. Marks

INTRODUCTION

The challenges inherent in early detection of developmental problems are many. Although health care providers have abundant contact with young children and their families, well-visits have many competing demands including physical examination immunizations, safety and injury prevention counseling, and anticipatory guidance. Thus, there may be actual little time to devote to screening for developmental disabilities. Other primary care barriers to early detection include limited third-party reimbursement, a lack of awareness of available referral resources, misconceptions that problems are likely to be obvious without measurement, a sense that many children will simply outgrow their delays (i.e. maturational lags), and a reluctance to give parents difficult news. For these reasons, health care providers tend to use problematic approaches to early detection including a dependence on clinical observation rather than measurement, a deployment of informal checklists of milestones that lack objective validation and distinct cutoffs, or the use of screening tests with limited accuracy (Sices 2004, Rydz et al. 2005). As a consequence, only 30% of children with developmental disabilities are identified prior to school entrance, at which point all opportunities for effective early intervention are lost (King and Glascoe 2003, Halfon et al. 2004, Silverstein et al. 2005). In contrast, when professionals routinely use quality instruments, early identification rates soar, and in a single administration can detect 70–80% of children with developmental disabilities (First and Palfrey 1994, Silverstein et al. 2005).

Because accurate screening tools, rather than informal methods, carry the burden of proof, the first critical questions are:

1 How can we identify a good measure?
2 Are there tools that can work in busy medical settings?
3 What is available for those professionals beyond primary care service delivery with more time to devote to the process with different information needs (e.g. for program evaluation, progress tracking)?

RATIONALE FOR SCREENING

Early intervention (e.g. rehabilitation services, quality preschool programs) have a known positive impact on children's development, behavior, and subsequent school performance (Reynolds et al. 2001). As a consequence, the American Academy of Pediatrics (AAP) and other professional groups related to child health recommend that health care providers screen *routinely and repeatedly*. This begs the question of why is it necessary to repeatedly rescreen patients. There are two essential reasons.

1 **Development is pliant, particularly in the earliest years.** Academic, language, social, and other developmental skills are readily influenced in positive directions by environments that promote, foster, and encourage learning. When parents engage children's interests; respond by talking, listening, and modeling; implement discipline rather than punishment as an approach to teaching; and have few evident risk factors, their children tend to perform in the average to above-average range on measures of intelligence, a strong predictor of later school success (Sameroff et al. 1987, Aylward 1990). In contrast, when parents' interaction styles are characterized largely by commands, or limited verbal expansions on child-initiated topics of conversation, children fare less well.

   Possession of four of the more known risk factors, which include parental substance abuse, mental health problems, limited social support, single parent status, more than three children in the home, numerous stressful life events (i.e. job loss, deaths in the family, physical illness, parental disruption), minority, and low occupational status, place children at 24 times the risk of having IQs below 85, roughly the point above which typical classroom instruction is effective (Sameroff et al. 1987).

   Young children with risk factors tend to demonstrate at least mild developmental delays by age 2, particularly in the area of language, which is also a strong predictor of later school success. Such weakened acquisition of higher order developmental skills creates a risk for subsequent school failure. Problematic school performance is associated with in-grade retention, dropping out of secondary school, teen pregnancy, unemployment, and adjudication (Reynolds et al. 2001).

   Despite the bleakness of this picture, early risk factors can change during childhood (e.g. due to divorce or marriage, acquisition or loss of employment, fluctuations in mental health status, addition of new siblings, involvement in early intervention). Thus, developmental progress can change, for better or for worse. To monitor changes in developmental status, repeated screening is necessary for accuracy and detection.

2 **Development develops. Developmental problems develop too.** We cannot know, for example, that a typically developing 9-month-old will remain on a positive trajectory. What if she is not using words by 18 months or two-word

utterances by 24 months? Even if language emerges well and progresses adequately, we cannot know that she will be a successful reader at age 5 until she reaches the age when most children have some facility with letter and word recognition. The term 'age-related developmental manifestations' (Bell 1986) captures the emerging nature of development and developmental problems. This phenomenon results in an emerging risk of disabilities across the lifespan. Of the many types of neuro-developmental disabilities, the most common are speech-language impairment, learning disabilities and global developmental delay/mental retardation/intellectual disability, followed by the autism spectrum disorders. Only 2–3% of children between 0 and 24 months of age have developmental problems, while the prevalence increases to 8% when children up to age 5 are added (Algozinne and Korinek 1985, Yeargin-Allsopp et al. 1992, Newacheck et al. 1998).

Public school special education programs serve almost 12% of the school-age population, a figure considered low by epidemiologists who generally find prevalence rates of 16–18% in population-based surveys (Yeargin-Allsopp et al. 1992, Newacheck et al. 1998) for developmental disabilities alone. When mental health problems are also included, the combined prevalence is 22%, quite similar to high school drop-out rates in the United States (Lavigne et al. 1993, www.uscensus.gov 2005).

HOW TO SELECT A GOOD SCREENING TEST

Because of development's pliability and age-related manifestations, there is a clear need for systematic screening. Given problematic suboptimal detection rates when using informal methods such as checklists and clinical observation, the need is not only for screening, but screening with quality instruments, and screening repeatedly. What are the most accurate screen tools? Which ones are suitable for busy primary care clinics? Which ones are more appropriate for early intervention programs and other settings where professionals have more time to work with children directly? While there are many published tests, it is important to recognize that their publication is not regulated, particularly in the United States. In contrast, the Canadian Psychological Association (CPA) requires publishers to report specific indicators of accuracy and avoid misleading findings such as overall hit-rates (CPA 1996). Even so, the CPA guidelines regulate only reporting requirements and do not deter inaccurate measures from being actively marketed. Thus, professionals involved in testing should become knowledgeable about the basics of test psychometry so they can select measures that are well-constructed and accurate.

Screening test standards and related terms are defined below. These were drawn from several sources including *Standards for Educational and Psychological Tests* published by the American Psychological Association et al. (1999) and from the recommendations of researchers in screening (Barnes 1982, Lichtenstein & Ireton 1984, Squires et al. 1996).

Screening is a brief method for sorting those who probably have problems from those who probably do not. Screening measures are meant to be given to the asymptomatic, those with subclinical non-apparent (i.e. non-overt) difficulties. The group with probable problems are typically referred for further diagnostic work-up and, if formally diagnosed, referred for treatment. It is worth noting that often a specific diagnosis is not necessary for young children to enter early intervention. Rather, the presence of quantifiable delays serves as an acceptable eligibility criterion for services and complete detailed diagnostic evaluations are typically provided later.

Screens may be broad-band (i.e. they tap all or most developmental domains) or narrow-band (i.e. they focus on a single domain of development such as motor skills or on a specific recognizable condition such as autism or attention deficit hyperactivity disorder). The focus of this particular paper is on broad-band screens although the psychometric precepts underlying their construction also apply to narrow-band tools.

Developmental screens, even the most accurate ones, are not error free. This is not surprising given the moving target that is development itself. Nevertheless, screens should be as accurate as possible in order to minimize the costs (financial and non-financial) associated with both overreferrals and underdetection. The components of screening accuracy include the following features.

SENSITIVITY

Sensitivity is the percentage of children with disabilities correctly detected by a screening test. Sensitivity is computed by test authors by administering diagnostic tests to a randomly selected group of children. Some will be found to have disabilities. If screening tests are then given to the same group, researchers can then look at the number of children with disabilities correctly detected (e.g. by failing, abnormal or positive results). Standards for sensitivity are the identification of at least 70–80% of children with disabilities on a single point administration.

SPECIFICITY

Specificity is defined as the percentage of children without difficulties correctly identified by a screening test. In the above example in which diagnostic tests were given to a group of children, most would be found to have typical development. If a screening test is then administered, it should identify the typically developing children as such (e.g. by passing, typical or negative findings on screening). Because there are many more children with typical development than not, specificity should be closer to 80%, so as to minimize possible overreferrals.

POSITIVE PREDICTIVE VALUE

Positive predictive value is the percentage of children with failing scores on screening tests who are found to have a disability. When a child does poorly on a screening test, the results mean that he/she probably has a problem. Still, there is always a chance that the screening test is in error. How much of a chance? Put another way, what is the predictive value of a failing (or positive) test score in reflecting an actual problem? For example, if 4 out of 5 children with failing scores on screening tests are found to have developmental disabilities diagnoses, the test's positive predictive value is 4/5 or 80%, meaning that for any screening test failure, there would be an 80% chance that the child actually has a disability. In application, however, positive predictive value is rarely so high and values of 30–50% are typical (meaning that for every 2–3 children referred only one would result in a confirmatory diagnosis).

While this may seem troubling, what is of particular interest is the nature of false-positives. Research shows that children who fail screening tests, but are not found to have a developmental diagnosis, are those with numerous psychosocial risk factors and below average performance on the better predictors of school success: academics/pre-academics, language, and intelligence (Glascoe 2001). These are children for whom help is definitely needed. Although they will not qualify for special education, they benefit enormously from programs such as Head Start, quality daycare/preschool, developmental promotion, parent training, social services, and summer school. These findings indicate that screening tests followed by additional assessments, which are usually available through early intervention programs, are particularly helpful in identifying the at-risk child as well as those with undetected disabilities. For this reason, there is no agreed upon percentage standard for positive predictive value.

OTHER CHARACTERISTICS OF QUALITY SCREENING TESTS

Screening tests must first embody the same psychometric properties as all other tests (Majnemer & Limperopoulos 2002, Rydz et al. 2005). Thus, screens should be standardized on a large national and current sample whose characteristics reflect those of the country in which they are deployed (e.g. inclusion of ethnic minorities in proportion to their prevalence in the general population, correct proportions of parents with varying levels of education, correct percentage of children with disabilities in relation to the population as a whole). Typically, census information is used to determine current population parameters and thus the optimal standarization sample profile. The representativeness of this sample is critical because it is this performance sample from which normative information on test performance is derived (i.e. to construct the test's scores such as percentiles, quotients, age-equivalents). Standardization must be current and recommendations from the American Psychological Association call for the restandardization of measures every 10 years at a minimum. This is wise because populations parameters change and test stimuli become out of date (e.g. images of a rotary dial telephone no longer have any meaning for young children). Ideally, the standardization sample should also be naturalistically acquired (e.g. consecutive children seeking well-child care). In contrast, including groups with and without known disabilities will likely exclude those with subtle problems with a concomitant loss of gradations in developmental status in the range between atypical and typical. The result is tests that perform less than optimally in what will be real-life application situations.

Screening tests must also include proof of reliability. There are many types of reliability: (1) test–retest (i.e. retesting the same child by the same examiner a few weeks apart), and (2) inter-rater reliability (retesting the same child by a different examiner). These measures show that the directions are clear, the items tap relatively enduring developmental behaviors, and that different examiners can confidently use test norms to compare children's performance. Ideally, these reliability figures should approach 90% or higher. Internal consistency is another type of reliability which shows that the items cluster as expected into various domains. If, for example, motor items and language items have a great deal of overlap, test users cannot be confident that they are measuring each domain adequately and independently (e.g. a child with a language delay but excellent motor skills might do poorly on the latter items simply because the directions were too complicated).

Validity studies should be voluminous and include concurrent validity (i.e. high correlations between the screen and a broad range of diagnostic measures typically including test of language, intelligence, motor, social, self-help skills, etc). If broad-band screening is given only alongside a test of intelligence, users do not have adequate information that motor, language, pre-academic, social, or other skills are measured well. There should also be proof of discriminant validity, again expressed either as correlations or percent correctly detected, through which it can be seen how well a screen detects various and usually highly prevalent conditions (including language impairment, autism, specific learning disabilities, and mental retardation). Occasionally, screening tests are also studied for their predictive validity which means that the screen is administered and then, typically 1–2 years later, diagnostic measures are administered. High correlations, after adjusting for interval intervention, illustrate that the screen is measuring meaningful and relevant aspects of development.

Utility is the term used to describe other features of screens that are practical in nature:

1 Materials that are interesting to children but sufficiently minimal in number so that examiners can find them easily in the test kit
2 Easy to read and find direction for items
3 Clear scoring procedures of sufficient simplicity that computation errors are minimized
4 Clear information about the amount of training required and videos and/or training exercises included with the test manual to ensure consistent screen application

5 Directions for interpreting and conveying test results to families (e.g. examiners should be encouraged not to use diagnostic labels, to present the information and service referrals in a positive and practical way, and to offer ongoing support to families struggling with difficult news)
6 Guidance should be given for the kinds of referrals that may be needed based on various profiles (e.g. failing scores on motor domains but average performance in other areas should indicate a referral to a neurologist and/or physical therapist)
7 Alternative methods for administering items if needed to circumvent behavioral non-compliance, limited language proficiency, limited knowledge of the child's development on the part of the caretaker accompanying the child during screening, etc.

SPECIFIC SCREENING INSTRUMENTS

Table 7.1 provides information on the best developmental screening tests now available. These tests were selected because they (1) cover most or all developmental domains (although some emotional/behavioral screens are discussed separately because few developmental tests measure this domain), (2) meet standards for screening test accuracy – sensitivity and specificity were rated highly if they exceeded 70–80%, (3) had adequate and appropriate standardization samples, (4) had studies of reliability that met performance standards, and (5) included a range of validity studies showing high correlations between screening and a battery of diagnostic measures. Not included in Table 7.1 are measures that fail to meet standards or comply with basic psychometric values. Excluded tests are as follow:

1 Denver-II and its pre-screening derivative, the PDQ-R, because they were standardized only in Denver and lack validation of any kind. Research showed that the Denver-II consistently overrefers or underdetects depending on how a questionable score is handled (Glascoe et al. 1992)
2 Early Screening Profile, which, while nationally standardized and validated, has very poor sensitivity
3 CAT-CLAMS, which, although heavily language-oriented, was validated only against measures of intelligence on referred rather than general pediatric samples, thus rendering its sensitivity and specificity likely inflated (Hoon et al. 1993, Kube et al. 2000); and the DIAL-III and Nipossing because of limited sensitivity.
4 Battelle Developmental Inventory Screening Test-II, which fails to provide any assessment of its sensitivity and specificity.

Measures include those relying on parental report which are especially useful in busy general primary care clinics. Parent report measures can be completed in waiting or exam rooms or even prior to the scheduled appointment. They can be administered by self-report, or interview and most have multiple language translations.

TABLE 7.1
Behavioral and/or Developmental screens relying on information from parents

Developmental screen	Age range	Description	Scoring	Accuracy	Time frame/costs
Parents' Evaluations of Developmental Studies (PEDS) (2008) Ellsworth & Vandermeer Press Ltd, 1013 Austin Court, Nolensville, TN37135 (Phone: 615-776-4121; fax: 615-776-4119)). ($30.00)http://www.pedstest.com PEDS is also available online together with the Modified Checklist of Autism in Toddlers for electronic records. See www.pedstest.com for trial information	Birth to 8 years	10 questions eliciting parents' concerns. Written at the 5th grade level (varying from low 1st to 7th grade). Determines when to refer, provide a second screen, provide patient education, or monitor development, behavior/emotional, and academic progress. Provides longitudinal surveillance and triage. Available in 14+ languages including Spanish, Vietnamese and Somali.	Identifies children as low, moderate, or high risk for various kinds of disabilities and delays	Sensitivity ranging from 74% to 79% and specificity ranging from 70% to 80% across age levels	About 2 minutes (if interview needed) Print materials ~$0.31 Admin. ~$0.88 Total = ~$1.19
Ages and Stages Questionnaire (2009). Paul H Brookes Publishing Inc, PO Box 10624, Baltimore, Maryland 21285 (1-800-638-3755). ($199.50) http://www.pbrookes.com/ Online at www.patienttools.com	4–60 months	Parents indicate children's developmental skills on 25–35 items (4–5 pages) using a different form for each well visit. Average reading level is 4th grade varying across items from 3rd to 12th grade. Can be used in mass mail-outs for child-find programs. In English, Spanish, French, Korean and other languages	Single pass/fail score for developmental status	Sensitivity ranged 70–90% at all ages except the 4-month level. Specificity ranged from 76% to 91%	About 15 minutes (if interview needed) Materials ~$0.40 Admin. ~$4.20 Total = ~$4.60

Measure	Age	Description	Scoring	Accuracy	Time/Cost
PEDS- Developmental Milestones (PEDS-DM (2007)) Ellsworth & Vandermeer Press, Ltd. 1013 Austin Court, Nolensville, TN 37135. Phone: 615-776-4121; fax: 615-776-4119 http://www.pedstest.com ($275.00) To be online soon.	0–8 years	PEDS-DM consists of 6–8 items at each age level (spanning the well visit schedule). Each item taps a different domain (fine/gross motor, self-help, academics, expressive/receptive language, social-emotional). Items are administered by parents or professionals. Forms are laminated and marked with a grease pencil. It can be used to complement PEDS or stand alone. Administered by parent report or directly. Written at the 2nd grade level. A longitudinal score form tracks performance. Supplemental measures also included include the M-CHAT, Family Psychosocial Screen, PSC-17, the SWILS, the Vanderbilt, and a measure of parent-child interactions. An Assessment Level version is available for NICU follow-up and early intervention programs. In English and Spanish.	Cutoffs tied to performance above and below the 16th percentile for each item and its domain. On the Assessment Level, age equivalent scores are produced and enable users to compute percentage of delays.	Sensitivity (.75–.87); specificity (.71–.88 to performance in each domain. Sensitivity (.70–.94); specificity (.77–.93) across age	About 3–5 minutes Materials ~.$.02 Admin. ~$1.00 Total ~$1.02

Behavioral/emotional screens relying on information from parents

Measure	Age	Description	Scoring	Accuracy	Time/Cost
Pediatric Symptom Checklist. Jellinek et al. (1988) (the test is included in the article). Also can be freely downloaded at http://psc.partners.org/ or with factor scores at www.pedstest.com The Pictorial PSC, useful with low-income Spanish speaking families can be downloaded freely at www.dbpeds.org	4–16 years.	35 short statements of problem behaviors including both externalizing (conduct) and internalizing (depression, anxiety, adjustment, etc.) Ratings of never, sometimes or often are assigned a value of 0, 1, or 2. Scores totaling 28 or more suggest referrals. Factor scores identify attentional, internalizing and externalizing problems. Factor scoring is available for download at: http://www. pedstest.com/links/resources.html	Single refer/ non-refer score	All but one study showed high sensitivity (80% to 95%) but somewhat scattered specificity (68%–100%).	About 7 minutes (if interview needed) Materials ~$.10 Admin. ~$2.38 Total = ~$2.48
Ages & Stages Questionnaires: Social-Emotional (ASQ:SE) Paul H Brookes Publishers, PO Box 10624, Baltimore, Maryland 21285 (1-800-638-3775). ($149) http://www.pbrookes.com/	6–60 months	Designed to supplement the ASQ, the ASQ:SE consists of 30 item forms (4–5 pages long) for each of 8 visits between 6 and 60 months. Items focus on self-regulation, compliance, communication, adaptive functioning, autonomy, affect, and interaction with people	Single cutoff score indicating when a referral is needed	Sensitivity ranged from 71% to 85%. Specificity from 90% to 98%	10–15 minutes if interview needed. Materials ~$0.54 Admin. ~$4.20 Total = ~$4.94

TABLE 7.1 (continued)
Developmental screens relying on information from parents

Developmental screen	Age range	Description	Scoring	Accuracy	Time frame/costs
Brief Infant–Toddler Social–Emotional Assessment (BITSEA) Harcourt Assessment Inc, 19500 Bulverde Road, San Antonio, Texas 78259 (1-800-211-8378). ($105.00) harcourtassessment.com	12–36 months	42 item parent-report measure for identifying social–emotional/behavioral problems and delays in competence. Items were drawn from the assessment level measure, the ITSEA. Written at the 4–6th grade level. Available in Spanish, French, Dutch, Hebrew	Cut-points based on child age and sex show presence/absence of problems and competence	Sensitivity (80–85%) in detecting children with social emotional/behavioral problems and specificity 75–80%	5–7 minutes Materials ~$1.25 Admin. ~$0.88 Total = ~$2.13
Connors Rating Scale-Revised (CRS-R) Pearson Assessments Inc. 1-800-627-7271 ($276-00). http://www.pearsonassessment.com	3–17 years	Three versions are used for diagnosis: teacher report, parent report, and youth self-report. Produces 7 factor scores: Cognitive Problems/Inattention, Hyperactivity, Oppositional, Anxious-shy, Perfectionism, Social Problems, and Psychosomatic. Several subscales specific to ADHD are also included: DSM-IV symptom subscales (Inattentive, Hyperactive/Impulsive, and Total); Global Indices (Restless-Impulsive, Emotional Lability, and Total), and an ADHD index. The GI is useful for treatment monitoring. Also available in French	Cutoff tied to the 93rd percentile for each factor	Sensitivity 78–92% Specificity: 84–94%	About 20 minutes Materials ~$2.50 Admin. ~$20.15 Total = ~$22.65
Family screens					
Family Psychosocial Screening Kemper and Kelleher (1996) The measures are include in the article are downloadable at http://www.pedstest.com and are included in PEDS: Developmental Milestones	Screens parents and best used along with the above screens	A 2-page clinic intake from that identifies psychosocial risk factors associated with developmental problems including: (1) a 4-item measure of parental history of physical abuse as a child; (2) a 6-item measure of parental substance abuse; and (3) a 3-item measure of maternal depression	Refer/non-refer scores for each risk factor. Also has guides to referring and resource lists	All studies showed sensitivity and specificity to larger inventories greater than 90%	About 15 minutes (if interview needed) Materials ~$0.20 Admin. ~$4.20 Total = ~$4.40

Developmental screens relying on eliciting skills directly from children

Brigance Screens-II Curriculum Associates Inc. (2005), 153 Rangeway Road, N. Billerica, Massachusetts 01862 (1-800-225-0248). ($822.00) http://www.curriculumassociates.com/	0–90 months	Nine separate forms, one for each 12-month age range. Taps speech-language, motor, readiness, and general knowledge at younger ages and also reading and math at older ages. Uses direct elicitation and observation. In the 0–2 year age range, can be administered by parent report	Cutoff, quotients, percentiles, age equivalent scores in various domains and overall	Sensitivity and specificity to giftedness and to developmental and academic problems are 70–82% across ages	10–15 minutes Materials ~$2.33 Admin. ~$10.15 Total = ~$12.48
Bayley Infant Neurodevelopmental Screen (BINS) San Antonio Texas: The Psychological Corporation, 1995. 555 Academic Court, San Antonio, TX http://www.psychcorp.com	3–24 months	Uses 10–13 directly elicited items per 3–6 month age range assess neurologic processes (reflexes and tone); neurodevelopmental skills (movement symmetry) and developmental accomplishments (object permanence, imitation, and language)	Categorizes performance into low, moderate, or high risk via cut scores. Provides subtest cut scores for each domain	Specificity and sensitivity are 75–86% across ages	10–15 minutes Materials ~$0.30 Admin. ~$10.15 Total = ~$10.45

Academic screens

Comprehensive Inventory of Basic Skills-Revised Screener (CIBS-R Screener) (1985) Curriculum Associates Inc. 153 Rangeway Road, N. Billerica, Massachusetts 01862 (1-800-225-0248). ($224.00) http://www.curriculumassociates.com/	1–6th grade	Administration involves one or more of three subtests (reading comprehension, math computation, and sentence writing). Timing performance also enables on assessment of information processing skills, especially rate	Computerized or hand scoring produces percentiles, quotients, cutoffs	70–80% accuracy across all grades	Takes 10–15 minutes Materials ~$0.53 Admin ~$10.15 Total = ~$10.68
Safety Word Inventory and Literacy Screener (SWILS) Glascoe (2002). Items courtesy of Curriculum Associates Inc. The SWILS can be freely downloaded at: http://www.pedstest.com/ and is included in PEDS: Developmental Milestones	6–14 years	Children are asked to read 29 common safety words (e.g. High Voltage, Wait, Poison) aloud. The number of correctly read words is compared to a cutoff score. Results predict performance in math, written language and a range of reading skills. Test content may serve as a springboard to injury prevention counseling	Single cutoff score indicating the need for a referral	78–84% sensitivity and specificity across all ages	About 7 minutes (if interview needed) Materials ~$0.30 Admin. ~$2.38 Total = ~$2.68

TABLE 7.1 (continued)
Narrow-band screens for autism and attention-deficit–hyperactivity disorder (ADHD)

Developmental screen	Age range	Description	Scoring	Accuracy	Time frame/costs
Modified Checklist for Autism in toddlers (M-CHAT) (1997) Free download at the First Signs Web site: http://www.firstsigns.org/downloads/m-chat.PDF ($0.00) Online for parents and EMRS at www.forepath.org ($1.00)	18–60 months	Parent report of 23 questions modified for American usage at 4–6th grade reading level. Available in English and Spanish. Uses telephone follow-up for concerns. The M-CHAT is copyrighted but remains free for use on the First Signs website. The full text article appeared in the April 2001 issue of the *Journal of Autism and Developmental Disorders*	Cutoff based on 2 of 3 critical items or any 3 from checklist	Initial study shows sensitivity at 90%; specificity at 99%. Future studies are need for a full picture. Promising	About 5 minutes Print materials ~$0.10 Admin. ~$0.88 Total = ~$0.98
Connors Rating Scale Revised (CRSR) Multi-Health Systems Inc, PO Box 950, North Tonawanda, NY 14120-0950 (Tel: 1-800-456-3003 or 1-416-492-2627. Fax: 1-888-540-4484 or 1-416-492-3343). ($193.00) http://www.mhs.com/	3–17 years	Although the CRSR can screen for a range of problems, several subscales specific to ADHD are included: DSM-IV symptom subscales (Inattentive, Hyperactive/Impulsive, and Total), and an ADHD Index. The GI is useful for treatment monitoring. Also available in French	Cutoff tied to the 93rd percentile for each factor	Sensitivity 78–92% Specificity 84–94	About 20 minutes Materials ~$2.25 Admin. ~$20.15 Total = ~$22.40

© Glascoe FP (2005) *Collaborating with Parents.* Nashville, Tennessee: Ellsworth & Vandermeer Press, Ltd. Permission is given to reproduce this table.

Directly elicited measures of good quality are also listed. These take longer to administer and generally provide more in-depth information. As such, they can be considered second-stage screens in primary care (meaning that they would be administered only to a subset of patients identified by briefer measures as being at higher risk). Some primary care practices, depending on staffing patterns, may be able to administer directly elicited screens, although most opt to make this a referral question for early intervention programs to address. Outside of primary care, where there is often less reactive child behavior and often greater professional skill in establishing rapport and, if necessary, establishing behavioral control, directly elicited measures are more common (e.g. outreach screening clinics, child-find programs, behavioral practices, neonatal intensive care unit follow-up programs). Table 7.1 describes the selected measures including publisher contact information, time frames, scores produced, and recent costs.

IMPLEMENTATION ISSUES

It is generally insufficient to select a quality measure and then expect that it will be routinely deployed unless the primary care office is adequately prepared. Table 7.2 is a worksheet that lists the many issues requiring planning when considering the routine use of measures including preparing office staff, charting workflow, etc.

The introduction of screening measures alerts parents that developmental and behavioral issues are of interest and thus increases the need for routinely available patient education and support materials. Sources for addressing a range of behavioral and developmental issues that comprise the typical problems encountered by children and families (e.g. guidance on toileting, eating, sleeping, discipline) are listed in Table 7.3.

At the same time, providers also need skill in explaining screening results to parents. This is easiest when their concerns are elicited because affirmation is an effective springboard to thorough discussions about referrals. Otherwise, Table 7.4 includes guidance on how to explain screening test results without straying into uncharted, and not yet indicated, discussions of potential diagnoses.

Ultimately, one of the biggest challenges for primary care providers is knowledge of referral resources. Providers tend to refer only to those services they know well and programs that fail to confirm receipt of referrals, provide copies of test results, engage providers in collaborative decision-making about needed services are not likely to receive ongoing referrals (Forrest et al. 2002). Thus, non-medical providers need to respond and maintain close communication with primary care providers. Table 7.5 lists national referral resources that, with exploration of each website, can help providers find a range of services including early intervention, Head Start, parent training, and parenting information. An additional resource is the American Academy of Pediatrics' Section on Developmental and Behavioral Pediatrics' website (www.dbpeds.org) which provides information on disabilities, screening measures,

TABLE 7.2
Screening implementation worksheet

Action item	Time frame	Person(s) responsible	Date completed
1. Who will ensure that copies of screens are available each day for parents to complete?			
2. Who will ask whether parents can complete the forms on their own or need assistance?			
3. Who will help parents who need assistance?			
4. Who will collect screens from families?			
5. Who will score screens?			
6. Who will attach screens to the chart or otherwise make sure they are available to clinicians?			
7. Who will locate patient education materials and referral resources? Who will follow up if needed? How will this person know when to follow up?			
8. Who will explain results to families?			
9. Who will contact referral resources when a referral is needed? Who will locate referral resources when needed?			
10. What will you do with the screening materials once they've been discussed with families?			
11. If using electronic records or age-specific encounter forms, who will indicate and where, the fact that screening has been completed?			
12. Who will train staff and clinicians in the use of electronic screening?			
13. Who will keep track of billing/coding procedures when they vary by payer?			
14. Who will bill/code for completion of screens and for positive/negative results?			
15. What procedure and diagnosis codes will you use (if these are needed)?			
16. Who will explain to utilization review personnel your decision about CPT and DX codes?			
17. Where will you keep supplies of screens and patient education materials?			
18. Who will make sure enough screens on on-hand at all times?			
19. Who will lead staff through your rationale for deploying validated screening in your practice and otherwise inspire them about the value of screening?			
20. How will you handle things if staff is unwilling?			

TABLE 7.3
Organizing offices for detecting and addressing developmental and behavioral problems

1. Ask parents to complete parent-report instruments while in waiting or exam rooms
2. To avoid incomplete, incorrect, or non-returned parent-report screens, ask parents if they would like to complete the measure or on their own or have someone go through it with them. Almost all poor readers will select the latter
3. Mail parent-report tests in advance of well visits so that physicians need only score and interpret during the visit. This often improves the quality of parent-report because families may have sufficient time to respond thoughtfully. Advance mailings are also helpful with families whose English is limited because they can usually find someone in the community to help translate items
4. Set up a return visit devoted to screening when developmental concerns are raised unexpectedly toward the end of an encounter. A similar alternative is to have office staff call families after an incomplete encounter and administer a screen over the telephone
5. Train office staff to administer, score, and even interpret screening tests so that professional staff need only explain results to families and identify needed resources
6. Pool a portion of practice profits to fund a developmental specialist or a nurse practitioner. Such a person can administer screening tests (and perhaps provide parent counseling, run parent training groups, assist with group well-child visits, offer diagnostic evaluations and referrals)
7. Recruit education majors or train volunteers to administer screening tests on a periodic basis (e.g. set a regular screening day in your office)
8. Maintain a current list of telephone numbers for local service providers (e.g. speech-language centers, school psychologists, mental health centers, private psychologists and psychiatrists, parent training classes). The availability of brochures describing services may promote parental follow-through on referral suggestions. Giving families phone numbers when you make referrals eliminates this as a barrier to seeking services. We keep a list of our most common referral resources glued to the wall of each exam room
9. Encourage professionals involved in hospital-based care (e.g. child-life workers) to screen patients and refer to them when appropriate
10. Collaborate with local service providers (e.g. day care centers, Head Starts, public health clinics, department of human services workers) to establish community-wide child-find programs that use valid, accurate screening instruments
11. Keep parent information sheets handy. My clinic keeps them in plastic binders (so that originals are not lost). When an issue arises, I retrieve the original handout, copy it, read it on the way back to the exam room (in order to refresh myself on the contents) and then go through the highlights with parents
12. When using information handouts, go through them briefly with families and highlight the significant parts. Use of a highlighter pen (along with your oral description) should help parents (especially those with limited literacy) recall the more critical information
13. Use screens as designed, adhering to standard wording, scoring, and decision-making. Violating test standardization decreases validity and increases the chance of underdetection
14. Experienced physicians and nurses often memorize test items and internalize norms. This may lead them to rely heavily on clinical judgment. Because human reasoning is not infallible and judgment can drift over time, professionals should test their decisions at least periodically by comparing them with the results of standardized screening tests. This should help keep clinical skills honed and provide an appropriate model for less experienced professionals such as residents and medical students

© Adapted from Glascoe (2005). Permission is granted to reproduce this page for training purposes.

TABLE 7.4(a)
Sources for patient education materials

American Academy of Child and Adolescent Psychiatry: Facts for Families (www.aacap.org)
Has numerous handouts that can be downloaded for free. Written in multiple languages, they
   address such topics as divorce, disaster recovery and how to choose a psychiatrist.
American Academy of Pediatrics: You and Your Family (www.aap.org)
Describes child-care books, videos, hand-held health records, waiting room magazines, etc.
British Columbia Council for Families (www.bccf.bc.ca/)
Well maintained site with articles, online questionnaires and links to resources on a variety of
   parenting and family topics. Carries individual and bulk copies of books and brochures on
   such topics as adolescence, marriage, family cohesion, and child development, as well as a
   parenting program, Nobody's Perfect.
Children and Youth Health (www.cyh.sa.gov.au)
From the South Australian Department of Human Services, this site has extremely rich information for parents on a huge range of psychosocial issues for teens and young children. Diapers
   are "nappies" and ear infections are "glue ear," but other than that, the depth and quality of
   parenting advice is unparalleled.
First Signs (www.firstsigns.org)
This organization promotes early detection of autism and other developmental disorders
   through routine screening, and collaboration among medical and non-medical professionals.
   The organization assembled an information kit for physicians including a wonderful video
   showing the behaviors of children on and off the spectrum. States can contract with First
   Signs for local training. The website is a repository of information for both parents and
   professionals.
Kids' Health (www.kidshealth.org/)
From the Nemours Foundation, this site has excellent information on health and safety, emotional and social development and positive parenting, focused on teens and younger children.
Medem Smart Parents' Health Source (www.medem.com/)
Medem is an internet library of health information from a variety of medical societies, includ-
   ing the American Academy of Pediatrics. Smart Parents' Health Source is a monthly e-mail
   newsletter on children's health which can be customized to the age and gender of your child,
   and by topics of interest. Previous issues are archived on the site.
Early Childhood Connections (www.rch.org.au/ecconnections)
This website has sections for parents and professionals interested in developmental and behavioral issues in early childhood. It houses parent information sheets (Adobe Reader is required)
   in various languages including Arabic, Bosnian, Chinese, Croatian, Somali, Spanish, Turkish,
   Vietnamese and English.
United Kingdom Department of Health (www.dh.gov.uk)
Has an entire book on parenting and child-rearing on its website
Tufts University has a site housing downloadable handouts in various Asian languages on health,
   child-rearing and disabilities (http://spiral.tufts.edu/topic.html)
The U.S. Department of Education website houses information for Spanish-speaking families
   on how to promote child development, help school age children, etc.
   (http://www.ed.gov/parents/academic/help/partnership.html)
California First Five has child-rearing guidance for Spanish speaking parents
   (http://www.ccfc.ca.gov/parentinfo.htm)

TABLE 7.4(b)
Interpreting screening tests to families and encouraging follow through

---

1. Prepare parents for screening in a positive way. When making phone calls or sending reminder letters about upcoming well-visit appointments, explain in an encouraging manner that the visit represents an opportunity to view how children are coming along developmentally and behaviourally and to provide parents suggestions about addressing any difficulties children are experiencing. This should help families keep these critical appointments and better prepare for screening

2. For parents with expressed concerns for which additional screening or referral is the best response, prepare them by affirming the value of their worries and their careful observations for their child (e.g. 'Your concerns are important and we need to look further at how your child is doing. This will help us decide whether additional help is needed.')

3. Inform parents about the purpose for each test prior to administering screening tools. This should help ensure that parents understand what is happening and better preprare them for the results

4. Use euphemisms rather than diagnostic labels when interpreting screening tests. Phrases like 'may be delayed,' 'may be behind other kids,' 'seems to be learning more slowly,' 'could be having difficulty learning' do not connote a child in a wheelchair or one with multiple genetic anomalies. They are effective terms but not devastating ones. They seem to encourage families to seek additional evaluations without causing paralytic fear

5. Provide telephone numbers and descriptions of services. It is likely that families who have the necessary information to follow through are better able to do so. Descriptions of programs may enable families to visualize themselves participating and increase the chance they actually will

6. Write non-medical recommendations on a prescription pad or letterheaded paper. This is a powerful tool for affirming the importance of a recommendation and confirms the need for families to treat this as seriously as other medical interventions

7. Offer ongoing support. Parents will often be faced with family members who have minimal investment in your recommendations for further evaluations and services. This may be because they were not present during the original encounter and only hear the recommendation second-hand. It may also be a result of observing the problem but rationalizing its meaning (e.g. 'His dad was just like that as a boy and he's doing fine now.' 'It's just a phase, she'll grow out of it.'). One way to approach this is to help the parent who accompanied the child anticipate and deal with resistance. Acknowledge their fears and the likelihood that they will have a bout of wishful thinking (e.g. observing their child very carefully for signs that contradict delays). It is also helpful to invite parents to return with dissenting family members in tow so that you can re-explain your findings. Finally, you might let parents know that if they get 'cold feet' and decide not to go that you want to be informed (e.g. 'It's just as if I prescribed medicine and you decided not to give it to him, I'd want you to talk with me about it. Treat this prescription/recommendation in the same way. Don't be afraid to talk with me if you have reservations about following through.')

8. Consider referrals to parent support groups or give parents the names and phone numbers of parents who successfully experienced the process of developmental/behavioral screening and diagnosis. This is particularly important for parents who are observably anxious or have numerous other life stressors. However, parents may not always reveal when they are distressed and it is probably best to have a uniform approach to offering parents ongoing support

TABLE 7.4(b) (continued)
Interpreting Screening Tests to Families

9. Avoid giving screening results over the telephone. If this is not possible, alert parents that they may be confused and invite them to call back later if they have questions. This should reduce misinformation and resultant confusion and anxiety. Whether conveying results in person or over the phone, provide written information (e.g. a brochure about the referral source, a copy of the referral letter you write). This should help ensure that parents understand the results and implications

10. Provide accurate written and verbal information. Communication about positive screening test results should clearly indicate that screens only tell whether a child is more likely to have problems and that screens, while often correct, are not perfect. Children with true difficulties may not be identified and children who are coming along normally may fail a screen. Specifically, parents who raise significant concerns but whose children perform well on screening should benefit from being told that you will follow their children carefully for any emerging problems and that you will given them some suggestion about how to help in the interim (e.g. a parent education sheet on how to stimulate children's language). In this way, you have prepared parents for the possibility that screens may over- as well as under-identify difficulties, and you will have capitalized on a 'teachable moment' by giving parents guidance in how to promote their child's development

11. Find social workers to help families who are likely to have multiple barriers to following through with recommendations (e.g. single parents with low incomes and multiple life stressors)

© Adapted from Glascoe (2005). Permission is granted to reproduce this page for training purposes.

TABLE 7.5
Referral resources

http://www.nectac.org	For locating state, regional and local early intervention programs and testing services for young children with suspected or known disabilities
http://www.ehsnrc.org/	For help locating Head Start programs
http://www.naeyc.org/	For help locating quality preschool programs
http://www.patnc.org	For help locating parenting programs
http://www.mentalhealth.org	For help locating mental health services
http://www.firstsigns.org/	For services and information about autistic spectrum disorders
http://www.aap.org,	For links or copies of patient education materials
www.dbpeds.org, and	For locating services for school age children, call the school
www.pedstest.com	psychologist or speech-language pathologist in the child's school of zone

implementation guidance, and hosts a discussion list where primary care providers can post challenging cases and discuss these cases with developmental–behavioral and neurodevelopmental pediatricians.

Once children are identified as having special needs, the primary care provider often has the challenging role of making sure that medical care is not fragmented because the presence of subspecialty care can often distort or disrupt the vital services of primary care (e.g. ensuring that children with special needs are immunized). Ideally, the child's primary health care provider should be viewed by all as the central figure or 'hub' in the process of coordinating and authorizing referrals. The AAP's Medical Home model (www.medicalhomeinfo.org) offers helpful guidance on how primary care practices can best maintain the organization structure and communication skills needed to ensure necessary and thorough continuity of care to best meet the needs of children with disabilities and their families.

CONCLUSIONS

The availability and use of highly accurate screens is only the first step in the process of caring for the developmental and behavioral needs of children. Skill in delivering difficult news to families, access to patient education materials, awareness of referral resources, and locating support at various professional levels are also critical. Ideally, screening measures should be combined with the ongoing process of developmental surveillance; knowledge of medical history, family strengths and weaknesses, and determination of psychosocial risk factors. Incorporating such information into the results of screening measures ensures that referral resources are honed to those that will best meet children's and families' particular and individualized needs.

REFERENCES

Algozinne B, Korinek L (1985) Where is special education for students with high prevalence handicaps going? *Except Child* 51: 388–394.

American Psychological Association, National Council on Measurement in Education, American Educational Research Association (1999) *Standards for Educational and Psychological Tests (2nd edn)* Washington, DC: American Psychological Association.

Aylward GP (1990) Environmental influences on the developmental outcome of children at risk. *Infants Young Child* 2: 1–9.

Barnes KE (1982) *Preschool Screening: The Measurement and Prediction of Children At-Risk.* Springfield, Illinois: Charles C Thomas.

Bell RQ (1986) Age-specific manifestations in changing psychosocial risk. In: Farran DC, McKinney JC (eds) *Risk in Intellectual and Psychosocial Development.* Orlando, Florida: Academic Press.

Canadian Psychological Association (CPA) (1996) *Guidelines for Advertising Preschool Screening Tests.* Ottawa, Ontario: Canadian Psychological Association, 1996. (http://www.cpa.ca/guide11.html)

First LR, Palfrey JS (1994) The infant or young child with developmental delay. *N Engl J Med* 330: 478–483.

Forrest CB, Nutting PA, Starfield B, von Schrader S (2002) Family physicians' referral decisions: results from the ASPN referral study. *J Fam Pract* 51: 215–222.

Glascoe FP (2001) Are over-referrals on developmental screening tests really a problem? *Arch Pediatr Adolesc Med* 115: 54–59.

Glascoe FP (2005) *Collaborating With Parents: Using Parents' Evaluations of Developmental Status to Detect and Address Developmental and Behavioral Problems.* Nashville, Tennessee: Ellsworth & Vandermeer Press.

Glascoe FP, Byrne KE, Chang B, Strickland B, Ashford L, Johnson K (1992) The accuracy of the Denver-II in developmental screening. *Pediatrics* 89: 1221–1225.

Glascoe FP, Oberklaid F, Dworkin P, Trimm F (1998) Brief approaches to educating patients and parents in primary care. *Pediatrics* 101(6): E101–E108.

Halfon N, Regalado M, Sareen H, Inkelas M, Peck Reuland CH, Glascoe FP, et al. (2004) Assessing development in the pediatric office. *Pediatrics* 113: 1926–1933.

Hoon AH Jr, Pulsifer MB, Gopalan R, Palmer FB, Capute AJ (1993) Clinical Adaptive Test/ Clinical Linguistic Auditory Milestone Scale in early cognitive assessment. *J Pediatr* 23: S1–8.

Jelinek MS, Murphy JM, Robinson J, et al. (1988) Pediatric Symptom Checklist: Screening school age children for academic and psychosocial dysfunction. *J Pediatr* 112: 201–209.

King T, Glascoe F (2003) Developmental surveillance of infants and young children in pediatric primary care. *Curr Opin Pediatr* 15: 624–629.

Kemper KJ, Kelleher KJ (1996) Family psychosocial screening: instruments and techniques. *Ambul Child Health* 4: 325–339.

Kube DA, Wilson WM, Petersen MC, Palmer FB (2000) CAT/CLAMS: its use in detecting early childhood cognitive impairment. *Pediatr Neurol* 23: 208–215.

Lavigne JV, Binns JH, Christoffel KK, Rosenbaum D, Arend R, Smith K, et al. and the Pediatric Practice Research Group (1993) Behavioral and emotional problems among preschool children in pediatric primary care: prevalence and pediatrician's recognition. *Pediatrics* 91: 649–655.

Lichtenstein R, Ireton H (1984) *Preschool Screening: Identifying Young Children with Developmental and Educational Problems.* Orlando, Florida: Gruen & Stratton.

Majnemer A, Limperopoulos C (2002) Importance of outcome determinants in pediatric rehabilitation. *Dev Med Child Neurol* 47: 773–777.

Newacheck PW, Strickland B, Shonkoff JP, Perrin JM, McPherson M, McManus M, et al. (1998). An epidemiologic profile of children with special health care needs *Pediatrics* 102: 117–123.

Reynolds AJ, Temple JA, Robertson DL, Mann EA (2001) Long-term effects of an early childhood intervention on educational achievement and juvenile arrest: a 15-year follow-up of low-income children in public schools. *JAMA* 285: 2339–2346.

Rydz D, Shevell MI, Majnemer A, Oskoui M (2005) Developmental screening. *J Child Neurol* 20: 4–21.

Sameroff AJ, Seifer R, Barocas R, Zax M, Greenspan S (1987) Intelligence quotient scores of 4-year-old children: social–environmental risk factors. *Pediatrics* 79: 343–350.

Sices L (2004) How do primary care physicians manage children with possible developmental delays? *Pediatrics* 113: 274–282.

Silverstein M, Sand N, Glascoe FP, Gupta B, Tonniges T, O'Conner K (2005) Pediatricians' reported practices regarding developmental screening: Do guidelines work? And do they help? *Pediatrics* 116: 174–179.

Squires J, Nickel RE, Eisert D (1996) Early detection of developmental problems: strategies for monitoring young children in the practice setting. *J Dev Behav Pediatr* 17: 420–427.

Yeargin-Allsopp M, Murphy CC, Oakley GP, Sikes RK (1992) A multiple-source method for studying the prevalence of developmental disabilities in children: the Metropolitan Atlanta Developmental Disabilities Study. *Pediatrics* 89: 624–630.

8

ETIOLOGY AND EVALUATION IN NEURODEVELOPMENTAL DISABILITY

Michael Shevell

Etiology can be defined from a practical and pragmatic perspective as a 'specific diagnosis that can be transmitted into useful clinical information for the family, including providing information about prognosis, recurrence risk and preferred modes of available therapy' (Schaefer and Bodensteiner 1992). The clinical diagnosis of a neurodevelopmental disability is not an end point and should prompt asking an important and highly relevant question: Why this particular child? Finding an etiologic explanation provides information regarding prognosis, recurrent risk, possible therapeutic options, and additional requirements pertaining to ongoing medical and rehabilitation management (Shevell 1998). Finding a reason also empowers the family in their role as autonomous decision-makers acting in the best interests of their affected child. Indeed, the process of trying to find out why may be a necessary first step in accepting a 'less than perfect' child who faces, together with his/her family, a lifetime of challenges to optimizing activity and participation (Shevell 2005).

All children with neurodevelopmental disability have an underlying reason for their impairment (Fenichel 2001). Unfortunately, given present limitations in both our understanding of pathogenesis and the availability of investigative modalities, we may not be able to find this underlying reason despite our best efforts. Recent advances in neuroimaging and genetics have greatly enhanced our success rate in our etiologic search (Srour et al. 2006). Future improvements can be expected as novel technologies such as volumetric magnetic resonance imaging (MRI), diffuse tensor imaging, magnetic resonance spectroscopy, subtelomeric probing, comparative genomic hybridization (i.e. microarray), and selective mass gene screening move from the research sphere into the clinical world (Shevell and Sherr 2006, Shevell et al. 2008).

Success in determining an underlying etiology is a function of two variables: (1) the type of neurodevelopmental disability under study, and (2) the willingness to search for a cause which is reflected in the utilization of contemporary investigative technologies (Shevell et al. 2000b). Recent studies, both retrospective and prospective, have illustrated that etiologic yield in the neurodevelopmental disabilities is largely a dichotomous split between (1) those neurodevelopmental disabilities in which an etiology is 'more likely than not' (i.e. greater than 50%) to be determined; e.g. global developmental delay (Majnemer and Shevell 1995, Shevell et al.

2000b, 2003a, Ozmen et al. 2005, Srour et al. 2006), cerebral palsy (Shevell et al. 2003b), and gross motor delay (Shevell et al. 2000a), and (2) those in which an underlying etiology is 'rarely' (i.e. less than 5%) ascertained; e.g. developmental language impairment (Shevell et al. 2000a, Webster and Shevell 2004), and autistic spectrum disorders (Shevell et al. 2001b).

The failure to determine an underlying etiology in either developmental language impairment or the autistic spectrum disorders reflects our present lack of understanding of both normal language and social development and the processes at a basic biologic level by which this development can be rendered aberrant. The willingness to search for a cause requires interest on the part of the investigating practitioner, the co-operation of the patient and family who place value and meaning in the search, and in society's broader facilitation (e.g. through availability and third party financing) of applying relevant investigative modalities to this particular search (Shevell et al. 2001a).

The reported etiologic yield in global developmental delay has been highly variable; however, most recent studies suggest a yield of 50–65% in the absence of co-existing autistic features (Shevell et al. 2000b, Ozmen et al. 2005, Srour et al. 2006). Most etiologies appear to be accounted for by five broad diagnostic categories:

1 Cerebral dysgenesis
2 Intrapartum asphyxia
3 Antenatal toxin(s) exposure
4 Chromosomal anomalies/genetic syndromes
5 Profound psychosocial neglect (Srour et al. 2006)

A multitude of potential causes have been identified, some quite rare in occurrence, suggesting the ongoing need for and challenge of diagnostic vigilance. Causes span the traditional categorization of onset (i.e. prenatal, perinatal and postnatal) with the preponderance (about 60%) prenatal in origin, with the remaining timing of onset almost equally divided between perinatal and postnatal causes (Srour et al. 2006).

Almost half of identifiable causes have an element of preventability (e.g. intrapartum asphyxia, antenatal toxin(s) exposure, psychosocial neglect), suggesting potential future strategies for prevention (Srour et al. 2006). Sometimes a multiplicity of causes are apparent, suggesting interplay and a 'threshold effect' which results in the final phenotype of a global developmental delay. History and physical examination is often sufficient to suggest an etiologic diagnosis, and laboratory investigations in such a context are utilized to confirm this suspicion (Shevell et al. 2000b, Srour et al. 2006). However, in almost 20% of cases, investigations (typically, karyotyping and imaging) undertaken on a screening, rather than an indicated basis, may reveal a previously unsuspected etiology. Nevertheless, with an indication, laboratory investigations have a higher yield than when performed on a screening basis alone (Shevell et al. 2000b, Srour et al. 2006).

Studies have identified clinical features apparent in the detailed history and physical examination that may suggest that an underlying cause can be identified (Shevell et al. 2003a, Srour et al. 2006). These include female sex, abnormal prenatal/perinatal history, the absence of co-existing autistic features, the presence of microcephaly, documented dysmorphology, and an abnormal neurologic examination (typically, focal or lateralizing findings on motor assessment). Interestingly, the severity of observed delay has not been found to be a predictor of success in determining an underlying etiology (Shevell et al. 2003a). This suggests that an equally vigorous approach to assessment and investigation should be adopted regardless of how delayed a child is.

The inherent value of searching for a cause is manifested by the high compliance of affected families to requested investigations (Shevell et al. 2001a). The value of searching for a cause is further evident by the high frequency that finding an etiology modifies recurrent risk estimation, medical management, or therapeutic options. Debate and controversy currently exists on the precise approach to be utilized for etiologic diagnosis. Guidance for the practitioner is provided by the American Academy of Neurology/Child Neurology Society Joint Practice Parameter (Shevell et al. 2003a) and the recent technical commentary of the American Academy of Pediatrics (Moeschler and Shevell 2006). Laboratory testing in the setting of childhood developmental delay needs to be selective and rationally based as extensive non-directed testing is neither justified nor feasible on the basis of yield, invasiveness, associated risks, or overall costs.

It is also important to note that there are populations of children with an established statistically increased risk for subsequent neurodevelopmental sequelae (Msall et al. 1998). The identification of such risk factors has been important in implementing programs that regularly and systematically monitor such children and intervene where necessary to attempt to minimize adverse eventual outcome. However, these risk factors, in and of themselves, do not constitute etiologic causes.

Risk factors thus far identified include (but not limited to) preterm birth, small for gestational age, low birth weight, neonatal encephalopathy, congenital heart disease, bronchopulmonary dysplasia, failure to thrive, chronic medical conditions, low socioeconomic status, and familial disruption (Msall et al. 1998, Shevell and Sherr 2006). Thus, a not insignificant subset of the pediatric population can be considered as 'developmentally fragile,' meriting increased longitudinal attention for possible neurodevelopmental sequelae. Of interest will be determining the mechanisms by which these risk factors are channeled at the biologic level to result in aberrant developmental attainment. This may offer the opportunity for future preventative strategies.

EVALUATION

A specialty evaluation of the preschool aged child has a number of inter-digitating objectives (Shevell 1998, 2005):

1 Confirmation and categorization of the child's developmental delay
2 Identification of a possible underlying etiology
3 Referral to, and assurance of, the provision of appropriate rehabilitation services and resources
4 Counseling of the affected family regarding diagnosis, etiology, and prognosis
5 Identification of any possible co-existing conditions that may require medical intervention and ongoing management

The first objective of confirming and precisely categorizing the type of delay is predominant as this will then direct specific efforts focusing on the remaining non-hierarchical, and indeed equally important, objectives.

The specialty evaluation of the delayed child begins with a detailed and particular history and physical examination which is an essential precondition to realizing the objectives listed above (Shevell 1998, 2005, Shevell and Sherr 2006). With our increasing multicultural and multilinguistic practice environments, every effort should be made to obtain the history and conduct the examination in the language most familiar to the family unit.

HISTORY

A detailed background is necessary to situate precisely the child's particular story. This begins with a family history. A three-generation pedigree of the referred child's family is required which at a minimum ascertains health and developmental status of individual family members as well as the occurrence of specific neurologic conditions. Examples of such disorders (e.g. neuromuscular, mental retardation, epilepsies) may need to be overtly suggested so that relevant conditions are not inadvertently omitted by the parents. Maternal pregnancy losses or early neonatal or infantile deaths may be suppressed because of the emotional pain of their recall and also may need to be specifically asked for. The possibility of parental consanguinity, precise ethnic heritage, and geographic origin are relevant questions that, although sometimes uncomfortable to probe for, have to be asked.

The possibility of a prenatal or perinatal etiologic origin to the child's developmental delay requires that attention be devoted to obtaining details regarding the mother's pregnancy and delivery of the affected child. The provision of antenatal care should be documented as well as the occurrence of antenatal ultrasounds and amniocentesis procedures and their results. Specific questions concerning possible prenatal adverse events such as per vaginal bleeding, gestational diabetes, pregnancy-induced hypertension, intercurrent infections, intrauterine growth retardation, or maternal medical conditions should be directly asked. Maternal prescription medication, alcohol, tobacco, or illicit drug use should be documented. In the non-primigravida mother, the relative quantity of antenatal fetal movements compared with other pregnancies experienced may be of interest. The timing of labor (preterm or term), its onset (spontaneous or induced), duration, presentation (vertex or breech), and mode of delivery (vaginal, assisted, cesarean) should be determined. The reason for a cesarean is important to note as are suggestions of problems during the delivery process itself such as the prolonged rupture of membranes, maternal peripartum fever, meconium staining, and any abnormal fetal heart rate monitoring.

Birth weight, APGAR scores (especially beyond 5 minutes if low initially), requirement and specifics of caseroom resuscitation and possible admission to a neonatal intensive care unit are important indicators of an infant's immediate post-natal status. Determining the duration of a child's post delivery hospital stay is a simple way of ascertaining if there were any clinically significant neonatal concerns. If beyond that expected locally, the reason(s) thereof should be documented. In particular, possible postnatal signs of suspected encephalopathy or feeding difficulties are good markers of a possibly compromised newborn nervous system. Suggestions of adverse prenatal, perinatal, or neonatal events may require directly obtaining the maternal obstetric or the child's neonatal records for detailed review.

The child's postneonatal medical history then needs to be documented. This includes any chronic medical conditions, hospital admissions, or surgical procedures. Concurrent medication use, prior assessments, or provision of specialty services pertaining to developmental concerns, especially if rehabilitative in character, require documentation. In order to understand the child's social and family context, parental origin (i.e. foreign or domestic – if foreign current immigration standing), socioeconomic status (i.e. educational attainment, parental employment), marital situation, custody, and childcare arrangements should be determined.

Once this background is obtained, the evaluation can then move to a specific and detailed developmental history. This begins with determining the age and domain (i.e. motor, language, social) of initial parental concern. Developmental trajectory in each domain should be established although parental recall, especially in multiplex families, may be difficult to pin down precisely (Table 8.1) (Levy and Hyman 1993). Key milestones usually recalled well are walking independently and first meaningful specific words. Comparing a child with other children (their own or peers) or recalling a child's developmental performance at a personal specific chronologic milestone (i.e. first or second birthday) may provide a snapshot of developmental attainment. Essential in this elicitation is the careful probing for any possible loss of developmental skills or regression and establishing whether the child's delay is global, domain-specific (i.e. motor, language), or has evident autistic features. The latter is ascertained through specifically asking about eye contact, emotional awareness, and appropriateness, an obsessive desire for sameness, presence of repetitive behaviors

TABLE 8.1
Guide to early child development and functional milestones

Age (months)	Motor	Language	Social/play
2	Head up in prone		Smiles Fixes and follows
3	Head/chest up in prone Grasp placed object	Coos	Laughs
4	Rolls Reaches for objects		
6	Sits with support Transfers objects	Babbles Turns to sound	Mouthing objects
8	Sits without support Weight bears	Turns to name	
10	Pincer grasp Starting to cruise Crawling four points	'Bye-bye' wave	Drinks from cup
12	Walks but falls easily	First specific words	Finger feeds Objects in and out of containers
15	Walks steadily Scribbling	Pointing Multiple single words	Spoon use Assists in dressing
18	Up/down stairs with assistance Climbing Throws ball	Two-word phrases Pointing to body parts	Build towers Play with others
24	Up/down stairs – 1 step at a time Kicks ball	Three-word phrases Pronoun use	

or obsessive preoccupations, and the quality of social interactions especially pertaining to play behaviors. Current developmental attainment in all domains should be documented, subject to confirmation through the physical examination, as well as functional attainment pertaining to activities of daily living such as feeding skills, toileting, dressing, and self-hygiene which may or may not be age appropriate.

With a developmental profile established by history, a functional inquiry can then be pursued that targets co-existing conditions that occur frequently in the setting of developmental delay (Shevell and Sherr 2006). These include paroxysmal disorders that may be epileptic in origin, sleep disturbances (e.g. frequent nocturnal awakening, failure of sleep consolidation), behavioral concerns that are disruptive to the family unit, attentional deficits that may be reflected in hyperactivity and limit the effectiveness of rehabilitation interventions attempted, and feeding difficulties. In many families, it is these co-existing conditions that may be the greater familial challenge rather than the actual delay itself.

PHYSICAL EXAMINATION

The physical examination is an essential part of the comprehensive assessment of the child with delayed development. The physical examination comprises general physical, neurologic, and developmental elements. Results obtained may (1) confirm an etiologic suspicion suggested originally by history, (2) put forward a novel etiologic possibility previously unsuspected, or (3) document findings that may suggest a heightened probability of finding an etiology on screening tests. In addition, developmental elements of the examination will also allow precise categorization of the child's developmental delay.

The examination should be conducted in a child friendly environment in which age-appropriate playthings such as paper, crayons, blocks, picture books, puzzles, stuffed animals, dolls, and small pretend play situations (e.g. doll houses, work settings with figurines) are made available to the child. During the initial extensive history-taking, observation of the child's own spontaneous exploration of these play opportunities will provide insight into the child's neurodevelopmental profile, encompassing language, cognition, motor skills, play, and sociability in a detailed non-threatening manner. This also serves the purpose of putting the child at ease for the more formal aspects of the examination where co-operation may at times be tenuous.

Physical proximity of the child with a caregiver is reassuring and should be maximized. Thus, in the infant or toddler, much of the examination may take place with the child on the caregiver's lap. Establishing a rapport with the child is essential. Even the preverbal child needs to be told what to expect next. Fluidity of examination is required to take advantage of opportunities as they present themselves. Direct manipulation or the placing of hands on the child needs to be deferred to the end so that co-operation is maintained for as long as possible. These caveats, however, should not preclude the comprehensiveness of the physical examination.

The general physical examination requires obtaining and plotting current somatic measurements for height and weight. Possible dysmorphic features need to be looked for within the context of ethnic and familial variation. Possible stigmata of a neurocutaneous disorder (e.g. café-au-lait spots, hypomelanotic macules) or myelodysplasia mandates undressing the child fully and inspecting the skin and spine thoroughly. Hepatosplenomegaly and coarsening of the facies may indicate an underlying storage disorder.

Obtaining and plotting an occipital-frontal (i.e. head) circumference is essential to obtain a sex- and age-appropriate percentile. Documented microcephaly (less than the 2nd percentile) or macrocephaly (greater than the 98th percentile) requires obtaining and plotting prior measurements for the child and obtaining and plotting the head circumference for each biologic parent and the child's siblings if available.

Formal neurologic assessment includes cranial nerves to document any possible aberrant pupillary responses, visual field defects by gross confrontation, retinal abnormalities, nystagmus, facial paresis, excessive drooling, head tilt, dysphagia, or dysarthria. Primary sensory impairments affecting vision or hearing occur commonly in the child with delayed development and should be screened for in the office setting; however, 'normal' office results should not preclude a more detailed ophthalmologic and audiometric assessment by specialists. Motor examination targets by observation any evidence of lateralizing features, asymmetries, or dyskinesias (e.g. dystonia, athetosis, chorea, tremor, dysmetria). Formal testing of tone and stretch reflexes allow postulation of possible upper or lower motor unit pathology. Arising from a supine or squatting position, going up and down stairs, walking or running down an extended hallway, jumping and hopping in place all provide for observational assessment of the motor system's integrity. Copying figures and simple ball games provide an insight into motor planning, dexterity, and co-ordination skills. Cerebellar function can be assessed by the observation of gait and the smoothness and accuracy of reaching for objects.

A formal developmental assessment supplements and fills in the information obtained through initial observation of the child's integration and play in the examination setting. Fine motor skills are assessed through manipulation of blocks and pen and paper tasks (e.g. copying). Gross motor skills are revealed through ball playing, gait, running, and going up and down stairs. Spontaneous speech provides insight into vocabulary, grammatic, and semantic capabilities. Story telling and following complex commands provide an illustration of the child's comprehension. Language can also be assessed through picture, body part, color, shape, and item recognition, and the use of analogies and oppositional concepts (i.e. short/long, big/small, open/close, on/under) which also provide insight into cognitive capability.

Formal developmental measures have been developed for use in the office by physicians (Shevell and Sherr 2006). A number of such measures exist; however, the simple reality is that physician time is too limited in the busy office setting to utilize these measures on a regular basis. Essentially, allied health professionals in related disciplines (e.g. occupational therapy, physiotherapy, speech language pathology) have more experience, time, and skill in applying such standardized measures and their expertise, where available, on this aspect should be deferred too.

DIAGNOSIS

Once the history and physical examination is complete, sufficient information typically exists to provide a diagnosis of a specific neurodevelopmental disability. Such a diagnostic formulation is essential as it guides further testing and referral. If delay is apparent in more than one developmental domain (typically all domains are then affected) in a young child less than 5 years of age, a global developmental delay can be diagnosed (Kinsbourne 2001, Shevell et al. 2003a, Rydz et al. 2005, Shevell and Sherr 2006). If delay is restricted to a single domain (i.e. motor or speech/language), either a gross motor delay or developmental language impairment can be inferred (Shevell et al. 2000a). If in addition to motor delay, evidence for spasticity or dyskinesias is apparent, with or without co-existing cognitive and speech limitations, a cerebral palsy may be diagnosed (Shevell and Bodensteiner 2004). If qualitative impairments in either social and/or language skills are apparent, an autistic spectrum disorder can be diagnosed (Rapin and Tuchman 2006). Sometimes, a threshold for such a diagnosis may not be readily apparent in the clinical situation, as some children with global developmental delay may have some autistic features present but of insufficient quantity to merit an autistic spectrum diagnostic label.

LABORATORY INVESTIGATIONS AND CONSULTATIONS

If subsequent to the history and physical examination, a specific diagnosis is strongly suspected, laboratory investigations should selectively target this possibility (e.g. neuroimaging for intrapartum asphyxia, fluorescent *in situ* hybridization (FISH) for Prader–Willi or Angelman syndrome, FMR1 triplet repeat analysis for fragile X) (Shevell et al. 2003a). In the absence of a suspected diagnosis, at present high resolution banding karyotyping, FMR1 triplet repeat testing, and neuroimaging are suggested on a screening basis, with a positive yield in approximately one-sixth of cases (Shevell et al. 2003a). The yield of neuroimaging improves threefold if any microcephaly or lateralizing findings are present, while the yield of karyotyping is surprisingly consistent whether dysmorphology is documented or not (Srour et al. 2006). With respect to neuroimaging, MRI is preferable to computed tomography where readily available (Shevell et al. 2003a).

Routine metabolic testing (capillary blood gas, lactate, ammonia, liver function studies, serum amino and urine organic acids, very long chain fatty acids) at present cannot be justified except in certain clinical situations which include a prior family history of a similarly affected child, parental consanguinity, documented developmental regression, episodic decompensation, suggested dysmorphology, involvement of non-ectodermal derived organ systems, suggestion of white matter involvement on imaging, or non-screening as a newborn (Shevell et al. 2003a). Electroencephalography should be pursued only if there is a possibility of a paroxysmal event (e.g. seizures) based on the history obtained (Shevell et al. 2003a).

In the setting of isolated language delay, careful evaluation rarely yields a specific etiology (Webster and Shevell 2004). Routine laboratory testing in this clinical setting should be restricted to detailed audiometric assessment and perhaps an eletro-encephalogram (EEG) if suspicion regarding a possible acquired epileptic aphasia (e.g. Landau–Kleffner syndrome) exists and if strongly suspected this should include a sleep EEG study.

The above recommendations reflect our present knowledge and technology limitations. Advances in genetics such as comparative genomic hybridization/genomic microarray, subtelomeric probes, and proteonomics together with advances in neuro-imaging that provide complementary means of assessing brain structure or function such as volumetric MRI, diffusion tensor imaging, functional MRI, and magnetic resonance spectroscopy may radically alter the diagnostic approach to the delayed child in the near to intermediate future (Shevell and Sherr 2006).

The comprehensive and complete evaluation of the preschool child with delayed development does not take place in isolation (Shevell 2005). Ongoing management also requires that representatives of other disciplines become involved and actively engaged in providing assessments and services. Complementary expertise is required to evaluate developmental concerns, often through the application of standardized assessments which objectively document a child's developmental profile and apparent deficits in a more rigorous way than that which can be accomplished in the office evaluation. These health professionals include occupational therapists, physical therapists, speech-language pathologists, and psychologists. In addition to assessments, these professionals will typically assume responsibility for the provision of goal-directed therapeutic interventions, and the obtainment of appropriate relevant community resources, and will be useful adjuncts as information resources and counselors to the family as they adapt to their child's developmental concerns and limitations.

The high frequency of primary sensory impairments affecting either vision or hearing apparatus and their relative correctability, together with limitations in routine office screening for such impairments, mandates careful consideration of both formal audiometric (Rupa 1995) and ophthalmologic evaluations (Warburg 1994). The high frequency of genetic etiologies and concerns, together with the increasing complexity of molecular laboratory testing, often calls for the involvement of a genetic consultant. Specific care needs related to issues concerning behavior, feeding, respite care, financial concerns, or available programs may mandate the involvement of psychology, nursing, and social service expertise in this population.

SECOND VISIT

Not to be overlooked is the value of a second encounter with the child and family 3–9 months after the initial visit and assessment (Shevell 2005). Recent longitudinal studies have noted that developmental trajectories are not necessarily smooth or predictable, thus highlighting the dynamic nature of development across all domains (Darrah et al. 2003). A second visit serves to validate or correct initial impressions. It also serves to either support or refute the possibility of a progressive encephalopathy or a neurodegenerative process that would feature a loss of previously acquired skills and new findings on examination. The existence of such a possibility will call into play an especially vigorous etiologic search often involving quite rare disorders and esoteric investigations. A second visit allows for the review and integration of evaluations from allied health disciplines that provides precise specification of the child's developmental delay subtype. Results of laboratory investigations can be reviewed and issues of etiologic diagnosis addressed that may require further testing to be arranged. The provision, or lack thereof, of rehabilitation services can be confirmed together with a plan for long-term community-based resources. It also provides a forum for families to bring forth specific care needs related to issues of feeding, behavior, or sleep which may be more challenging to the family unit than the child's actual delay. Most importantly, it provides a forum for the family to bring forth questions concerning their child's present status, future prognosis, and realistic expectations.

CONCLUSIONS
The office evaluation of the young child with a developmental delay challenges the pediatric subspecialist on a number of levels that addresses both the science and art of medicine as a diagnostician, service provider, and counselor. A 'quick fix' is not possible and precious time is required to meet all the necessary objectives and goals attached to this evaluation. Personal satisfaction can be found in meeting these challenges and realizing one's integral role in facilitating a family's recognition and adaptation to their child's chronic disorder and thus optimizing the child's eventual functional attainment.

ACKNOWLEDGMENTS
MS is grateful for the support of the MCH Foundation and YCC during the writing of this manuscript. Alba Rinaldi provided the necessary secretarial assistance.

REFERENCES
Darrah J, Hodge M, Magill-Evans J, Kembhavi G (2003) Stability of serial assessments of motor and communication abilities in typically developing infants: implications for screening. *Early Hum Dev* 72: 97–110.
Fenichel GM (2001) *Psychomotor Retardation and Regression in Clinical Pediatric Neurology: A signs and symptoms approach (4th edn)*. Philadelphia, Pennsylvania: WB Saunders, pp 117–147.
Kinsbourne MGW (2001) Disorders of mental development. In: Sarnat B, Maria B (eds) *Child Neurology*. Baltimore, Maryland: Lippincott Williams & Wilkins, pp 1155–1211.
Levy SE, Hyman SL (1993) Pediatric assessment of the child with developmental delay. *Pediatr Clin North Am* 40: 465–477.

Majnemer A, Shevell MI (1995) Diagnostic yield of the neurologic assessment of the developmentally delayed child. *J Pediatr* 127: 193–199.

Moeschler JB, Shevell MI and the AAP Committee on Genetics (2006) Clinical genetic evaluation of the child with mental retardation or developmental delays. *Pediatrics* 117: 2304–2316.

Msall ME, Bier JA, Lagosse L, Tremont M, Lester B (1998) The vulnerable preschool child: the impact of biomedical and social risks on neurodevelopment function. *Semin Pediatr Neurol* 5: 52–61.

Ozmen M, Tatli B, Aydinli N, Caliskan M, Demirkol M, Kayserili H (2005) Etiologic evaluation in 247 children with global developmental delay at Istanbul, Turkey. *J Trop Pediatr* 51: 310–313.

Rapin I, Tuchman RF (2006) Where we are: overview and definitions. In: Tuchman R, Rapin E (eds) *Autism: A Neurological Disorder of Early Brain Development.* London: Mac Keith Press, pp 1–18.

Rupa V (1995) Dilemmas in auditory assessment of developmentally retarded children using behavioral observation audiometry and brainstem evoked response audiometry. *J Laryngol Otol* 109: 605–609.

Rydz D, Shevell MI, Majnemer A, Oskoui M (2005) Developmental screening. *J Chld Neurol* 20: 4–21.

Schaefer GB, Bodensteiner JB (1992) Evaluation of the child with idiopathic mental retardation. *Pediatr Clin North Am* 39: 929–943.

Shevell MI (1998) The evaluation of the child with a global developmental delay. *Semin Pediatr Neurol* 5: 21–26.

Shevell MI (2005) Diagnostic approach to developmental delay. In: Maria B (ed) *Current Management in Child Neurology (3rd edn).* Hamilton, Ontario: BC Decker, pp 246–250.

Shevell M, Ashwal S, Donley D, Flint J, Gingold M, Hirtz D, et al. (2003a) Practice parameter: evaluation of the child with global developmental delay. Report of the Quality Standards Subcommittee of the American Academy of Neurology and the Practice Committee of the Child Neurology Society. *Neurology* 60: 367–380.

Shevell M, Bejjani BA, Srour M, Rorem EA, Hall N, Shaffer LG (2008) Array comparative genomic hybridization in global developmental delay. *Am J Med Genet B Neuropsychiatr Genet* 147B: 1101–1108.

Shevell MI, Bodensteiner J (2004) Cerebral palsy: defining the problem. *Semin Pediatr Neurol* 1: 2–4.

Shevell MI, Majnemer A, Morin I (2003b) Etiologic yield of cerebral palsy: a contemporary case-series. *Pediatr Neurol* 28: 352–359.

Shevell MI, Majnemer A, Rosenbaum P, Abrahamowicz M (2001a) A profile of referrals for early childhood developmental delay to ambulatory sub-specialty clinics. *J Child Neurol* 16: 645–650.

Shevell MI, Majnemer A, Rosenbaum P, Abrahamowicz M (2001b) Etiologic yield of autistic spectrum disorders: a prospective study. *J Child Neurol* 16: 509–512.

Shevell MI, Majnemer A, Rosenbaum P, Abrahamowicz M (2000a) Etiologic yield in single domain developmental delay: a prospective study. *J Pediatr* 137: 633–637.

Shevell MI, Majnemer A, Rosenbaum P, Abrahamowicz M (2000b) Etiologic yield of sub-specialists evaluation of young children with global developmental delay. *J Pediatr* 136: 593–598.

Shevell MI, Sherr E (2006) Global developmental delay and mental retardation. In: Swaiman K, Ashwal S, Ferreiro D (eds) *Pediatric Neurology: Principles & Practice (4th edn).* Philadelphia: Mosby-Elsevier, pp 799–820.

Srour M, Mazer B, Shevell MI (2006) Analysis of clinical features predicting etiologic yield in the assessment of global developmental delay. *Pediatrics* 118: 139–145.

Warburg M (1994) Visual impairment among people with developmental delay. *J Intellect Disabil Res* 38: 423–32.

Webster R, Shevell MI (2004) The neurobiology of specific language impairment. *J Child Neurol* 19: 471–481.

9
NOVEL IMAGING TECHNIQUES
Jeff Neil and Terrie Inder

Neuroimaging has an important role in the assessment of children with neuro-developmental disabilities. The main imaging modalities available in children are cranial ultrasound (CUS), computed axial tomography (CT), and magnetic resonance imaging (MRI). Of these, MRI is the most widely used. CUS requires an open fontanel, and is not practical after the age of 6 months. Head CT does not require an open fontanel and provides more detailed information on central nervous system (CNS) structure than CUS. It provides excellent views of bone and is very sensitive for the detection of intracranial hemorrhage. However, its routine use outside the setting of evaluation for acute intracranial processes has been called into question because of potential problems related to radiation exposure. It has been suggested that cranial irradiation early in life may lead to impaired cognitive development (Ron et al. 1982, Hall et al. 2004) and/or predispose to cancer later in life (Karlsson et al. 1998, Brenner et al. 2003). These studies are far from conclusive, but raise concerns that perhaps require caution and further investigation.

MRI provides an even more detailed view of the CNS than CT and does not involve the use of ionizing radiation. However, the longer imaging times typical of MRI studies require that younger, less cooperative children be sedated for study. Unlike CUS and CT, MRI offers a remarkably varied and sometimes daunting array of image contrast types. 'Conventional' MRI, which provides information on macroscopic CNS structure, has a central role in the assessment of children with developmental delay.

Other contrast modalities, such as functional MRI, diffusion tensor MRI, magnetic resonance angiography, magnetic resonance spectroscopy, and magnetic resonance measures of blood flow, are not yet as widely used for the evaluation of subjects with developmental delay. These methods continue to undergo rapid technical development. The first half of this chapter focuses on conventional and newer MRI methods, with an emphasis on newer methods. This is followed by a review of the application of MRI to some more common etiologies and subtypes of neuro-developmental disability.

MAGNETIC RESONANCE METHODS
CONVENTIONAL MAGNETIC RESONANCE IMAGING
Conventional MRI is based on the detection of the ^{1}H nuclei of ordinary water (^{1}H$_2$O). Because the concentration of ^{1}H in water is in the order of 100M, magnetic

resonance detection of water allows acquisition of data with a high signal:noise ratio, particularly compared with detection of metabolites such as lactate, which have concentrations in the millimolar range. While other nuclides – such as ^{23}Na, ^{31}P, ^{2}H, and ^{3}H – are magnetic resonance detectable, their use for MRI is very rare because of their low concentrations and other technical considerations. For this reason, the discussion of imaging in this chapter is confined to ^{1}H-based magnetic resonance.

Contrast in conventional images of brain water is based upon differing physical characteristics (T1 and T2 relaxation time constants, hereafter referred to as 'T1' and 'T2') of ^{1}H$_2$O in different tissues. This contrast is present because the T1 and T2 values for ^{1}H vary with the immediate chemical environment. For example, the T2 of water ^{1}H in cerebrospinal fluid (CSF) is greater than that of water in white or gray matter. Image acquisition parameters can be adjusted to emphasize different forms of contrast. When an image is obtained with timing optimized for T2-based contrast, the magnetic resonance signal from water in CSF is greater (i.e. appears brighter) than that for white or gray matter because of its greater T2.

Magnetic resonance image acquisition parameters must be optimized for the age of the patient undergoing study and the field strength at which the images are obtained. Values for T1 and T2 (measured in milliseconds) vary not only with tissue type, but also with age and the field strength at which the images are obtained. In fact, the bright–dark contrast between white and gray matter on conventional MRI during the first months of life is opposite to that of images obtained from the age of 1 year through adulthood. As a result of the temporal evolution of these values, it is critical to optimize magnetic resonance sequence acquisition parameters to the specific age of the subject being studied. Without doing so, image contrast (and particularly, contrast:noise ratio) may be inherently poor. For example, the optimum echo time for T2-weighted images obtained from preterm infants is significantly longer (~100ms) than for images obtained from older children (~50ms). Further, image acquisition parameters that work well at one field strength (e.g. 1.5T) must be readjusted for images acquired at a different field strength (e.g. 3.0T).

In addition to image contrast based on water T1 and T2, it is possible to obtain images of ^{1}H$_2$O in which image contrast is based upon the homogeneity of the local magnetic field. The magnetic field strength within the tissue is generally homogeneous, but the presence of regions of differing magnetic susceptibility causes distortions in the local magnetic field. In a clinical setting, such effects are greatest at the interfaces between tissue and air or metal. While conventional magnetic resonance images are usually obtained in a fashion that minimizes these distortion effects, they can be maximized by employing a gradient echo imaging pulse sequence. Metal dental braces provide an extreme example of such effects. Distortions of the local magnetic field can extend posteriorly to the brainstem and superiorly through the frontal lobes of subjects wearing braces, causing poor image quality (e.g. signal

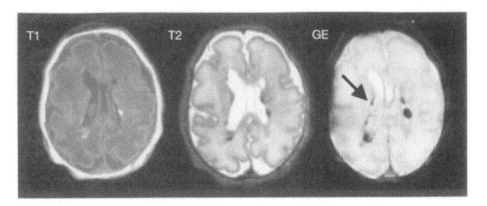

Fig. 9.1. Axial images from a preterm infant with multiple subependymal hemorrhages. The image on the left is T1-weighted, the one in the center is T2-weighted, and the one on the right is a gradient echo (GE) image. Note the relatively flat gray–white contrast in the GE Image. While many hemorrhages are visible on all three images (bright on T1, dark on T2 and GE), some are only visible on the GE image (arrow), which is more sensitive to the presence of blood.

drop-out and image distortion) in these areas. Less severe distortions occur near the air–tissue interfaces of sinuses. It is possible to exploit these effects to detect hemorrhage. The reduced iron of deoxyhemoglobin is paramagnetic, which causes distortions to the local magnetic field. As a result, areas of hemorrhage are readily detected as areas of low signal which 'bloom' on gradient echo images (Fig. 9.1).

Such sensitivity to local magnetic field distortions also provides the basis of functional magnetic resonance imaging (fMRI). In this modality, brain activation is associated with a local decrease in deoxyhemoglobin concentration. This is detected as a small increase in MRI signal (usually less than 5%) which identifies the areas of activation. Magnetic susceptibility affects scale with varying field strength and is stronger at higher magnetic fields. This can be both an advantage and a disadvantage. It is more difficult to obtain good images using a 3T scanner from a child wearing braces, but the contrast available for fMRI studies is better.

DIFFUSION MAGNETIC RESONANCE IMAGING

Diffusion MRI has its basis in methods developed in the mid-1960s. Stejskal and Tanner (1965) discovered that it is possible to make the magnetic resonance measurement sensitive to molecular motion. In its first application, the method was used to measure the diffusion of solvents. In the 1980s, a variation of this method was introduced as a novel means by which to obtain contrast from human brain tissue (LeBihan et al. 1986). In this case, image contrast is based not on the T1 or T2 of water, but on the displacements of water molecules. These displacements are typically tens of micrometers, and measuring such small displacements in living tissue is a remarkable technologic achievement. One parameter describing these displacements is the 'apparent' diffusion coefficient (ADC). The word 'apparent' is used in recognition of the fact that tissue water displacements are affected by a variety of factors in addition to Brownian motion, such as the hindrance of displacements by membranes and macromolecules.

The diffusion MRI method was initially proposed as a means of evaluating cerebral blood flow, but it quickly became apparent that although it does not provide useful measures of blood flow, it has a myriad of other uses. Its most common clinical use is for the acute detection of cerebral injury. Water ADC values decrease very quickly following stroke, providing a reliable means for detecting early brain injury (Moseley et al. 1990). Subsequently, ADC values have been shown to fall after a variety of cerebral insults including trauma, excitotoxic injury, and status epilepticus. It is also important to be aware that the ADC changes following injury are dynamic. While ADC values are decreased for the first few days following injury, they return to normal about 1 week after injury (pseudo-normalization). This is followed by a persistent increase in local ADC values, probably brought about by tissue breakdown (Fig. 9.2). Thus, the sensitivity of diffusion images for detecting injury varies with the actual time after injury (McKinstry et al. 2002a).

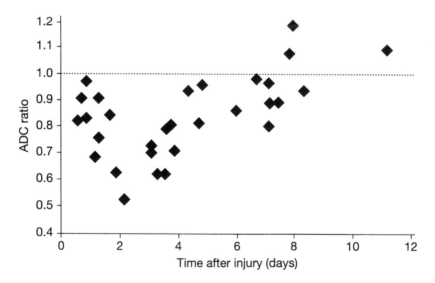

Fig. 9.2. Time course of 'apparent' diffusion coefficient (ADC) changes following brain injury in term infants. The abscissa is the time after injury in days; the ordinate is the normalized ADC value (1.0 is normal, <1.0 represents a low ADC, >1.0 represents a high ADC). Note that ADC values are lowest, and injury most readily detected on diffusion images, 2–4 days after injury.

Source: McKinstry et al. (2002a), with permission from Lippincott Williams & Wilkins.

Another intriguing aspect of diffusion imaging is diffusion anisotropy. This refers to the condition in which ADC values are not the same in all directions in space. In myelinated white matter, for example, ADC values are higher when measured parallel to axons than perpendicular to them. This is a consequence of tissue microstructure. For water molecules to move perpendicular to myelinated axons, they must cross the membrane layers of myelin that hinders their displacement. When moving parallel to axons, they need not cross membrane layers and thus have relatively greater ADC values. When diffusion images are obtained, the orientation along which water displacements are measured can be selected from within the magnetic resonance pulse sequence.

In diffusion tensor imaging (DTI), a series of diffusion images are obtained to measure water ADC values in a variety of different directions. These images can be combined to provide a 3D representation of water displacements for each element (voxel) in the image. For isotropic diffusion, which is equal in all direction in space, such a presentation would be a sphere. For myelinated white matter, such a representation would be shaped more like a rugby ball or cigar, with the long axis parallel to the orientation of the axons. These representations from white matter are sometimes evaluated with respect to their long axis (known as 'axial diffusivity') and their short axes (perpendicular to the orientation of the fibers, known as 'radial diffusivity'). Data from animal studies show that a primary injury to myelin is associated with an increase in radial diffusivity, presumably because there are fewer myelin membranes to hinder water displacements in this direction. Conversely, primary injury to axons, such as Wallerian degeneration, is associated with a decrease in axial diffusivity, presumably because of disruption of the long fiber tracts along which water molecules can diffuse (Song et al. 2002, 2005, Sun et al. 2006).

DTI data can be used for tracing white matter tracts. The direction of greatest ADC in white matter corresponds to the direction along which the white matter fiber tracts are oriented. By following these orientations from region to region, it is possible to trace white matter tracts. Although this method is certainly not a substitute for histologic evaluation of white matter connectivity, it has the enormous advantage of being non-destructive, non-invasive, and accessible *in vivo* (Mori and Van Zijl 2002).

Anisotropy values from developing cerebral cortex reflect changes in tissue microstructure that accompany cortical maturation. In the adult human brain, water displacements in cortical gray matter are isotropic, meaning they are equal in all directions. This reflects the organization for mature cortex, in which the collection of glia, neurons, axons, and dendrites provides relatively homogeneous restriction to water displacement in all directions. In developing cortex, the cellular architecture is dominated by the radial orientation of the apical dendrites of the pyramidal cells and the radial glial cells (Marin-Padilla 1988). As a result, water displacements are greatest radially (McKinstry et al. 2002b), which is parallel to these processes

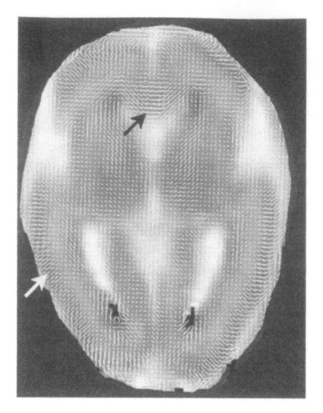

Fig. 9.3. An axial, T2-weighted image of an infant at 26 weeks' gestational age. Superimposed on the image are lines representing the direction of greatest water diffusion for each voxel (orientation of the principal eigenvector). The orientation of lines in the corpus callosum shows crossing fibers (black arrow). There is a strong radial orientation of diffusion in developing cortex (white arrow).

(Fig. 9.3). The loss of anisotropy associated with maturation can be used to assess cortical development and reflects varying rates of development among different cortical areas (Deipolyi et al. 2005). Currently, these diffusion anisotropy methods are available mainly as research tools. Their application to developmental abnormalities is only just beginning.

Functional Connectivity Magnetic Resonance Imaging

Functional MRI studies are based on an MRI acquisition method in which contrast is based on distortions induced in the local magnetic field by the presence of deoxyhemoglobin. When a brain region is activated during a task, cerebral blood flow (oxygen delivery) increases with little or no change in oxygen consumption. As a result, local deoxyhemoglobin levels decrease and magnetic resonance signal increases. This methodology is widely known, and a variety of fMRI studies have been carried out on subjects with developmental disorder. However, a variant of fMRI, functional connectivity (fcMRI), deserves special mention. For fcMRI, the subject does not perform a task during scanning – fMRI data are collected with the subject at rest. The 'noise' in fMRI date is of physiologic origin, and this aspect of the 'resting' signal is then analyzed. Correlations are sought between low frequency (<0.1Hz) signal fluctuations in the fMRI signal from a seed region (e.g. motor cortex) and other brain regions. For regions that are functionally connected, the signal fluctuations are temporally correlated (Biswal et al. 1995). When the signal in the seed area shows a positive fluctuation, the signal in the connected area does so too. Thus, fcMRI provides information regarding neural networks.

The precise neural network evaluated depends upon the seed region chosen for analysis. Correlations have been detected between regions commonly modulated together by task paradigms such as somatomotor, visual, and language systems (Biswal et al. 1995, Lowe et al. 1998, Cordes et al. 2000, Hampson et al. 2002). Further, it is well known that fMRI studies show task-related activation in some brain areas, whereas others undergo task-related deactivation. In a study of attention-demanding cognitive tasks, it has been shown that the fcMRI signal fluctuations in regions that undergo task-related deactivation are temporally anticorrelated with those of regions that undergo task-related activation (Fox et al. 2005). When the signal in the seed area shows a positive fluctuation, the signal in the connected area shows a negative fluctuation. In this fashion, fcMRI shows both correlations within neural networks and anticorrelations between neural networks. Finally, fcMRI effects persist under a variety of conditions. During the performance of low-level tasks, correlations corresponding to neural networks can be detected during both the rest and stimulus epochs (Arfanakis et al. 2000, Greicius and Menon 2004). The effects are also present, and become more prominent under midazolam sedation (Kiviniemi et al. 2005).

FcMRI overcomes two major hurdles for applying fMRI to developmental disorders. Because no task is required of the subject, fcMRI studies can be carried out in any subject who can undergo an MRI scan, making this imaging modality available to subjects of all ages. Secondly, the absence of an activation paradigm makes it much simpler to compare data across different imaging environments.

MAGNETIC RESONANCE SPECTROSCOPY

The concentration of metabolites in the brain is considerably less than that of water, which makes their detection via magnetic resonance spectroscopy challenging. Typically, spatial resolution for spectroscopy is much less than that for routine imaging, with spectroscopy voxels 1–2cm on a side as opposed to 1–2mm for imaging voxels. There are two basic approaches to magnetic resonance spectroscopy. The first is to choose a single region of interest in the brain and obtain a spectrum for this area; a method known as single-voxel spectroscopy. The second involves obtaining spectra from a series of voxels in the image. This is usually carried out by selection of a section of brain from which to obtain spectra from a grid of voxels in the section. This method is often referred to as a chemical shift imaging (CSI). While it is possible to measure absolute metabolite concentrations using magnetic resonance spectroscopy, this is technically demanding. As a result, many authors simply report ratios of metabolite resonance amplitudes rather than the absolute concentrations.

Most clinical spectroscopy involves acquisition of spectra from ^1H nuclei in non-water molecules. In general, it is necessary to suppress the very strong signal from ^1H in water in order to detect the smaller ^1H signal from metabolites, and a variety of water suppression methods are available to accomplish this task. A typical ^1H spectrum from brain is shown in Fig. 9.4. Note the improvements in signal:noise ratio and spectral dispersion present for spectra obtained at a higher field strength. Note also that, although a vast number of ^1H-containing molecules are present in the brain, a limited number of resonance peaks are detectable in spectra obtained at currently clinically available field strengths – choline (Cho), creatine (Cr), N-acetyl aspartate (NAA), and lactate (Lac). Increased levels of choline tend to be associated with a rapid turnover of lipid membranes such as that which occurs during brain development or in tumors. Creatine levels are relatively constant, and the amplitude of this resonance is sometimes used as a denominator or 'normalizing' factor when metabolite ratios are reported rather than absolute metabolite concentrations. N-acetyl aspartate is found primarily in neurons, and decreases in N-acetyl aspartate levels are often used as a marker for the loss of neurons in gray matter or the loss of axons in white matter. Lactate is a well-known by-product of anaerobic metabolism. It is ordinarily present at low levels in the brain, and its presence at higher levels is associated with poor neurologic outcome in some clinical settings and as a marker of disorders of anaerobic substrate utilization and energy production. It is important to remember that while lactate may be present as a consequence of a local lack of oxygen with anaerobic metabolism in neurons and glia (e.g. an ischemic penumbra), it may also be present as a normal by-product of anaerobic metabolism in infiltrating white blood cells. The ^1H signal from other brain metabolites may be detectable either at high field, as shown in Fig. 9.4, or by modifying the magnetic resonance spectroscopy acquisition in such a manner as to suppress the major resonances, allowing resonances of lower amplitude to emerge and be detected. This approach is known as spectral editing. If high field scanners (i.e. 7T) become more widely available, it will open more avenues for both research and clinical applications of magnetic resonance spectroscopy because many more metabolites will then be more reliably detectable.

VOLUMETRIC MEASUREMENTS THROUGH MAGNETIC RESONANCE
Conventional MRI can be used to measure cerebral volumes. Images of different contrasts, such as T1, T2, and proton-density weighted, are analyzed to classify

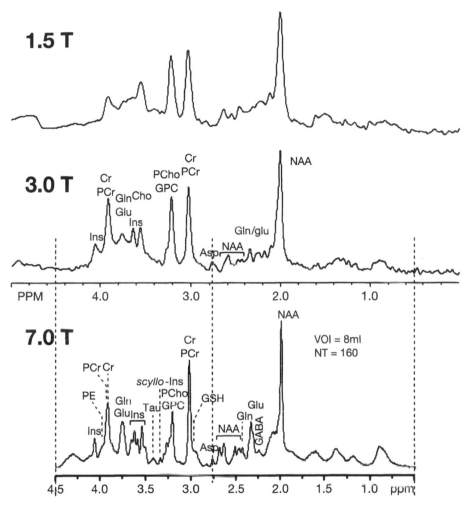

Fig. 9.4. ^{1}H magnetic resonance spectra from a single, 8ml voxel. The data were obtained from normal volunteers at the three magnetic field strengths indicated. Note the improvements in signal:noise ratio and spectral dispersion present at higher magnetic field strengths. Abbreviations: Asp, aspartate; GABA, gamma-aminobutyric acid; Gln, glutamine; Glu, glutamate; GPC, glycerophosphocholine; GSH, glutathione; Ins, inositol; NAA, N-acetyl aspartate; PE, phosphoethanolamine; (P)Cho, (phospho)choline; (P)Cr, (phospho)creatine; Tau, taurine.

Spectra provided by Drs. Peter van Zijl (Kennedy Krieger Institute), Peter Barker (Johns Hopkins University, 1.5 and 3T), and Ivan Tkac (University of Minnesota, 7T).

tissue as CSF, gray or white matter in a process referred to as 'segmentation.' The number of image elements, or voxels, corresponding to each class can be summed to compute volumes in units of milliliters. There is not yet a consensus as to the precise optimal means of assessing and comparing these volumes. Furthermore, there is not yet agreement on how these volumes should be normalized. For example, should gray matter be expressed as an absolute volume (ml), as a percentage of total brain volume or as a percentage of intracranial volume? While it has proven useful to measure total intracranial volumes for tissue types, it is also desirable to evaluate volumes on a regional basis because injuries affecting cerebral volumes may preferentially affect some brain areas. One approach is to apply arbitrary boundaries for regions, similar to lines for latitude and longitude on a map. Although this approach is fairly simple and relatively straightforward to implement, it tends to group brain regions of disparate function and physiology, such as brainstem and temporal lobe, together in the same volume. It also may miss volume abnormalities that involve small brain regions that are split by the borders of adjacent areas chosen for analysis. A more sophisticated approach, sometimes called voxel-based optometry, consists of applying statistical methods to compare the volume of the brain of interest with that of a 'standard' brain on a voxel-by-voxel bass (Sowell et al. 1999). A variety of methods has also been developed to assess the surface of the brain and quantify specific gyral development using conventional images (Rettmann et al. 2005, Van Essen 2005, Luders et al. 2006).

APPLICATIONS

The clinical application of neuroimaging in pediatrics is optimally related to the underlying content and object: What question is being asked? Neuroimaging is most frequently applied to determine the nature and extent of the alteration in brain structure resulting from acquired injury or cerebral dysgenesis. However, it may be used clinically to assist in prognosis, guide treatment programs, and assess recurrence risk. To illustrate the clinical application of neuroimaging in pediatric brain disorders we describe the most common applications in the clinical syndromes of the very preterm infant, the term born infant with encephalopathy, the infant and child with neurodevelopmental disorders, and the infant and child with cerebral palsy. It is worth noting explicitly two potential limitations to the utility of MRI in these conditions – sedation and image interpretation.

SEDATION

MRI generally requires that children under the age of about 6 years be sedated for study (Committee on Drugs 2002, Committee on Drugs, American Academy of Pediatrics 2002). This is critical to obtaining images not degraded by motion artefact. For the infant up to 6 weeks of age, it is possible to undertake MRI with feeding 30 minutes prior to scanning and swaddling the infant with a vacuum cushion support wrapped around the infant's head and body. For older infants and young children, chloral hydrate is often used, while general anesthesia may be occasionally required for very uncooperative children. Familiarization of subjects with magnetic resonance scanning equipment using mock MRI units with play therapists has also been employed to reduce anxiety and fear and the need for sedation or anesthesia in young children. As with all forms of sedation, there is a risk to the subject, and this risk may vary from institution to institution. Although the risk of a serious adverse event resulting in long-term sequelae is very small (Malviya et al. 1997), this risk must be balanced against the potential benefit of the information to be obtained from the imaging study.

IMAGE INTERPRETATION

Image interpretation requires knowledge of the normal brain anatomy and development, recognition of the nature of findings in specific disorders, and an awareness of study artefacts (Anupindi and Jaramillo 2002). Evaluation of images from preterm infants, for example, requires specialized knowledge for consistent and accurate interpretation. An interdisciplinary communicative relationship between the radiologist and the clinician is essential to the accurate interpretation of the images in the setting of the patient's clinical history and examination findings.

PRETERM INFANTS

Conventional magnetic resonance imaging

The earliest studies of conventional MRI in ex-preterm infants showed areas of abnormal signal intensity in periventricular white matter, ventriculomegaly, varying degrees of cerebral atrophy, thinning of the corpus callosum, and delayed myelination (Wilson and Steiner 1986, De Vries et al. 1987, Flodmark et al. 1989). These findings have been confirmed to be very common in preterm children (Barkovich and Truwit 1990, Truwit et al. 1992) and suggest that MRI can be used to detect the sequelae of the most common neuropathology in the white matter in older, ex-preterm children. However, MRI abnormalities consistent with white matter lesions detected in ex-preterm children (Olsen et al. 1997, Cooke and Abernethy 1999) have shown only moderate correlation with long-term cognitive and motor deficits, highlighting the limitations of this qualitative structural–functional link in early childhood.

Magnetic resonance images obtained at term equivalence in preterm infants show stronger correlations with eventual outcome than those obtained at later ages. In a study of 51 infants, 11 of whom had neurologic deficit at follow-up, the presence of parenchymal MRI lesions at term gave a sensitivity of 100% and specificity of 79% for a later motor abnormality (Valkama et al. 2000). However, the most common abnormality found on MRI in preterm infants at term is that of qualitative abnormalities in white matter with up to 70% of infants showing such abnormalities (Inder et al. 2003). These abnormalities were also associated with alterations in cognitive and motor development assessed at 2 years of age (Table 9.1) (Woodward et al. 2006). White matter abnormality at term equivalence is the strongest independent predictor of impaired neurodevelopment at 2 years of age when

TABLE 9.1
Cerebral white matter abnormalities on term equivalent magnetic resonance imaging (MRI) and neurodevelopmental outcomes at age 2 years (corrected).

2-year outcome	White matter abnormality at term				
	None (N = 47)	Mild (N = 85)	Moderate (N = 29)	Severe (N = 6)	p
Severe (<–2 SD) cognitive delay (%)	6.5	15.3	29.6	50.0	0.008
Severe (<–2 SD) motor delay (%)	4.3	4.7	25.9	66.7	<0.001
Cerebral palsy (%)	2.1	5.9	24.1	66.7	<0.001

TABLE 9.2
Cerebral gyral delay on term equivalent magnetic resonance imaging (MRI) and neurodevelopmental outcomes at age 2 years (corrected).

2-year outcome	Gyral abnormality at term		
	Normal (N = 85)	Abnormal (N = 82)	p
Severe (<–2 SD) cognitive delay (%)	9.5	23.8	0.01
Severe (<–2 SD) psychomotor delay (%)	4.8	16.3	0.02
Cerebral palsy (%)	4.7	15.9	0.02

compared with other perinatal factors. Even after controlling for the effects of perinatal factors including intraventricular hemorrhage and white matter lesions on CUS, children with moderate to severe white matter injury are 3.5 times more likely to exhibit severe cognitive impairment, 10.3 times more likely to have severe motor impairment, and 9.5 times more likely to have cerebral palsy. In addition, a qualitative delay in gyral development is very common, occurring in 50% of the infants, and is associated with a fourfold increase in significant cognitive difficulties, motor delay, and cerebral palsy (Table 9.2). It is not clear why MRI studies obtained at term equivalence have a stronger correlation with outcome than those obtained later in life. This question can be addressed by longitudinal MRI studies in which magnetic resonance images obtained at term equivalence can be compared with those obtained later in life.

Diffusion magnetic resonance imaging
Diffusion weighted imaging has also proven effective for evaluating the preterm infant brain. Abnormalities in ADC are associated with white matter injury on

conventional MRI. Abnormally high ADC values have been found for white matter in subjects with diffuse signal abnormalities on T2-weighted images (Counsell et al. 2003) and focal white matter signal abnormalities on T1- and T2-weighted images (Miller et al. 2003).

While evaluation of ADC values is proving useful for detecting acute injury, measures of diffusion anisotropy have the potential to provide additional information regarding specific tissue microstructure. Diffusion anisotropy is present in both white and gray matter. For white matter, anisotropy values are relatively low until myelination takes place (Huppi et al. 1998, Neil et al. 1998, Mukherjee et al. 2002). For gray matter, diffusion anisotropy values are highest during early development, because of the radial organization of developing cortex, and decrease steadily up to term (McKinstry et al. 2002b). Thus, anisotropy values change with development for both tissues and this allows the *in vivo* evaluation of the microstructural changes associated with maturation.

To date, there have been relatively few studies of anisotropy in the injured preterm brain. However, alterations in white matter anisotropy values and tissue organization have been described in infants with white matter injury (Huppi et al. 2001). Measures of axial and radial diffusivity have been shown in animal studies to reflect the disruption of axons and myelin, respectively. This approach has been applied to preterm infants imaged at term equivalence. Preterm infants with diffuse high signal intensity on T2-weighted imaging (Counsell et al. 2006) have been evaluated. When compared with values from term infants and preterm infants with normal-appearing white matter, radial diffusivity was elevated in the posterior portion of the posterior limb of the internal capsule and the splenium of the corpus callosum. In addition, both axial and radial diffusivity were elevated in the white matter at the level of the centrum semiovale, and frontal, periventricular, and occipital white matter. There was no significant difference between term comparison group infants and preterm infants with normal-appearing white matter in any region studied. The authors interpreted the change observed in radial diffusivity as suggesting a disturbance of oligodendrocyte function. They also suggested that the increase in axial diffusivity indicated an abnormality of axons, although this finding is difficult to interpret because axial diffusivity was increased rather than decreased as it is in animal studies of axonal disruption.

Finally, DTI analysis has been used to evaluate cortico-thalamic connectivity in preterm infants imaged at age 2 years (Counsell et al. 2007). This method involves using DTI tract tracing to follow white matter tracts between the thalamus and cerebral cortex, thereby generating a map of cortico-thalmic connectivity. Cortico-thalamic connectivity appeared normal for 11 former preterm children with normal MRI and cognitive outcome, but appeared disrupted in a single child with marked white matter abnormalities on conventional MRI and later neurodevelopmental delay. Although these data were published as proof of principle, the method offers promise for the evaluation of children with a variety of cognitive impairments in addition to those of children born preterm.

Volumetric magnetic resonance analysis

Conventional magnetic resonance images have also been evaluated for tissue volumes in the preterm infant. Preterm infants with periventricular leukomalacia have a marked reduction in cerebral cortical gray matter volume when imaged at term equivalence compared with either preterm infants without periventricular leukomalacia or normal term infants. A reduction in the volume of total brain myelinated white matter is also present, with an apparent compensatory increase in total CSF volume (Inder et al. 1999). In addition, reductions in deep nuclear gray matter volume are present (Inder et al. 2005). The volume reductions detected at term equivalence age are region-specific and correlate with later clinical course. White matter injury and intrauterine growth restriction were both shown to be associated with a reduction in more posterior brain volumes, whereas bronchopulmonary dysplasia was associated with a more global reduction across all regions (Thompson et al. 2007). In contrast, the degree of immaturity was not related to regional brain structure among preterm infants (Thompson et al. 2007). Preterm infants imaged during adolescence showed a lower whole brain volume, cortical gray matter volume, and hippocampal volume; they also had larger lateral ventricles (Nosarti et al. 2002). Thus, the alterations in cerebral volumes that appear at term equivalence are also present in adolescence, suggesting the ongoing persistence throughout maturation of these changes in cerebral structure.

Correlations have also been identified between cognitive outcome and brain volumes. Scores of the Mental Developmental Index of the Bayley Scales of Infant Development for preterm infants assessed at 18–20 months chronologic age correlated with right-sided sensorimotor and mid-temporal white matter volumes measured near term (Peterson et al. 2003). In addition, the volume of the corpus callosum correlated with verbal skills in boys (Nosarti et al. 2004), hippocampal volume correlated with memory function (Isaacs et al. 2000), and cerebellar volume was associated with executive, visuospatial, and language function (Allin et al. 2005). While the interactions between volumes and other indicators of injury (e.g. white matter injury and reduced cerebellar volume) are complex, the presence of outcome correlates for measured volume disturbances is interesting and suggests that this methodology may eventually find clinical utility for evaluating children with cognitive deficits related to causes other than preterm birth.

TERM INFANTS WITH HYPOXIC–ISCHEMIC ENCEPHALOPATHY

MRI of the term infant with suspected hypoxic–ischemic encephalopathy (HIE) is useful for establishing the diagnosis, understanding the potential timing of an insult, and predicting the long-term neurodevelopmental outcome from the nature of the cerebral injury imaged. The MRI findings vary in relation to the type of injury and the timing of MRI relative to the occurrence of the insult. Magnetic resonance spectroscopy abnormalities are detectable within the first 12 hours of injury, ADC abnormalities most conspicuous between 2 and 4 days, and conventional MRI shows injury best from 5–9 days onward.

Conventional magnetic resonance imaging
Three main patterns of injury have been described in term infants with HIE on conventional T1- and T2-weighted MRI studies between postnatal days 2 and 8 (Kuenzle et al. 1994, Leth et al. 1997, Aida et al. 1998, Barkovich et al. 1998, Rutherford et al. 1998, Mercuri et al. 2000, Biagioni et al. 2001, Roelants-Van Rijn et al. 2001a). These include (1) injury to the thalami +/− posterolateral putamen with variable involvement of the subcortical white matter, (2) injury to the parasagittal gray matter and subcortical white matter, and (3) focal or multifocal injury. Thalamic and basal ganglia damage, characterized by hyperintensity on T1-weighted imaging, is the most common form of MRI abnormality reported, accounting for over half of all abnormalities reported and occurring in over one-third of all infants studied. This is often accompanied by a loss of signal intensity in the posterior limb of the internal capsule on fluid-attenuated inversion recovery (FLAIR) T2-weighted imaging by day 5 of life. The prognostic significance of such basal ganglia injury and/or the loss of signal intensity in the posterior limb of the internal capsule is profound, with close to 90% of infants with moderate to severe abnormalities developing cerebral palsy, mental retardation, and seizures at 1–2 years of age (Barkovich et al. 1998, Rutherford et al. 1998, Mercuri et al. 2000, Biagioni et al. 2001, Roelants-Van Rijn et al. 2001a).

Diffusion magnetic resonance imaging
Interpretation of ADC values from diffusion imaging following injury is complicated by the dynamic nature of the decrease in ADC, particularly with regards to the nature of the injury. In animal studies, occlusion of the middle cerebral artery is associated with a rapid decline in the ADC values in the brain area supplied by this artery. If the occlusion is removed and blood flow restored with 30 minutes, ADC values return quickly to normal. However, ADC values then show a secondary decline, most apparent at 2–4 days after injury. This secondary decline reflects the evolution of tissue caused by the transient reduction in blood flow which was sufficient to cause ischemic injury. If the occlusion persists for 90 minutes, ADC values do not return to normal when blood flow is restored, but rather stay low (Dijkhuizen et al. 1998, Li et al. 2000, Lin et al. 2001). It should be noted that, in both cases, ADC values eventually return to normal after about 7 days, a process known as pseudo-normalization, and remain higher than normal thereafter. This difference in the time course of ADC changes following injury explains some of the difference

between the findings in infant and adult injury. With adult stroke, vascular occlusion typically persists for longer than 12 hours and ADC values rarely return to normal in the hours following the injury. Thus, the incidence of 'diffusion negative' stroke (stroke in which ADC values are normal during the first day after injury) in adults is only on the order of 6% (Schlaug et al. 1997, Oppenheim et al. 2000). In contrast, the duration of ischemic injury in infants with complications at delivery may be relatively brief if the infant is delivered quickly and resuscitated effectively or the insult is of a repeated 'partial' nature. The incidence of 'diffusion negative' injury in term infants has been estimated at 30% (McKinstry et al. 2002a). Thus, while diffusion imaging shows injury early in about 70% of infants, it is most reliable at 2–4 days after injury. At 7–10 days after injury, when ADC values undergo pseudo-normalization and injury is not readily detected on diffusion images, injury is typically detectable by more conventional imaging approaches.

Diffusion abnormalities also vary regionally within the brain following an ischemic insult in term infants. It has been suggested that the regional variation in diffusion MRI may reflect secondary injury to descending white matter fiber tracts which precedes Wallerian degeneration, although the time course and evolution of such changes remains poorly understood at present (Mazumdar et al. 2003). Diffusion abnormalities in one case showed the expected pseudo-normalization in cortical gray matter but persistence of low ADC values in white matter, which was then attributed to Wallerian degeneration (Neil and Inder 2006). In addition to these observations, the presence of a sustained reduction in ADC in the posterior limb of the internal capsule has been correlated with poor outcome consistent with injury to the corticospinal tracts by primary or secondary Wallerian degeneration in term infants (Hunt et al. 2004).

Proton Magnetic Resonance Spectroscopy
A number of authors have explored the utility of ^{1}H magnetic resonance spectroscopy for the evaluation of term infants with HIE (Penrice et al. 1996, Barkovich et al. 1999). For infants studied at any time during the first 2 postnatal weeks, lactate:creatine ratios of >1.5 are associated not only with high neonatal encephalopathy scores, but also with an elevated risk for later adverse neurodevelopmental outcome of 50–89% (Barkovich et al. 1999, Robertson et al. 1999, Roelants-Van Rijn et al. 2001b). Elevated lactate:N-acetyl aspartate, lactate:creatine and lactate:choline ratios are also more common in infants with suspected neonatal encephalopathy than age-matched controls. In these studies, elevated ratios of lactate:N-acetyl aspartate, lactate:choline or lactate:creatine in the region of the basal ganglia are significantly associated with later cerebral palsy and mental retardation/intellectual disability. These data suggest the utility of magnetic resonance spectroscopy strategies for assessment of encephalopathic term infants, with lactate:creatine levels >1 in the first 18 hours being strongly predictive of a poor outcome. However, more studies are required

to determine the upper limits of these ratios in the normal population, their sensitivity and specificity, and their positive and negative predictive values. Further longitudinal studies are also needed to determine the optimal timing of magnetic resonance spectroscopy evaluation of term infants with neonatal encephalopathy.

DEVELOPMENTAL DISORDERS OF INFANCY AND CHILDHOOD

These disorders include autistic spectrum disorder (ASD), attention-deficit–hyperactivity disorder (ADHD), developmental language disorder (DLD), and reading disorder (dyslexia). Unlike preterm birth and HIE, they typically do not have abnormalities detectable by conventional neuroimaging. As a result, MRI does not aid significantly in their diagnosis. Nevertheless, more advanced MRI acquisition and analysis methods have been applied in a wide variety of research studies in an effort to understand their underlying neuropathology. At the outset, it is worth noting that differences in cohort selection, magnetic resonance scanning protocols, analysis methods, and (for fMRI) specific activation paradigms between studies often lead to apparently contradictory results and make it difficult to directly compare studies carried out at different centers. Filipek (1999) likens the research in this area to an unrelated collection of 'apples and camels.' The discussion of these disorders below is not comprehensive; rather, examples are given to illustrate recent applications of the more novel of the imaging methods outlined in this chapter.

Autistic Spectrum Disorder

Autistic spectrum disorder (ASD) has long been associated with macrocephaly (Lainhart 2003). Retrospective analysis of head size suggests that the average head circumference is smaller than normal at birth, with infants with ASD undergoing abnormally high rates of head growth during the first year of life such that the average head circumference is greater than normal by 12 months of age (Courchesne et al. 2003). A number of magnetic resonance volumetry studies have been undertaken to determine if brain enlargement is caused by an increase in gray matter volume, white matter volume, or both (Lainhart 2006). During very early childhood, both volumes appear to be increased, with the greatest increase in white matter in the frontal lobes (Carper et al. 2002). Later in childhood, when mean total brain volume is less increased than typically developing infants, elevated white matter volume is present, out of proportion to the total brain volume. Cerebral cortical gray matter volume is also decreased at this age (Herbert et al. 2003). Changes in other volumes, such as limbic structures and the cerebellum, are more controversial, with conflicting results from various research groups (Filipek 1999).

A variety of conventional fMRI studies have suggested that subjects with ASD utilize different cognitive strategies and different brain areas to process information (Lainhart 2006). Further, studies suggest 'functional underconnectivity' in anterior–posterior connections compared with typically developing subjects (Cherkassky et al.

2006). The precise relationship between these findings and the pathophysiology underlying ASD has yet to be precisely determined.

ATTENTION-DEFICIT–HYPERACTIVITY DISORDER

A number of volumetry studies have been carried out in those with ADHD. Discordant results have been found for hemisphere size, caudate volume, and callosal volumes. However, these studies do not provide a unified theory of the neuropathology of this disorder, but fcMRI and DTI tract tracing methods have been applied with interesting results.

On the basis of behavioral, neuroimaging, lesion, and electrophysiologic studies, a model for attention has emerged suggesting that different attentional operations during sensory orienting are carried out by two separate frontal parietal systems: (1) a bilateral dorsal attention system involved in the top-down orienting of attention, and (2) a right-lateralized ventral attention system involved in reorienting attention in response to salient sensory stimuli (Corbetta and Shulman 2002). These systems were evaluated in a recently published fcMRI study in which both systems were identified solely on the basis of spontaneous activity in 10 typically developing subjects (Fox et al. 2006). The systems are widely segregated in their spatial topography with only small regions of overlap in the prefrontal cortex. While this study does not address whether these neural circuits are abnormal in those with ADHD, it elegantly confirms their presence, highlighting the potential utility of this imaging approach.

In a preliminary study, white matter diffusion anisotropy was evaluated in 18 individuals with ADHD and 15 individuals without the disorder (Ashtari et al. 2005). Investigators detected lower anisotropy values in the right premotor, right striatal, right cerebral peduncle, left middle cerebellar peduncle, left cerebellum, and left parieto-occipital areas in those with the disorder. Although the study's findings are preliminary, the data can be cautiously interpreted as supporting the hypothesis that alterations in brain white matter integrity in frontal and cerebellar regions occur in ADHD, implicating the cortico-ponto-cerebellar circuit in the pathophysiology of this disorder.

DEVELOPMENTAL LANGUAGE AND READING DISORDER (DYSLEXIA)

Most imaging studies in DLD or reading disorder point to anomalous structure and function in the traditional language regions of the brain, including the primary auditory and auditory association cortices in the temporal and adjacent posterior parietal regions of the brain (Filipek 1999). The discussion below is focused on two studies – one in which diffusion anisotropy measures are compared against reading ability, and one in which cortical folding is assessed in subjects with Williams syndrome.

Klingberg et al. (2000) studied white matter anisotropy in six adults with poor reading ability and 11 with normal reading ability. Anisotropy of white matter in the left temporal-parietal area was compared with the subject's reading score on the Woodcock word identification test. A striking linear relationship was identified between these two parameters when all subjects, both normal and poor readers, were included in the analysis. This relationship persisted when the groups were analyzed separately. The authors postulate that the anisotropy changes reflect abnormalities of white matter tract microstructure, which may contribute to reading ability by determining the 'strength of communication' between cortical areas involved in visual, auditory, and language processing. Whether such changes are related to direct disruption of white matter or are secondary to developmental abnormalities of the cortex to which the white matter is connected is not known. This study is the first of its kind in which localized values of white matter diffusion anisotropy show a strong direct correlation with a measurable clinical function.

Surface-based analysis, also known as cortical cartography, has recently been applied to subjects with a developmental disturbance of language function. This method entails generating detailed maps of the cortical surface from conventional T1- and/or T2-weighted images. Statistical methods are then used to compare features of the cortical surface, such as sulcal depth, between populations. This method has been applied to subjects with Williams syndrome (Van Essen et al. 2006). Williams syndrome is associated with an unusual pattern of strengths and weaknesses. Subjects show relative strengths in language and facial processing with a profound impairment in spatial cognition. The overall cognitive abilities (IQs) of individuals with Williams syndrome are typically in the mild–moderate range of mental retardation/intellectual disability with variations between different cognitive domains (Bellugi et al. 2000). Surface-based analysis shows discrete cortical folding abnormalities extending across a broad swath from dorso-posterior to ventro-anterior regions of each hemisphere, in cortical areas associated with multiple sensory modalities as well as regions implicated in cognitive and emotional behavior. Furthermore, hemispheric asymmetry in the temporal cortex is reduced in subjects with Williams syndrome compared with control subjects.

The authors of this particular study postulated a number of structure–function relationships based on these data. Among them, folding abnormalities in the dorsal parietal cortex were suggested to explain impairment in visuospatial tasks, which could be related to altered circuitry of these parietal lobe regions. Alterations in the cortical topography of the planum temporal were postulated to help account for the relatively intact language with a rich vocabulary and heightened emotional response to music found in those with Williams syndrome. Although these relationships await confirmation, this study highlights the potential utility of cortical cartography for evaluating and detecting cortical folding abnormalities that are too subtle to be detected on qualitative (i.e. visual inspection) analysis of conventional magnetic resonance images. One can foresee application of their technique in the near future to a variety of neurodevelopmental disability etiologic subtypes.

CEREBRAL PALSY

Cerebral palsy can be defined as a disorder of aberrant control of movement or posture, appearing early in life secondary to a CNS lesion or dysfunction that is not the result of a recognized progressive or degenerative brain disease (Nelson and Ellenberg 1978). This definition clearly encapsulated considerable clinico-pathologic heterogeneity and cerebral palsy encompasses a variety of different neuropathologies. Despite considerable evidence to the contrary (Nelson 1989), cerebral palsy has been attributed to perinatal asphyxia since the first use of the term. As Little wrote in 1862, 'the act of birth does occasionally imprint upon the nervous and muscular systems of the nascent infantile organism very serious and peculiar evils' (Little 1862). Despite the obvious heterogeneity of cohorts identified as having cerebral palsy, the term remains in widespread use.

The American Academy of Neurology recommends that conventional MRI be obtained to evaluate children with cerebral palsy (Ashwal et al. 2004). As a generality, children with spastic syndromes often show white matter injury, whereas those with an extrapyramidal syndrome frequently have basal ganglia abnormalities on imaging (Hoon 2005). Neuroimaging can be very important in distinguishing these disorders, with implications for treatment, prognosis, and recurrence risk. The utility of neuroimaging in cerebral palsy is linked to whether the test is performed for a specific indication (e.g. microcephaly), with diagnostic yield being three times higher than when carried out on a screening basis (Shevell et al. 2000) and is clearly of greatest utility in combination with a thorough history and neurologic examination.

Neuroimaging in cerebral palsy associated with preterm birth and HIE is discussed extensively above. Cerebral palsy is also associated with developmental CNS anomalies. The application of DTI tractography to cortical and white matter dysplasia in cerebral palsy has been reported (Lee et al. 2005). Areas of dysplastic gray matter in heterotopias showed high diffusion anisotropy, consistent with primitive poorly developed gray matter. White matter showed low anisotropy near areas of malformed cortex and aberrant courses in areas of dysplasia. Callosal agenesis was associated with abnormal hemispheric fiber connections. It is clear from this remarkably comprehensive study that DTI methods can provide a great deal of information about cerebral microstructure. Further research is required to establish the developmental consequences of these specific observed alterations.

CONCLUSIONS

MRI, in its various forms, has two primary roles in assessing infants and children with neurodevelopmental disabilities. The first is diagnostic, and conventional MRI still remains the mainstay of this clinical application. The second is a more research-related role in which MRI is employed to improve our understanding of the pathophysiology underlying specific neurodevelopmental disorders. An improved understanding of the anatomic basis for the disabilities faced by children, and insight into the pathways to such clinical impairments, may help with the development of new interventions and rehabilitative strategies. With time, many of the currently 'novel' methods will no doubt find their way into standard clinical practice, improving our understanding of the individual affected child.

REFERENCES

Aida N, Nishimura G, Hachiya Y, Matsui K, Takeuchi M, Itani Y (1998) MR imaging of perinatal brain damage: comparison of clinical outcome with initial and follow-up MR findings. *AJNR Am J Neuroradiol* 19: 1909–1921.

Allin MP, Salaria S, Nosarti C, Wyatt J, Rifkin L, Murray RM (2005) Vermis and lateral lobes of the cerebellum in adolescents born very preterm. *Neuroreport* 16: 1821–1824.

Anupindi S, Jaramillo D (2002) Pediatric magnetic resonance imaging techniques. *Magn Reson Imaging Clin N Am* 10: 189–207.

Arfanakis K, Cordes D, Haughton VM, Moritz CH, Quigley MA, Meyerand ME (2000) Combining independent component analysis and correlation analysis to probe interregional connectivity in fMRI task activation datasets. *Magn Reson Imaging* 18: 921–930.

Ashtari M, Kumra S, Bhaskar SL, Clarke T, Thaden E, Cervellione KL, et al. (2005) Attention-deficit/hyperactivity disorder: a preliminary diffusion tensor imaging study. *Biol Psychiatry* 57: 448–455.

Ashwal S, Russman BS, Blasco PA, Miller G, Sandler A, Shevell M, et al. (2004) Practice parameter: diagnostic assessment of the child with cerebral palsy: report of the Quality Standards Subcommittee of the American Academy of Neurology and the Practice Committee of the Child Neurology Society. *Neurology* 62: 851–863.

Barkovich AJ, Baranski K, Vigneron D, Partridge JC, Hallam DK, Hajnal BL, et al. (1999) Proton MR spectroscopy for the evaluation of brain injury in asphyxiated, term neonates. *AJNR Am J Neuroradiol* 20: 1399–1405.

Barkovich AJ, Hajnal BL, Vigneron D, Sola A, Partridge JC, Allen F, et al. (1998) Prediction of neuromotor outcome in perinatal asphyxia: evaluation of MR scoring systems. *AJNR Am J Neuroradiol* 19: 143–149.

Barkovich AJ, Truwit CL (1990) Brain damage from perinatal asphyxia: correlation of MR findings with gestational age. *AJNR Am J Neuroradiol* 11: 1087–1096.

Bellugi U, Lichtenberger L, Jones W, Lai Z, St George M (2000) The neurocognitive profile of Williams syndrome: a complex pattern of strengths and weaknesses. *J Cogn Neurosci* 12 (Suppl 1): 7–29.

Biagioni E, Mercuri E, Rutherford M, Cowan F, Azzopardi D, Frisone MF, et al. (2001) Combined use of electroencephalogram and magnetic resonance imaging in full-term neonates with acute encephalopathy. *Pediatrics* 107: 461–468.

Biswal B, Yetkin FZ, Haughton VM, Hyde JS (1995) Functional connectivity in the motor cortex of resting human brain using echo-planar MRI. *Magn Reson Med* 34: 537–541.

Brenner DJ, Doll R, Goodhead DT, Hall EJ, Land CE, Little JB, et al. (2003) Cancer risks attributable to low doses of ionizing radiation: assessing what we really know. *Proc Natl Acad Sci U S A* 100: 13761–13766.

Carper RA, Moses P, Tigue ZD, Courchesne E (2002) Cerebral lobes in autism: early hyperplasia and abnormal age effects. *Neuroimage* 16: 1038–1051.

Cherkassky VL, Kana RK, Keller TA, Just MA (2006) Functional connectivity in a baseline resting-state network in autism. *Neuroreport* 17: 1687–1690.

Committee on Drugs (2002) Practice guidelines for sedation and analgesia by non-anesthesiologists. *Anesthesiology* 96: 1004–1017.

Committee on Drugs, American Academy of Pediatrics (2002) Guidelines for monitoring and management of pediatric patients during and after sedation for diagnostic and therapeutic procedures: addendum. *Pediatrics* 110: 836–838.

Cooke RW, Abernethy LJ (1999) Cranial magnetic resonance imaging and school performance in very low birth weight infants in adolescence. *Arch Dis Child Fetal Neonatal Ed* 81: F116–F121.

Corbetta M, Shulman GL (2002) Control of goal-directed and stimulus-driven attention in the brain. *Nat Rev Neurosci* 3: 201–215.

Cordes D, Haughton VM, Arfanakis K, Wendt GJ, Turski PA, Moritz CH, et al. (2000) Mapping functionally related regions of brain with functional connectivity MR imaging. *AJNR Am J Neuroradiol* 21: 1636–1644.

Counsell SJ, Allsop JM, Harrison MC, Larkman DJ, Kennea NL, Kapellou O, et al. (2003) Diffusion-weighted imaging of the brain in preterm infants with focal and diffuse white matter abnormality. *Pediatrics* 112: 1–7.

Counsell SJ, Dyet LE, Larkman DJ, Nunes RG, Boardman JP, Allsop JM, et al. (2007) Thalamo-cortical connectivity in children born preterm mapped using probabilistic magnetic resonance tractography. *Neuroimage* 34: 896–904.

Counsell SJ, Shen Y, Boardman JP, Larkman DJ, Kapellou O, Ward P, et al. (2006) Axial and radial diffusivity in preterm infants who have diffuse white matter changes on magnetic resonance imaging at term-equivalent age. *Pediatrics* 117: 376–386.

Courchesne E, Carper R, Akshoomoff N (2003) Evidence of brain overgrowth in the first year of life in autism. *JAMA* 290: 337–344.

De Vries LS, Connell JA, Dubowitz LM, Oozeer RC, Dubowitz V, Pennock JM (1987) Neurological, electrophysiological and MRI abnormalities in infants with extensive cystic leuko-malacia. *Neuropediatrics* 18: 61–66.

Deipolyi AR, Mukherjee P, Gill K, Henry RG, Partridge SC, Veeraraghavan S, et al. (2005) Comparing microstructural and macrostructural development of the cerebral cortex in premature newborns: diffusion tensor imaging versus cortical gyration. *Neuroimage* 27: 579–586.

Dijkhuizen RM, Knollema S, van der Worp HB, Ter Horst GJ, De Wildt DJ, Berkelbach van der Sprenkel JW, et al. (1998) Dynamics of cerebral tissue injury and perfusion after temporary hypoxia-ischemia in the rat: evidence for region-specific sensitivity and delayed damage. *Stroke* 29: 695–704.

Filipek PA (1999) Neuroimaging in the developmental disorders: the state of the science. *J Child Psychol Psychiatry* 40: 113–128.

Flodmark O, Lupton B, Li D, Stimac GK, Roland EH, Hill A, et al. (1989) MR imaging of periventricular leukomalacia in childhoood. *AJNR Am J Neuroradiol* 10: 111–118.

Fox MD, Corbetta M, Snyder AZ, Vincent JL, Raichle ME (2006) Spontaneous neuronal activity distinguishes human dorsal and ventral attention systems. *Proc Natl Acad Sci U S A* 103: 10046–10051.

Fox MD, Snyder AZ, Vincent JL, Corbetta M, Van Essen DC, Raichle ME (2005) The human brain is intrinsically organized into dynamic, anticorrelated functional networks. *Proc Natl Acad Sci U S A* 102: 9673–9678.

Greicius MD, Menon V. (2004) Default-mode activity during a passive sensory task: uncoupled from deactivation but impacting activation. *J Cogn Neurosci* 16: 1484–1492.

Hall P, Adami HO, Trichopoulos D, Pedersen NL, Lagiou P, Ekbom A, et al. (2004) Effect of low doses of ionising radiation in infancy on cognitive function in adulthood: Swedish population based cohort study. *BMJ* 328: 19.

Hampson M, Peterson BS, Skudlarski P, Gatenby JC, Gore JC (2002) Detection of functional connectivity using temporal correlations in MR images. *Hum Brain Mapp* 15: 247–262.

Herbert MR, Ziegler DA, Deutsch CK, O'Brien LM, Lange N, Bakardjiev A, et al. (2003) Dissociations of cerebral cortex, subcortical and cerebral white matter volumes in autistic boys. *Brain* 126: 1182–1192.

Hoon AH Jr (2005) Neuroimaging in cerebral palsy: patterns of brain dysgenesis and injury. *J Child Neurol* 20: 936–939.

Hunt RW, Neil JJ, Coleman LT, Kean MJ, Inder TE (2004) Apparent diffusion coefficient in the posterior limb of the internal capsule predicts outcome following perinatal asphyxia. *Pediatrics* 114: 999–1003.

Huppi PS, Murphy B, Maier SE, Zientara GP, Inder TE, Barnes PD, et al. (2001) Microstructural brain development after perinatal cerebral white matter injury assessed by diffusion tensor magnetic resonance imaging. *Pediatrics* 107: 455–460.

Huppi PS, Warfield S, Kikinis R, Barnes PD, Zientara GP, Jolesz FA, et al. (1998) Quantitative magnetic resonance imaging of brain development in premature and mature newborns. *Ann Neurol* 43: 224–235.

Inder TE, Huppi PS, Warfield S, Kikinis R, Zientara GP, Barnes PD, et al. (1999) Periventricular white matter injury in the premature infant is followed by reduced cerebral cortical gray matter volume at term. *Ann Neurol* 46: 755–760.

Inder TE, Warfield SK, Wang H, Huppi PS, Volpe JJ (2005) Abnormal cerebral structure is present at term in premature infants. *Pediatrics* 115: 286–294.

Inder TE, Wells SJ, Mogridge NB, Spencer C, Volpe JJ (2003) Defining the nature of the cerebral abnormalities in the premature infant: a qualitative magnetic resonance imaging study. *J Pediatr* 143: 171–179.

Isaacs EB, Lucas A, Chong WK, Wood SJ, Johnson CL, Marshall C, et al. (2000) Hippocampal volume and everyday memory in children of very low birth weight. *Pediatr Res* 47: 713–720.

Karlsson P, Holmberg E, Lundell M, Mattsson A, Holm LE, Wallgren A. (1998) Intracranial tumors after exposure to ionizing radiation during infancy: a pooled analysis of two Swedish cohorts of 28 008 infants with skin hemangioma. *Radiat Res* 150: 357–364.

Kiviniemi VJ, Haanpaa H, Kantola JH, Jauhiainen J, Vainionpaa V, Alahuhta S, et al. (2005) Midazolam sedation increases fluctuation and synchrony of the resting brain BOLD signal. *Magn Reson Imaging* 23: 531–537.

Klingberg T, Hedehus M, Temple E, Salz T, Gabrieli JD, Moseley ME, et al. (2000) Microstructure of temporo-parietal white matter as a basis for reading ability: evidence from diffusion tensor magnetic resonance imaging. *Neuron* 25: 493–500.

Kuenzle C, Baenziger O, Martin E, Thun-Hohenstein L, Steinlin M, Good M, et al. (1994) Prognostic value of early MR imaging in term infants with severe perinatal asphyxia. *Neuropediatrics* 25: 191–200.

Lainhart JE (2003) Increased rate of head growth during infancy in autism. *JAMA* 290: 393–394.

Lainhart JE (2006) Advances in autism neuroimaging research for the clinician and geneticist. *Am J Med Genet C Semin Med Genet* 142: 33–39.

LeBihan D, Breton E, Lallemand D, Grenier P, Cabanis E, Laval-Jeantet M. (1986) MR imaging of intravoxel incoherent motions: application to diffusion and perfusion in neurologic disorders. *Radiology* 161: 401–407.

Lee SK, Kim DI, Kim J, Kim DJ, Kim HD, Kim DS, et al. (2005) Diffusion-tensor MR imaging and fiber tractography: a new method of describing aberrant fiber connections in developmental CNS anomalies. *Radiographics* 25: 53–65; discussion 66–58.

Leth H, Toft PB, Herning M, Peitersen B, Lou HC (1997) Neonatal seizures associated with cerebral lesions shown by magnetic resonance imaging. *Arch Dis Child Fetal Neonatal Ed* 77: F105–110.

Li F, Silva MD, Liu KF, Helmer KG, Omae T, Fenstermacher JD, et al. (2000) Secondary decline in apparent diffusion coefficient and neurological outcomes after a short period of focal brain ischemia in rats. *Ann Neurol* 48: 236–244.

Lin S-P, Song SK, Miller JP, Ackerman JJ, Neil JJ (2001) Direct longitudinal comparison of ^{1}H and ^{23}Na MRI after transient focal cerebral ischemia. *Stroke* 32(4): 925–932.

Little WJ (1862) On the influence of abnormal parturition, difficult labours, premature birth, and asphyxia neonatorum, on the mental and physical condition of the child, especially in relation to deformities. *Trans Obstet Soc Lond* 3: 293–344.

Lowe MJ, Mock BJ, Sorenson JA (1998) Functional connectivity in single and multislice echo-planar imaging using resting-state fluctuations. *Neuroimage* 7: 119–132.

Luders E, Thompson PM, Narr KL, Toga AW, Jancke L, Gaser C (2006) A curvature-based approach to estimate local gyrification on the cortical surface. *Neuroimage* 29: 1224–1230.

Malviya S, Voepel-Lewis T, Tait AR (1997) Adverse events and risk factors associated with the sedation of children by non-anesthesiologists. *Anesth Analg* 85: 1207–1213.

Marin-Padilla M (1988) Early ontogenesis of the human cerebral cortex. In: Peters A, Jones EG (eds) *Development and Maturation of Cerebral Cortex*. New York: Plenum Press, pp 1–34.

Mazumdar A, Mukherjee P, Miller JH, Malde H, McKinstry RC (2003) Diffusion-weighted imaging of acute corticospinal tract injury preceding Wallerian degeneration in the maturing human brain. *AJNR Am J Neuroradiol* 24: 1057–1066.

McKinstry RC, Miller JH, Snyder AZ, Mathur A, Schefft GL, Almli CR, et al. (2002a) A prospective, longitudinal diffusion tensor imaging study of brain injury in newborns. *Neurology* 59: 824–833.

McKinstry RC, Mathur A, Miller JP, Ozcan AO, Snyder AZ, Schefft GL, et al. (2002b) Radial organization of developing human cerebral cortex revealed by non-invasive water diffusion anisotropy MRI. *Cereb Cortex* 12: 1237–1243.

Mercuri E, Ricci D, Cowan FM, Lessing D, Frisone MF, Haataja L, et al. (2000) Head growth in infants with hypoxic-ischemic encephalopathy: correlation with neonatal magnetic resonance imaging. *Pediatrics* 106: 235–243.

Miller SP, Cozzio CC, Goldstein RB, Ferriero DM, Partridge JC, Vigneron DB, et al. (2003) Comparing the diagnosis of white matter injury in premature newborns with serial MR imaging and transfontanel ultrasonography findings. *AJNR Am J Neuroradiol* 24: 1661–1669.

Mori S, van Zijl PC. (2002) Fiber tracking: principles and strategies: a technical review. *NMR Biomed* 15: 468–480.

Moseley ME, Cohen Y, Mintorovitch J, Chileuitt L, Shimizu H, Kucharczyk J, et al. (1990) Early detection of regional cerebral ischemia in cats: comparison of diffusion- and T2-weighted MRI and spectroscopy. *Magn Reson Med* 14: 330–346.

Mukherjee P, Miller JH, Shimony JS, Philip JV, Nehra D, Snyder AZ, et al. (2002) Diffusion-tensor MR imaging of gray and white matter development during normal human brain maturation. *AJNR Am J Neuroradiol* 23: 1445–1456.

Neil JJ, Inder TE (2006) Detection of Wallerian degeneration in a newborn by diffusion MR imaging. *J Child Neurol* 21: 115–118.

Neil JJ, Shiran SI, McKinstry RC, Schefft GL, Snyder AZ, Almli CR, et al. (1998) Normal brain in human newborns: apparent diffusion coefficient and diffusion anisotropy measured using diffusion tensor imaging. *Radiology* 209: 57–66.

Nelson KB (1989) Relationship of intrapartum and delivery room events to long-term neurologic outcome. *Clin Perinatol* 16: 995–1007.

Nelson KB, Ellenberg JH (1978) Epidemiology of cerebral palsy. *Adv Neurol* 19: 421–435.

Nosarti C, Al-Asady MH, Frangou S, Stewart AL, Rifkin L, Murray RM (2002) Adolescents who were born very preterm have decreased brain volumes. *Brain* 125: 1616–1623.

Nosarti C, Rushe TM, Woodruff PW, Stewart AL, Rifkin L, Murray RM (2004) Corpus callosum size and very preterm birth: relationship to neuropsychological outcome. *Brain* 127: 2080–2089.

Olsen P, Paakko E, Vainionpaa L, Pythinen J, Jarvelin M-J (1997) Magnetic resonance imaging of periventricular leukomalacia and its clinical correlation in children. *Ann Neurol* 41: 754–761.

Oppenheim C, Stanescu R, Dormont D, Crozier S, Marro B, Samson Y, et al. (2000) False-negative diffusion-weighted MR findings in acute ischemic stroke. *AJNR Am J Neuroradiol* 21: 1434–1440.

Penrice J, Cady EB, Lorek A, Wylezinska M, Amess PN, Aldridge RF, et al. (1996) Proton magnetic resonance spectroscopy of the brain in normal preterm and term infants, and early changes after perinatal hypoxia-ischemia. *Pediatr Res* 40: 6–14.

Peterson BS, Anderson AW, Ehrenkranz R, Staib LH, Tageldin M, Colson E, et al. (2003) Regional brain volumes and their later neurodevelopmental correlates in term and preterm infants. *Pediatrics* 111: 939–948.

Rettmann ME, Tosun D, Tao X, Resnick SM, Prince JL (2005) Program for assisted labeling of sulcal regions (PALS): description and reliability. *Neuroimage* 24: 398–416.

Robertson NJ, Cox IJ, Cowan FM, Counsell SJ, Azzopardi D, Edwards AD (1999) Cerebral intracellular lactic alkalosis persisting months after neonatal encephalopathy measured by magnetic resonance spectroscopy. *Pediatr Res* 46: 287–296.

Roelants-van Rijn AM, Groenendaal F, Beek FJ, Eken P, van Haastert IC, de Vries LS. (2001a) Parenchymal brain injury in the preterm infant: comparison of cranial ultrasound, MRI and neurodevelopmental outcome. *Neuropediatrics* 32: 80–89.

Roelants-Van Rijn AM, van der Grond J, de Vries LS, Groenendaal F. (2001b) Value of ¹H-MRS using different echo times in neonates with cerebral hypoxia-ischemia. *Pediatr Res* 49: 356–362.

Ron E, Modan B, Floro S, Harkedar I, Gurewitz R. (1982) Mental function following scalp irradiation during childhood. *Am J Epidemiol* 116: 149–160.

Rutherford MA, Pennock JM, Counsell SJ, Mercuri E, Cowan FM, Dubowitz LM, et al. (1998) Abnormal magnetic resonance signal in the internal capsule predicts poor neurodevelopmental outcome in infants with hypoxic-ischemic encephalopathy. *Pediatrics* 102: 323–328.

Schlaug G, Siewert B, Benfield A, Edelman RR, Warach S (1997) Time course of the apparent diffusion coefficient (ADC) abnormality in human stroke. *Neurology* 49: 113–119.

Shevell MI, Majnemer A, Rosenbaum P, Abrahamowicz M (2000) Etiologic yield of subspecialists' evaluation of young children with global developmental delay. *J Pediatr* 136: 593–598.

Song SK, Sun SW, Ramsbottom MJ, Chang C, Russell J, Cross AH. (2002) Dysmyelination revealed through MRI as increased radial (but unchanged axial) diffusion of water. *Neuroimage* 17: 1429–1436.

Song SK, Yoshino J, Le TQ, Lin SJ, Sun SW, Cross AH, et al. (2005) Demyelination increases radial diffusivity in corpus callosum of mouse brain. *Neuroimage* 26: 132–140.

Sowell ER, Thompson PM, Holmes CJ, Batth R, Jernigan TL, Toga AW (1999) Localizing age-related changes in brain structure between childhood and adolescence using statistical parametric mapping. *Neuroimage* 9: 587–597.

Stejskal EO, Tanner JE. (1965) Spin diffusion measurements: Spin echoes in the presence of time-dependent field gradients. *J Chem Phys* 42: 288–292.

Sun SW, Liang HF, Le TQ, Armstrong RC, Cross AH, Song SK. (2006) Differential sensitivity of in vivo and ex vivo diffusion tensor imaging to evolving optic nerve injury in mice with retinal ischemia. *Neuroimage* 32: 1195–1204.

Thompson DK, Warfield SK, Carlin JB, Pavlovic M, Wang HX, Bear M, et al. (2007) Perinatal risk factors altering regional brain structure in the preterm infant. *Brain* 130: 667–677.

Truwit CL, Barkovich AJ, Koch TK, Ferriero DM (1992) Cerebral palsy: MR findings in 40 patients. *AJNR Am J Neuroradiol* 13: 67–78.

Valkama AM, Paakko EL, Vainionpaa LK, Lanning FP, Ilkko EA, Koivisto ME (2000) Magnetic resonance imaging at term and neuromotor outcome in preterm infants. *Acta Paediatr* 89: 348–355.

Van Essen DC (2005) A population-average, landmark- and surface-based (PALS) atlas of human cerebral cortex. *Neuroimage* 28: 635–662.

Van Essen DC, Dierker D, Snyder AZ, Raichle ME, Reiss AL, Korenberg J (2006) Symmetry of cortical folding abnormalities in Williams syndrome revealed by surface-based analyses. *J Neurosci* 26: 5470–5483.

Wilson DA, Steiner RE (1986) Periventricular leukomalacia: evaluation with MR imaging. *Radiology* 160: 507–511.

Woodward LJ, Anderson PJ, Austin NC, Howard K, Inder TE (2006) Neonatal MRI to predict neurodevelopmental outcomes in preterm infants. *N Engl J Med* 355: 685–694.

10
NEUROBIOLOGY OF SPECIFIC LANGUAGE IMPAIRMENT

Richard I Webster

Despite the complexity of language, normally developing children acquire language through environmental exposure with little explicit instruction (Bishop 2000). In most children, the potential for language appears to be present at birth. However, for some children with otherwise normal development, the acquisition of language proves disproportionately difficult. Despite relatively normal non-linguistic cognitive function and normal hearing, their language development is impaired. These children are considered to have specific language impairment (SLI).

With an estimated prevalence of 7.4% in kindergarten children, SLI is one of the most common childhood neurodevelopmental disorders (Tomblin et al. 1997). In a high proportion of children, SLI is associated with ongoing impairments which involve not only communication skills, but also academic and social skills (Aram et al. 1984, Stothard et al. 1998, Snowling et al. 2000). As such, SLI represents a major challenge for our society's public health and education systems. However, it is uncommon for clinicians to be able to identify an underlying cause for language impairment in children who have SLI (Shevell et al. 2000).

Over the past 20 years there has been increasing research investigating the biologic causes of SLI. This research has followed several different lines. Initial research aimed to accurately characterize the nature of the language disorder seen in children with SLI and to identify psycholinguistic markers that could be used to identify such children. This research found evidence of impairments in verbal working memory (Gathercole and Baddeley 1990, Bishop et al. 1996, Adams and Gathercole 2000, Botting and Conti-Ramsden 2001) and difficulties processing rapidly changing sounds (Tallal and Piercy 1974, 1975, Merzenich et al. 1996, Benasich et al. 2002) in children with SLI. It has also become clear that the impairments seen in children with SLI extend to developmental domains beyond language and cannot be explained simply as a consequence of the language disorder (Johnston 1994, Hill 1998, Manor et al. 2001, Bishop 2001, Webster et al. 2005, 2006).

Evidence that there are strong genetic determinants of language development has come from epidemiologic and twin studies (Bishop et al. 1995, Kovas et al. 2005). Genome-wide searches have identified several possible genetic loci associated with SLI (Bartlett et al. 2002, 2004, SLI Consortium 2002, 2004). With the recent progress in brain imaging technologies, evidence has emerged that the brain morphology of some children with SLI differs from children without language disorders (Plante et al. 1991, Jernigan et al. 1991, Gauger et al. 1997, Trauner et al. 2000, Herbert et al. 2004, 2005, De Fosse et al. 2004). Evidence of abnormalities in auditory processing in children with SLI has come from electrophysiologic studies (Ors et al. 2002a, McArthur and Bishop 2004) and more recently functional MRI (fMRI) has identified differing patterns of brain activation in adolescents with SLI (Weismer et al. 2005). This chapter aims to summarize what is presently known about the neurobiologic basis of SLI.

DEFINITION OF SPECIFIC LANGUAGE IMPAIRMENT

There continues to be considerable debate about how SLI should be defined (Lahey 1990, Aram et al. 1993, Bishop 1997, Tomblin et al. 1997). Arriving at a consistent consensus definition is obviously important when comparing studies that aim to identify the biologic causes of a disorder. Most authors would agree that SLI is a developmental disorder in which an individual's impairment in language is disproportionately greater than impairments evident in other non-linguistic domains. SLI is generally conceptualized as a neurodevelopmental disorder and, as such, children with an acquired language disorder (e.g. aphasia following a left hemispheric cerebrovascular accident or Landau–Kleffner syndrome) are usually not considered to have SLI, even though they may show problems that are indeed specific and restricted to language. There is also agreement that children do not have SLI if they have (1) a language disorder resulting from a neurologic disease, (2) a significant hearing impairment, (3) a significant impairment in other non-linguistic developmental domains (e.g. global developmental delay, autistic spectrum disorder), or (4) a speech/language disorder associated with a cleft palate (World Health Organization 1992, Aram et al. 1993, Tomblin et al. 1997, Leonard 1998, American Psychiatric Association – Taskforce on DSM-IV 2000).

Experienced speech-language pathologists usually have little difficulty identifying individuals who they would consider to have a language disorder; however, operationalizing this clinical intuition and recognition is challenging. M t definitions of SLI rely on a discrepancy between tests of non-verbal cognitive function and language (Lahey 1990, World Health Organization 1992, Tomblin et al. 1996, 1997, Leonard 1998, American Psychiatric Association – Taskforce on DSM IV 2000), with scores on language tests falling markedly below scores on non-verbal cognitive tests. However, children with language disorders can have a range of difficulties in differing areas of language. Should a child with a relatively limited language disorder (e.g. restricted expressive vocabulary) be considered to have the same disorder as a child who is impaired in all areas of language? Most studies have addressed this issue by using a composite measure of language which combines scores in a number of different areas of language to identify language impairment (Tomblin et al. 1996, 1997).

Similarly, deciding how the discrepancy between non-verbal cognition and language is measured and what objectively measured degree of discrepancy is required has also been the subject of considerable debate (Lahey 1990, Bishop 1997, Tomblin et al. 1997). Some of the disagreement in this area results from the differing needs of clinicians and researchers. For research, there is a need for an objective definition of SLI preferably based on statistical criteria, whereas for clinicians the functional significance of a disorder and its disablement of language is the most important issue. However, given the complexity of language, a child with a significant functional impairment may not readily be identified on standard tests of language (Aram et al. 1993). Conversely, a child with a statistically abnormal performance on a language test may not have any functional impairment or disablement.

The International Classification of Diseases-10 (ICD-10) classifies children with SLI within the category of Specific Developmental Disorders of Speech and Language and requires that a child's language skills (i.e. receptive and/or expressive) have been impaired from the early stages of development and fall markedly below the level expected on the basis of mental age (World Health Organization 1992). The Diagnostic and Statistical Manual of Mental Disorders IV-TR (DSM-IV) requires that there is a *substantial* discrepancy between language and non-verbal skills (American Psychiatric Association – Taskforce on DSM-IV 2000). Neither the ICD-10 nor the DSM-IV specifically defines what objective measurable degree of discrepancy is required between non-verbal and language skills. However, in contrast to the ICD-10, the DSM-IV also includes a requirement that the abnormality on testing is associated with a functional language impairment (i.e. disablement). It should be noted that neither definition requires that the child's non-verbal cognitive scores fall within the normal range.

The need of epidemiologic researchers for more precise criteria to identify children with SLI resulted in what is probably the presently most widely accepted definition (Tomblin et al. 1996, 1997). According to these criteria, SLI is defined as a combination of normal intelligence (i.e. performance IQ greater than 85) and language impairment (i.e. score on a composite language measure falling more than 1.25 SD below the mean). A −1.25 SD cutoff for language impairment (equivalent to the 10th centile or below) was chosen by Tomblin et al. (1996, 1997) to reflect the level at which experienced speech-language pathologists clinically readily identified language impairment in a child (Records and Tomblin 1994, Tomblin et al. 1996).

The current definitions of SLI have been criticized for a number of reasons. Bishop (1994) has pointed out that measures of verbal/non-verbal discrepancy potentially have poor reliability. Bishop (1994, 1997) also notes that children with non-verbal cognitive scores that fall below the cutoff for SLI can have language problems identical to children who otherwise meet criteria for SLI.

SLI has been considered to be 'specific' because there is preservation of non-verbal cognitive function, usually assessed using tests of visuospatial skills. However, on detailed testing children with SLI show visuospatial deficits (Johnston 1994). A recently published longitudinal study of children who met criteria for SLI at 7 years of age found that there was a significant drop-off in non-verbal IQ by the time these children reached 14 years of age (Botting 2005). Thus, a number of children diagnosed with SLI at the time of their original assessments would no longer be considered to have SLI at the time of later assessments. This finding has significant implications for researchers aiming to identify and study older children with SLI.

Finally, there continues to be debate about the use of the label 'specific' when applied to children with SLI. SLI is associated with a range of other developmental co-morbidities and thus a number of authors have suggested that the term 'specific' should no longer be applied to children with SLI (Ors 2002, Webster et al. 2006). Because of the lack of 'specificity' of impairments in SLI, a number of authors have preferred the use of terms such as developmental language disorder (Herbert et al. 2004), developmental language impairment (Trauner et al. 2000, Webster et al. 2006) or language-learning impaired (Tallal et al. 1996, Merzenich et al. 1996) to refer to children who would otherwise meet criteria for SLI.

LANGUAGE IMPAIRMENTS IN SLI

Parents of children with SLI commonly become concerned about their child's language development towards the end of their second year of life (Webster et al. 2004). When compared with their normally developing peers, children with SLI utter their first words later, combine words later, achieve intelligible speech later, and their language development reaches a perceptible plateau earlier (Rapin 1996a, Leonard 1998). While it was originally suggested that SLI represented a 'maturational' lag in language development, the profile of language development in children with SLI differs from that seen in normally developing children. Moreover, when compared with normally developing younger children matched for measures of language development, children with SLI show an uneven profile in the development of language skills, an abnormal frequency of errors, and different types of errors than those seen in children who subsequently develop normal language (Leonard 1998).

While impairments can be identified in all areas of language in children with SLI, some areas cause greater problems than others (Leonard 1998). In the English language, morphosyntax (from: morphology, the structure of words; syntax, the relationship between words and other units within a sentence) is the area that causes the greatest evident difficulty. The use of grammatical inflections (the units of language appended to words that express an attribute, e.g. possessive s as in Jane's dog) causes children with SLI particular difficulty. The grammatical function of an inflection also influences the difficulty that children with SLI experience with the use of that particular inflection. Thus, children with SLI have greater difficulty using the third person singular inflection −s (he runs) and the possessive inflection −s (Michael's dog), than the plural inflection −s (three dogs).

Children with SLI commonly have problems with phonology (i.e. the system of sounds of a language). Phonologic problems can either be receptive (difficulty identifying or differentiating individual speech sounds) or expressive (producing the correct sounds for words). Isolated impairments in phonology are usually not considered to be sufficient to make a diagnosis of a language disorder; however, young children with SLI frequently have difficulties with expressive phonology or articulation (Bishop and Edmundson 1987a, Leonard 1998). Vocabulary is the area that tends to cause the least difficulty for children with SLI (Rice 1994, Bishop 1997, Leonard 1998, Webster et al. 2004) and so screening tests based predominantly on measures of vocabulary may fail to identify children with significant language impairments.

Difficulties with the social use of language (pragmatics) are not uncommon in children with SLI. In some children with SLI, difficulties with social communication are entirely explained by the effects of their language disorder and the resulting social limitations; however, there are a group of children with SLI in whom pragmatic impairment appears to be distinct and more severe than would be expected on the basis of their skills in other areas of language (Bishop and Norbury 2002). Given that pragmatic language impairments are a cardinal feature of autism, this is a group of children whose language disorder is similar to that seen in children with autism, which may pose diagnostic and nosologic challenges (Bishop and Norbury 2002).

While there are areas of language that commonly cause greater difficulties for children with SLI, the profiles of language performance in different children with SLI show considerable heterogeneity. Researchers have hoped that this phenotypic heterogeneity might reflect underlying biologic heterogeneity and so attempts have been made to identify similar profiles of language performance among children with SLI (Wilson and Risucci 1986, Rapin and Allen 1988, Korkman and Hakkinen-Rihu 1994, Conti-Ramsden et al. 1997, Van Weerdenburg et al. 2006). Conti-Ramsden and Botting (1997, 1999) used cluster analysis to identify children with similar profiles of language performance among 242 seven- and eight-year-olds with SLI. They identified five profiles of performance on language testing with features that were broadly similar to the categories originally proposed by Rapin and Allen (1988) based on clinical observation. However, when these children were retested a year after the original assessment, only 55% of children showed a similar performance profile. More recently, Van Weerdenburg et al. (2006) identified four different patterns of language impairment using cluster analysis which seemed to differentiate children with SLI both at 6 and 8 years of age. The proportion of 8-year-olds in particular clusters was much lower than in the 6-year-old group. These studies suggest that the language profiles of a relatively high proportion of children with SLI are not inherently stable.

Moreover, language impairments sometimes appear to resolve in younger children (Stothard et al. 1998, Bishop and Edmundson 1987a, 1987b). Bishop and

Edmundson (1987a, 1987b) found that 44% of children with a diagnosis of SLI at 4 years of age had normal language when retested 18 months later. However, when these children were reviewed 10 years later they were found to have subtle deficits in language, suggesting that some children may find ways of compensating for an underlying deficit (Stothard et al. 1998). The issue of phenotypic hetero-geneity and the observation that individual language profiles are not stable with time is a major issue for research. This suggests that a given deficit may lead to different problems with language at differing ages over the lifespan.

LACK OF 'SPECIFICITY' OF SLI: IMPAIRMENTS IN NON-LINGUISTIC DOMAINS

Impairments in areas of development unrelated to language are common in chil-dren with SLI. There is an increased incidence of attention-deficit disorders among children with SLI (Manor et al. 2001) and an increased incidence of language impair-ment among children with attention-deficit disorders (Tannock and Brown 2000). Fein et al. (1996) found significant impairments in attention and memory involving both visual and verbal domains in children classified as having a developmental language disorder.

Motor impairments (gross and fine motor) are common co-morbidities in chil-dren with language disorders. Several studies have reported that children with SLI have an increased incidence of motor abnormalities such as synkinesia and hyperreflexia (Trauner et al. 2000), dysdiadochokinesia (Johnston et al. 1981), poor praxis (Hill 1998), and slow performance of motor tasks (Bishop 2001). Rapin found that 17% of preschool age children with developmental language disorder had evidence of limb apraxia, although this percentage was significantly lower than in children with autistic spectrum disorders and children with both language and cognitive impairment who were examined concurrently (Rapin 1996b). Among a cohort of 43 children diagnosed with developmental language impairment prior to school entry, slightly more than half had evidence of fine and/or gross motor impairments on a standardized measure of motor function when followed up in early elementary school (Webster et al. 2005). This study also found that children's scores on tests of motor function correlated strongly with their performance on tests of communication, but were less strongly correlated with their objective cog-nitive skills. This finding suggests that factors required both for communication and motor skills contribute to the language deficits seen in SLI.

While most definitions of SLI require that a child's non-verbal IQ falls within the normal range, a number of studies of children with SLI have reported a skewed distribution of non-verbal IQs with a tendency for non-verbal IQ scores to cluster at the lower limits of the normal range (Stothard et al. 1998, Catts et al. 2002). Recently, Botting (2005) reported longitudinal data on performance IQ (PIQ) in 82 children with SLI followed from 7 to 14 years of age. Over a period of 7 years, the mean PIQ of these children fell from 106 to 83 (23 points). Thus, a high per-centage of children with SLI at 7 years of age would not meet generally accepted criteria for SLI in adolescence. While it is possible that these deficits result from covert requirements for adequate verbal processing skills in tests of non-verbal IQ, tests that attempt to assess purely visuospatial skills have also shown impairments in children with SLI (Johnston 1994).

The co-existence of SLI and a reading disability is common (Stothard et al. 1998, Snowling et al. 2000, Catts et al. 2002). Indeed, Snowling et al. (2000) found that 43% of children with SLI had a specific reading disability when assessed at 15 years of age. Conversely, in a study of 102 children identified as having a specific reading disabil-ity, McArthur et al. (2000) found that 52 (51%) would meet criteria for SLI. More recently, Catts et al. (2002) reported a lower incidence of co-morbid reading and language impairments in a longitudinal study of children with language impairments. This study found that 25% of children who met criteria for SLI in kindergarten had dyslexia in second, fourth and eighth grade, and that 20% of the children found to have dyslexia in these grades were originally classified as having SLI in kindergarten.

There is strong evidence that a child's phonologic skills (the ability to identify sounds within words) contribute to their ability to decode written words (Shaywitz 1998). Phonologic deficits are a common problem in children with SLI and hence the co-existence of SLI and dyslexia is not surprising. Bishop and Snowling (2004) argue that children with SLI are further disadvantaged by having a limited vocabu-lary and a poor understanding of grammar and discourse. These skills allow children to identify novel words on the basis of their context and also are critical to comprehending the meaning of written passages. For children with SLI, impair-ments in phonologic skills make it difficult to map written words to stored phono-logic codes and a poor understanding of grammatical structure with vocabulary limitations makes it difficult to derive meaning from written passages and hence to identify an unfamiliar word based on its context. Bishop and Snowling (2004) and Snowling and Hayiou-Thomas (2006) propose a model in which reading skills are determined by a combination of phonologic and language skills. Children with isolated phonologic impairments have pure dyslexia and have problems predomin-antly with decoding words, whereas children with phonologic deficits and language impairments have both difficulties with decoding words and a poor understand-ing of what they are actually reading.

In summary, factors that lead to language impairment are frequently not specific to language and also affect other neurologic and cognitive processes. Language may be the function that is most sensitive to the underlying deficit or may be more easily recognized than other impairments. Theoretical accounts of SLI need to explain a range of developmental deficits that extend well beyond language. SLI is rarely specific and for this reason it is has been argued that there is a need for a change in our terminology (Ors 2002).

IMPAIRMENTS IN PHONOLOGIC WORKING MEMORY IN SLI

In young children there is a strong correlation between language development and tests of phonologic working memory (Gathercole and Baddeley 1989, Gathercole et al. 1994, Adams and Gathercole 2000). Tests of non-word repetition are considered to assess the adequacy of a child's phonologic working memory (Gathercole and Baddeley 1989). Non-word repetition involves the repetition of nonsense words with varying numbers of syllables. Nonsense words with more syllables require more resources for storage in phonologic short-term memory than nonsense words with fewer syllables. Gathercole and Baddley found that children with SLI performed in a similar manner to comparison group children on one and two syllable non-words; however, on longer non-words their performance objectively deteriorated. This suggests that working memory limitations rather than articulatory impairments limited their performance (Gathercole and Baddeley 1990). A number of other studies have since confirmed the observation that non-word repetition is impaired in SLI (Gathercole and Baddeley 1990, Bishop et al. 1996, Snowling et al. 2000, Bishop 2001, Botting and Conti-Ramsden 2001). Indeed, it is uncommon for children with SLI to perform well on standardized tests of non-word repetition (Botting and Conti-Ramsden 2001). Even children with 'resolved' SLI have evidence of poor performance on later tests of non-word repetition (Bishop et al. 1996). These findings suggest that impairments in phonologic working memory may be a core deficit in SLI.

AUDITORY PROCESSING IN SLI

It has been known for some time that children with SLI have difficulty differentiating syllables that are acoustically similar, particularly stop consonant/vowel combinations (e.g. /ba/ and /da/). These sounds are characterized by acoustic waveforms that change within a very short time intervals – roughly 50ms or less (Tallal and Piercy 1974). These difficulties raised the possibility that some of the impairments seen in SLI might be caused by limitations in the brain's capacity to process rapidly changing sounds (rapid auditory processing). In a series of experiments, Tallal and Piercy (1973, 1974, 1975) investigated the auditory processing abilities of a small group of children with SLI using synthesized verbal and non-verbal sounds. They found that children with SLI had difficulty discriminating between sounds if the sounds had rapid transitions in frequency or if the sounds were separated by very short intervals (Tallal and Piercy 1974, 1975). If the period during which the change in frequency occurred was lengthened or the intervals between sounds was extended, then the performance of children with SLI normalized. It was considered that this resulted from an intrinsically impaired perception of sounds with a short acoustic duration. These results formed the basis of a program for treating children with SLI using acoustically modified sound (Merzenich et al. 1996, Tallal et al. 1996). The initial results of this program were very promising, with children showing dramatic gains in language after training for only a month (Merzenich et al. 1996, Tallal et al. 1996). A recent randomized controlled trial evaluating the effects of a commercial version of this program (Fast ForWord) in 6- to 10-year-old children with SLI, however, failed to find any significant difference between the treated group and control groups (Cohen et al. 2005).

While a number of researchers have found auditory processing deficits in children with SLI, the findings are by no means universal (McArthur and Bishop 2001). Bishop et al. (1999) found no link between the presence of language impairment and poor performance on tests of auditory temporal processing among a group of 14 twin pairs. Difficulties with auditory processing also appear to extend to tasks that require discriminating sounds of different frequencies (McArthur and Bishop 2004). It has been suggested that difficulties with frequency discrimination may account for poor performance in tests of rapid auditory processing that require a frequency discrimination judgment (e.g. which tone is higher?). It has also been argued that some of the impairments identified in the auditory processing skills of children with SLI may not result from primary deficits in the processing of sounds, but may actually be secondary to attention and memory limitations commonly seen in children with SLI (McArthur and Bishop 2004).

In summary, while difficulties in auditory processing (rapid auditory processing, frequency discrimination) occur more commonly in children with SLI, it is unclear whether these problems actually contribute to the language impairment seen in SLI. Impairments in rapid auditory processing do not appear to be necessary for a child to have a specific language impairment (Bishop et al. 1999) although they may contribute to the disorder.

NEUROPHYSIOLOGY OF SLI

Children with SLI more commonly have abnormalities on electroencephalogram (EEG) than children with normal language. Picard et al. (1998) reported the EEG findings during wakefulness and sleep in a series of 52 children with developmental dysphasia. Half of these children (26/52) were found to have epileptiform activity. Sleep recordings most frequently identified epileptiform activity. In the majority of children these abnormalities were not present during EEG recordings performed during wakefulness.

Most definitions of SLI exclude children with seizure disorders (Leonard 1998) and so children with language disorders and epilepsy (Staden et al. 1998, Berroya et al. 2004) or Landau–Kleffner syndrome are generally not considered to have SLI (Bishop 1997). In a cohort of 210 children identified as having a developmental language disorder (criteria broadly consistent with SLI), Rapin (1996a) found that approximately 5% had epilepsy.

Landau–Kleffner syndrome (acquired epileptic aphasia) is usually characterized by language regression, a profound impairment in receptive language (verbal auditory agnosia) which is often much greater than difficulties with expressive language, and behavioral difficulties. These features are not typically seen in SLI and so it is unlikely that the two disorders would be clinically confused (Bishop 1997).

The question of whether epileptiform discharges contribute to language impairment in SLI has not yet been resolved. Maccario et al. (1982) reported the EEG findings in seven children referred for investigation of verbal–non-verbal discrepancy; five of these children had no history of seizures and the remaining two only had seizures with fever. All children had focal epileptiform activity and four had periods of generalized epileptiform activity. The authors report that treatment with antiepileptic medication failed to influence epileptiform activity or the course of the language disorder and concluded that language impairment and the associated EEG findings represent an epiphenomenon associated with an unidentified neurophysiologic abnormality.

AUDITORY EVENT-RELATED BRAIN POTENTIALS

There is an increasing body of research examining electrophysiologic responses to acoustic stimuli in SLI. These studies have reported abnormalities both in children with SLI (Ors et al. 2002a, Uwer et al. 2002) and also in affected parents (Ors et al. 2002b). Ors et al. (2002a) studied auditory event-related potentials (ERP) in a group of 10 children with SLI using a paradigm in which children were asked to respond to an infrequently presented target tone or speech stimulus that differed from a more frequently presented stimulus. They found that children with SLI performed more poorly and had longer reaction times than did the comparison group in identifying discrepant tone and speech stimuli. In children with SLI, the P3 potential (a long latency positive potential occurring 300–800ms after the original stimulus) was found to have a prolonged latency and a lower amplitude than in the comparison group. Ors et al. (2002a) attributed these findings to an underlying deficit in the neuronal network of children with SLI. A subsequent study of the parents of children with SLI also found prolonged P3 latencies to speech stimuli in those parents with a history of language delay in childhood (Ors et al. 2002b).

McArthur and Bishop (2004) found that there were significant differences between the waveforms of ERP following a 600Hz tone in children with SLI when compared with controls. These differences were noted throughout the ERP starting with the immediate responses to auditory stimuli within the primary auditory cortex. Interestingly, these findings were not confined to those children with SLI with demonstrable difficulties with auditory processing.

Uwer et al. (2002) used mismatch negativity, an auditory event-related potential produced in response to a deviant sound, to study the processing of tone and speech stimuli in children with SLI. They found children with SLI had reduced mismatch negativity amplitudes in response to speech stimuli but not to pure tones. They hypothesized that these changes reflected an abnormal sensory memory for speech stimuli (Uwer et al. 2002).

NEUROPATHOLOGIC FINDINGS IN SLI

Given that SLI is not a fatal illness, pathologic studies are limited to children who have died of other causes, and hence are relatively rare. There are two studies that have reported neuropathologic findings in SLI (Landau et al. 1960, Cohen et al. 1989). Landau et al. (1960) reported the autopsy findings in a 10-year-old boy with congenital heart disease associated with severe language impairment and normal non-verbal intelligence. The child was found to have a bilateral loss of cortical tissue and underlying white matter in a region that extended back from the central sulci, involving the insulae and the region bordering the sylvian fissures. The medial geniculate nuclei also showed signs of severe degeneration. Cohen et al. (1989) described the neuropathologic findings in a 7-year-old girl with developmental dysphasia who died of Epstein–Barr virus infection. The girl was found to have a dysplastic gyrus in the left inferior frontal cortex with an abnormal symmetry of the auditory association cortex (planum temporale).

The overlap between dyslexia and SLI raises the possibility that some of the neuropathologic factors that contribute to dyslexia may also be relevant to SLI (Galaburda et al. 2006). Galaburda et al. (1985) described neuronal ectopia and cyto-architectonic dysplasia of the perisylvian cortex with an associated symmetry of the planum temporale (this is normally asymmetrical) in four young adults with dyslexia.

NEUROIMAGING IN SLI

Neuroimaging research in SLI has attempted to identify morphometric and functional factors that differentiate individuals with SLI from people with normal language. In most normal adults, the planum temporale (primary auditory cortex) has a leftward asymmetry (Geschwind and Levitsky 1968). This asymmetry is considered to be one of the factors underlying the lateralization of language to the left hemisphere and so there has been considerable research investigating patterns of brain asymmetry in children with SLI. A number of studies have reported evidence of atypical patterns of brain asymmetry in children with SLI involving perisylvian regions (Plante et al. 1991, Gauger et al. 1997, Leonard et al. 2002, Herbert et al. 2005), frontal regions (Jernigan et al. 1991), the pars triangularis (Gauger et al. 1997), and regions of the parietal lobe (Jernigan et al. 1991, Herbert et al. 2005). The findings of these studies are summarized in Table 10.1. The inconsistent regions identified may reflect differences in how regions of interest were defined and evaluated and the relatively small sample sizes in the studies thus far reported. However, it should be noted that a single study using a well-defined sample of children with SLI found normal patterns of cerebral asymmetry in children with SLI (Preis et al. 1998b). In this study, the only factor differentiating children with SLI from control children was a 7% reduction in forebrain volume.

There is also evidence that children with SLI are more likely to have focal CNS pathology. Trauner et al. (2000) reported that more than one-third of children with

TABLE 10.1
Volumetric magnetic resonance imaging (MRI) findings in children with specific language impairment (SLI)

Author	Sample	Methods	Findings
Plante et al. (1991)	8 SLI/8 controls	Region of interest, identified anatomically. Volumetric analysis	Significantly different pattern of asymmetry of the perisylvian region (frontal and parietal operculae, superior temporal gyrus and the planum temporale) when compared with controls. No other regions significantly different. Perisylvian asymmetry R = L or R>L (6/8 boys with SLI)
Jernigan et al. (1991)	20 LLI/12 controls	Brain parcelled into six regions of interest according to anatomical landmarks. Volumetric analysis	Total brain volumes not significantly different. Posterior perisylvian volume relatively smaller in children with SLI. Prefrontal asymmetry R>L Superior parietal L>R
Gauger et al. (1997)	11 SLI/19 controls	Measured surface of area of planum temporale, posterior ascending ramus, and pars triangularis	Children with SLI had significantly smaller right hemispheres and smaller plana temporale. Combination of surface area of the planum temporale and posterior ascending ramus R>L No significant differences in the surface areas of individual structures
Preis et al. (1998b)	21 SLI/21 controls	Regions of interest surface area of the palnum temporale and the palnum parietale	Children with SL had 7% less forebrain volume than control children. No difference in asymmetry in children with SLI
Bollich (2002)	17 SLI/18 controls	Regions of interest: primary auditory cortex (Heschl gyrus), planum temporale, posterior ascending ramus, superior temporal gyrus. Volumetric MRI	Right-handed children with SLI had no asymmetry of primary auditory cortex (Heschl gyrus) (controls leftward asymmetry). Left-handed children with SLI had leftward asymmetry (controls no asymmetry)
Leonard et al. (2002)	Three studies SLI/DRD/good readers/ adults and children	Measures of surface area and volume based on manual identification of regions of the cortex	Children with SLI tended to have significantly smaller volumes of the brain regions measured. Children with SLI had more symmetry of brain measures than children with DRD or controls
Herbert et al. (2004)	21 DLD/13 autism/29 controls	Semi-automated parcellation of white matter. Volumetric analysis	Children with DLD (and autism) had significantly greater volumes of white matter in the frontal temporal and occipital lobes than controls
De Fosse (2004)	9 SLI/22 autism/11 controls	Manual cortical parcellation	Boys with SLI and autism (with language impairment) had abnormal (rightward asymmetry of frontal language areas (inferior frontal gyrus, pars opercularis, pars triangularis). Exaggerated leftward asymmetry of the planum temporale in boys with SLI and language impaired boys with autism
Herbert et al. (2005)	15 DLD/16 autism/15 controls	Cortical parcellation with volumetric analysis	Boys with DLD (and autism) had more rightward asymmetrical cortex than controls. Boys with DLD had significantly less leftward asymmetrical cortex than either group

DLD, developmental language disorder; DRD, developmental reading disorder; LLI, language/learning impaired.

developmental language impairment (i.e. these children would meet criteria for SLI) had abnormalities on MRI, whereas no comparison group child was found to have an abnormality. The study found evidence of white matter lesions (including periventricular leukomalacia), white matter volume loss, and ventricular enlargement in 12 children drawn from a series of 35 children with developmental language impairment. Similarly, we found two children with significant structural brain abnormalities on MRI among nine children with SLI (Webster et al. 2008). One child had an area of left temporo-parietal porencephaly with white matter volume loss and the other child had a large left fronto-temporal arachnoid cyst with mass effect. None of 12 comparison group children had a significant structural brain abnormalitiy. Preis et al. (1998a) reported twins with SLI who were found to have focal gray matter heterotopia within the right and left parieto-temporal white matter. Other abnormal neuroimaging findings reported in SLI include abnormal morphology of the inferior frontal gyrus (Clark and Plante 1998) and an increased thickness of the corpus callosum (Njiokiktjien et al. 1994).

Newly developed techniques for morphometric analysis of the brain, such as voxel-based morphometry, have the potential to identify previously unsuspected structural brain abnormalities and allow for more robust statistic interpretation of findings than approaches that rely on non-standardized manual identification of regions of interest (Ashburner and Friston 2000). Herbert et al. (2004) used semi-automated white matter parcellation to examine localized white matter volumes in 21 children with a developmental language disorder and compared these with both autistic children and a healthy comparison group. White matter was divided into two compartments labeled the superficial/radiate white matter (corona radiata and subcortical U fibres reflecting almost all the subcortical white matter) and the sagittal and bridging system (deeper white matter and the corpus callosum). Children with a developmental language disorder were found to have significantly greater volumes of radiate and bridging white matter in the frontal, temporal, and occipital lobes than controls. A similar pattern was seen in children with autism although they also had greater white matter volumes than controls in the parietal lobe. As noted above, one other study that reported white matter volumes in children with SLI found that the total volume of white matter was decreased in the frontal lobes (Preis et al. 1998b).

Herbert et al. (2005) reported abnormal patterns of brain asymmetry in boys with either developmental language disorder or autism when compared with age and sex matched controls. The study found that these boys had substantially more rightward asymmetrical cortex than controls. Boys with developmental language disorder were also found to have less leftward asymmetrical cortex than either the autistic or control groups. These changes were noted mostly in the unimodal and higher order association cortex. In unimodal cortex, the degree of asymmetry was only significant if regions of unimodal cortex associated with language processing were included (e.g. the planum temporale). For higher order association cortex, there were statistically significant different patterns of asymmetry even if the areas predominantly involved in language were excluded from the analysis. They hypothesized that language was particularly vulnerable to these widespread abnormalities in the association cortex because it is heavily reliant on processing within association cortex.

In a study using voxel-based morphometry, Watkins et al. (2002a) identified significant reductions in gray matter within the caudate nucleus, sensorimotor cortex, and cerebellum in 10 related individuals with a familial speech-language disorder secondary to a mutation in the FOXP2 gene (Lai et al. 2001). The volume of the left caudate nucleus correlated directly with overall performance on tests of praxis, fine motor function, and non-word repetition. While this family has a more severe motor speech disorder than that usually seen in children with SLI, bordering on verbal dyspraxia (Vargha-Khadem et al. 1995; Watkins et al. 2002b), the study raises the possibility that abnormalities of subcortical gray matter structures might contribute to language impairment in SLI.

Thus, there is reasonably strong evidence that children with SLI have brains that are structurally different from children with normal language. To date, the most consistent finding is that children with SLI have abnormal patterns of cerebral asymmetry predominantly involving regions of language cortex. However, given the different regions of asymmetry identified, there is still remaining uncertainty as to whether methodologic differences or underlying true biologic heterogeneity have contributed to the discrepant findings.

FUNCTIONAL MAGNETIC RESONANCE IMAGING
Functional MRI (fMRI) uses changes in blood oxygen level dependent (BOLD) signal as a surrogate marker of neuronal activation. It offers better spatial resolution for studying language processing than electrophysiologic tests (e.g. ERP) and allows regional patterns of brain activation to be studied. FMRI has proved to be a useful tool for examining abnormalities in neural systems in children with dyslexia (Shaywitz et al. 2002) and more recently studies investigating language processing in children with SLI have appeared.

Weismer et al. (2005) studied eight adolescents with SLI and compared their behavioral and fMRI findings with eight controls. The tasks used for fMRI specifically targeted verbal working memory and involved tests requiring yes/no responses to sentences of varying length and grammatical complexity (encoding) followed by a task requiring the correct identification of the word at the end of these sentences after an interval (recognition). Adolescents with SLI activated similar brain regions to controls and did not show significant differences in lateralization. However, during the encoding task, the adolescents with SLI showed hypoactivation of the left parietal region and the left precentral sulcus. Both of these regions are normally activated by the memory requirements and attentional demands of these tasks. During the recognition task, these adolescents were found to have hypo-activation of the insular portion of the left inferior frontal gyrus, an area import-ant for language processing and retention of verbal information. Moreover, the children with SLI showed abnormal co-ordination of activity between the brain regions activated in the encoding and recognition tasks. The authors note that the areas of hypoactivation during the encoding tasks occurred in brain regions responsible for general attention and memory processes and were not restricted to regions involved in language processing.

GENETIC INFLUENCES ON THE DEVELOPMENT OF SLI

There is strong evidence to suggest that genetic factors influence the development of SLI. Stromswold (1998) reviewed 14 studies that reported the incidence of a positive family history of language impairment, usually a first degree relative with language impairment, or a history of language impairment, in children with develop-mental language impairment. In these studies, the median incidence of a positive family history of SLI was 39% (range 24–77%). In those studies that compared probands and controls, there was a significantly higher incidence of language impair-ment among the families of the probands.

Most studies have found a higher incidence of SLI in boys, with reported male:female ratios ranging from 1.3:1 to 5.9:1 (Tallal et al. 1989, Stromswold 1998, Stanton-Chapman et al. 2002). This finding suggests that either genetic (e.g. X-linked) or early hormonal factors may influence the development of SLI. However, Tomblin et al. (1997) found no significant difference between male and female prevalence of SLI in a systematically screened population sample, which raises the possibility that an ascertainment bias (i.e. a higher referral rate of affected boys for evaluation) may contribute to the higher reported incidence in boys (Tomblin et al. 1997, Stromswold 1998).

While an increased familial incidence of SLI could be explained by either environmental or genetic factors, twin studies have shown that genetic factors are probably more important. Bishop et al. (1995) reported a concordance rate for SLI of 72% for monozygotic twins compared with 49% for dizygotic twins based on an observed threshold 20-point non-verbal–verbal discrepancy in IQ. When more liberal criteria for language impairment were used, the concordance rate increased to 90% in monozygotic twins and 62% in dizygotic twins. Bishop (2001) also reported evidence of common genetic factors leading to an observed impairment on tests of motor performance and of spoken language (non-word repetition).

A more recent twin study (173 twin pairs) investigated the genetic influences on verbal working memory and grammar (i.e. verb tense marking) in a cohort in which children with language impairment were over-represented (Bishop et al. 2006). The study examined two behavioral markers of SLI: (1) non-word repetition, and

(2) verb tense marking (e.g. the use of third person singular 'she walks to school'). Both of these traits proved to have significant heritability, with genetic factors accounting for a large proportion of the variance in both measures. Interestingly, these traits appeared to be influenced by different genetic factors. This argues against the hypothesis that grammatical impairments can be explained on the basis of impairments in sound processing. These findings suggest that two of the most important recognized psycholinguistic markers of SLI have independent genetic origins.

In one family, a dominant mutation in the FOXP2 gene (a transcription factor) has been found to be associated with a severe speech and language disorder (Vargha-Khadem et al. 1995, Lai et al. 2001, Watkins et al. 2002a, 2002b). A different mutation in FOXP2 was subsequently found in another family with a dominantly inherited speech-language disorder (MacDermot et al. 2005). However, individuals with mutations in FOXP2 have a more severe speech disorder than that usually seen in SLI, and mutations in FOXP2 do not appear to be a common cause of SLI when populations of sporadic cases are screened for this gene (Newbury et al. 2002, O'Brien et al. 2003).

Two groups have performed genome-wide scans on families containing individuals with SLI, looking for evidence of linkage to specific chromosomal loci (Bartlett et al. 2002, 2004, SLI Consortium 2002, 2004). The SLI Consortium (2002) found linkage between quantitative measures of language impairment and two separate loci on chromosomes 16 and 19. The locus on chromosome 16 was associated with poor performance on a non-word repetition test, whereas the locus on chromosome 19 was linked to poor performance on an expressive language test (SLI Consortium 2002). When data from this original study were combined with those derived from a new cohort of families with language disorders, the locus on chromosome 16 proved to have highly significant linkage with performance on non-word repetition and also with performance on tests of reading and spelling (SLI Consortium 2004). However, the locus on chromosome 19 was no longer significant. These findings suggest that a region of chromosome 16 is important for phonologic working memory.

Bartlett et al. (2002) used a genome-wide screen to identify regions associated with language impairment, reading impairment, or a history of language difficulty in five Canadian families with a history of language or reading impairment. In contrast to the studies cited above, a categoric approach was used in which individuals were classified as being either impaired or normal. The study found that a locus on chromosome 13 (i.e. 13q21) was strongly linked to a phonologic measure of reading impairment (non-word reading more than 1 SD below performance IQ). In a subsequent study, using an independent sample of US families with a history of language impairment, reading impairment was again found to be linked to the same locus (Bartlett et al. 2004). However, the authors note that this evidence of linkage was found in less than 30% of the families and thus this region may not be a general risk factor for SLI.

Regions of chromosome 7 on either side of the FOXP2 gene were found to be linked to language impairment in a large sample of North American families where the proband was identified as having SLI (O'Brien et al. 2003). However, no mutations were identified when exon 14 of the FOXP2 gene (the abnormal exon in the original KE family) was sequenced in children with SLI. Bartlett et al. (2004) also found evidence of linkage to this chromosome 7 region.

In summary, there is strong evidence from converging methodologies (epidemiologic studies, twin studies, linkage studies, and genome-wide screens) that various genetic factors are important determinants of language impairment seen in SLI. The distinct and differing regions of chromosomes identified by the European and North American studies likely reflect differing approaches to identifying language impairment (quantitative trait locus versus categorical identification of impairment), different methods used to recruit the populations studied, and underlying genetic differences between the groups studied.

ENVIRONMENTAL INFLUENCES ON THE DEVELOPMENT OF LANGUAGE

There is evidence that antenatal and perinatal factors may contribute to the development of SLI. In an epidemiologic study, Stanton-Chapman et al. (2002) examined risk factors at birth which were associated with being identified as having SLI in early elementary school. A total of 5862 children with SLI aged 6–7 years were studied drawn from a population of 244 619 school students. Adjusted odd ratios showed that 5-minute Apgar score less than 3, low birth weight <2500g (particularly very low birth weight <1500g), high birth order (third or greater), a shorter duration of maternal education, maternal marital status (single opposed to coupled), and late commencement of antenatal care were associated with a significant increase in the risk of SLI. It is clear that some of these factors reflect various attributes of maternal socioeconomic status and may relate at a basic level to either genetic or environmental influences on the development of language. However, the increased risk associated with low birth weight and a low 5-minute Apgar score suggests that chronic prenatal or acute perinatal adversity may lead to or at least predispose to later SLI. Unfortunately, this paper provides few data about the objective criteria used to identify SLI in elementary school. In contrast, Rapin (1996a) found no evidence that preschool children with developmental language disorders were more likely to have been born preterm, have a low birthweight, or have had perinatal complications than children with autistic spectrum disorder or children with more global cognitive impairments.

Two further studies have provided evidence that prenatal or perinatal insults may specifically impair language development (Singer et al. 2001, Bandstra et al. 2002). Singer et al. (2001) found evidence of language impairment that was independent of cognitive function in 3-year-old children with a history of bronchopulmonary dysplasia. A longitudinal study of the effects of prenatal cocaine exposure found evidence of language impairment in children with prenatal cocaine exposure (Bandstra et al. 2002). This effect persisted when the effect of co-variates, such as IQ and the adequacy of the language exposure at home, were controlled for.

THEORETICAL ACCOUNTS OF SLI

Theoretical accounts of SLI reflect how researchers view the psychobiologic basis of language, in particular, whether they consider language to be 'modular' (largely independent of other cognitive systems) or mainly dependent upon factors that are also important for other cognitive systems. Supporters of a modular view of language would argue that the fact that language can be specifically impaired implies that some biologic factors are unique to language. Disorders such as Williams syndrome, in which children have language skills that are significantly better than their non-verbal cognitive function skills, demonstrate that language performance can be dissociated from other aspects of cognitive function (Marcus and Rabagliati 2006).

However, SLI is frequently associated with a range of other developmental impairments (Bishop and Edmundson 1987b, Johnston 1994, Hill 1998, Tannock and Brown 2000, Trauner et al. 2000, Bishop 2001, Manor et al. 2001). This suggests that the factors that lead to language impairment are also important for the function of other neurologic processes. Marcus and Rabagliati (2006) propose that a large part of the neurobiologic substrate which permits language also contributes to other cognitive processes. However, there are specific factors that are critical for language which have little effect on other cognitive processes. This model suggests that language will usually be impaired along with other cognitive processes; however, it also permits the possibility of relatively specific language impairment.

Several theories have been proposed to explain the problems with morpho-syntax seen in SLI. On the basis of a study of a large family with autosomal dominant language impairment that was subsequently found to have a mutation in the FOXP2 gene, Gopnik and Crago (1991) hypothesized that affected individuals within the family were unable to learn the rules that allow the generation of inflections (e.g. the past tense inflection *ed* as in walk*ed*) and so learned inflected forms of words as new words. They further theorized that a single gene controlled the ability to generate the inflected forms of these words. Subsequent research on members of this family found a broader phenotype than among affected individuals with intellectual, linguistic, and motor impairments (Vargha-Khadem et al. 1995, Watkins et al. 2002b). Moreover, affected family members were found to overregularize irregular verbs suggesting that they did have an awareness of grammatical rules; however, sometimes these rules were applied inappropriately.

The 'surface' hypothesis proposed by Leonard (1998) also addressed the particular difficulty that children with SLI have with grammatical infections, particularly third person singular –s, possessive –s, and past tense –ed. These inflections are of short duration and children with SLI have been shown to have difficulties processing rapidly changing sounds. Leonard hypothesized that as a result of processing limitations, perhaps from inadequate representation in verbal working memory, these inflections were more often omitted. However, Leonard (1998) notes that this theory is unable to account for the range of linguistic problems encountered in children with SLI.

A number of authors have suggested that the fundamental deficit in SLI is a limitation in the brain's capacity to process information rapidly (Bishop 1997, Leonard 1998, Miller et al. 2001, Montgomery 2002). Evidence for processing limitations is seen in studies showing that children with SLI have longer response times associated with performing linguistic and non-linguistic tasks (Ors et al. 2002a, Uwer et al. 2002, Miller et al. 2001, Montgomery 2002). More complex grammatical structures may take longer to process than simpler structures. With increasing sentence complexity, structures that place greater demands on processing resources such as grammatical inflections may be omitted. Other factors that increase processing demands, such as phonologic complexity and even prosodic difficulty, can impair comprehension and speech production in children with SLI (Leonard 1998). Limitations in the amount of information that can be stored in verbal working memory may further constrain language processing capability (Weismer et al. 1999, Montgomery 2002).

Recently, Ullman and Pierpont (2005) hypothesized that the range of linguistic and non-linguistic impairments could be accounted for by deficits in the 'procedural memory' system. This system is involved in learning new skills and procedures. The anatomic substrate for the procedural memory system is the frontal cortex (especially premotor cortex and Broca area) and the basal ganglia (especially the caudate and the putamen) with some contribution from regions of the parietal and temporal cortices and the cerebellum. They posited that damage to this region could explain the greater difficulties that children with SLI have with linguistic processes that require the consistent application of rules (e.g. grammatical structure), when compared with word retrieval tasks which largely rely on declarative memory (i.e. the memory for facts). They also contend that deficits in the neurologic network underlying the procedural memory system could account for impairments both in working memory and in temporal processing which are reported in SLI.

FUTURE RESEARCH DIRECTIONS IN SLI

Our understanding of the neurobiology of SLI has advanced considerably and is likely to progress rapidly with the development of new genetic and imaging technologies. Given the wide range of co-morbidities seen in SLI, it would seem likely that the biologic factors that lead to 'specific' language impairment are also important for other brain functions. Language researchers have spent considerable time attempting to classify a child's language phenotype; however, little research has been conducted into establishing the broader phenotype. For example, does the presence or absence of motor impairments or attentional deficits change the language phenotype? Such information may allow the development of a more detailed phenotype, perhaps identifying biologic heterogeneity which is not obvious solely on applying tests restricted to an evaluation of language.

A better understanding of the broader developmental profile of SLI has obvious relevance for genetic studies. It is likely that genes that affect language are also important for other neurologic functions. Detailed clinical and imaging studies have delineated a complex language, cognitive, and motor phenotype associated with the FOXP2 mutation (Vargha-Khadem et al. 1995, Watkins et al. 2002a, 2002b). Similar studies in broader groups of children with SLI would potentially allow the identification of genetic factors that influence not only language but also other neurologic functions. Newer approaches to identifying chromosomal loci that quantitatively influence the core psycholinguistic features of SLI have the potential to avoid some of the difficulties inherent in deciding who has SLI as well as identifying traits that independently contribute to language impairment (SLI Consortium 2002, 2004).

New techniques for structural imaging have great potential to improve our understanding of SLI. There is strong evidence that children with SLI have abnormal patterns of cerebral asymmetry (Jernigan et al. 1991, Plante et al. 1991, Gauger et al. 1997, De Fosse et al. 2004, Herbert et al. 2005). However, the underlying factors that cause these abnormal patterns of asymmetry remain to be delineated. For example, is abnormal asymmetry the cause of the language disorder or is it secondary to abnormal use of language cortex during development? Longitudinal studies might help resolve this issue. There is evidence that SLI is associated with an increase in white matter volume although only one study to date has addressed this (Herbert et al. 2004) and there is a need for this finding to be replicated. If white matter volume is increased, then its cause remains to be delineated. New technologies that allow the mapping of fiber tracts such as diffusion tensor imaging may cast light on abnormalities in white matter.

Despite suggestions that subtle cortical dysplasias may contribute to SLI, an analysis of cortical thickness has not yet been reported although studies that have used cortical parcellation suggest that there is asymmetry of gray matter in language cortex (De Fosse et al. 2004). There are limited data on the morphometry of subcortical structures involved in language (e.g. the cerebellum and basal ganglia) in SLI.

The potential for functional studies to further our understanding of the causes of SLI is considerable. ERP studies have provided strong evidence that the brains of children with SLI show different electrical responses to acoustic stimuli than typically developing children (Ors et al. 2002a, Uwer et al. 2002, McArthur and Bishop 2004). Abnormalities of brain activation have also been shown using fMRI

(Weismer et al. 2005). There are very few data on the use of magnetoencephalo-graphy in children with SLI; however, its temporal resolution is superior to that of fMRI and provides better spatial localization than ERP. Studies using a combination of these measures are likely to further delineate abnormalities of language processing which differentiate children with SLI from children with normal language. These techniques may demonstrate both spatial and temporal abnormalities in the way that language is processed in children with SLI. They may also reveal functional differences associated with the phenotypic heterogeneity seen in SLI and serve to document how interventions influence language processing. Functional studies may also show how other networks are recruited to compensate for language processing difficulties.

CAN KNOWLEDGE OF NEUROBIOLOGY INFLUENCE TREATMENT?

A better understanding of the neurobiology of SLI is not only of academic interest. While most studies show language intervention is effective (Nye et al. 1987), it is common for children with SLI to be left with a significant language disability despite optimal present therapy (Leonard 1998). Therapy for children with SLI tends to be empiric. Better understanding of the basis of a child's language impairment potentially would allow more specifically targeted therapy, avoidance of therapy that is ineffective, an ability to predict associated co-morbidity, and a better ability to prognosticate regarding eventual outcome. It also may allow the identification of markers indicating a young child at risk of developing SLI, allowing earlier commencement of therapy and a greater likelihood of an improved outcome, emphasizing broader community participation for the affected individual.

CONCLUSIONS

Despite its designation, SLI is not truly 'specific.' While language is the function that is most obviously impaired in SLI, non-verbal cognition, motor skills, and attention are frequently affected. Given the range of co-morbidities seen in SLI, it would seem that some children might be more appropriately considered to have specific *preservation* of non-verbal cognition.

Receptive language is characterized by a need to store and analyze a stream of acoustic information followed by rapid sequential processing as sounds are decoded and meaning is extracted using grammatical rules and an understanding of context and social rules (Bishop 1997). Speech requires the initial conceptualization of an idea to be expressed, the retrieval of words from a lexical store, and the rapid generation of appropriate grammatical structures followed by the activation of motor programs (Indefrey and Levelt 2000). The impairment of a general cognitive process (e.g. working memory) may produce what appears to be a relatively specific language impairment because of the heavy reliance of language on this function.

Current theories of SLI hold that the language and cognitive impairments seen in SLI result from limitations in the capacity for, and the speed with which, information can be processed (Bishop 1997, Leonard 1998). Understanding of speech may be constrained further by limitations in verbal short-term memory (Gathercole and Baddeley 1990, Bishop et al. 1996, Botting and Conti-Ramsden 2001) and in difficulties differentiating acoustic stimuli (Tallal and Piercy 1973, 1974, 1975, McArthur and Bishop 2001). Electrophysiologic studies have provided evidence that the early phases of auditory processing are abnormal in children with SLI (Ors et al. 2002a, Uwer et al. 2002). Neuroimaging studies suggest that atypical patterns of asymmetry of language cortex and an increase in the volume of more peripheral cerebral white matter are indeed risk factors for SLI (Jernigan et al. 1991, Plante et al. 1991, Gauger et al. 1997, Leonard et al. 2002, De Fosse et al. 2004, Herbert et al. 2004, 2005). Focal damage or dysgenesis of perisylvian cortex is also associated with a phenotype consistent with SLI (Landau et al. 1960, Cohen et al. 1989, Preis et al. 1998a).

SLI is perhaps a description of a cognitive phenotype rather than a single unique biologic disorder. When the phenotypic heterogeneity of SLI is considered, it is perhaps not surprising that there is evidence of biologic heterogeneity. It is likely that both genetic (Bishop et al. 1995, 2006, SLI Consortium 2002, Bartlett et al. 2002, 2004) and environmental (Singer et al. 2001, Bandstra et al. 2002, Stanton-Chapman et al. 2002) risk factors contribute and often interact, leading to the development of SLI. It is hoped that future research into the causes of SLI will identify biologic factors that limit language processing and also influence other cognitive processes. A better understanding of the neurobiology of SLI is critical for the rational development of therapeutic strategies to treat this common disorder.

REFERENCES

Adams A, Gathercole SE (2000) Limitations in working memory: implications for language development. *Int J Lang Commun Disord* 35: 95–116.

American Psychiatric Association – Taskforce on DSM-IV (2000) *Diagnostic and Statistical Manual of Mental Disorders IV-TR.* American Psychiatric Association: Washington.

Aram DM, Ekelman BL, Nation JE. (1984) Preschoolers with language disorders: 10 years later. *J Speech Hear Res* 27: 232–244.

Aram DM, Morris R, Hall NE (1993) Clinical and research congruence in identifying children with specific language impairment. *J Speech Hear Res* 36: 580–591.

Ashburner J, Friston KJ (2000) Voxel-based morphometry: the methods. *Neuroimage* 11: 805–821.

Bandstra ES, Morrow CE, Vogel AL, Fifer RC, Ofir AY, Dausa AT, et al. (2002) Longitudinal influence of prenatal cocaine exposure on child language functioning. *Neurotoxicol Teratol* 24: 297–308.

Bartlett CW, Flax JF, Logue MW, Smith BJ, Vieland VJ, Tallal P, et al. (2004) Examination of potential overlap in autism and language loci on chromosomes 2, 7, and 13 in two independent samples ascertained for specific language impairment. *Hum Hered* 57: 10–20.

Bartlett CW, Flax JF, Logue MW, Vieland VJ, Bassett AS, Tallal P, et al. (2002) A major susceptibility locus for specific language impairment is located on 13q21. *Am J Hum Genet* 71: 45–55.

Benasich AA, Thomas JJ, Choudhury N, Leppanen PHT (2002) The importance of rapid auditory processing abilities to early language development: evidence from converging methodologies. *Dev Psychobiol* 47: 278–292.

Berroya AG, McIntyre J, Webster R, Lah S, Sabaz M, Lawson J, et al. (2004) Speech and language deterioration in benign rolandic epilepsy. *J Child Neurol* 19: 53–58.

Bishop DV (1994) Is specific language impairment a valid diagnostic category? Genetic and psycholinguistic evidence. *Philos Trans R Soc Lond B Biol Sci* 346: 105–111.

Bishop DVM (1997) *Uncommon Understanding: Development and Disorders of Language Comprehension in Children.* Hove: Psychology Press.

Bishop DV (2000) How does the brain learn language? Insights from the study of children with and without language impairment. *Dev Med Child Neurol* 42: 133–142.

Bishop DV (2001) Motor immaturity and specific speech and language impairment: evidence for a common genetic basis. *Am J Med Genet* 114: 56–63.

Bishop DV, Adams CV, Norbury CF (2006) Distinct genetic influences on grammar and phonological short-term memory deficits: evidence from 6-year-old twins. *Genes Brain Behav* 5: 158–169.

Bishop DV, Edmundson A (1987a) Language-impaired 4-year-olds: distinguishing transient from persistent impairment. *J Speech Lang Hear Dis* 52: 156–173.

Bishop DV, Edmundson A (1987b) Specific language impairment as a maturational lag: evidence from longitudinal data on language and motor development. *Dev Med Child Neurol* 29: 442–459.

Bishop DVM, North T, Donlan C (1995) Genetic basis of specific language impairment: evidence from a twin study. *Dev Med Child Neurol* 37: 56–71.

Bishop DVM, North T, Donlan C (1996) Nonword repetition as a behavioral marker for inherited language impairment: evidence from a twin study. *J Child Psychol Psychiatry* 37: 391–403.

Bishop DV, Carlyon RP, Deeks JM, Bishop SJ (1999) Auditory temporal processing impairment: neither necessary nor sufficient for causing language impairment in children. *J Speech Lang Hear Res* 42: 1295–1310.

Bishop DVM, Norbury C (2002) Exploring the borderlands of autistic disorder and specific language impairment: a study using standardized diagnostic instruments. *J Child Psychol Psychiatry* 43: 917–929.

Bishop DVM, Snowling MJ (2004) Developmental dyslexia and specific language impairment: same or different? *Psychol Bull* 130: 858–886.

Bollich AM, Leonard CM, Knaus T, Corey DM, Lombardino LJ, Fennell EB, et al. (2002) Atypical anatomy of primary auditory cortex in children with specific language impairment. *Neurology* 58: 7 (Suppl 3): A269.

Botting N (2005) Non-verbal cognitive development and language impairment. *J Child Psychol Psychiatry* 46: 317–326.

Botting N, Conti-Ramsden G (2001) Non-word repetition and language development in children with specific language impairment (SLI). *Int J Lang Commun Disord* 36: 421–432.

Catts HW, Fey ME, Tomblin JB, Zhang X (2002) A longitudinal investigation of reading outcomes in children with language impairments. *J Speech Lang Hear Res* 45: 1142–1157.

Clark MM, Plante E (1998) Morphology of the inferior frontal gyrus in developmentally language-disordered adults. *Brain Lang* 61: 288–303.

Cohen M, Campbell R, Yaghmai F (1989) Neuropathological abnormalities in developmental dysphasia. *Ann Neurol* 25: 567–570.

Cohen W, Hodson A, O'Hare A, Boyle J, Durrani T, McCartney E, et al. (2005) Effects of computer-based intervention through acoustically modified speech (Fast ForWord) in severe mixed receptive-expressive language impairment: outcomes from a randomized controlled trial. *J Speech Lang Hear Res* 48: 715–729.

Conti-Ramsden G, Botting N (1999) Classification of children with specific language impairment: longitudinal considerations. *J Speech Lang Hear Res* 42: 1195–1204.

Conti-Ramsden G, Crutchley A, Botting N (1997) The extent to which psychometric tests differentiate subgroups of children with SLI. *J Speech Lang Hear Res* 40: 765–777.

De Fosse L, Hodge SM, Makris N, Kennedy DN, Caviness VSJr, McGrath L, et al. (2004) Language-association cortex asymmetry in autism and specific language impairment. *Ann Neurol* 56: 757–766.

Fein D, Dunn M, Allen DA, Aram DM, Hall N, Morris R, et al. (1996) Language and neuropsychological findings. In: Rapin I (ed) *Preschool Children with Inadequate Communication.* London: Mac Keith Press, pp 123–154.

Galaburda AM, LoTurco J, Ramus F, Fitch RH, Rosen GD (2006) From genes to behavior in developmental dyslexia. *Nat Neurosci* 9: 1213–1217.

Galaburda AM, Sherman GF, Rosen GD, Aboitiz F, Geschwind N (1985) Developmental dyslexia: four consecutive patients with cortical anomalies. *Ann Neurol* 18: 222–233.

Gathercole SE, Baddeley AD (1989) Evaluation of the role of phonological STM in the development of vocabulary in children: a longitudinal study. *J Mem Lang* 28: 200–213.

Gathercole SE, Baddeley AD (1990) Phonological memory deficits in language disordered children: is there a causal connection? *J Mem Lang* 29: 336–360.

Gathercole SE, Willis C, Baddeley AD, Emslie H (1994) The children's test of nonword repetition: a test of phonological working memory. *Memory* 2: 103–127.

Gauger LM, Lombardino LJ, Leonard CM (1997) Brain morphology in children with specific language impairment. *J Speech Lang Hear Res* 40: 1272–1284.

Geschwind N, Levitsky W (1968) Human brain: left–right asymmetries in temporal speech region. *Science* 161: 186–187.

Gopnik M, Crago MB (1991) Familial aggregation of a developmental language disorder. *Cognition* 39: 1–50.

Herbert MR, Ziegler DA, Deutsch CK, O'Brien LM, Kennedy DN, Filipek PA, et al. (2005) Brain asymmetries in autism and developmental language disorder: a nested whole-brain analysis. *Brain* 128: 213–226.

Herbert MR, Ziegler DA, Makris N, Filipek PA, Kemper TL, Normandin JJ, et al. (2004) Localization of white matter volume increase in autism and developmental language disorder. *Ann Neurol* 55: 530–540.

Hill EL (1998) A dyspraxic deficit in specific language impairment and developmental coordination disorder? Evidence from hand and arm movements. *Dev Med Child Neurol* 40: 388–395.

Indefrey P, Levelt WJM (2000) The neural correlates of language production. In: Gazzaniga MSE (ed) *The New Cognitive Neurosciences.* Cambridge, MA: MIT Press, pp 845–958.

Jernigan TL, Hesselink JR, Sowell E, Tallal PA (1991) Cerebral structure on magnetic resonance imaging in language- and learning-impaired children. *Arch Neurol* 48: 539–545.

Johnston JR (1994) Cognitive abilities of children with language impairment. In: Watkins RV, Rice ML (eds) *Specific Language Impairments in Children.* Baltimore: Paul H. Brookes, pp 107–121.

Johnston RB, Stark RE, Mellits ED, Tallal P (1981) Neurological status of language-impaired and normal children. *Ann Neurol* 10: 159–163.

Korkman M, Hakkinen-Rihu P (1994) A new classification of developmental language disorders (DLD). *Brain Lang* 47: 96–116.

Kovas Y, Hayiou-Thomas ME, Oliver B, Dale PS, Bishop DV, Plomin R (2005) Genetic influences in different aspects of language development: the etiology of language skills in 4.5-year-old twins. *Child Dev* 76: 632–651.

Lahey M (1990) Who shall be called language disordered? Some reflections and one perspective. *J Speech Hear Dis* 55: 612–620.

Lai CS, Fisher SE, Hurst JA, Vargha-Khadem F, Monaco AP (2001) A forkhead-domain gene is mutated in a severe speech and language disorder. *Nature* 413: 519–523.

Landau WM, Goldstein R, Kleffner FR (1960) Congenital aphasia: a clinicopathologic study. *Neurology* 10: 915–921.

Leonard CM, Lombardino LJ, Walsh K, Eckert MA, Mockler JL, Rowe LA, et al. (2002) Anatomical risk factors that distinguish dyslexia from SLI predict reading skill in normal children. *J Commun Dis* 35: 501–531.

Leonard LB (1998) *Children with Specific Language Impairment.* Cambridge, MA: MIT Press.

Maccario M, Hefferen SJ, Keblusek SJ, Lipinski KA (1982) Developmental dysphasia and electroencephalographic abnormalities. *Dev Med Child Neurol* 24: 141–155.

MacDermot KD, Bonora E, Sykes N, Coupe AM, Lai CS, Vernes SC, et al. (2005) Identification of FOXP2 truncation as a novel cause of developmental speech and language deficits. *Am J Hum Genet* 76: 1074–1080.

Manor O, Shalev RS, Joseph A, Gross-Tsur V (2001) Arithmetic skills in kindergarten children with developmental language disorders. *Eur J Ped Neurol* 5: 71–77.

Marcus G, Rabagliati H (2006) What developmental disorders can tell us about the nature and origins of language. *Nat Neurosci* 9: 1226–1229.

McArthur GM, Bishop DV (2001) Auditory perceptual processing in people with reading and oral language impairments: current issues and recommendations. *Dyslexia* 7: 150–170.

McArthur GM, Bishop DVM (2004) Which people with specific language impairment have auditory processing deficits? *Cogn Neuropsychol* 21: 79–94.

McArthur GM, Hogben JH, Edwards VT, Heath SM, Mengler ED (2000) On the 'specifics' of specific reading disability and specific language impairment. *J Child Psychol Psychiatry* 41: 869–874.

Merzenich MM, Jenkins WM, Johnston P, Schreiner C, Miller SL, Tallal P (1996) Temporal processing deficits of language-learning impaired children ameliorated by training. *Science* 271: 77–81.

Miller CA, Kail R, Leonard LB, Tomblin JB (2001) Speed of processing in children with specific language impairment. *J Speech Lang Hear Res* 44: 416–433.

Montgomery JW (2002) Information processing and language comprehension in children with specific language impairment. *Top Lang Disord* 22: 62–90.

Newbury DF, Bonora E, Lamb JA, Fisher SE, Lai CS, Baird G, et al. International Molecular Genetic Study of Autism Consortium (2002) FOXP2 is not a major susceptibility gene for autism or specific language impairment. *Am J Hum Genet* 70: 1318–1327.

Njiokiktjien C, de Sonneville L, Vaal J (1994) Callosal size in children with learning disabilities. *Behav Brain Res* 64: 213–218.

Nye C, Foster S, Seaman D (1987) Effectiveness of language intervention with the language/learning disabled. *J Speech Hearing Disord* 52: 348–357.

O'Brien EK, Zhang X, Nishimura C, Tomblin JB, Murray JC (2003) Association of specific language impairment (SLI) to the region of 7q31. *Am J Hum Genet* 72: 1536–1543.

Ors M (2002) Time to drop 'specific' in 'specific language impairment'. *Acta Paediatr* 91: 1025–1030.

Ors M, Lindgren M, Blennow G, Nettelbladt U, Sahlen B, Rosen I (2002a) Auditory event-related brain potentials in children with specific language impairment. *Eur J Ped Neurol* 6: 47–62.

Ors M, Lindgren M, Blennow G, Rosen I (2002b) Auditory event-related brain potentials in parents of children with specific language impairment. *Eur J Ped Neurol* 6: 242–249.

Picard A, Cheliout HF, Bouskraoui M, Lemoine M, Lacert P, Delattre J (1998) Sleep EEG and developmental dysphasia. *Dev Med Child Neurol* 40: 595–599.

Plante E, Swisher L, Vance R, Rapcsak S (1991) MRI findings in boys with specific language impairment. *Brain Lang* 41: 52–66.

Preis S, Engelbrecht V, Huang Y, Steinmetz H (1998a) Focal grey matter heterotopias in monozygotic twins with developmental language disorder. *Eur J Ped Neurol* 157: 849–852.

Preis S, Lancke L, Schittler P, Huang Y, Steinmetz H (1998b) Normal intrasylvian anatomical asymmetry in children with developmental language disorder. *Neuropsychologia* 36: 849–855.

Rapin I (1996a) Historical data. In: Rapin I (ed) *Preschool Children with Inadequate Communication*. London: Mac Keith Press, pp 53–97.

Rapin I (1996b) Neurological examination. In: Rapin I (ed) *Preschool Children with Inadequate Communication*. London: Mac Keith Press, pp 98–122.

Rapin I, Allen D (1988) Syndromes in developmental dysphasia and aphasia. In: Plum F (ed) *Language Communication and the Brain*. New York: Raven Press.

Records NL, Tomblin JB (1994) Clinical decision making: describing the decision rules of practicing speech-language pathologists. *J Speech Lang Hear Res* 37: 144–156.

Rice ML (1994) Grammatical categories of children with specific language impairment. In: Watkins RV, Rice ML (eds) *Specific Language Impairments in Children*. Baltimore: Paul H Brookes Publishing, pp 69–88.

Shaywitz BA, Shaywitz SE, Pugh KR, Mencl WE, Fulbright RK, Skudlarski P, et al. (2002) Disruption of posterior brain systems for reading in children with developmental dyslexia. *Biol Psychiatry* 52: 101–110.

Shaywitz SE (1998) Dyslexia. *N Engl J Med* 338: 307–312.

Shevell MI, Majnemer A, Rosenbaum P, Abrahamowicz M (2000) Etiologic yield of single domain developmental delay: a prospective study. *J Pediatr* 137: 633–637.

Singer LT, Siegel AC, Lewis B, Hawkins S, Yamashita T, Baley J (2001) Preschool language outcomes of children with history of bronchopulmonary dysplasia and very low birth weight. *J Dev Behav Pediatr* 22: 19–26.

SLI Consortium (2002) A genomewide scan identifies two novel loci involved in specific language impairment. *Am J Hum Genet* 70: 384–398.

SLI Consortium (2004) Highly significant linkage to the SLI1 locus in an expanded sample of individuals affected by specific language impairment. *Am J Hum Genet* 41: 407–418.

Snowling M, Bishop DVM, Stothard SE (2000) Is preschool language impairment a risk factor for dyslexia in adolescence? *J Child Psychol Psychiatry* 41: 587–600.

Snowling MJ, Hayiou-Thomas ME (2006) The dyslexia spectrum: continuities between reading, speech, and language impairments. *Top Lang Disord* 26: 110–126.

Staden U, Isaacs E, Boyd SG, Brandl U, Neville BG (1998) Language dysfunction in children with Rolandic epilepsy. *Neuropediatrics* 29: 242–248.

Stanton-Chapman, Chapman DA, Bainbridge NL, Scott KG (2002) Identification of early risk factors for language impairment. *Res Dev Disabil* 23: 390–405.

Stothard SE, Snowling MJ, Bishop DV, Chipchase BB, Kaplan CA (1998) Language-impaired preschoolers: a follow-up into adolescence. *J Speech Lang Hear Res* 41: 407–418.

Stromswold K (1998) Genetics of spoken language disorders. *Hum Biol* 70: 297–324.

Tallal P, Miller SL, Bedi G, Byma G, Wang X, Nagarajan SS, et al. (1996) Language comprehension in language-learning impaired children improved with acoustically modified speech. *Science* 271: 81–84.

Tallal P, Piercy M (1973) Developmental aphasia: impaired rate of non-verbal processing as a function of sensory modality. *Neuropsychologia* 11: 389–398.

Tallal P, Piercy M (1974) Developmental aphasia: rate of auditory processing and selective impairment of consonant perception. *Neuropsychologia* 12: 83–93.

Tallal P, Piercy M (1975) Developmental aphasia: the perception of brief vowels and extended stop consonants. *Neuropsychologia* 13: 69–74.

Tallal P, Ross R, Curtiss S (1989). Unexpected sex-ratios in families of language/learning-impaired children. *Neuropsychologia* 27: 987–998.

Tannock R, Brown TE (2000) Attention-deficit disorders with learning disorders in children and adolescents. In: Brown TE (ed) *Attention-Deficit Disorders and Comorbidities in Children, Adolescents, and Adults.* Washington, DC: American Psychiatric Publishing, pp 231–295.

Tomblin JB, Records NL, Buckwalter P, Zhang X, Smith E, O'Brien M (1997) Prevalence of specific language impairment in kindergarten children. *J Speech Lang Hear Res* 40: 1245–1260.

Tomblin JB, Records NL, Zhang X (1996) A system for the diagnosis of specific language impairment in kindergarten children. *J Speech Lang Hear Res* 39: 1284–1294.

Trauner D, Wulfeck B, Tallal P, Hesselink J (2000) Neurological and MRI profiles of children with developmental language impairment. *Dev Med Child Neurol* 42: 470–475.

Ullman MT, Pierpont EI (2005) Specific language impairment is not specific to language: the procedural deficit hypothesis. *Cortex* 41: 399–433.

Uwer R, Albrecht R, von Suchodeletz W (2002) Automatic processing of tones and speech stimuli in children with specific language impairment. *Dev Med Child Neurol* 44: 527–532.

Van Weerdenburg M, Verhoeven L, van Balkom H (2006) Towards a typology of specific language impairment. *J Child Psychol Psychiatry* 47: 176–189.

Vargha-Khadem F, Watkins K, Alcock K, Fletcher P, Passingham R (1995) Praxic and non-verbal cognitive deficits in a large family with a genetically transmitted speech and language disorder. *Proc Natl Acad Sci U S A* 92: 930–933.

Watkins KE, Dronkers NF, Vargha-Khadem F (2002b) Behavioural analysis of an inherited speech and language disorder: comparison with acquired aphasia. *Brain* 125: 452–464.

Watkins KE, Vargha-Khadem F, Ashburner J, Passingham RE, Connelly A, Friston KJ, et al. (2002a) MRI analysis of an inherited speech and language disorder: structural brain abnormalities. *Brain* 125: 465–478.

Webster RI, Erdos C, Evans K, Majnemer A, Kehayia E, Thordardottir E, et al. (2006) The clinical spectrum of developmental language impairment in school-aged children: language, cognitive, and motor findings. *Pediatrics* 118: e1541–e1549.

Webster RI, Erdos C, Evans K, Majnemer A, Saigal G, Kehayia E, et al. (2008) Neurological and magnetic resonance imaging finding in children with developmental language impairment. *J Child Neurol* 23: 870–877.

Webster RI, Majnemer A, Platt R, Shevell MI (2004) The predictive value of a preschool diagnosis of developmental language impairment. *Neurology* 63: 2327–2331.

Webster RI, Majnemer A, Platt RW, Shevell MI (2005) Motor function at school age in children with a preschool diagnosis of developmental language impairment. *J Pediatr* 146: 80–85.

Weismer S, Evans J, Hesketh LJ (1999) An examination of verbal working memory capacity in children with specific language impairment. *J Speech Lang Hear Res* 42: 1249–1260.

Weismer S, Plante E, Jones M, Tomblin JB (2005) A functional magnetic resonance imaging investigation of verbal working memory in adolescents with specific language impairment. *J Speech Lang Hear Res* 48: 405–425.

Wilson BC, Risucci DA (1986) A model for clinical-quantitative classification. Generation I: Application to language-disordered preschool children. *Brain Lang* 27: 281–309.

World Health Organization (1992) *The ICD-10 Classification for Mental and Behavioral Disorders: Diagnostic Criteria for Research.* WHO: Geneva.

11

EFFECTS OF NEUROLOGIC DISORDERS AT THE SYNAPSE

Brian R Christie, Brennan D Eadie, Carl Ernst, Andrea K Titterness, Cristina O Vasuta and Alina J Webber

THE SYNAPSE

The term synapse was introduced just over 100 years ago and appears to be a combination of two Greek words: 'syn' meaning together and 'haptein' meaning to clasp. Synaptogenesis refers to the formation of synapses and can involve a number of processes:

1 Neuronal and glial signaling
2 Axonal and dendritic guidance cues
3 Cell adhesion molecules
4 Electrochemical activity

Indeed, the complexity of the synapse partially gives strength to the belief that all of our mental faculties are the result of the chemical and electrical signals that are transmitted between neurons in the central nervous system. There are two basic types of synapses: (1) electrochemical synapses, and (2) gap junctions. Gap junctions are rare in the mammalian nervous system but common in lower vertebrates. They are formed at sites of contact between two neurons, where a small pore forms which can directly propagate electrical activity between the neurons. Electrochemical synapses use neurotransmitter molecules for intracellular communication. In the mammalian central nervous system, the majority of neuronal communication occurs via electrochemical synapses and for the most part when reference is made to synapses it is in reference to the electrochemical subtype.

The basic electrochemical synapse has three components: the presynaptic bouton, the synaptic cleft, and the post-synaptic density. The presynaptic bouton contains hundreds to thousands of synaptic vesicles which each carry packets of neurotransmitter molecules. When an action potential reaches the bouton, it causes synaptic vesicles to fuse with the neuron's plasma membrane and release neurotransmitter into the synaptic cleft. In addition to synaptic vesicles, the presynaptic bouton is also populated by a variety of other organelles, including mitochondria, neurofilaments, microtubules, smooth endoplasmic reticulum, and the molecule glycogen. The synaptic cleft separates the presynaptic and post-synaptic membranes and is about 20–30 nanometers (nm) wide. Filaments appear to traverse the synapse and contribute to the formation of a dense plaque that occupies the intervening space between the contacts. The post-synaptic density is the region of a cell that is primarily concerned with translating these arriving chemical signals into electrical events. Here, neurotransmitter molecules bind to specific receptor proteins where they can exert their effects. The post-synaptic density is a dense network of proteins that extends across the synaptic cleft to the active zone of the presynaptic bouton as well as into the cytoplasm of the post-synaptic cell itself (Palay 1956, Sheng 2001). This structure seems dependent upon the existence of a presynaptic bouton and, if these boutons degenerate, the post-synaptic density will also disappear. Typically, the presynaptic bouton is on an axon, and the post-synaptic density is on a dendritic spine (axo-dendritic synapse), but it is also possible for transmitter to be released from dendrites on to dendrites (dendro-dendritic synapse) (Schoppa and Urban 2003) and for axons to synapse on other axons (axo-axonic synapse) (Andersen 1990). While by far the majority of synaptic connections are made between different neurons in the brain, it should also be noted that synapses can be made by neurons on to themselves, a type of synapse referred to as an 'autapse' (Bekkers 2003). Thus, it should be apparent that the constituents of both the presynaptic boutons and the post-synaptic density can congregate in cell bodies, axonal processes, and dendritic processes, and it is these constituents that actually determine the physical structure of the synapse. Thus, it is not really accurate to assume that a neurotransmitter is only released from axons and that all processing is performed by dendrites. Nevertheless, for the remainder of this chapter the traditional axo-dendritic synapse will be utilized to describe neurotransmission.

SYNAPTIC COMMUNICATION

The following highlights some of the activity that normally occurs at a synapse, but a more in-depth discussion complete with illustrations can be obtained from any of a number of recent neuroscience textbooks (Kandel et al. 2000, Bear et al. 2001, Pinel 2006).

When neurons fire action potentials, it leads to a series of events that result in the release of neurotransmitters from the presynaptic boutons. There are two basic categories of neurotransmitter which can be distinguished by the size of the vesicle in the presynaptic bouton. The largest molecules are peptides, which are proteins composed of 10 or fewer amino acids. These are assembled in the cytoplasm of the cell body on ribosomes before being packaged into vesicles by the cell's Golgi apparatus. They are then transported to the presynaptic bouton by microtubules at a rate of about 40cm a day. There are numerous varieties of smaller molecule neurotransmitters, and these are typically synthesized in the cytoplasm of the terminal bouton before being packaged into vesicles by the local Golgi apparatus. Both classes of vesicles can be released when an action potential invades the presynaptic bouton and opens voltage-gated calcium channels. The influx of extracellular Ca^{2+} causes the synaptic vesicles to fuse to the presynaptic membrane and empty their contents into the synaptic cleft.

Once released, the contents of the vesicles can then have an effect on the post-synaptic neuron by binding to specific receptor proteins that are located on the post-synaptic membrane. Ionotropic receptors are proteins that, when activated, result in the flux of ions into or out of the post-synaptic cell. When these receptors are activated, the associated ion channel opens or closes, immediately resulting in a post-synaptic potential change (either depolarizing or hyperpolarizing). For example, in some instances, excitatory post-synaptic potentials will be produced by an influx of sodium flowing into the cell (depolarizing potential), while different receptors might allow either potassium to flow out, or chloride to flow in, producing an inhibitory post-synaptic potential (hyperpolarizing). Unlike inotropic receptors, the activation of metabotropic receptors does not directly result in ion channel activity, but rather results in the activation of intracellular signaling cascades such as those triggered by G proteins. These cascades in turn can influence the activity of cell surface voltage-gated calcium channels and other ion channels, including inotropic receptors.

DISORDERS OF THE SYNAPSE AND TREATMENT POSSIBILITIES

The sequence of steps involved in establishing a functional synapse represent points at which various pathologic processes can have an effect and disrupt normal inter-neural communication. Indeed, it also appears that a number of pharmacologic treatments that are normally used in the treatment of various disorders also have their effects at the synapse. In the following sections, we give a brief overview of how disorders with complex etiologies, as well as a variety of familial (genetic) and environmental-based disorders (i.e. teratogen exposure), can alter synaptic communication in the brain. In each section we discuss what is currently known of how the disorder affects the synapse, and what, if any, therapies are targeted at producing changes in synaptic communication.

FRAGILE X SYNDROME

The most common cause of autism and inherited intellectual disability is fragile X syndrome (FXS). Herbert Lubs first observed the genetic defect in 1969, when he noticed a constriction in the X chromosome. It was later found that this constriction, or fragile site, marked the site of a 'loss of function' mutation in the FMR1 gene, causing FXS. The first clinical sign is typically the delay of one or more developmental milestones particularly in language and social domains. Common symptoms include autistic behaviors, attentional difficulties, and mood instability. Physical features include a dysmorphic phenotype characterized by a long narrow face, large ears, an arched palate, and connective tissue irregularities, such as hyperextensible joints (Wattendorf and Muenke 2005). The FXS phenotype becomes more prominent with age, and affected males can have IQ values in the range of 20–70. As FXS is an X-linked disorder, symptoms are milder in females and only one-third of females carrying the mutation exhibit mild to severe mental retardation reflecting lyonization. Around 20% of patients with FXS also experience epileptic seizures (Incorpora et al. 2002).

The brains of patients with FXS do not exhibit gross cortical abnormalities; however, magnetic resonance imaging (MRI) studies indicate a decrease in the size of the posterior vermis of the cerebellum, while the size of the hippocampus and caudate nucleus is increased (Hessl et al. 2004). Interestingly, the measured volumes of the cerebellum, caudate nucleus, and ventricles correlate with cognitive functioning (Reiss et al. 1995, Mostofsky et al. 1998). Caudate volumes also correlate to the methylation status of the FMR1 gene (Reiss et al. 1995). Although these changes are linked to gene expression and cognitive function, perhaps a more striking difference can be seen at the cellular level in these patients.

The first report that there were changes at the synapse in FXS came in a case study by Rudelli et al. (1985). Dendritic spine abnormalities linked to synaptic immaturity were seen, similar to those observed in trisomic chromosomal disorders. These long thin spines had prominent heads that resembled filopodia or immature spine-like structures. The appearance of these immature spines has been confirmed in subsequent studies (Hinton et al. 1991, Irwin et al. 2001). It appeared that a lack of fragile X mental retardation protein (FMRP), as seen in FXS, causes an increase in spine density, particularly of spines with an immature phenotype. It should be noted that most of the patients in these studies have been on numerous medications for a significant portion of their lives; therefore, the development of an animal model for FXS was an important step in being able to determine the effects of the loss of FMRP on the synapse.

FMRP is highly conserved throughout species, and the gene can be selectively knocked out in both mice and *Drosophila*. A greater number of spines with an immature phenotype, characterized by an elongated shape, and a decreased number of mature spines are also found in these animal models, resembling the microscopic findings in humans (Irwin et al. 2001, McKinney et al. 2005). Research also suggests that the spine defects may develop as mice age, although further quantification is required (Galvez and Greenough 2005), and, interestingly, human patients with FXS have cognitive deficits that appear to increase with age. A potential area of future research could be to link the severity of observed symptoms to the spine morphology. Research with the *Drosophila* model of FXS shows that the analogous protein to human FMRP is involved in the regulation of synaptogenesis. FMRP has been shown to increase in regions of the rat brain undergoing active synaptogenesis.

N-methyl-D-aspartate (NMDA) receptor dependent long-term potentiation (LTP) is unaltered in the FXS animal model (Godfraind et al. 1996, Huber et al.

2002); however, synaptic plasticity involving group 1 metabotropic glutamate receptors (Grp1 mGluR) is dramatically affected by the loss of FMRP. In the mouse model of FXS, mGluR-dependent long-term depression (LTD) is significantly increased (Huber et al. 2002). LTD is thought to be involved in synapse maturation and synaptic pruning during certain points in the lifespan. LTD that is mGluR dependent has been shown to cause a reduction in synaptic strength and subsequent synapse elimination (i.e. pruning) (Shinoda et al. 2005).

An increase in mGluR-dependent LTD, in combination with other observations, has led to a theory that many of the effects of FXS are mediated by increased mGluR signaling (Bear et al. 2004). The mGluR theory of fragile X pathogenesis was based on observations of altered LTD, but also notes that other mGluR-mediated effects are seen in FXS. Interestingly, prolonged Grp1 mGluR activation can trigger epileptiform bursts in hippocampal slices (NB epilepsy occurs in a portion of FXS cases). FXS can also be associated with loose bowels, and mGluR agonists increase intestinal motility. FXS also involves a hypersensitivity to tactile stimulation, and mGluR5 receptors are involved in nociception. Several other parallels between the symptoms of FXS and overactivation of Grp1 mGluRs also support this pathogenetic theory (Bear et al. 2004).

In summary, the lack of FMRP causes structural and functional changes at the synapse. Of crucial importance to FXS is understanding the mechanism of how FMRP functions. FMRP is an RNA binding protein, and a point mutation that prevents FMRP from associating with mRNA protein complexes has been sufficient enough to result in a severe human case of FXS, suggesting the clinical importance of this association (Feng et al. 1997). FMRP interacts with approximately 4% of human fetal mRNA (Ashley et al. 1993). With a growing lists of mRNA associations in mice (Brown et al. 2001), the role FMRP may have in transcriptional regulation is therefore quite complex and treating the disease may not be as simple as treating a few of the biochemical abnormalities by increased mGluR signaling.

Group 1 mGluR antagonists have been proposed as potential therapeutic targets in FXS (Bear et al. 2004). Antagonists of mGluR1 can cause cerebellar ataxia; therefore, mGluR5, and its antagonist, 2-methyl-6-(phenylethynyl)-pyridine (MPEP), have received the most attention as putative therapeutic agents. MPEP has been tested on animal models of FXS and was able to rescue two of three disease phenotypes including audiogenic seizure susceptibility and anxiety-related behavior (Yan et al. 2005). Another study looked at the *Drosophila* model of FXS. In the FXS *Drosophila* model, there are some learning and memory defects, along with brain morphology defects. These defects were rescued by LiCl (linked to mGluR signaling) and MPEP, yet little is known of how these treatments affect the synapse.

Interestingly, some behavioral abnormalities have been reversed and increased dendritic branching observed after animals have been raised in enriched environments.

In addition, the long characteristic immature spines seen in FXS appeared more mature in the treated knockout mice. Anxiety levels of the treated FMR1 knockout mice were still above normal as was spine density. Even so, the fact that several features of the disease were reversed is promising. Previous studies have shown that environmental enrichment and voluntary exercise can benefit the brain at the level of the synapse, and in these mice, a simple plastic running wheel plus some brightly colored balls, tubes, and bells to play with made quite a difference (Restivo et al. 2005). It is not clear how much of a benefit such a therapy might have for humans, who normally live in a much more enriched environment, and these findings may indicate that the animal model is insufficient to explain all of the symptoms of FXS in humans.

RETT SYNDROME

Andreas Rett, an Austrian pediatrician, first described this novel neurodevelopmental disorder in 1966. For almost two decades following Rett's observations, clinicians remained unaware or skeptical of the existence of this unique disorder. However, in 1983 Hagberg et al. reported on 35 female patients with a similar constellation of symptoms to those that Rett had described (Haas 1988). Hagberg suggested that this is in fact a unique syndrome inherited in an X-linked dominant manner resulting in affected females and non-viable homozygous males conceptuses. In 1999, American investigators found several mutations in the X-linked gene MeCP2 encoding methyl-CpG-binding protein 2 in a proportion of Rett patients (Amir et al. 1999, Gura 1999, Willard and Hendrich 1999). It is now accepted that the large majority of patients who meet the clinical diagnosis of Rett syndrome also present with a sporadic mutation in the MeCP2 gene (Miltenberger-Miltenyi and Laccone 2003).

Rett syndrome is now well accepted as a unique monogenic neurodevelopmental disorder. The current necessary criteria for a diagnosis of classic Rett syndrome include the following:

1 Apparently normal prenatal and perinatal history
2 Psychomotor development largely normal through the first 6 months of life
3 Normal head circumference at birth
4 Postnatal deceleration of head growth (i.e. secondary microcephaly)
5 Loss of achieved purposeful hand skill (i.e. fine motor apraxia) between 6 months and 2 years 6 months of age
6 Stereotypic hand movements such as hand-wringing/squeezing, clapping/tapping, mouthing and washing/rubbing automatisms
7 Emerging social withdrawal communication dysfunction (i.e. autistic features, loss of learned words, and cognitive impairment)
8 Impaired (dyspraxic) or failing locomotion

The ability to probe the neuropathology of Rett syndrome was further advanced by the generation of a mouse model of Rett syndrome in 2001. Amazingly, MeCP2 deficient mice showed a delayed onset of hind limb clasping reminiscent of hand-wringing characteristically observed in patients with Rett syndrome. Symptomatic female MeCP2$^{+/-}$ mice were also significantly less mobile in an open field maze (Guy et al. 2001). MeCP2 mutant mice have recently been utilized to probe the abnormal neuronal and synaptic functioning that may underlie the motor and cognitive impairment in Rett syndrome beyond what has historically been possible with clinical postmortem and antemortem neuroimaging studies.

Interestingly, patients with Rett syndrome exhibit cognitive and motor ability regression during the postnatal period which is normally characterized by intense synaptic remodeling, suggesting that MeCP2 expression and its cellular functions are associated with synapse formation and/or maintenance. In fact, it has been shown that MeCP2 expression and synaptogenesis normally occur in synchrony in various brain regions including the cortex, hippocampus, and cerebellum across development (Mullaney et al. 2004). Further, in one study of isolated olfactory neurons, induction of neurogenesis led to a gradual increase in the expression of MeCP2 to normal levels in the presence of target cells and to subnormal levels in isolation, suggesting that synapse formation and MeCP2 expression possesses an intimate relationship within single neurons (Cohen et al. 2003).

Clinical observations and rare autopsies of patients with Rett syndrome have shown that head circumference and brain weight plateau at an abnormally low level (Nomura et al. 1984, Jellinger and Seitelberger 1986). It is likely that this overall reduction of head and brain growth is a function of abnormal development of the constituent cells. Because MeCP2 is preferentially expressed in well-differentiated neurons and not neuroblasts or glial cells, the morphology of the mature neuron is of prime interest (Kishi and Macklis 2004). Neuropathologic findings from autopsies describe significant reductions in cortical thickness, neuronal size, and dendritic arborization with relative preservation of actual neuronal number (Jellinger et al. 1988, Bauman et al. 1995, Armstrong 1997, Belichenko et al. 1997). A paucity of dendritic spines and a marked reduction in synaptic density has also been reported (Naidu 1997). Further, the density of neurons has been reported to be increased (Bauman et al. 1995). The abnormal neuronal morphology is diffuse and it may be that decreased synaptogenesis allows an increase in the ability of neurons to become concentrated and/or a cessation of head and brain growth.

Electroencephalography recordings obtained from patients with Rett syndrome first revealed a possible abnormality in neurotransmission, suggesting that synaptic communication may be altered in addition to morphology (Niedermeyer et al. 1997). Furthermore, cerebrospinal fluid obtained from symptomatic patients with Rett syndrome contained increased amounts of glutamate, the major excitatory neurotransmitter in the brain, suggesting that the levels of glutamate may also be elevated at the synapse (Hamberger et al. 1992). Corroborating this notion was the magnetic resonance spectroscopy finding that patients with Rett syndrome exhibit elevations in the glutamate:glutamine ratio (Pan et al. 1999). Postmortem autoradiographic studies further revealed that the NMDA-type glutamate receptor is elevated in young patients with Rett syndrome and reduced in older patients compared to controls (Blue et al. 1999a). It has been suggested that elevated NMDA receptor levels may reflect a persistence of an immature developmental state in light of the fact that normal infants show elevated NMDA receptor levels for several postnatal months. Interestingly, α-amino-5-hydroxy-3-methyl-4-isoxazole propionic acid (AMPA) and gamma-aminobutyric acid (GABA) receptors showed similar trends particularly in the basal ganglia (Blue et al. 1999b).

Recently, electrophysiologic recordings obtained from a mouse model of Rett syndrome has been reported (Asaka et al. 2006). LTP, which is dependent upon glutamatergic activation of NMDA receptors, was shown to be progressively impaired in the CA_1 region of the hippocampus of MeCP2$^{+/-}$ mice. Further, NMDA-dependent LTD is absent in symptomatic MeCP2$^{+/-}$ mice. Presynaptic glutamate release was also found to be impaired, as revealed by a significant reduction in paired-pulse facilitation. Basal neurotransmission was otherwise normal. Interestingly, immuno-blot analyses showed that the expression of the NR2A-type NMDA receptor was down-regulated and the NR2B-type NMDA receptor was up-regulated in MeCP2$^{+/-}$ mice (Asaka et al. 2006).

The current therapies for patients with Rett syndrome are aimed at treating symptoms such as seizures and poor motor control. There are currently no drug trials in progress that specifically target the glutamatergic system in Rett syndrome. Further research into the relationship between the NMDA receptor and MeCP2 may elucidate novel drug targets for this unusual developmental disorder of the synapse.

FETAL ALCOHOL SYNDROME

Fetal alcohol syndrome (FAS) is a disorder that results from maternal consumption of alcohol during pregnancy. As the leading preventable cause of mental retardation/intellectual disability, approximately 1000–6000 infants are born with FAS each year in North America. It is increasingly seen as a major health care concern as the annual cost of care for individuals affected by FAS has reached $4 billion (Lupton et al. 2004). Diagnostic criteria for FAS include:

1 Very specific facial abnormalities (e.g. smooth philtrum, small palpebral fissure, and thin vermillion border)
2 Growth deficits (defined as both height and weight in the lower 10th percentile)
3 At least one of three central nervous system disorders which fall into three categories: (a) structural – the size of the head and smaller brain structures such

as the corpus callosum and cerebellum, (b) functional – delayed development decreased IQ, problems with social skills and behavioral disorders, and (c) neurologic problems with coordination, visual motor skills, and motor control that are outside normal ranges (Bertrand et al. 2005)

To further elucidate the effects of prenatal ethanol exposure, several animal models have been developed in which the fetus is exposed to ethanol at various time points of gestation. These models have provided significant insights into structural, functional, and neurologic impairments that result from prenatal ethanol exposure. Indeed, there are alterations to the size of brain structures such as the corpus callosum, basal ganglia, and the hippocampus in particular (Mattson et al. 1994, Byrnes et al. 2001, Qiang et al. 2002, Livy et al. 2003), deficits in behavioral learning (Kim et al. 1997, Richardson et al. 2002), and growth deficits (Schapiro et al. 1984, Lopez-Tejero et al. 1986). Therefore, animal models of FAS provide a means through which the effects of prenatal ethanol exposure that affect cognition, behavior, and structural abnormalities can be assessed.

Prenatal ethanol exposure can affect spine morphology throughout the brain. Spines can be thin and elongated in the sensory cortex (Galofre et al. 1987), but there is evidence of an increase in stubby spines within the hippocampus along with a decrease in the expression of thin spines (Tarelo-Acuna et al. 2000). The effects within the hippocampus imply alterations in neuronal firing as thin spines enhance synaptic communication. In addition to alterations in spine shape, dendritic branching is also decreased following prenatal ethanol exposure (Lopez-Tejero et al. 1986). Synaptic stability is also affected by prenatal ethanol exposure as there is a delay in synaptic turnover because the development of complex spines is delayed (Hoff 1988). Overall, there appears to be a decrease in the number of spines and their functional capability as a result of prenatal ethanol exposure.

Another way in which the synapse is affected by prenatal ethanol exposure is through neurogenesis or the creation of new neurons in the brain. Animals with prenatal ethanol exposure show a decrease in the amount of hippocampal neurogenesis (Redila et al. 2006), effectively limiting the number of new synaptic contacts that can be established. Additionally, ethanol can trigger widespread apoptosis during brain growth spurts (Olney et al. 2000) which are periods of immense innate synaptogenesis. Together with decreased neurogenesis, alterations in spine morphology, and the aberrant development of mature synaptic connections, it would appear that synaptic communication would also be expected to be affected by prenatal ethanol exposure.

Major changes within the glutamate system occur following prenatal ethanol exposure. There are fewer glutamate-binding sites, a decrease in the expression of NMDA receptor subunits, and altered NMDA channel properties (Savage et al. 1991, Abdollah and Brien 1995, Diaz-Granados et al. 1997, Hughes et al. 1998,

Costa et al. 2000a, 2000b, Nixon et al. 2004). It is interesting to note, however, that excessive activity derived from NMDA receptors might actually contribute to problems that result from prenatal ethanol exposure (Thomas et al. 2004). However, it is undisputed that changes to NMDA receptors may contribute to cognitive deficits incurred by prenatal ethanol exposure. There is a decrease in the induction of LTP (Swartzwelder et al. 1988, Sutherland et al. 1997, Richardson et al. 2002), which is a neuronal model of learning and memory. Taken together, changes in synaptic connectivity and glutamate receptors might contribute to the varying cognitive deficits that result from prenatal ethanol exposure.

Within the human population, much attention has been focused on the prevention of FAS by educating women on the dangers of drinking during pregnancy. Management of FAS consists of preventing secondary disorders through a variety of measures such as early diagnosis and having a stable home environment (Burd et al. 2003). Exciting research with animal models of FAS has provided insight into possible additional treatments. Environmental enrichment, where an animal is housed in a socially and physically enriched environment, improves performance on behavioral learning tasks (Hannigan et al. 1993). Additionally, voluntary exercise can increase hippocampal neurogenesis (Redila et al. 2006), enhance hippocampal LTP, and improve performance on behavioral learning tasks (Christie et al. 2005). Taken together, these postnatal environmental manipulations indicate that it is still possible to improve cognitive capacity following prenatal ethanol exposure and that these behavioral therapies might be an effective treatment for enhancing synaptic communication in individuals with FAS.

Epilepsy

Epilepsy is a condition characterized by recurrent seizures, unprovoked by any immediately identifiable cause (i.e. intercurrent central nervous system infections or metabolic disturbances). Seizures result from abnormal excessive and hypersynchronous discharge patterns in neuronal populations, and can produce a number of clinical symptoms which include alterations in consciousness as well as motor, sensory, autonomic, and psychic events. Epilepsy occurs frequently in individuals with neurodevelopmental disabilities and indeed is a co-morbid condition that may affect and modulate eventual outcome.

Seizure discharges in mesial temporal lobe epilepsy (MTLE) can initiate in the hippocampus, enthorinal cortex, and/or amygdala. Ongoing seizures result in these limbic structures undergoing histopathologic changes, while in the neocortex morphologic abnormalities frequently remained undetected. The brain of patients with MTLE is characterized by a type of brain injury known as mesial temporal sclerosis (MTS), which may result from status epilepticus or prolonged febrile seizures in early childhood. MTS is characterized by the loss of neurons in the layer 3 of the enthorinal cortex, in the dentate hilus, and areas CA_3 and CA_1 of the hippocampus.

In patients with MTLE, a phenomenon known as 'mossy fiber sprouting' has also been described. This phenomenon is characterized by the mossy fibers of the dentate hilus branching out to abnormally innervate other cells in the dentate inner molecular layer, instead of converging into the dentate hilus and synapsing with hilar and CA_3 neurons (Koyama and Ikegaya 2004). It is believed that the loss of hippocampal neurons leaves synapses open in target neurons; thus sprouting of fibers occurs in the dentate hilus and CA_1 to replace the afferent lost fibers (Babb et al. 1991). This reorganization consists of aberrantly sprouted granule cell axons projecting to the granule cell or molecular layers in the way of recurrent excitation (Houser et al. 1990). After sprouting, mossy fibers form exclusively asymmetric synapses in the supragranular region and granule cell layer (van Gelder et al. 1983).

As would be expected, synaptic mechanisms are not normal in epilepsy. Dentate granule cells generate prolonged NMDA-dependent currents (Isokawa et al. 1997). The electrophysiologic findings are correlated with a loss of spine density and changes in ionotropic glutamate mRNA levels. Short-term plasticity is disturbed in the sclerotic hippocampi as revealed by studies of evoked field potentials. There is an increased inhibition in hippocampal inputs and a decreased inhibition in the hippocampus, suggesting a hypersynchronizing drive for further seizure generation. LTP is also severely reduced (Beck et al. 2000).

Reduced inhibition in neuronal networks causes hyperexcitability which leads to the occurrence of seizures (Calcagnotto et al. 2000, Avoli et al. 2005). The number of $GABA_A$ receptor subunits is reduced, and GABAergic interneuronal loss is noted in the hippocampus. Sclerotic hippocampus in patients with MTLE is characterized by reorganization of chandelier cells, a type of interneuron, in both the dentate gyrus and hippocampal formation. Recently, spontaneous synchronous events were observed in the subiculum in preparations from patients with MTLE. These discharges are dependent on both glutamatergic and GABAergic transmission (Cepeda et al. 2002, Cohen et al. 2002).

The goals of therapies for epilepsy are directed towards reducing neuronal excitation ('braking' excitability). Towards this end, many of the more common pharmacologic treatments increase inhibitory synaptic transmission in the central nervous system.

CONCLUSIONS
Our understanding of the complexity of the synapse has increased greatly over the past 20 years, and we are now recognizing how a number of different neuropathologic disorders might impact on this delicate node in neuronal communication. While pharmacologic treatments have had a positive impact in disorders such as epilepsy and may provide a source of hope for attenuating the development of FXS, it is also clear that a better understanding of how synapses develop will be crucial in creating specific targeted therapies that will enable us to control the growth and

development of synapses. Indeed, the dendritic spine pathology that is often observed in neurologic disorders may in fact be primarily the result of a loss of excitatory input to dendritic spines during development, and not directly caused by the underlying disease itself. Gaining a clear understanding of how each disorder impacts the synapse, both directly and indirectly, will ultimately provide the soundest basis for the development of effective medically based and rational treatment options.

REFERENCES

Abdollah S, Brien JF (1995) Effect of chronic maternal ethanol administration on glutamate and N-methyl-D-aspartate binding sites in the hippocampus of the near-term fetal guinea pig. *Alcohol* 12: 377–382.

Amir RE, Van den Veyver IB, Wan M, Tran CQ, Francke U, Zoghbi HY (1999) Rett syndrome is caused by mutations in X-linked MECP2, encoding methyl-CpG-binding protein 2. *Nat Genet* 23: 185–188.

Andersen P (1990) Synaptic integration in hippocampal CA1 pyramids. Prog Brain Res 83: 215–222.

Armstrong DD (1997) Review of Rett syndrome. *J Neuropathol Exp Neurol* 56: 843–849.

Asaka Y, Jugloff DG, Zhang L, Eubanks JH, Fitzsimonds RM (2006) Hippocampal synaptic plasticity is impaired in the Mecp2-null mouse model of Rett syndrome. *Neurobiol Dis* 21: 217–227.

Ashley CT Jr, Wilkinson KD, Reines D, Warren ST (1993) FMR1 protein: conserved RNP family domains and selective RNA binding. *Science* 262: 563–566.

Avoli M, Louvel J, Pumain R, Kohling R (2005) Cellular and molecular mechanisms of epilepsy in the human brain. *Prog Neurobiol* 77: 166–200.

Babb TL, Kupfer WR, Pretorius JK, Crandall PH, Levesque MF (1991) Synaptic reorganization by mossy fibers in human epileptic fascia dentata. *Neuroscience* 42: 351–363.

Bauman ML, Kemper TL, Arin DM (1995) Pervasive neuroanatomic abnormalities of the brain in three cases of Rett's syndrome. *Neurology* 45: 1581–1586.

Bear MF, Connors BW, Paradiso MA (2001) *Neuroscience: Exploring the Brain, 2nd edn.* Baltimore, Maryland: Lippincott Williams & Wilkins.

Bear MF, Huber KM, Warren ST (2004) The mGluR theory of fragile X mental retardation. *Trends Neurosci* 27: 370–377.

Beck H, Goussakov IV, Lie A, Helmstaedter C, Elger CE (2000) Synaptic plasticity in the human dentate gyrus. *J Neurosci* 20: 7080–7086.

Bekkers JM (2003) Synaptic transmission: functional autapses in the cortex. Curr Biol 13: R433–435.

Belichenko PV, Hagberg B, Dahlstrom A (1997) Morphological study of neocortical areas in Rett syndrome. *Acta Neuropathol (Berl)* 93: 50–61.

Bertrand J, Floyd LL, Weber MK (2005) Guidelines for identifying and referring persons with fetal alcohol syndrome. *MMWR Recomm Rep* 54: 1–14.

Blue ME, Naidu S, Johnston MV (1999a) Development of amino acid receptors in frontal cortex from girls with Rett syndrome. *Ann Neurol* 45: 541–545.

Blue ME, Naidu S, Johnston MV (1999b) Altered development of glutamate and GABA receptors in the basal ganglia of girls with Rett syndrome. *Exp Neurol* 156: 345–352.

Brown V, Jin P, Ceman S, Darnell JC, O'Donnell WT, Tenenbaum SA, et al. (2001) Microarray identification of FMRP-associated brain mRNAs and altered mRNA translational profiles in fragile X syndrome. *Cell* 107: 477–487.

Burd L, Cotsonas-Hassler TM, Martsolf JT, Kerbeshian J (2003) Recognition and management of fetal alcohol syndrome. *Neurotoxicol Teratol* 25: 681–688.

Byrnes ML, Reynolds JN, Brien JF (2001) Effect of prenatal ethanol exposure during the brain growth spurt of the guinea pig. *Neurotoxicol Teratol* 23: 355–364.

Calcagnotto ME, Barbarosie M, Avoli M (2000) Hippocampus-entorhinal cortex loop and seizure generation in the young rodent limbic system. *J Neurophysiol* 83: 3183–3187.

Cepeda C, Crawford CA, Margulies JE, Watson JB, Levine MS, Cohen RW (2002) Enhanced epileptogenic susceptibility in a genetic model of reactive synaptogenesis: the spastic Han-Wistar rat. *Dev Neurosci* 24: 262–271.

Christie BR, Swann SE, Fox CJ, Froc D, Lieblich SE, Redila V, et al. Voluntary exercise rescues deficits in spatial memory and long-term potentiation in prenatal ethanol-exposed male rats. *Eur J Neurosci* 21: 1719–1726.

Cohen DR, Matarazzo V, Palmer AM, Tu Y, Jeon OH, Pevsner J, Ronnett GV (2003) Expression of MeCP2 in olfactory receptor neurons is developmentally regulated and occurs before synaptogenesis. *Mol Cell Neurosci* 22: 417–429.

Cohen I, Navarro V, Clemenceau S, Baulac M, Miles R (2002) On the origin of interictal activity in human temporal lobe epilepsy *in vitro. Science* 298: 1418–1421.

Costa ET, Savage DD, Valenzuela CF (2000a) A review of the effects of prenatal or early postnatal ethanol exposure on brain ligand-gated ion channels. *Alcohol Clin Exp Res* 24: 706–715.

Costa ET, Olivera DS, Meyer DA, Ferreira VM, Soto EE, Frausto S, Savage DD, Browning MD, Valenzuela CF (2000b) Fetal alcohol exposure alters neurosteroid modulation of hippocampal N-methyl-D-aspartate receptors. *J Biol Chem* 275: 38268–38274.

Diaz-Granados JL, Spuhler-Phillips K, Lilliquist MW, Amsel A, Leslie SW (1997) Effects of prenatal and early postnatal ethanol exposure on [3H]MK-801 binding in rat cortex and hippocampus. *Alcohol Clin Exp Res* 21: 874–881.

Feng Y, Absher D, Eberhart DE, Brown V, Malter HE, Warren ST (1997) FMRP associates with polyribosomes as an mRNP, and the I304N mutation of severe fragile X syndrome abolishes this association. *Mol Cell* 1: 109–118.

Galofre E, Ferrer I, Fabregues I, Lopez-Tejero D (1987) Effects of prenatal ethanol exposure on dendritic spines of layer V pyramidal neurons in the somatosensory cortex of the rat. *J Neurol Sci* 81: 185–195.

Galvez R, Greenough WT (2005) Sequence of abnormal dendritic spine development in primary somatosensory cortex of a mouse model of the fragile X mental retardation syndrome. *Am J Med Genet A* 135: 155–160.

Godfraind JM, Reyniers E, De Boulle K, D'Hooge R, De Deyn PP, Bakker CE, et al. (1996) Long-term potentiation in the hippocampus of fragile X knockout mice. *Am J Med Genet* 64: 246–251.

Gura T (1999) Gene defect linked to Rett syndrome. *Science* 286: 27.

Guy J, Hendrich B, Holmes M, Martin JE, Bird A (2001) A mouse Mecp2-null mutation causes neurological symptoms that mimic Rett syndrome. *Nat Genet* 27: 322–326.

Haas RH (1988) The history and challenge of Rett syndrome. *J Child Neurol* 3 (Suppl): S3–5.

Hamberger A, Gillberg C, Palm A, Hagberg B (1992) Elevated CSF glutamate in Rett syndrome. *Neuropediatrics* 23: 212–213.

Hannigan JH, Berman RF, Zajac CS (1993) Environmental enrichment and the behavioral effects of prenatal exposure to alcohol in rats. *Neurotoxicol Teratol* 15: 261–266.

Hessl D, Rivera SM, Reiss AL (2004) The neuroanatomy and neuroendocrinology of fragile X syndrome. *Ment Retard Dev Disabil Res Rev* 10: 17–24.

Hinton VJ, Brown WT, Wisniewski K, Rudelli RD (1991) Analysis of neocortex in three males with the fragile X syndrome. *Am J Med Genet* 41: 289–294.

Hoff SF (1988) Synaptogenesis in the hippocampal dentate gyrus: effects of in utero ethanol exposure. *Brain Res Bull* 21: 47–54.

Houser CR, Miyashiro JE, Swartz BE, Walsh GO, Rich JR, Delgado-Escueta AV (1990) Altered patterns of dynorphin immunoreactivity suggest mossy fiber reorganization in human hippocampal epilepsy. *J Neurosci* 10: 267–282.

Huber KM, Gallagher SM, Warren ST, Bear MF (2002) Altered synaptic plasticity in a mouse model of fragile X mental retardation. *Proc Natl Acad Sci U S A* 99: 7746–7750.

Hughes PD, Kim YN, Randall PK, Leslie SW (1998) Effect of prenatal ethanol exposure on the developmental profile of the NMDA receptor subunits in rat forebrain and hippocampus. *Alcohol Clin Exp Res* 22: 1255–1261.

Incorpora G, Sorge G, Sorge A, Pavone L (2002) Epilepsy in fragile X syndrome. *Brain Dev* 24: 766–769.

Irwin SA, Patel B, Idupulapati M, Harris JB, Crisostomo RA, Larsen BP, et al. (2001) Abnormal dendritic spine characteristics in the temporal and visual cortices of patients with fragile-X syndrome: a quantitative examination. *Am J Med Genet* 98: 161–167.

Isokawa M, Levesque M, Fried I, Engel J Jr (1997) Glutamate currents in morphologically identified human dentate granule cells in temporal lobe epilepsy. *J Neurophysiol* 77: 3355–3369.

Jellinger K, Seitelberger F (1986) Neuropathology of Rett syndrome. *Am J Med Genet Suppl* 1: 259–288.

Jellinger K, Armstrong D, Zoghbi HY, Percy AK (1988) Neuropathology of Rett syndrome. *Acta Neuropathol (Berl)* 76: 142–158.

Kandel ER, Schwartz JH, Jessell TM (2000) Principles of neural science, 4th Edition. New York: McGraw-Hill, Health Professions Division.

Kim CK, Kalynchuk LE, Kornecook TJ, Mumby DG, Dadgar NA, Pinel JP, et al. (1997) Object-recognition and spatial learning and memory in rats prenatally exposed to ethanol. *Behav Neurosci* 111: 985–995.

Kishi N, Macklis JD (2004) MECP2 is progressively expressed in post-migratory neurons and is involved in neuronal maturation rather than cell fate decisions. *Mol Cell Neurosci* 27: 306–321.

Koyama R, Ikegaya Y (2004) Mossy fiber sprouting as a potential therapeutic target for epilepsy. *Curr Neurovasc Res* 1: 3–10.

Livy DJ, Miller EK, Maier SE, West JR (2003) Fetal alcohol exposure and temporal vulnerability: effects of binge-like alcohol exposure on the developing rat hippocampus. *Neurotoxicol Teratol* 25: 447–458.

Lopez-Tejero D, Ferrer I, M LL, Herrera E (1986) Effects of prenatal ethanol exposure on physical growth, sensory reflex maturation and brain development in the rat. *Neuropathol Appl Neurobiol* 12: 251–260.

Lupton C, Burd L, Harwood R (2004) Cost of fetal alcohol spectrum disorders. *Am J Med Genet C Semin Med Genet* 127: 42–50.

Mattson SN, Riley EP, Jernigan TL, Garcia A, Kaneko WM, Ehlers CL, et al. (1994) A decrease in the size of the basal ganglia following prenatal alcohol exposure: a preliminary report. *Neurotoxicol Teratol* 16: 283–289.

McKinney BC, Grossman AW, Elisseou NM, Greenough WT (2005) Dendritic spine abnormalities in the occipital cortex of C57BL/6 Fmr1 knockout mice. *Am J Med Genet B Neuropsychiatr Genet* 136B: 98–102.

Miltenberger-Miltenyi G, Laccone F (2003) Mutations and polymorphisms in the human methyl CpG-binding protein MECP2. *Hum Mutat* 22: 107–115.

Mostofsky SH, Mazzocco MM, Aakalu G, Warsofsky IS, Denckla MB, Reiss AL (1998) Decreased cerebellar posterior vermis size in fragile X syndrome: correlation with neurocognitive performance. *Neurology* 50: 121–130.

Mullaney BC, Johnston MV, Blue ME (2004) Developmental expression of methyl-CpG binding protein 2 is dynamically regulated in the rodent brain. *Neuroscience* 123: 939–949.

Naidu S (1997) Rett syndrome: a disorder affecting early brain growth. *Ann Neurol* 42: 3–10.

Niedermeyer E, Naidu SB, Plate C (1997) Unusual EEG theta rhythms over central region in Rett syndrome: considerations of the underlying dysfunction. *Clin Electroencephalogr* 28: 36–43.

Nixon K, Hughes PD, Amsel A, Leslie SW (2004) NMDA receptor subunit expression after combined prenatal and postnatal exposure to ethanol. *Alcohol Clin Exp Res* 28: 105–112.

Nomura Y, Segawa M, Hasegawa M (1984) Rett syndrome: clinical studies and pathophysiological consideration. *Brain Dev* 6: 475–486.

Olney JW, Ishimaru MJ, Bittigau P, Ikonomidou C (2000) Ethanol-induced apoptotic neurodegeneration in the developing brain. *Apoptosis* 5: 515–521.

Palay SL (1956) Synapses in the central nervous system. J Biophys Biochem Cytol 2: 193–202.

Pan JW, Lane JB, Hetherington H, Percy AK (1999) Rett syndrome: 1H spectroscopic imaging at 4.1 Tesla. *J Child Neurol* 14: 524–528.

Pinel JPJ (2006) *Biopsychology, 6th edn.* Boston: Pearson Allyn and Bacon.

Qiang M, Wang MW, Elberger AJ (2002) Second trimester prenatal alcohol exposure alters development of rat corpus callosum. *Neurotoxicol Teratol* 24: 719–732.

Redila VA, Olson AK, Swann SE, Mohades G, Webber AJ, Weinberg J, Christie BR (2006) Hippocampal cell proliferation is reduced following prenatal ethanol exposure but can be rescued with voluntary exercise. *Hippocampus.* 16(3): 305–11.

Reiss D, Hetherington EM, Plomin R, Howe GW, Simmens SJ, Henderson SH, et al. (1995) Genetic questions for environmental studies. Differential parenting and psychopathology in adolescence. *Arch Gen Psychiatry* 52: 925–936.

Restivo L, Ferrari F, Passino E, Sgobio C, Bock J, Oostra BA, et al. (2005) Enriched environment promotes behavioral and morphological recovery in a mouse model for the fragile X syndrome. *Proc Natl Acad Sci U S A* 102: 11557–11562.

Richardson DP, Byrnes ML, Brien JF, Reynolds JN, Dringenberg HC (2002) Impaired acquisition in the water maze and hippocampal long-term potentiation after chronic prenatal ethanol exposure in the guinea-pig. *Eur J Neurosci* 16: 1593–1598.

Rudelli RD, Brown WT, Wisniewski K, Jenkins EC, Laure-Kamionowska M, Connell F, et al (1985) Adult fragile X syndrome: clinico-neuropathologic findings. *Acta Neuropathol* 67: 289–295.

Savage DD, Montano CY, Otero MA, Paxton LL (1991) Prenatal ethanol exposure decreases hippocampal NMDA-sensitive [3H]-glutamate binding site density in 45-day-old rats. *Alcohol* 8: 193–201.

Schapiro MB, Rosman NP, Kemper TL (1984) Effects of chronic exposure to alcohol on the developing brain. *Neurobehav Toxicol Teratol* 6: 351–356.

Schoppa NE, Urban NN (2003) Dendritic processing within olfactory bulb circuits. Trends Neurosci 26: 501–506.

Sheng M (2001) Molecular organization of the postsynaptic specialization. Proc Natl Acad Sci U S A 98: 7058–7061.

Shinoda Y, Kamikubo Y, Egashira Y, Tominaga-Yoshino K, Ogura A (2005) Repetition of mGluR-dependent LTD causes slowly developing persistent reduction in synaptic strength accompanied by synapse elimination. *Brain Res* 1042: 99–107.

Sutherland RJ, McDonald RJ, Savage DD (1997) Prenatal exposure to moderate levels of ethanol can have long-lasting effects on hippocampal synaptic plasticity in adult offspring. Hippocampus 7: 232–238.

Swartzwelder HS, Farr KL, Wilson WA, Savage DD (1988) Prenatal exposure to ethanol decreases physiological plasticity in the hippocampus of the adult rat. Alcohol 5: 121–124.

Tarelo-Acuna L, Olvera-Cortes E, Gonzalez-Burgos I (2000) Prenatal and postnatal exposure to ethanol induces changes in the shape of the dendritic spines from hippocampal CA1 pyramidal neurons of the rat. Neurosci Lett 286: 13–16.

Thomas JD, Garcia GG, Dominguez HD, Riley EP (2004) Administration of eliprodil during ethanol withdrawal in the neonatal rat attenuates ethanol-induced learning deficits. Psychopharmacology (Berl) 175: 189–195.

van Gelder NM, Siatitsas I, Menini C, Gloor P (1983) Feline generalized penicillin epilepsy: changes of glutamic acid and taurine parallel the progressive increase in excitability of the cortex. Epilepsia 24: 200–213.

Wattendorf DJ, Muenke M (2005) Diagnosis and management of fragile X syndrome. Am Fam Physician 72: 111–113.

Willard HF, Hendrich BD (1999) Breaking the silence in Rett syndrome. Nat Genet 23: 127–128.

Yan QJ, Rammal M, Tranfaglia M, Bauchwitz RP (2005) Suppression of two major Fragile X Syndrome mouse model phenotypes by the mGluR5 antagonist MPEP. Neuropharmacology 49: 1053–1066.

12

MOLECULAR BASIS OF LEARNING AND MEMORY

François Bolduc and Tim Tully

The last decade has seen an explosion in our understanding of the biologic basis of cognitive diseases. Better knowledge of the cellular and molecular mechanisms of learning and memory has come from 'model systems,' wherein simple learning tasks are studied in whole animals or in cellular ensembles shown to underlie specific and modifiable behavior. This neurobiologic knowledge more recently has begun to yield pharmaceuticals targeting molecules underlying learning and memory, thereby promising more effective therapies for the treatment of cognitive dysfunction and mental retardation/intellectual disability.

In the late 19th century, psychologic studies revealed memory formation to be a time-dependent process. Ribot (1882) showed that memories were 'plastic' initially present in a labile state that could become stable with time. Ebbinghaus (1885) showed that the proficiency of memory consolidation improved with repeated training sessions separated by a rest interval ('spaced' or 'distributed' training). James (1890) observed that short-term memory (lasting minutes to hours) could be distinguished functionally from long-term memory (LTM) (lasting days to years). Muller and Pilzecker (1900) coined the term 'consolidation' to reflect the observation that memory took time to become fixed (Fig. 12.1). Ramon y Cajal (1894) was among the first to provide a neurobiologic explanation for memory consolidation, suggesting that LTM might be stored in newly grown neuronal connections.

Early 20th century physiologic investigations formalized these initial observations and conceptualizations with systematic study of animal learning and memory.

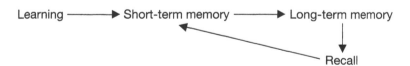

Fig. 12.1. Phases of memory. After a single exposure to a given experience, a transient and unstable memory of the event is formed. A longer lasting form of memory requires repeated exposures. In addition, a mental process known as consolidation will allow the long-term memory to become stable and long-lasting.

Pavlov (1927) established experimental paradigms to study 'associative' learning, a change in a behavioral response caused by the temporal association of two stimuli. In contrast to forms of non-associative learning, which include sensitization (an increased behavioral response to a stimulus) and habituation (a decreased response after repeated presentation of a stimulus), Pavlov's associative learning can be considered an elemental building block of more complex forms of 'contingency' learning (Rescorla 1982). In the canonical form of associative learning, an animal is presented with a neutral 'conditioned stimulus' which in itself does not elicit a behavioral response. When the presentation of the conditioned stimulus is paired for several trials with an 'unconditioned stimulus,' which has an inherent reward or punishment value and accordingly elicits an 'unconditioned response,' the conditioned stimulus independently comes to elicit a response similar to the unconditioned response. From this basic observation, Pavlov derived the general principle of stimulus substitution, which we now can think of as an elemental component of more complex forms of learning.

By mid-century, neuroscientists were attempting to localize various cognitive functions to distinct neuroanatomic sites. Milner (2005) pioneered the characterization of a distinct site involved in the storage of declarative memory by studying individual patients (those who developed memory deficits after localized cortical resection to control intractable epilepsy). Milner's work revealed that the hippocampus, a structure of the temporal lobe, was involved selectively in explicit memory (i.e. facts and knowledge that are expressed verbally) and not in implicit memory (i.e. skills and behavior).

These case studies suggested a more general correlation between various cognitive abilities and neuroanatomic locations leading to the fundamental question, 'Where is memory?' Attempts to address this question ushered in two generations of scientists looking for the cellular and molecular signatures of memory. Hebb (1949) formulated theoretical models of 'cellular plasticity' that underlay memory. He hypothesized that 'learning' reflected a change in the strength of synaptic connections (synaptic plasticity) among neurons that fired together (Fig. 12.2) and 'memory' then resulted in the recruitment of additional ensembles of neurons (neuronal networks) that respond to the original stimulus (experience) (Fig. 12.3). To date, this hypothesis has generated an enormous amount of supportive experimental data. Nowadays, studies of memory have explored both presynaptic and post-synaptic mechanisms that contribute to the process of synaptic plasticity.

This body of work can be summarized by stating that learning and memory reflect changes at three levels of biologic organization. First, the neural activity which registers a new experience induces biochemical (molecular) changes within the active neurons. Second, these biochemical events lead to changes in the connectivity of these neurons (synaptic plasticity). And third, changes in synaptic connectivity produce changes in the function of neural networks. In the remainder of this

Cellular model for learning and memory

1. Synaptic level

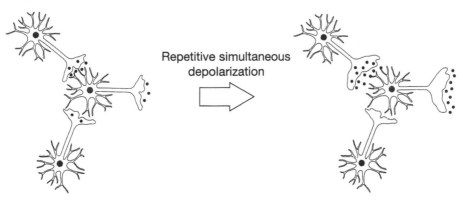

Repetitive simultaneous depolarization

Fig. 12.2. Hebb's model for synaptic plasticity. Monosynaptic reinforcement occurs after repetitive coincident activity. When the presynaptic neuron fires synchronously with the post-synaptic neuron repeatedly, a persistent increase in net output from the post-synaptic neuron is observed. Both structural and physiologic changes underlie this enhancement.

Cellular model for learning and memory

2. Network level

Cellular model for learning and memory

2. Network level

Post-conditioning

US

CS

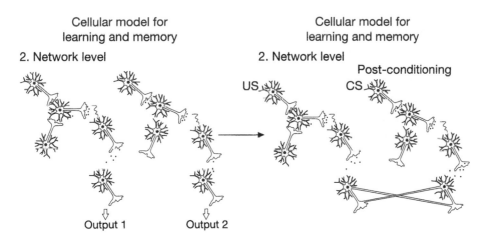

Output 1   Output 2

Fig. 12.3. Hebb's theory of network plasticity. In addition to synaptic plasticity observed after repetitive firing of two neurons, Hebb conceptualized the need for neuronal circuitry plasticity as part of learning and memory. In this example, conditioning will create structural or functional changes that will allow cross-talk between neuronal circuits previously independent. CS, odor; US, footshock.

article, we review the basic molecular and cellular changes which have been shown to underlie learning and memory in simple experimental paradigms. We include a discussion of how this knowledge has begun to inform our understanding of various neurologic diseases.

LEARNING AND SHORT-TERM MEMORY REFLECT TRANSIENT BIOCHEMICAL AND CELLULAR CHANGES

Learning is generally defined as a rapid change in a behavioral response following a new experience. Similarly, initial biochemical events involved in learning are usually fast and involve post-translational changes in already existing proteins (e.g. phosphorylation, dephosphorylation, translocation).

cAMP Pathway

In the latter half of the 20th century, several groups sought a cellular or molecular understanding of learning in animals with simpler nervous systems including *Limax hermissenda*, leech and even paramecium. Of these, the most well-developed and informative has been work on the sea snail, *Aplysia californica*, by Kandel and colleagues (Kandel 2001, 2006). Using a sensitization procedure for the gill withdrawal reflex, where an electric shock to the tail provokes a withdrawal of the gill, Kandel and co-workers were able to isolate identified neurons in the abdominal ganglion, which at least in part mediates an observed behavioral response (Castellucci et al. 1970, Kupfermann et al. 1970). In this abdominal ganglion, serotonin and dopamine were released after electrical stimulation of the tail. Of note, a minimal monosynaptic neural circuitry appeared to be involved in sensitization of the gill withdrawal reflex, which then allowed the demonstration that this simple form of learning produced an increase of the second messenger cyclic adenosine monophosphate (cAMP) which then led to a cAMP-dependent protein kinase A (PKA)-dependent presynaptic enhancement of neurotransmitter release at this synapse (Brunelli et al. 1976) (Fig. 12.4). The mechanism of increased neurotransmitter release was later shown to depend on phosphorylation of two potassium channels: (1) phosphorylation of the S-type K^+ channel caused increased excitability, and (2) phosphorylation of the delayed-rectifier K^+ channel caused broadening of the presynaptic depolarization current (Klein et al. 1982). After such changes in potassium channel currents, a given stimulus produced a stronger calcium influx in the presynaptic (sensory) neuron thereby increasing the release probabilities of neurotransmitter to the post-synaptic (motor) neuron (Kandel and Schwartz 1982). In *Aplysia*, it is worth noting that the molecular changes described above were presynaptic. Importantly though, associative learning in *Aplysia* involves an NMDA-dependent post-synaptic response. This suggested that molecular events implicated in learning had a rapid onset and took advantage of proteins already present in the neurons.

Work on a different animal model suggested an evolutionarily conserved role for cAMP signaling. *Drosophila melanogaster* (fruit fly) was capable to associate odors with footshock punishment (Benzer 1967, 1973, Hotta and Benzer 1973). Flies were exposed to two odors successively, with footshock associated with one of the odors. Odor avoidance then was quantified by exposing the trained flies to each odor

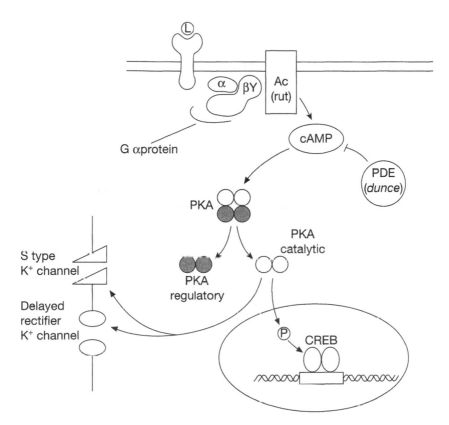

Fig. 12.4. Learning and short-term memory depend on cyclic adenosine monophosphate (cAMP) pathway. After activation of a G-protein-coupled receptor by a ligand (L), adenylyl cyclase (AC) synthesizes cAMP, which in turn is hydrolyzed by phosphodiesterase (PDE). The *Drosophila* mutants *rutabaga* (AC) and *dunce* (PDE) were among the first mutants isolated with heritable defects in learning/memory. Increased levels of cAMP lead to activation of protein kinase A (PKA). After dissociation from its regulatory subunit, the catalytic subunit phosphorylates many targets: (1) potassium channels, which regulate neural activity during short-term memory phases; and (2) the cAMP responsive element binding protein (CREB) transcription factor, which regulates the expression of other genes during long-term memory formation.

successively in the absence of footshock (Quinn et al. 1974). Later, this operant odor-shock avoidance task was modified into a classic conditioning task by: (1) trapping flies into the training chamber, and (2) presenting both odors simultaneously to trained flies in a T-maze (Tully and Quinn 1985). Memory retention measured immediately after one of these Pavlovian training sessions is robust. With repetitive training, flies show memory retention lasting more than a week (Tully et al. 1994).

The development of a learning and memory task in *Drosophila* brought to bear the power of genetics to discover genes and their coded proteins involved with behavioral plasticity. In fact, the first two biochemical defects identified for the single-gene mutants, *dunce* and *rutabaga*, both participated in the cAMP intracellular signaling pathway. The *dunce* mutations produced defects in cAMP-specific phosphodiesterase (PDE), an enzyme that is responsible for the degradation of cAMP (Dudai et al. 1976, Davis and Davidson 1984), and the *rutabaga* mutations produced defects in Ca^{2+} calmodulin-sensitive adenylyl cyclase (AC), an enzyme that is responsible for the synthesis of cAMP (Livingstone et al. 1984, Levin et al. 1992). Because these single-gene mutations were generated randomly and screened independently for defects in the same behavioral task (olfactory learning/memory), these two 'hits' in the same biochemical pathway most certainly could not have occurred by chance. Thus, cAMP signaling clearly appeared to underlie associative learning in *Drosophila*. Interestingly, basal cAMP levels were near-normal in *dnc/rut* double-mutants but the memory deficit was worse than either single-gene mutant. This observation suggested either that *modulation* of cAMP levels was necessary for associative learning/memory or that *dnc* and *rut* functioned in different cAMP signaling pathways distinguished in time or place rather than together.

As in *Aplysia*, the cAMP-dependent PKA also has been shown to be involved in *Drosophila* olfactory memory. PKA is a tetramer, composed of two regulatory subunits and two catalytic subunits. In the absence of cAMP, the regulatory dimer binds the catalytic dimer and inhibits its kinase activity. In the presence of cAMP, the regulatory subunits fail to bind the catalytic dimer and thus the kinase is in an activated state. An inducibly overexpressed transgenic construct encoding a mutant form of the regulatory subunit which no longer was able to bind cAMP had a dominant-negative effect on PKA activity. When expression was induced in adult flies, a defect in memory ensued (Drain et al. 1991).

Neurotransmitters activate cAMP signaling by binding to seven transmembrane domain G-protein-coupled receptors (Simon et al. 1991, Spiegel 1994). In *Aplysia*, the catecholaminergic transmitter serotonin is the relevant ligand for cAMP signaling that underlies behavioral and synaptic plasticity. However, in different neurons dopamine could also trigger increased cAMP synthesis. The gill withdrawal reflex can also be potentiated by dopamine. In *Drosophila*, recent studies have shown dopamine to mediate footshock (punishment) and octopamine to mediate sucrose (reward) stimuli during classic conditioning (Schwaerzel et al. 2003). When a ligand binds a receptor, guanosine triphosphatase (GTP)-bound G_α protein is free to interact with AC (Fig. 12.5). Such an interaction then is terminated when the intrinsic GTPase activity of G protein hydrolyzes GTP to guanosine diphosphate (GDP). Reassociation of GDP-bound G protein with a receptor then leads to the exchange of GDP for GTP. G proteins are composed of three subunits (α, β, γ), and the α subunit can either be stimulatory (G_s) or inhibitory (G_i). *Drosophila* genetics was utilized to test whether G-protein-mediated signaling was involved in Pavlovian olfactory learning (Connolly et al. 1996). Transgenic flies carrying a mutant

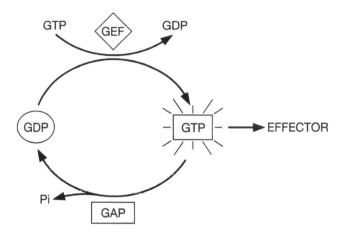

Fig. 12.5. Small GTPase oscillate between active, guanosine triphosphatase (GTP) bound and inactive, guanosine diphosphate (GDP) bound. Oscillation between GTP and GDP bound state is regulated by guanine exchange factor protein (GEF) and guanine activating protein (GAP).

TABLE 12.1
Disease-related genes involved in associative learning

Disease name	Gene name	Locus	OMIM
Albright osteodystrophy	Gs	20q13.2	103580
Neurofibromatosis	NF1	17q11.2	162200
CRASH	L1	Xq28	308840

CRASH, corpus callosum hypoplasia, retardation, adducted thumbs, spastic paraplegia, and hydrocephalus; OMIM, Online Mendelian Inheritance in Man (number).

G_s subunit was generated, which no longer could hydrolyze GTP to GDP. Thus, this mutant G protein would bind irreversibly to AC rendering it constitutively active. Associative learning was completely abolished in these transgenic flies.

In humans, an imprinting defect for a gene encoding G_s is known to cause Albright hereditary osteodystrophy (Online Mendelian Inheritance in Man [OMIM] 103580) (Farfel et al. 1999). This syndrome is characterized by short stature, obesity, round facies, subcutaneous ossifications, brachydactyly, and other skeletal anomalies. Some patients also have mental retardation/intellectual disability (Table 12.1) (Fitch 1982).

Although the degree of conservation across species appears impressive, activation of the cAMP pathway in mammalian brain is quite complex. Regional variations in ligands and effectors produce a variety of cAMP-mediated cellular responses. Other neurotransmitters affecting cAMP signaling include glucocorticoid and norepinephrine. Increased norepinephrine from the locus ceruleus seems to preferentially impair prefrontal lobe functions, such as attention, rather than hippocampus-dependent function, such as working memory. Alternatively, application of the α2A-adrenoreceptor agonist, guanfacine, improved working memory performance in the monkey and rat. Interestingly, this effect is on presynaptic receptors and mediated through the inhibition of the cAMP synthesis. Also, norepinephrine stimulation produced long-term potentiation (LTP) in the dentate gyrus. Thus, norepinephrine agonists appear to enhance plasticity in the hippocampus, but may suppress plasticity in other areas such as the frontal lobe.

NEUROPEPTIDES AND LEARNING

Another noteworthy memory mutant identified from a behavioral screen and highlighting another biochemical pathway was selected by looking for flies with normal learning but defective 45-minute memory (Quinn et al. 1979). Behavioral analyses of memory formation suggests that this mutation affected a functionally distinct phase of memory, middle-term memory (MTM), which appears later and lasts longer than short-term memory (STM) and which is disrupted by some forms of anesthesia. Interestingly, another *amnesiac* mutation, *cheapdate*, also was identified from a mutant screen for flies with defective responses to ethanol intoxication (Moore et al. 1998). The *amnesiac* gene encodes a putative fly homolog to mammalian pituitary adenylate cyclase activating peptide (PACAP), although the amino acid sequence similarity between the fly and mammalian genes is low and no biochemical assay has yet to show that *amnesiac* stimulates AC (Feany and Quinn 1995, Moore et al. 1998).

Using a synthetic human PACAP peptide (PACAP38), a link between PACAP and cAMP signaling was established at the larval neuromuscular junction (NMJ), a common location at which synaptic plasticity is studied (Zhong 1995). PACAP stimulated cAMP synthesis via two different pathways: (1) the *rutabaga* AC (above), and (2) the Ras-Raf pathway. Ras and its effector molecules involved in the active-GTP/inactive-GDP oscillation of G proteins (Fig. 12.5). Using 'genetic dissection' it was shown that separate stimulation of the cAMP and Ras-Raf pathways each were capable to enhance potassium (K^+) current independently at the NMJ, resulting in a net increase in neurotransmitter release probability.

This work on PACAP signaling also led to a study of the *neurofibromatosis 1* (*NF1*) gene in *Drosophila*. Neurofibromatosis type 1 (OMIM 162200) is clinically characterized by multiple tumors (optic neuroma, schanomas, plexiform neurofibroma), skin anomalies (café au lait spots, axillary freckling), and learning disability (Swaiman 2006). Molecularly, the neurofibromin protein contains a Ras-specific guanosine triphosphatase-activating (Ras-GAP) domain. GAP proteins enhance the intrinsic hydrolytic activity of Ras proteins, rendering them in an inactive GDP bound state. Flies mutant for *NF1* have decreased body size and deficits in Pavlovian olfactory learning (Guo et al. 2000). Ras1 signaling appeared normal in these *NF1* mutants but, curiously, transgenic overexpression of the catalytic subunit of PKA 'rescued' both their body size and learning defect, suggesting an interaction between NF1 and cAMP signaling (Guo et al. 2000). In addition, muta-tion of *NF1* blocked the PACAP-induced enhancement of potassium current at the larval NMJ (Zhong 1995). Further biochemical dissection of NF1 protein showed that a region outside of the GAP-related domain is responsible for the growth defect present in *NF1* mutant mice (Li et al. 2005, Hannan et al. 2006, Ho et al. 2007). Recently, an HMG-CoA inhibitor, lovastatin, was shown in mouse to reverse the learning deficit observed in *NF1* mutant mice (Krab et al. 2008) (Fig. 12.6).

14-3-3 and learning
Molecular characterization of a learning mutant *leonardo* reveals this to be a disruption of a gene encoding the fly homolog of 14-3-3 (Skoulakis and Davis 1996). In general, 14-3-3 is an 'adapter' protein known to interact with other proteins involved in a variety of cellular processes (regulation of tyrosine and tryptophan hydroxylase, calcium-regulated exocytosis, cell cycle control, protein kinase C [PKC] regulation, Raf-1, and phosphoinositide 3-kinase [PI-3] signal transduction). 14-3-3 has been identified as a constituent in Pick bodies in brains of patients with Pick bodies dementia, and the sigma isoform of 14-3-3 is a marker of a prion med-icated disorder (Creutzfeldt–Jakob disease). Obviously, the involvement of 14-3-3 in Ras-Raf signaling might provide a molecular explanation for the learning deficit of *leonardo* mutants. Recently, another possible mechanism has been suggested based on 14-3-3's interaction with PKC, because modulation of PKC zeta affects memory in *Drosophila*.

CELL ADHESION MOLECULES
Although originally noted for their role in cell–cell contact in cancerous tissues, cell adhesion molecules also appear to mediate physical contact and commun-ication at the synapse (Grotewiel et al. 1998). The prototypical vertebrate cell adhesion molecule is neural cell adhesion molecule (NCAM). In the mammalian hippocampus, LTP, a cellular model of synaptic plasticity (Lomo 2003, Bliss and Lomo 2004), is induced normally but decays away more rapidly than normal in mice with mutant NCAM. In *Aplysia*, the NCAM homolog, ApCAM, is down-regulated rapidly via endocytosis in presynaptic neurons after exposure to serotonin (Bailey et al. 2004). In *Drosophila*, it has been shown that mutants of *fasciclin II* (*fasII*), the *Drosophila* homolog of NCAM, display defects in short-term memory, thereby linking cell adhesion molecules to mechanisms of behavioral plasticity.

Some cell adhesion molecules may also signal between presynaptic and post-synaptic neurons. Integrins, for instance, are cell adhesion molecules that form heterodimers containing α and β subunits and promote cell adhesion and/or

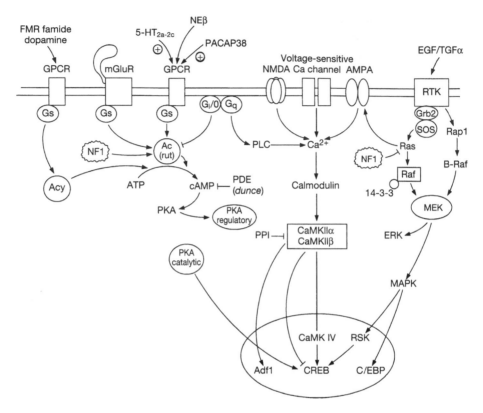

Fig. 12.6. Several signal transduction pathways involved in short-term memory lead to cyclic adenosine monophosphate (cAMP) responsive element binding protein (CREB) modulation. In addition to the cAMP pathway described above (Fig. 12.4), increase in intracellular calcium concentration leads to phosphorylation of the calcium-calmodulin kinase (CaMKII) which, when phosphorylated, can autophosphorylate, thus maintaining its enzymatic activity after the disappearance of the initial signal (calcium entry). CaMKII will phosphorylate CaMKIV resulting in CREB phosphorylation. This persistent activity is thought of as a molecular trace for memory. In parallel, stimulation of receptor tyrosine kinase can activate the ras-MEK pathway that will also lead to CREB phosphorylation, which then interact with the mitogen kinase (MEK) pathway.

extracellular matrix interactions. PKC and Ras signaling molecules family (H-Ras, R-Ras, and Rap) have been shown to influence these interactions. In *Drosophila*, α integrin and short-term memory are defective in *Voldao* mutants (Grotewiel et al. 1998).

L1 is another cell adhesion molecule that is involved in mammalian memory formation (Luthl et al. 1994, Bliss et al. 2000). Here again a link to the human condition exists. L1 originally was identified in patients with X-linked hydro-cephalus. Further investigation of these patients has revealed a more complex disorder known as CRASH syndrome (corpus callosum hypoplasia, mental retardation, adducted thumbs, spastic paraplegia, and hydrocephalus) (OMIM 308840) (Swaiman 2006).

LONG-TERM MEMORY

In general, LTM is defined as a change in behavior that persists for more than a day after training. The 'consolidation' of a new experience into LTM usually requires repeated training sessions with a rest interval in between. LTM appears initially to be disruptible by anesthesia or interference, but eventually becomes resistant to disruption. A growing body of neurobiologic evidence suggests that the appearance of a stable LTM is associated with long-lasting changes in the structure and function of synapses in neural circuits subserving the particular behavioral response.

LONG-TERM MEMORY REQUIRES PROTEIN SYNTHESIS

Early on, characterizations of LTM formation were phenomenologic. LTM was defined as memory retention of 1 day or more, resistant to disruption (anesthesia) or distraction (anterograde interference). LTM for most experiences required repeated practice with a rest in between practice sessions (Ebbinghaus 1885). One of the earliest biochemical characteristics was discovered to be its dependence on the synthesis of new proteins. Although the basic claim remained controversial for years, Flexner et al. (1963) was the first to show that 1-day memory after avoidance discrimination learning was lost in rats injected with puromycin, a protein synthesis inhibitor.

The *Aplysia* model system built upon this observation. Four repeated trials per day spaced over 4 days was required to produce a memory of the siphon withdrawal reflex that lasted for weeks. These behavioral results were encoded at the cellular level by showing electrophysiologically that long-term facilitation (LTF) at a sensorimotor synapse underlying the gill withdrawal response also required four applications of serotonin spaced in time. Using this reduced preparation, it was observed that application of the protein synthesis inhibitors, anisomycin, emetine (translational blockers), actinomycin D or α-amanitin (transcriptional blockers) inhibited the LTF normally induced by repeated application of serotonin (Montarolo et al. 1986). Interestingly, it was also determined that there existed a 3-hour 'critical period' immediately after serotonin application for the effects of protein synthesis inhibitors on LTF (Fig. 12.7).

In mammals, LTP is a electrophysiologic measure of cellular plasticity. Initially described for a specific circuit in the hippocampus, synaptic transmission in the perforant pathway of the dendate gyrus (a region of the hippocampus) was facilitated after a high frequency tetanic stimulation (Bliss and Lomo 1973, Lomo 2003). LTP – and its complementary phenomenon, long-term depression (LTD) – have become established as a more global cellular phenomenon in the brain, and

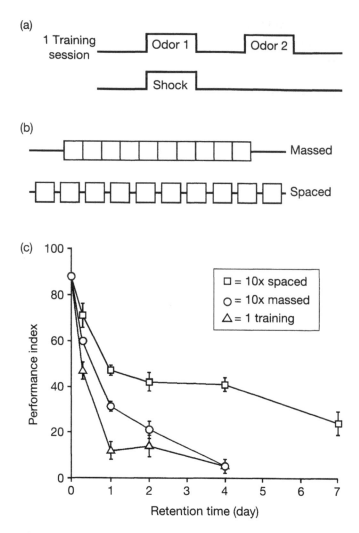

Fig. 12.7. Olfactory classic conditioning in *Drosophila* requires for spaced training for long-term memory. *Drosophila* can be trained to remember the association between an odor (CS) and a footshock (US). Single training (triangle) leads to a memory that decay rapidly but persist to low level for up to 4 days. Repeated training without rest interval leads to a higher level of performance but also last approximatively 4 days. In contrast, the same amount of repeated training separated by rest interval leads to a memory lasting for at least 1 week at higher performance level. (After Tully et al. 1994).

recently hippocampal LTP has been shown to be induced directly by behavioral plasticity. Similar evidence for the requirement for *de novo* protein synthesis came from the study of LTP. It was shown that intraventricular administration of ani- somycin during tetanization of the perforant path did not affect the induction of LTP, but rather blocked its persistence (Krug et al. 1984). It was also shown that the late phase of LTP (from 3 to 5 hours onward) specifically was blocked by anisomycin in the hippocampal CA1 region (Frey et al. 1988). Thus, the appearance of a long-lasting LTP also depends on protein synthesis.

In *Drosophila*, LTM after Pavlovian olfactory learning requires both repetitive spaced training and protein synthesis (Tully et al. 1994). Ten training sessions (with 12 'trials' in a session) with a 15-minute rest interval between each (i.e. spaced training) are sufficient to induce a memory (i.e. learned behavior) lasting more than 1 week. In contrast, the same 10 training sessions with no rest intervals (i.e. massed training) induces a memory that decays away within 4 days. One-day memory after spaced training usually is greater than that after massed training (Fig. 12.8). When flies were trained in the presence of the protein synthesis inhibitor, cycloheximide (CXM), 1-day memory after spaced training was reduced significantly to a level similar to 1-day memory after massed training. Moreover, CXM did not affect 1-day memory after massed training.

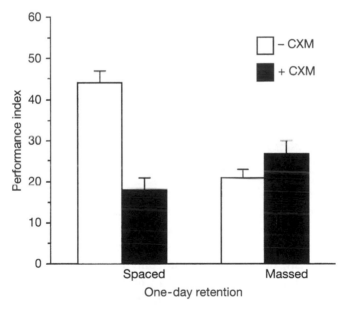

Fig. 12.8. Long-term memory requires new protein synthesis. In *Drosophila* as well as in most model systems, protein synthesis is required for long-term memory. Indeed, performance index 1 day after repeated training spaced by rest interval usually leads to a performance around 45 in wild-type flies. However, feeding cycloheximide (a protein synthesis inhibitor) to flies before training and during the consolidation interval leads to a score of around 20. Interestingly, cycloheximide feeding has no effect on the memory formed after massed training. Also, the residual level of performance in flies fed cycloheximide and trained in a spaced manner is similar to the score of massed training. Various protein synthesis inhibitors (cycloheximide, puromycin, and rapamycin) have been used to block long-term memory.

Together these data suggest a 'pharmacologic dissection' of 1-day memory into a CXM-sensitive LTM component and an CXM-insensitive memory component, referred to as 'anesthesia-resistant memory' (ARM). It remains unclear whether these functionally distinct memory phases represent different biochemical pathways or anatomic circuits or both during memory formation.

Recent studies in mammals suggest that LTM becomes unstable again each time it is recalled. This transient period has been shown recently in chick and rodents to require a somewhat similar molecular mechanism as initial memory storage, but interesting differences in biochemistry and anatomy may exist (Mileusnic et al. 2005).

TRANSLATIONAL CONTROL AND SYNAPSE SPECIFICITY

The requirement for protein synthesis is present across multiple *in vivo* and *in vitro* models of LTM. This observation immediately posed a conceptual conflict, because of another widespread observation that LTM was accompanied by synapse-specific structural and therefore functional changes (Matsuzaki et al. 2004). How then do transcription and translation, which were assumed to occur in and near the nucleus, lead to specific changes in limited remote synaptic sites? Four mechanisms have been suggested to explain how synapse specificity might result from a common cellular event (Fig. 12.9):

1 'Mail' hypothesis
2 Local protein synthesis hypothesis
3 Synaptic tag hypothesis
4 Perisynaptic pool activation
5 Synaptic capture

According to the mail hypothesis, proteins required for long-term changes are synthesized away from the synapse but are sent to activated synapses via a transport and address system (Satpute-Krishnan et al. 2006).

The local protein synthesis hypothesis, in contrast, postulates that mRNA is transported generally, but translated locally only in response to specific synaptic signals. Protein synthesis may occur at the base of the dendritic spine from material contained in mRNA granules similarly to previously observed in the growth cone (Crino and Eberwine 1996). The presence of mRNA (Kleiman et al. 1990, Glanzer and Eberwine 2003), ribosomes, and translation factors (Tiedge and Brosius 1996, Crino et al. 1998, Krichevsky and Kosik 2001) at the synapse support this hypothesis.

The synaptic tag hypothesis involves the construction of a tag at an activated synapse that then sequesters proteins made elsewhere in the neuron (Martin et al. 1997). Using a minimal cellular model with co-cultured sensory and motor neurons, long-term plasticity was sustained by functional and structural changes at recently activated synapses. Two mechanistic characteristics were identified to be required

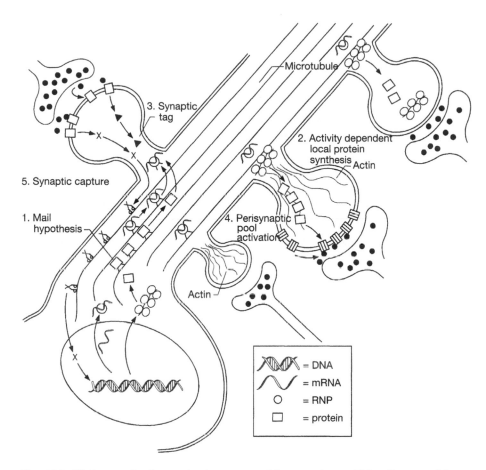

Fig. 12.9. Various molecular mechanisms can explain synaptic specificity. Some models are summarized here to explain how post-training changes could occur at specific synapses only in contrast to cell-wide phenomenon. 1. The mail hypothesis where a specific cargo of protein is delivered at a synapse marked after activation. 2. The local protein synthesis hypothesis suggests the presence of mRNA under the synapse ready to be translated into protein upon presentation of the appropriate signal. 3. The synaptic tag hypothesis suggest the marking of a synapse following its activation. Although the molecular nature of the tag is unknown, its postulated function would be to anchor the appropriate building blocks for the potentiated synapse. 4. The perisynaptic pool hypothesis refer to the observation of 'silent' synapses where receptors have been localized outside of the synatic space in the dendrite. These receptors are thought to be mobilized to the synaptic space rapidly after long-term potentiation (LTP). 5. Finally, the synaptic capture hypothesis suggests an interplay between the activated synapse and the nucleus, either via sequestration of RNA or localization of proteins.

for maintenance of this long-term plasticity. First, protein synthesis was necessary because the persistence of functional and structural changes was blocked by local application of the protein synthesis inhibitor, rapamycin. Second, PKA activity at the synapse also was necessary for the maintenance of these long-term changes.

Finally, the sensitization hypothesis suggests that proteins necessary for long-term changes are present at variable levels throughout the cell. Upon stimulation, the level of protein at a given location will influence the nature of the plasticity change.

In summary, multiple non-exclusive alternative mechanisms could create synapse specificity but the need for nucleus–synapse communication remains. Indeed, cAMP response element binding protein (CREB) activation has been shown to be required for the maintenance of the local structural changes elicited by long-term facilitation. By injecting anti-CREB2 (the CREB repressor), structural changes were observed, as well as the prevention of further change by future serotonin application. In addition, isolation of the nucleus from the synapse abolished the maintenance of the long-term changes observed (Martin et al. 1997).

One common aspect of these hypotheses is the transport of mRNA from the nucleus to the activated synapse either before or after training. Staufen is required for microtubule-dependent transport of RNA in rat. A role for Staufen has been postulated in LTM after spaced training in *Drosophila*. Taking advantage of a temperature-sensitive allele of *staufen*, the formation of LTM was blocked in staufen mutants, simply by keeping the flies at a restrictive temperature during the retention interval, but not during training or testing. Interestingly, developmental studies have shown that Staufen associates with the 3' untranslated region of mRNA (*bicoid* and *oscar*) and with microtubule-dependent molecular motors (St Johnston et al. 1991).

Furthermore, two mutant alleles within the *oskar* gene also showed LTM defects. *Pumilio* is another 'developmental gene' which appears to be required for LTM formation. Pumilio is involved in translational repression of *hunchback* (*hb*) and recognizes a specific nucleotide sequence, Nanos responsive element (NRE), within the 3' untranslated region of mRNA. Upon binding to an NRE, Nanos binds to Pumilio and represses translation of *hb*. Aside from its defect in LTM, *pumilio* mutants also present increased neuronal excitability (Stern et al. 1995). Previous studies have shown that overexpression of *oskar* rescues the increased neuronal excitability of *pumilio*. That *pumilio* and *staufen* mutants both disrupt LTM formation suggests a mechanistic link between these two genes (Smith et al. 1992).

Another protein involved in the regulation of mRNA translation is the fragile X mental retardation protein (FMRP). In fragile X syndrome (OMIM 309550), FMRP expression is absent as a result of transcriptional silencing of the *FMR1* gene. Most patients with fragile X syndrome have an increased number of CGG trinucleotide repeats in the FMR1 promoter region (>200) (Verkerk et al. 1991,

Fragile X syndrome pathogenesis

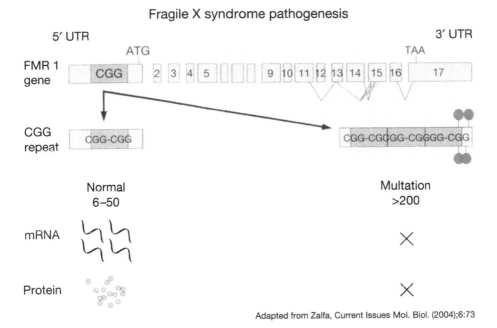

Adapted from Zalfa, Current Issues Mol. Biol. (2004);6:73

Fig. 12.10. Molecular basis of the fragile X syndrome. The fragile X syndrome gene is localized on the X chromosome. The region upstream of FMR coding region contains trinucleotid (CGG) repeats. In unaffected human, the number of repeats is 6–50. Affected individuals have an expansion of the repeat above 200 copies. This triggers DNA methylation of the promoter and the coding region downstream. Finally, this leads to lack of the fragile X mental retardation protein (FMRP).

Oostra et al. 1993). Methylation of these repeats as well as the downstream promoter appear to cause transcriptional silencing. Some individuals with trinucleotide repeats beyond 200, but with a defect in methylation, remain asymptomatic. A few cases of fragile X syndrome have been reported with either deletions or point mutations (De Boulle 1993) within the *FMR1* gene itself (Hegde et al. 2001). A patient with a severe form of fragile X syndrome has been reported who had a normal repeat region but a single amino acid substitution in an important RNA binding domain, the KH2 domain, of FMR1 (De Boulle et al. 1993) (Fig. 12.10).

Several biochemical studies have suggested a role for FMRP in translational control. Furthermore, several studies have identified possible FMRP target mRNA, but little overlap among the candidates has been observed. One target identified in both *in vitro* and *in vivo* studies is the microtubule-associated protein (MAP1B) (aka Futsch in *Drosophila*). FMRP has been shown to suppress MAP1B translation in adult flies and during mouse brain development. Genetic disruption of *FMR1* in mouse produces learning and memory defects (Mineur et al. 2002, Zhao et al. 2005). Enhanced LTD in the hippocampus of *FMR1* knockout mouse has been noted. Application of a glutamate metabotropic receptor antagonist, but not a NMDA receptor antagonist, blocked this effect. Metabotropic glutamate receptor-dependent LTD requires p38 mitogen-activated protein kinase (MAPK), PKC, phosopholipase C, and early onset protein synthesis (Malenka and Bear 2004). NMDA receptor-dependent LTD, however, is thought to involve protein phosphatase 1 (PP1), calcineurin, the Rap-p38MAPK pathway, and removal of AMPA receptor containing the subunit GluR2/R3 in a clathrin/AP2-dependent manner. Interestingly, the application of a metabotropic receptor agonist leads to spine elongation, a defect previously observed in both patients with fragile X and *FMR1* knockout mice. Alternatively, McBride et al. (2005) used a competitive antagonist of mGluR receptors (MPEP) to rescue a memory defect in *FMR1* mutants flies. Together, these observations suggest that FMRP regulates plasticity specifically at glutamatergic synapses.

Classically, translation is divided into initiation, elongation, and termination. At each of these steps, protein synthesis is regulated by both general (cell-wide) and specific (local) factors (Sutton and Schuman 2005). Cytoplasmic polyadenylation element binding protein (CPEB) favors translation of a subset of mRNAs (CaMKII, for instance) in response to synaptic activity (Wu et al. 1998). After NMDA receptor activation at the synapse, a rapid rise in intracellular calcium is observed which triggers phosophorylation of CaMKII, Aurora kinase, and finally CPEB. CPEB binds only to mRNAs that contain a specific nucleic acid sequence, the cytoplasmic polyadenylation element (CPE). When activated, CPEB promotes polyadenylation of nascent mRNAs, which enhances overall translation of mRNA (Paris and Richter 1990).

A more general regulatory pathway for translation involves mTOR (target of rapamycin) and S6Kinase. Translation is initiated by the assembly of several eukarotic initiation factors (eIFs). eIF-4E binds the 5′ end of mRNA, but its interaction with other eIFs is repressed by 4E binding protein (4E-BP). mTOR inhibits 4E-BP leading to increased translation. Interestingly, *TSC1* and *TSC2*, genes responsible for tuberous sclerosis complex syndrome 1 and 2 (OMIM 191100), respectively, function upstream in this pathway as inhibitors of mTOR. Tuberous sclerosis complex syndrome is characterized by various cortical malformations, epilepsy, and variable degrees of mental retardation/intellectual disability. Loss of function of either *TSC1* or *TSC2* results in the loss of complex formation, which then leads to loss of mTOR repression and increased mTOR repression of 4E-BP. The net effect is an increase in translation (Fig. 12.11).

So far, experimentally, local protein synthesis can be triggered *in vitro* by stimulation of NMDA receptors, metabotropic glutamate receptor (mGluR), and neurotrophic tyrosine kinase (TrKB) receptors.

In addition to modulation of 4E-BP, phosphorylation of translation initation factors also has a role in plasticity-induced translation. Recently, it was shown that

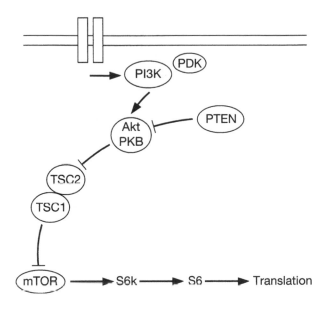

Fig. 12.11. Tuberous sclerosis proteins are involved in the control of protein synthesis. Control of translation occurs via S6 ribosomal subunit phosphorylation. Growth factor receptors activate the phosphoinositol 3-kinase (PI-3K) that phosphorylate Akt. Phosphorylated AKT then inhibits tuberous sclerosis protein 1 and 2. TSC1 and 2 form a complex that in turns inhibit a protein known as target of rapamycine (TOR). S6K phosphorylate the subunit 6 of the ribosome which in turn activate translation of the mRNA.

phosphorylation of eIF4α is required for LTP which is under bi-directional modulation with GCN2 (Costa-Mattioli et al. 2007). In the presence of a pharmacologic agonist of GCN, a single volley of stimulation lead to late LTP, compared to the four volleys normally required.

LONG-TERM MEMORY REQUIRES TRANSCRIPTION FACTOR CREB AND ADF-1

De novo mRNA synthesis (transcription) seems to be necessary for LTM formation. Transcription factors regulate this process. Guided by early studies in *Drosophila* which used mutant screens to identify the memory mutants *dunce* (phosphodiesterase) and *rutabaga* (AC) and by subsequent reverse-genetics methods to dissect other components of the cAMP signaling pathway, disruption of the CREB protein confirmed the hypothesis that protein synthesis-dependent LTM formation specifically would be blocked (Yin et al. 1994). In mammals, partial knockout of CREB impairs memory and injections of antisense oligonucleotides to CREB into the hippocampus or amygdala of normal rats also produces apparent memory deficits (Guzowski and McGaugh 1997). More recently, it was shown that CREB was required presynaptically for synaptic enhancement (Wagastuma et al. 1996).

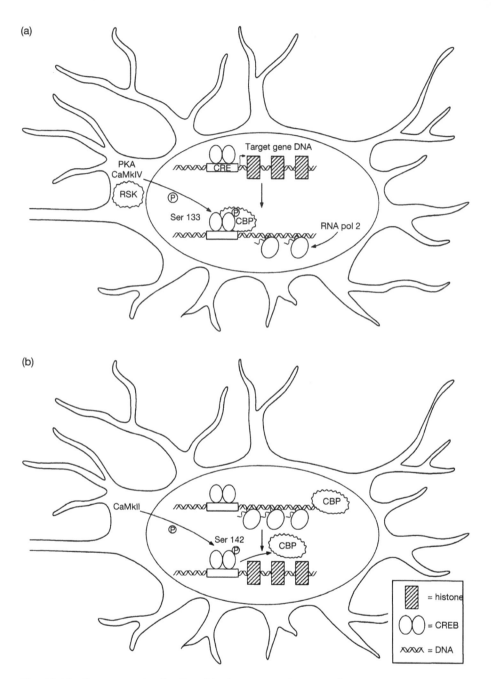

Fig. 12.12. Gene expression is affected by histone acetylation regulation. (a) DNA is wrapped around molecules known as histones (dashed rectangles). In order to transcribe a CRE containing gene, given signaling molecules (CaMKIV, RSK, or PKA) must phosphorylate CREB at serine 133 thus allowing conformation change and association to CREB binding protein (CBP) which in turn causes acetylation of histones. Once acetylated, histone allow transcription of DNA. (b) However, phosphorylation of CREB at serine 142 causes the release of CBP which leads to transcription repression.

The CREB-dependent gene transcription was induced after protocols that yielded late LTP but not early LTP (Impey et al. 1996). With the sensorimotor co-culture system in *Aplysia*, LTF is enhanced when cells are injected with antibodies to CREB repressor (Fig. 12.12).

CREB is a transcription factor that binds as a dimer to a specific DNA sequence (TGACGTCA) known as cAMP response element (CRE) in the promoter/enhancer regions of 'downstream' CREB-regulated genes. Several genes with CRE sites are involved in neuronal plasticity (Table 12.2). CREB is thought to be constituitively bound to DNA, but inactive until phosphorylated. Several kinases are known to target serine 133 of CREB for phosphorylation, among which are PKA, CaMKIV, and MAPK-activated ribosomal S6 kinase (Rsk). Phosphorylation at serine 133 promotes transcription (Hunter and Karin 1992). Interestingly, mutation of Rsk is known to cause Coffin–Lowry syndrome (OMIM 303600). This syndrome is characterized by mental retardation, a peculiar 'pugilistic' nose, large ears, tapered fingers, drumstick terminal phalanges on X-ray, and pectus carinatum (Swaiman 2006). Interestingly, phosphorylation by CaMKII at serine 142 leads to the opposite effect of CREB dimer dissociation and decreased transcription (Sun et al. 1994).

Once phosphorylated at serine 133, CREB recruits CREB binding protein (CBP). CBP is involved in histone acetylation which opens chromatin, exposing DNA to polymerase II dependent transcription. Deletions within CBP are responsible for Rubinstein–Taybi syndrome (OMIM 180849). This syndrome is characterized by mental retardation/intellectual disability (IQ average 51), seizures (one-quarter of patients), microcephaly, and various dysmorphismic features, such as downward-slanting palpebral fissures, a hypoplastic maxilla with narrow palate, small mouth opening, broad thumb with radial angulation, and broad great toes (Swaiman 2006). A mouse model (Oike et al. 1999a, 1999b) of Rubinstein–Taybi syndrome shows behaviorally defective LTM in passive avoidance and fear conditioning tasks and goes on to show that mutant CBP mice had a selective deficit in LTM but normal STM (Bourtchouladze et al. 2003). In accordance with the previously established cAMP pathway (Fig. 12.2), phosphodiesterase inhibitors ameliorated this LTM defect, presumably by increasing cAMP levels and CREB phosphorylation after training. Importantly, this outcome in the mouse model of Rubinstein–Taybi syndrome suggests that: (1) some forms of mental retardation/intellectual disability result from functional (biochemical) rather than structural (developmental) deficits in brain function, and (2) the former may respond to a traditional drug therapy approach.

CREB acts in parallel with the adhesion molecule Fas II (Davis and Laroche 2006). Indeed, the expression of CREB in a mutant deficient for Fas II recovered normal synaptic structure. However, expression of CREB repressor in a *dunce* background recovered the synaptic activity, but not the structural defects observed at the NMJ, thus indicating the presence of parallel pathway downstream of initial cAMP signaling. *Naylot* mutants, found in a behavioral screen for *Drosophila* LTM

TABLE 12.2

Genes containing cyclic adenosine monophosphate (cAMP) response element (CRE) motif involved in synaptic plasticity

Gene name	Function
Adenylate cyclase VIII	Production cAMP
AMPA receptor GluR1 subunit	Glutamate receptor subunit
BDNF	Growth factor
CREM	CREB negative regulation
CRF	Cortisol/stress modulation
Dynorphin	Opioid-like neuropeptide
Fos	Immediate–early gene
Tyrosine hydroxylase	Neurotransmitter production

CREB, cAMP responsive element binding protein.

defects, identified another transcription factor, *Adf-1*. *Adf-1* is a myeloblastosis viral oncogene homolog (myb)-related transcription factor. Although no gross dysmorphism of the adult central nervous system was observed, developmental plasticity at the larval NMJ revealed microscopic evident defects in synaptic structure (DeZazzo et al. 2000).

MAP KINASE SIGNALING

Linking neural activity to gene transcription involves neurotransmitter receptors and intracellular second-messenger pathways. One important signal transduction pathway includes MAPK. This family of genes originally was found to regulate cell division and differentiation and is known to be crucial for LTM (Sharma and Carew 2004, Sweatt 2004, Davis and Laroche 2006). Initially known as microtubule-associated protein kinases, they have important interaction with microtubules. They are also responsible for intracellular signaling necessary for LTM, influencing several key aspects such as transcription factors (CREB, Elk-1), protein synthe ˙ ˙, cytoskeletal proteins, and post-synaptic glutamate receptors. Three major families are known: ERK, p38MAPK, and cJunk. First, nerve growth factor (NGF) signals to both MAPK and ERK. Glutamate signals through two isoforms, ERK1 and ERK2 (p44MAPK and p42MAPK). Second, NMDA receptor and SynGAP signals through the p38MAPK pathway. The third member of MAPK is c-junk amino-terminal kinase for which little is known at present in relation to memory.

NOTCH SIGNALING AND LONG-TERM MEMORY

Notch is another 'developmental gene' previously known to be involved in cellular differentiation during neuronal development which serves both as a transmembrane receptor and a transcription factor. Notch is known to be cleaved by a furin-like convertase and to insert in the cellular membrane. Binding with DSL (Delta, Serrate, or Lag-2) then triggers a gamma secretase-dependent cleavage, thereby releasing an intracellular fragment which then translocates to the nucleus. Presenilin, for which mutations have been identified in some patients with Alzheimer's disease, is a component of gamma-secretase (Verdile et al. 2007). Recently, a role for *Notch* in *Drosophila* LTM formation has been reported (Ge et al. 2004, Presente et al. 2004). Similarly, mouse *Notch* mutants displayed memory defects in a water maze task (Costa et al. 2003). *Notch* antisense transgenic mice exhibited normal development but have a decreased level of LTP (Wang et al. 2004). Mutations in *Notch 3* have been identified in CADASIL (cerebral arteriopathy, autosomal dominant with subcortical infarcts and leukodystrophy) (OMIM 125310). CADASIL is characterized clinically by recurrent migraines, strokes featuring progressive focal neurologic signs (including pseudobulbar signs), seizures, and dementia.

NMDA Receptors, Long-term Potentiation, and Long-term Memory
Following the clinical observation that the hippocampus was crucial for declarative memory formation, electrophysiologic methods were utilized to measure synaptic plasticity in the hippocampus. LTP was delineated as a cellular analog of memory (Lomo 1973). After high frequency tetanic stimulation of the perforant pathway to the dentate (a region of the hippocampus) facilitation in synaptic transmission was observed. This type of plasticity is spike timing dependent. Indeed, depolarization 5–15ms before tetanic stimulation causes LTP. In the CA1 region of the hippocampus, LTP was discovered to require NMDA receptors (Collingridge et al. 1983). A key finding was that pharmacologic inhibitors of NMDA receptors imported both LTP and memory. NMDA receptor conductance is blocked at resting potential by magnesium ions. Cellular depolarization is required to remove the Mg^{2+} block. This property suggested that the NMDA receptor might function as a coincidence detector where depolarization from a unconditioned stimulus for example, and neurotransmitter release (from a conditioned stimulus, are both required for its activation. Indeed, this was shown to be true. More recently, a role for NDMA receptors in *Drosophila* memory has been demonstrated, again emphasizing the evolutionarily conserved nature of molecular mechanisms of associative learning (Xia and Yang 2005).

NMDA receptors are composed of an obligatory NR1 subunit and a variable NR2 subunit (NR2A–D) (Paoletti and Nexton 2007). During development, a progressive switch from NR2B to NR2A has been observed in the visual, somatosensory, and motor cortex (Barth and Malinka 2001, Lu et al. 2001). Because NR2A promotes a faster kinetic and an increased temporal resolution of synaptic depolarizations, higher stimulation frequencies are required to induce LTP in older animals. This may constitute a homeostatic mechanism whereby synaptic overexcitation is prevented and stimulus resolution is optimized. Notably, NR2B appears to be constituvely present at the synapse, while neural activity drives incorporation of the NR2A into NMDA receptors (Barria and Malinow 2002). NMDA receptor activation, and the concommittant rise in intracellular calcium, leads to Ras activation and signaling through PI-3 kinase and AKT. AKT activation then induces the mTOR pathway.

The mediators and modulators of NMDA receptor-dependent LTP are being investigated currently. NMDA-dependent LTP is considered now to be largely postsynaptic and has been induced by a variety of protocols. With NMDA receptor activation, a rise in intracellular calcium is followed by the activation of calmodulin and calcium/calmodulin kinase 2 (CaMKII). So far, all protocols used to induce LTP require CaMKII. Activated CaMKII phosphorylates serine 831 of the GluR1 subunit of AMPA receptor (Roche et al. 1996, Barria et al. 1997). Phosphorylation at serine 831 potentiates channel activity by increasing the probability of channel opening and therefore conductance through the channel (Brenke 1998). An NMDA receptor independent form of LTP can be induced in the mossy fiber-CA3 region by glutamatergic activation of kainate receptors. This form of LTP is cAMP dependent and appears presynaptic in origin.

INSERTION OF AMPA RECEPTORS AT SILENT SYNAPSES AND MAINTANCE OF LONG-TERM PLASTICITY

Following NMDA activation, a cascade of second messenger pathways eventually leads to modification of the subunit composition of AMPA receptor (Bredt and Nicoll 2003). This change in the ratio of various subunits is thought to be necessary for the persistence of memory. AMPA receptors are composed of two subunits of variable type (GluR1–R4). Subunits can be grouped according to the length of the C terminal region. It was shown that fluorescent protein (GFP)-tagged AMPA receptor moved from the dendritic shaft to the spine after high frequency stimulation and that this movement was blocked upon application of NMDA antagonists (Shi et al. 2001). Use of an electrophysiologic tag similarly showed *de novo* insertion of AMPA receptors. Activation of NMDA receptor stimulates the Ras-Gap and p42-MAPK pathways resulting in the addition of AMPA receptors with subunit GluR1/GluR2 (Zhu et al. 2001, Malinow and Malinka 2002, Malenka and Bear 2004). Fast addition of GluR2 subunit to the synapse is dependent on N-ethylmaleimide-sensitive fusion protein (NSF), which binds GluR2 and is an ATPase involved in membrane fusion. Interestingly, NSF was initially identified in a screen for genes involved in seizures in rodents and was called epilepsy-related gene 1 (ERG-1). Mutant NSF mice later were found to have defective spatial memory in the Morris water maze.

NMDA receptor-dependent addition of AMPA receptors to synapses previously devoid of them (known as the silent synapse) is thought to be a major mechanism of LTP (Isaac 2003). Insertion of new receptors to the synapse would require

SNARE-dependent exocytosis and actin. Mutation of the CaMKII phosphory-lation site on GluR1 did not prevent the delivery of AMPA receptor. However, mutation in the PDZ domain binding blocked the delivery of the receptor (Hayashi et al. 2007).

In vivo expression of CREB and CaMKIV increased NMDA-dependent synaptic transmission and LTP (Marie et al. 2005). In addition, there was evidence of silent synapses being populated after CREB expression. During NMDA-dependent LTP, two protein kinases are involved in increasing conductance and delivering AMPA receptors to the synapse. Serine 831 phosphorylation on GluR1 by CaMKII increased conductance, but mutation of that site did not prevent delivery at the synapse. Conversely, serine 845 phosphorylation by PKA is necessary for targeting to the synapse. PKA activity may be mediated by AKAP-mediated binding to cytoskeleton, thus bringing PKA to the GluR1 subunit.

All forms of LTD thus far seem to involve decreased post-synaptic AMPA signaling (Malenka 2003, Malinow 2003, Malenka and Bear 2004). Long-term synaptic depression (LTD) has been associated with loss of AMPA receptors via endocytosis. The process is associated with clathrin-coated vesicles and is dependent on dynamin (Fig. 12.13).

Neuronal Structure and Plasticity

Modifications in neuronal shape, especially at the synapse, occur during long-term plasticity. Most of the work so far has focused on dendritic changes. Dendrites contain extensions of smaller caliber known as spines. Various lines of evidence link dendritic spine morphology to memory formation. First, syndromes associated with mental retardation (i.e. fragile X syndrome) are associated with histologic evidence of spine anomalies either in density or morphology. Second, LTP causes a rapid increase in extension of filipodia and formation of new synapses at the site of stimulation in a NMDA- and calcium-dependent manner (Matsuzaki et al. 2004). Indeed, dendritic arbor maturation was demonstrated to be NMDA receptor-dependent in *Xenopus* (Sin et al. 2002). Finally, there seems to be a strong correlation between spine size (volume) and synaptic strength. For instance, larger spines have been shown to contain more AMPA receptors (Nusser et al. 1998, Takumi et al. 1999). Also, local synaptic stimulation via a caged glutamate technique has shown that larger spines yield larger excitatory post-synaptic potentials (Matsuzaki et al. 2001).

The structure of dendritic spines emerges from the organization of the cytoskeleton, which is composed of actin polymer and microtubule bundles. Thus, regulators of actin or microtubules are likely to underlie long-term structural changes observed at the synapse (Fig. 12.14). A known regulator of actin is the Ras super-family which includes the Ras, Rho, and Rab families. Multiple genes in these pathway have recently been identified as responsible for mental retardation when disrupted. As a GTPase, Ras molecules oscillate between the GTP and

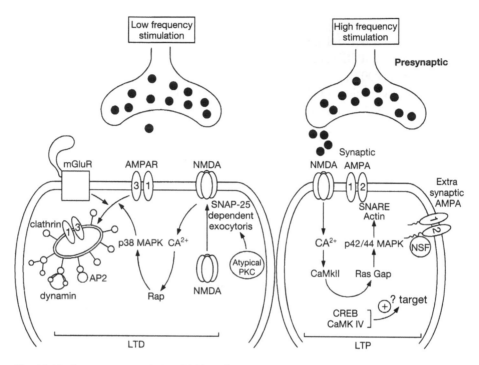

Fig. 12.13. Long-term potentiation (LTP) or depression is caused by differential signaling according to level of intracellular calcium raise. (a) Long-term depression is induced after mild intracellular raise from NMDA receptor. This mild entry of calcium usually result from low-frequency stimulation of the synapse. A reduction in the number of AMPA receptors containing the subunit 1–3 is then observed causing a decrease in synaptic strength. (b) However, a high frequency stimulation will lead to massive calcium entry through NMDA receptors leading to de novo AMPA receptors. The addition of these new receptors will cause a net increase in synaptic strength. The N-ethylmaleimide-sensitive fusion protein (NSF) factor is required for rapid insertion of the AMPA receptors during LTP.

GDP bound forms. Ras molecules, however, possess little intrinsic activity and are therefore influenced by these modulating factors:

1 Guanine exchange factor (GEF) will promote the binding of GTP
2 GTPase activating protein (GAP) will enhance GTP hydrolysis to GDP

Several mutations in Rho-GTPase-dependent signaling have been found in non-syndromic mental retardation. For instance, oligophrenin-1 (OPHN 1) (OMIM 300127) which encodes a RhoGTPase activating protein (GAP), has been linked to mental retardation and cerebellar hypoplasia (Billuart et al. 1998). An OPHN1 knockdown in the mouse hippocampus CA1 region leads to a reduction in spine length (Govek et al. 2004). Another gene involved in severe mental retardation

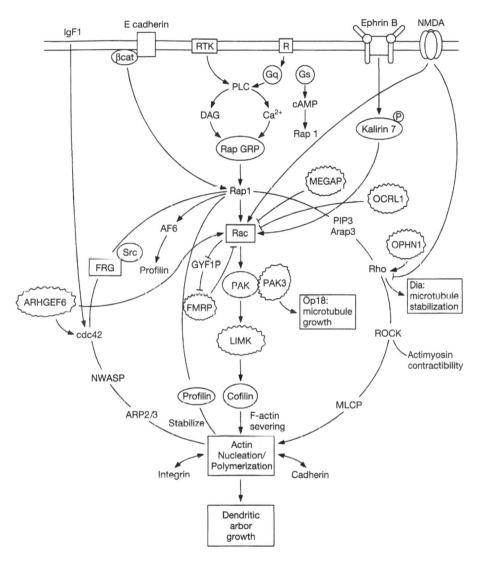

Fig. 12.14. The RAS pathway influence cell shape via cytoskeleton reorganization. Three major component of the RAS family include the cdc42, rac, and rho family of signaling. In addition to molecules involved in intracellular cytoskeleton structure, the ras pathway interacts interact with integrin and cadherin which mediates cell–cell interaction.

and hypotonia is MEGAP (Endris et al. 2002). MEGAP functions as a GAP protein and has been shown to be involved in the slit-robo pathway during axonal branching and neuronal migration.

Other cases of mental retardation have been linked to PAK3 (OMIM 300142) (Allen et al. 1998) and ARHGEF6 (OMIM 300267) (Kutsche et al. 2000) both involved in the Rac pathway. NMDA and growth factor receptors also have an impact on the Rac pathway. Among growth factor receptors, the Ephrin family has been investigated the most with respect to learning and memory. Mice mutant for all three Ephrin B subunits have abnormal dendritic spines (Ethell et al. 2001). Culture of neurons from these mutants fail to form spines or post-synaptic specializations and show decreased levels of expression of AMPA and NMDA receptors (Klein 2004). Moreover, actin appears to accumulate in the dendritic shaft. The ephrin B receptor is localized post-synaptically and signals through kalirin 7, a RhoGEF that binds PDZ. Kalirin 7 activates Rac 1 that then activates CDK 5 and p21-activating-kinase 1/3 (PAK1/3). PAK is a serine/threonine protein kinase that acts downstream of Rac. An up-regulation of PAK after LTP has been demonstrated (Boda et al. 2002). These ultimately impinge on LIMK1 and CDC 42. However, ARHGEF6 serves as a Rac GEF putting a brake on this pathway. Finally, mutations in transmembrane 4 superfamily 2 (TM4SF2) have also been linked to X-linked mental retardation 58 (MRX58) (OMIM 300096) initially reported in a single Austrian family (Holinski-Feder et al. 1999). TM4SF2 is a member of the tetraspanin family of genes, which is involved in β_1-integrin pathway. α-integrin mutants show impaired short-term memory in *Drosophila* (Grotewiel et al. 1998).

LIMK1 (Fig. 12.14) is a serine/threonine kinase that is among a cluster of heterozygously contiguously deleted genes in Williams–Beuren syndrome (OMIM 194050). LIMK1 phosphorylates and inactivates cofilin. Cofilin promotes filamentous actin (F-actin) disassembly. Profilin stabilizes actin filaments. LIMK1 may be regulated by Wit signaling. The wit pathway is activated with glass-bottom boat (Gbb). Gbb is thought to be secreted post-synaptically and is inhibited by CaMKII. The role of wit has been mostly investigated using the neuromuscular junction in *Drosophila*. *Drosophila* wit mutants present with: (1) a decreased number of synaptic boutons, (2) reduced quantal content to 15% of wild-type, and (3) detachment of the pre–post synaptic membrane especially in the active zone region (Baines 2004). Utilizing a *Drosophila* CNS interneuron to motoneuron system post-synaptic expression of *rutabaga* was shown to lead to synaptic strengthening. This effect was dependent on presynaptic TGF-B receptor and postsynaptic TGF-B receptor ligand Gbb (Baines 2004) (Fig. 12.15).

PSD95 is the most concentrated adhesion molecule and is present in the post-synaptic side of the synapse. It links various post-synaptic receptors with their chaperone molecules. In addition, some molecules such as integrin and NCAM bridge between presynaptic and post-synaptic cells.

In addition to PSD-95, another important protein is shank. Shank binds metabotropic glutamate receptors, NMDA receptors, and AMPA receptors. With Densin and AKAP79/150 (a kinase-associated protein of molecular mass 79 and 150KDa), shank couples the cell membrane of the dendritic spine with the

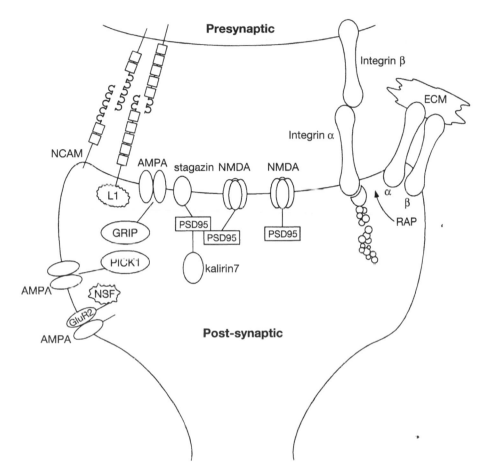

Fig. 12.15. Adhesion molecules form synaptic contact between the presynaptic and post-synaptic cells.

underlying actin cytoskeleton. Some proteins control the interaction of the intra-cellular secondary messenger. For instance, AKAP 79/150 has the ability to bind PKC, PKA, and calcineurin.

Another class of scaffolding proteins includes G-protein-coupled receptor kinase interacting protein (GTI) and intersectin. These control the local formation and branching of actin filaments. GTI is thought to be responsible for the localization of activated Rac. In addition to binding Rac, GTI also binds to Rac modifying proteins such as PIX (RacGEF) and PAK (Fig. 12.14). Intersectin associates with activated Ephrin B receptors and CDC42, N-WASP, ARP2/3. N-WASP up-regulates GEF activity of intersectin for CDC42 resulting in increased CDC42GFP (Table 12.3).

TABLE 12.3
Genes associated with human cognitive diseases and long-term memory

Disease	Gene symbol	Locus	OMIM
Fragile X syndrome	FMR1	Xq27.3	309550
Tuberous sclerosis	TSC1/2	9q34; 16p3	605284; 191092
Coffin–Lowry	RSK2	Xp22.2	303600
Rubinstein–Taybi	CBP	22q13	180849
MRX60	OPHN1	Xq12	300127
MRX30	PAK3	Xq21.3	300142
MRX46	ARHGEF6	Xq26	300267
MRX58	TM4SF2	Xq11	300096
Williams–Beuren	ELN, LIMK (+ others)	7q11.23	194050

CONCLUSIONS

With the growing number of genes and molecular pathways revealed by model organisms and human genetics, important links between synaptic plasticity, memory, and mental retardation are emerging. First, experimental dissection of the developmental from the acute physiologic role of genes has illustrated that genes are reused at multiple levels to accomplish multiple functions within the adult nervous system. Consequently, we can suppose that the same gene networks with differential modulation are involved to accomplish different functions. This opens up an interdigitated cascade-like biochemical complexity, but at the same time gives us clues as to how specificity can be accomplished *in vivo*. Understanding the mechanisms underlying this specificity is what will be needed to translate our knowledge of the molecular pathway to eventual target therapeutical intervention.

REFERENCES

Allen KM, Gleeson JG, Bagrodia S, Partington MW, MacMillan JC, Cerione RA, et al. (1998) PAK3 mutation in nonsyndromic X-linked mental retardation. *Nat Genet* 20: 25–30.

Bailey CH, Kandel ER, Si K (2004) The persistence of long-term memory: a molecular approach to self-sustaining changes in learning-induced synaptic growth. *Neuron* 44: 49–57.

Baines RA (2004) Synaptic strengthening mediated by bone morphogenetic protein-dependent retrograde signaling in the *Drosophila* CNS. *J Neurosci* 24: 6904–6911.

Barria A, Derkach V, Soderling T (1997) Identification of the Ca^{2+}/calmodulin-dependent protein kinase II regulatory phosphorylation site in the alpha-amino-3-hydroxyl-5-methyl-4-isoxazole-propionate-type glutamate receptor. *J Biol Chem* 272: 32727–32730.

Barria A, Malinow R (2002) Subunit-specific NMDA receptor trafficking to synapses. *Neuron* 35: 345–353.

Barth AL, Malenka RC (2001) NMDAR EPSC kinetics do not regulate the critical period for LTP at thalamocortical synapses. *Nat Neurosci* 4: 235–236.

Benzer S (1967) Behavioral mutants of *Drosophila* isolated by countercurrent distribution. *Proc Natl Acad Sci U S A* 58: 1112–1119.

Benzer S (1973) Genetic dissection of behavior. *Sci Am* 229: 24–37.

Billuart P, Bienvenu T, Ronce N, des Portes V, Vinet MC, Zemni R, et al. (1998) Oligophrenin-1 encodes a rhoGAP protein involved in X-linked mental retardation. *Nature* 392: 923–926.

Bliss T, Errington M, Fransen E, Godfraind JM, Kauer JA, Kooy RF, et al. (2000) Long-term potentiation in mice lacking the neural cell adhesion molecule L1. *Curr Biol* 10: 1607–1610.

Bliss TV, Lomo T (1973) Long-lasting potentiation of synaptic transmission in the dentate area of the anaesthetized rabbit following stimulation of the perforant path. *J Physiol* 232: 331–356.

Boda B, Mas C, Muller D (2002) Activity-dependent regulation of genes implicated in X-linked non-specific mental retardation. *Neuroscience* 114: 13–17.

Bourtchouladze R, Lidge R, Catapano R, Stanley J, Gossweiler S, Romashko D, et al. (2003) A mouse model of Rubinstein–Taybi syndrome: defective long-term memory is ameliorated by inhibitors of phosphodiesterase 4. *Proc Natl Acad Sci U S A* 100: 10518–10522.

Bredt DS, Nicoll RA (2003) AMPA receptor trafficking at excitatory synapses. *Neuron* 40: 361–379.

Brunelli M, Castellucci V, Kandel ER (1976) Synaptic facilitation and behavioural sensitization in Aplysia: possible role od serotonin and cyclic AMP. *Science* 194: 1178–1181.

Castellucci V, Pinsker H, Kupfermann I, Kandel ER (1970) Neuronal mechanisms of habituation and dishabituation of the gill-withdrawal reflex in *Aplysia*. *Science* 167: 1745–1748.

Collingridge GL, Kehl SJ, McLennan H (1983) Excitatory amino acids in synaptic transmission in the Schaffer collateral-commissural pathway of the rat hippocampus. *J Physiol* 334: 33–46.

Connolly JB, Roberts IJ, Armstrong JD, Kaiser K, Forte M, Tully T, et al. (1996) Associative learning disrupted by impaired Gs signaling in *Drosophila* mushroom bodies. *Science* 274: 2104–2107.

Costa RM, Honjo T, Silva AJ (2003) Learning and memory deficits in Notch mutant mice. *Curr Biol* 13: 1348–1354.

Costa-Mattioli M, Gobert D, Stern E, Gamache K, Colina R, Cuello C, et al. (2007) eIF2alpha phosphorylation bidirectionally regulates the switch from short- to long-term synaptic plasticity and memory. *Cell* 129: 195–206.

Crino P, Khodakhah K, Becker K, Ginsberg S, Hemby S, Eberwine J (1998) Presence and phosphorylation of transcription factors in developing dendrites. *Proc Natl Acad Sci U S A* 95: 2313–2318.

Crino PB, Eberwine J (1996) Molecular characterization of the dendritic growth cone: regulated mRNA transport and local protein synthesis. *Neuron* 17: 1173–1187.

Davis RL, Davidson N (1984) Isolation of *Drosophila melanogaster* dunce chromosomal region and recombinational mapping of dunce sequences with restriction site polymorphisms as genetic markers. *Mol Cell Biol* 4: 358–367.

Davis S, Laroche S (2006) Mitogen-activated protein kinase/extracellular regulated kinase signalling and memory stabilization: a review. *Genes Brain Behav* 5: 61–72.

De Boulle K, Verkerk AJ, Reyniers E, Vits L, Hendrickx J, Van Roy B, et al. (1993) A point mutation in the FMR-1 gene associated with fragile X mental retardation. *Nat Genet* 3: 31–35.

DeZazzo J, Sandstrom D, de Belle S, Velinzon K, Smith P, Grady L, et al. (2000) Nalyot, a mutation of the *Drosophila* myb-related Adf1 transcription factor, disrupts synapse formation and olfactory memory. *Neuron* 27: 145–158.

Drain P, Folkers E, Quinn WG (1991) cAMP-dependent protein kinase and the disruption of learning in transgenic flies. *Neuron* 6: 71–82.

Dudai Y, Jan YN, Byers D, Quinn WG, Benzer S (1976) Dunce, a mutant of Drosophila deficient in learning. *Proc Natl Acad Sci U S A* 73: 1694–1688.

Ebbinghaus H (1885) *On Memory.* Leipzig: Duncker ans Humblot.

Endris V, Wogatzky B, Leimer U, Bartsch D, Zatyka M, Latif F, et al. (2002) The novel Rho-GTPase activating gene MEGAP/srGAP3 has a putative role in severe mental retardation. *Proc Natl Acad Sci U S A* 99: 11754–11759.

Ethell IM, Irie F, Kalo MS, Couchman JR, Pasquale EB, Yamaguchi Y (2001) EphB/syndecan-2 signaling in dendritic spine morphogenesis. *Neuron* 31: 1001–1013.

Farfel Z, Bourne HR, Iiri T (1999) The expanding spectrum of G protein diseases. *N Engl J Med* 340: 1012–1020.

Feany MB, Quinn WG (1995) A neuropeptide gene defined by the *Drosophila* memory mutant amnesiac. *Science* 268: 869–873.

Fitch N (1982) Albright's hereditary osteodystrophy: a review. *Am J Med Genet* 11: 11–29.

Flexner JB, Flexner LB, Stellar E (1963) Memory in mice as affected by intracerebral puromycin. *Science* 141: 57–59.

Frey U, Krug M, Reymann KG, Matthies H (1988) Anisomycin, an inhibitor of protein synthesis, blocks late phases of LTP phenomena in the hippocampal CA1 region *in vitro. Brain Res* 452: 57–65.

Ge X, Hannan F, Xie Z, Feng C, Tully T, Zhou H, et al. (2004) Notch signaling in *Drosophila* long-term memory formation. *Proc Natl Acad Sci U S A* 101: 10172–10176.

Glanzer JG, Eberwine JH (2003) Mechanisms of translational control in dendrites. *Neurobiol Aging* 24: 1105–1111.

Govek EE, Newey SE, Akerman CJ, Cross JR, Van der Veken L, Van Aelst L (2004) The X-linked mental retardation protein oligophrenin-1 is required for dendritic spine morphogenesis. *Nat Neurosci* 7: 364–372.

Grotewiel MS, Beck CD, Wu KH, Zhu XR, Davis RL (1998) Integrin-mediated short-term memory in *Drosophila. Nature* 391: 455–460.

Guo HF, Tong J, HannanF, Luo L, Zhong Y (2000) A neurofibromatosis-1-regulated pathway is required for learning in *Drosophila. Nature* 403: 895–898.

Guzowski JF, McGaugh JL (1997) Antisense oligodeoxynucleotide-mediated disruption of hippocampal cAMP response element binding protein levels impairs consolidation of memory for water maze training. *Proc Natl Acad Sci U S A* 94: 2693–2698.

Hannan F, Ho I, Tong JJ, Zhu Y, Nurnberg P, Zhong Y (2006) Effect of neurofibromatosis type I mutations on a novel pathway for adenylyl cyclase activation requiring neurofibromin and Ras. *Hum Mol Genet* 15: 1087–1098.

Hayashi ML, Rao BS, Seo JS, Choi HS, Dolan BM, Choi SY, et al. (2007) Inhibition of p21-activated kinase rescues symptoms of fragile X syndrome in mice. *Proc Natl Acad Sci U S A* 104: 11489–11494.

Hayashi Y, Shi SH, Esteban JA, Piccini A, Poncer JC, Malinow R (2000) Driving AMPA receptors into synapses by LTP and CaMKII: requirement for GluR1 and PDZ domain interaction. *Science* 287: 2262–2267.

Hebb DO (1949) *The Organization of Behavior.* New York: Wiley.

Hegde MR, Chong B, Fawkner M, Lambiris N, Peters H, Kenneson A, et al. (2001) Microdeletion in the FMR-1 gene: an apparent null allele using routine clinical PCR amplification. *J Med Genet* 38: 624–629.

Ho IS, Hannan F, Guo HF, Hakker I, Zhong Y (2007) Distinct functional domains of neurofibromatosis type 1 regulate immediate versus long-term memory formation. *J Neurosci* 27: 6852–6857.

Holinski-Feder E, Chahrockh-Zadeh S, Rittinger O, Jedele KB, Gasteiger M, Lenski C, et al. (1999) Nonsyndromic X-linked mental retardation: mapping of MRX58 to the pericentromeric region. *Am J Med Genet* 86: 102–106.

Hotta Y, Benzer S (1973) Mapping of behavior in *Drosophila* mosaics. *Symp Soc Dev Biol* 31: 129–167.

Hunter T, Karin M (1992) The regulation of transcription by phosphorylation. *Cell* 70: 375–387.

Impey S, Mark M, Villacres EC, Poser S, Chavkin C, Storm DR (1996) Induction of CRE-mediated gene expression by stimuli that generate long-lasting LTP in area CA1 of the hippocampus. *Neuron* 16: 973–982.

Isaac JT (2003) Postsynaptic silent synapses: evidence and mechanisms. *Neuropharmacology* 45: 450–460.

James W (1890) *The Principles of Psychology*. New York: Holt.

Kandel ER (2001) The molecular biology of memory storage: a dialogue between genes and synapses. *Science* 294: 1030–1038.

Kandel ER (2006) *In Search of Memory*. New York/London: WW Norton.

Kandel ER, Schwartz JH (1982) Molecular biology of learning: modulation of transmitter release. *Science* 218: 433–443.

Kleiman R, Banker G, Steward O (1990) Differential subcellular localization of particular mRNAs in hippocampal neurons in culture. *Neuron* 5: 821–830.

Klein R (2004) Eph/ephrin signaling in morphogenesis, neural development and plasticity. *Curr Opin Cell Biol* 16: 580–589.

Klein M, Camardo J, Kandel ER (1982) Serotonin modulates a specific potassium current in the sensory neurons that show presynaptic facilitation in *Aplysia*. *Proc Natl Acad Sci U S A* 79: 5713–5717.

Krab LC, de Goede-Bolder A, Aarsen FK, Pluijm SM, Bouman MJ, van der Geest JN, et al. Effect of simvastatin on cognitive functioning in children with neurofibromatosis type 1: a randomized controlled trial. *JAMA* 300: 287–294.

Krichevsky AM, Kosik KS (2001) Neuronal RNA granules: a link between RNA localization and stimulation-dependent translation. *Neuron* 32: 683–696.

Krug M, Lossner B, Ott T (1984) Anisomycin blocks the late phase of long-term potentiation in the dentate gyrus of freely moving rats. *Brain Res Bull* 13: 39–42.

Kutsche K, Yntema H, Brandt A, Jantke I, Nothwang HG, Orth U, et al. (2000) Mutations in ARHGEF6, encoding a guanine nucleotide exchange factor for Rho GTPases, in patients with X-linked mental retardation. *Nat Genet* 26: 247–250.

Kupfermann I, Castellucci V, Pinsker H, Kandel E (1970) Neuronal correlates of correlates of habituation and dishabituation of the gill-withdrawal reflex in Aplysia. *Science* 167: 1743–1745.

Levin LR, Han PL, Hwang PM, Feinstein PG, Davis RL, Reed RR (1992) The *Drosophila* learning and memory gene rutabaga encodes a Ca^{2+}/Calmodulin-responsive adenylyl cyclase. *Cell* 68: 479–489.

Li W, Cui Y, Kushner SA, Brown RA, Jentsch JD, Frankland PW, et al. (2005) The HMG-CoA reductase inhibitor lovastatin reverses the learning and attention deficit ina mouse model of neurofibromatosis type 1. *Curr Biol* 15: 1961–1967.

Livingstone MS, Sziber PP, Quinn WG (1984) Loss of calcium/calmodulin responsiveness in adenylate cyclase of rutabaga, a *Drosophila* learning mutant. *Cell* 37: 205–215.

Lomo T (2003) The discovery of long-term potentiation. *Phil Trans R Soc Lond B Biol Sci* 358: 617–620.

Lu HC, Gonzalez E, Crair MC (2001) Barrel cortex critical period plasticity is independent of changes in NMDA receptor subunit composition. *Neuron* 32: 619–634.

Luthl A, Laurent JP, Figurov A, Muller D, Schachner M (1994) Hippocampal long-term potentiation and neural cell adhesion molecules L1 and NCAM. *Nature* 372: 777–779.

Malenka RC (2003) Synaptic plasticity and AMPA receptor trafficking. *Ann N Y Acad Sci* 1003: 1–11.

Malenka RC, Bear MF (2004) LTP and LTD: an embarrassment of riches. *Neuron* 44: 5–21.

Malinow R (2003) AMPA receptor trafficking and long-term potentiation. *Phil Trans R Soc Lond B Biol Sci* 358: 707–714.

Malinow R, Malenka RC (2002) AMPA receptor trafficking and synaptic plasticity. *Annu Rev Neurosci* 25: 103–126.

Marie H, Morishita W, Yu X, Calakos N, Malenka RC (2005) Generation of silent synapses by acute *in vivo* expression of CaMKIV and CREB. *Neuron* 45: 741–752.

Martin KC, Casadio A, Zhu H, Yaping E, Rose JC, Chen M, et al. (1997) Synapse-specific, long-term facilitation of aplysia sensory to motor synapses: a function for local protein synthesis in memory storage. *Cell* 91: 927–938.

Matsuzaki M, Ellis-Davies GC, Nemoto T, Miyashita Y, Iino M, Kasai H (2001) Dendritic spine geometry is critical for AMPA receptor expression in hippocampal CA1 pyramidal neurons. *Nat Neurosci* 4: 1086–1092.

Matsuzaki M, Honkura N, Ellis-Davies GC, Kasai H (2004) Structural basis of long-term potentiation in single dendritic spines. *Nature* 429: 761–766.

McBride SM, Choi CH, Wang Y, Liebelt D, Braunstein E, Ferreiro D, et al. (2005) Pharmacological rescue of synaptic plasticity, courtship behaviour, and mushroom body defects in a Drosophila model of fragile X syndrome. *Neuron* 45: 753–764.

Mileusnic R, Lancashire CL, Rose SP (2005) Recalling an aversive experience by day-old chicks is not dependent on somatic protein synthesis. *Learn Mem* 12: 615–619.

Milner B (2005) The medial temporal lobe amnesiac syndrome. *Psychiatr Clin North Am* 28: 599–611.

Mineur YS, Sluyter F, de Wit S, Oostra BA, Crusio WE (2002) Behavioral and neuroanatomical characterization of the Fmr1 knockout mouse. *Hippocampus* 12: 39–46.

Montarolo PG, Goele P, Castellucci VF, Morgan J, Kandel ER, Schacher S (1986) A critical period for macromolecular synthesis in long-term heterosynaptic facilitation in *Aplysia*. *Science* 234: 1249–1254.

Moore MS, DeZazzo J, Luk AY, Tully T, Singh CM, Heberlein U (1998) Ethanol intoxication in *Drosophila*: genetic and pharmacological evidence for regulation by the cAMP signaling pathway. *Cell* 93: 997–1007.

Müller GE, Pilzecker A (1900) *Experimentelle Beitrage zur Lehre vom Gedachtnis*. Berlin: Gerdes.

Nusser Z, Lujan R, Laube G, Roberts JD, Molnar E, Somogyi P (1998) Cell type and pathway dependence of synaptic AMPA receptor number and variability in the hippocampus. *Neuron* 21: 545–559.

Oike Y, Hata A, Mamiya T, Kaname T, Noda Y, Suzuki M, et al. (1999a) Truncated CBP protein leads to classical Rubinstein–Taybi syndrome phenotypes in mice: implications for a dominant-negative mechanism. *Hum Mol Genet* 8: 387–396.

Oike Y, Takakura N, Hata A, Kaname T, Akizuki M, Yamaguchi Y, et al. (1999b) Mice homozygous for a truncated form of CREB-binding protein exhibit defects in hematopoiesis and vasculo-angiogenesis. *Blood* 93: 2771–2779.

Oostra BA, Jacky PB, Brown WT, Rousseau F (1993) Guidelines for the diagnosis of fragile X syndrome. National Fragile X Foundation. *J Med Genet* 30: 410–413.

Paoletti P, Neyton J (2007) NMDA receptor subunits: function and pharmacology. *Curr Opin Pharmacol* 7: 39–47.

Paris J, Richter JD (1990) Maturation-specific polyadenylation and translational control: diversity of cytoplasmic polyadenylation elements, influence of poly(A) tail size, and formation of stable polyadenylation complexes. *Mol Cell Biol* 10: 5634–5645.

Pavlov IP (1927) *Conditioned Reflexes*. Oxford, England: Oxford University Press.

Presente A, Boyles RS, Serway CN, de Belle JS, Andres AJ (2004) Notch is required for long-term memory in *Drosophila*. *Proc Natl Acad Sci U S A* 101: 1764–1768.

Quinn WG, Harris WA, Benzer S (1974) Conditioned behavior in *Drosophila melanogaster*. *Proc Natl Acad Sci U S A* 71: 708–712.

Quinn WG, Sziber PP, Booker R (1979) The *Drosophila* memory mutant amnesiac. *Nature* 277: 212–214.

Ramon y Cajal S (1894) *Les Nouvelles Idées sur la Fine Anatomie de Système Nerveux*. Paris.

Rescorla RA (1982) Effect of a stimulus intervening between CS and US in autoshaping. *J Exp Pyschol Anim Behav Process* 8: 131–141.

Ribot TA (1882) *Diseases of Memory: An Essay in the Positive Psychology*. New York: Appleton D.

Roche KW, O'Brien RJ, Mammen AL, Bernhardt J, Huganir RL (1996) Characterization of multiple phosphorylation sites on the AMPA receptor GluR1 subunit. *Neuron* 161: 1179–1188.

Satpute-Krishnan P, DeGiorgis JA, Conley MP, Jang M, Bearer EL (2006) A peptide zipcode sufficient for anterograde transport within amyloid precursor protein. *Proc Natl Acad Sci U S A* 103: 16532–16537.

Schwaerzel M, Monastirioti M, Scholz M, Friggi-Grelin F, Birman S, Heisenberg M (2003) Dopamine and octopamine differentiate between aversive and appetitive olfactory memories in *Drosophila*. *J Neurosci* 23: 10495–10502.

Sharma RP, Grayson DR, Guidotti A, Costa E (2005) Chromatin, DNA methylation and neuron gene regulation: the purpose of the package. *J Psychiatry Neurosci* 30: 257–263.

Sharma SK, Carew TJ (2004) The roles of MAPK cascades in synaptic plasticity and memory in *Aplysia*: facilitatory effects and inhibitory constraints. *Learn Mem* 11: 373–378.

Shi S, Hayashi Y, Esteban JA, Malinow R (2001) Subunit-specific rules governing AMPA receptor trafficking to synapses in hippocampal pyramidal neurons. *Cell* 105: 331–343.

Simon MI, Strathmann MP, Gautam N (1991) Diversity of G proteins in signal transduction. *Science* 252: 802–808.

Sin WC, Haas K, Ruthazer ES, Cline HT (2002) Dendrite growth increased by visual activity requires NMDA receptor and Rho GTPases. *Nature* 419: 475–480.

Skoulakis EM, Davis RL (1996) Olfactory learning deficits in mutants for leonardo, a *Drosophila* gene encoding a 14-3-3 protein. *Neuron* 17: 931–944.

Smith JL, Wilson JE, Macdonald PM (1992) Overexpression of oskar directs ectopic activation of nanos and presumptive pole cell formation in *Drosophila* embryos. *Cell* 70: 849–859.

Spiegel A (1994) *G proteins: Molecular Biology Intelligence Unit*. Austin, Texas: RG Landes.

St Johnston D, Beuchle D, Nusslein-Volhard C (1991) Staufen, a gene required to localize maternal RNAs in the *Drosophila* egg. *Cell* 66: 51–63.

Stern M, Blake N, Zondlo N, Walters K (1995) Increased neuronal excitability conferred by a mutation in the *Drosophila* bemused gene. *J Neurogenet* 10: 103–118.

Sun P, Enslen H, Myung PS, Maurer RA (1994) Differential activation of CREB by Ca^{2+}/calmodulin-dependent protein kinases type II and type IV involves phosphorylation of a site that negatively regulates activity. *Genes Dev* 8: 2527–2539.

Sutton MA, Schuman EM (2005) Local translational control in dendrites and its role in long-term synaptic plasticity. *J Neurobiol* 64: 116–131.

Swaiman KF (2006) *Pediatric Neurology, Principles and Practice, 4th edn.* Philadelphia: Mosby.

Sweatt JD (2004) Mitogen-activated protein kinases in synaptic plasticity and memory. *Curr Opin Neurobiol* 14: 311–317.

Takumi Y, Ramirez-Leon V, Laake P, Rinvik E, Ottersen OP (1999) Different modes of expression of AMPA and NMDA receptors in hippocampal synapses. *Nat Neurosci* 2: 618–624.

Tiedge H, Brosius J (1996) Translational machinery in dendrites of hippocampal neurons in culture. *J Neurosci* 16: 7171–7181.

Tully T, Preat T, Boynton SC, Del Vecchio M (1994) Genetic dissection of consolidated memory in *Drosophila. Cell* 79: 35–47.

Tully T, Quinn WG (1985) Classical conditioning and retention in normal and mutant *Drosophila melanogaster. J Comp Physiol [A]* 157: 263–277.

Verdile G, Gandy SE, Martins RN (2007) The role of presenilin and its interacting proteins in the biogenesis of Alzheimer's beta amyloid. *Neurochem Res* 32: 609–623.

Verkerk AJ, Pieretti M, Sutcliffe JS, Fu YH, Kuhl DP, Pizzuti A, et al. (1991) Identification of a gene (FMR-1) containing a CGG repeat coincident with a breakpoint cluster region exhibiting length variation in fragile X syndrome. *Cell* 65: 905–914.

Wagatsuma A, Azami S, Sakura M, Hatakeyama D, Aonuma H, Ito E (2006) *De novo* synthesis of CREB in a presynaptic neuron is required for synaptic enhancement involved in memory consolidation. *J Neurosci Res* 84: 954–960.

Wang Y, Chan SL, Miele L, Yao PJ, Mackes J, Ingram DK, et al. (2004). Involvement of Notch signaling in hippocampal synaptic plasticity. *Proc Natl Acad Sci U S A* 101: 9458–9462.

Wu L, Wells D, Tay J, Mendis D, Abbott MA, Barnitt A, et al. (1998) CPEB-mediated cytoplasmic polyadenylation and the regulation of experience-dependent translation of alpha-CaMKII mRNA at synapses. *Neuron* 21: 1129–1139.

Xia S, Miyashita T, Fu TF, Lin WY, Wu CL, Pyzocha L, et al. (2005) NMDA receptors mediate olfactory learning and memory in *Drosophila. Curr Biol* 15: 603–615.

Xia HJ, Yang G (2005) Inositol 1,4,5-trisphosphate 3-kinases: functions and regulations. *Cell Res* 15: 83–91.

Yin JC, Wallach JS, Del Vecchio M, Wilder EL, Zhou H, Quinn WG, et al. (1994) Induction of a dominant negative CREB transgene specifically blocks long-term memory in *Drosophila. Cell* 79: 49–58.

Zhao MG, Toyoda H, Ko SW, Ding HK, Wu LJ, Zhuo M (2005) Deficits in trace fear memory and long-term potentiation in a mouse model for fragile X syndrome. *J Neurosci* 25: 7385–7392.

Zhong Y (1995) Mediation of PACAP-like neuropeptide transmission by coactivation of Ras/Raf and cAMP signal transduction pathways in *Drosophila. Nature* 375: 588–592.

Zhu JJ, Qin Y, Zhao M, Van Aelst L, Malinow R (2002) Ras and Rap control AMPA receptor trafficking during synaptic plasticity. *Cell* 110: 443–455.

13

NEURONAL PLASTICITY AND DEVELOPMENTAL DISABILITIES

Sheryl L Rimrodt and Michael V Johnston

Plasticity is a one of the defining features of the child's nervous system, and many neurologic disabilities of childhood result from altered plasticity. Although clinicians are familiar with concrete examples of plasticity, such as the ability of infants to acquire different languages depending on their environment or to recover function after serious brain injuries, defining the concept of plasticity has proven challenging.

The word plasticity comes from the Greek 'plastikos' meaning 'to form.' Neuronal plasticity refers to the nervous system's capacity to reorganize after changes in sensory input and to be shaped or molded by ongoing experience (Greenough et al. 1987, Johnston et al. 2001, Chen et al. 2002, Johnston 2003). Typical brain development is manifested behaviorally by the acquisition and execution of an increasing array of specialized skills. In this context plasticity can be defined as 'the state of still having several options for specialization left within the developmental process' (Johnson 1999). Plasticity during development is characterized by relatively enhanced malleability in children and advancing age is associated with increasing 'restriction of fate' or specialization. For example, young infants can distinguish between distinct speech sounds occurring in many languages that are not their own native tongue, but by 6–9 months they show a preference for sounds of their native language and by adulthood many individuals have difficulty distinguishing distinct speech sounds of other languages (Kuhl 2004).

Nevertheless, there is also evidence that plasticity, manifested as the development and enhancement of specialized skills, is a prolonged process in humans which extends well beyond early postnatal life and into adulthood (Greenough et al. 1987, Buonomano and Merzenich 1998). For example, adults retain the ability to learn, remember and forget, to think creatively, and learn new motor tasks. Disruption of the fundamental processes involved in plasticity are implicated in childhood disorders including intellectual and learning disabilities, developmental language disorders, epilepsy, motor and behavioral disorders.

TYPES OF CLINICAL PLASTICITY

We find it is useful to distinguish four major types of plasticity as seen in clinical settings:

1 Adaptive plasticity
2 Impaired plasticity
3 Excessive plasticity
4 Plasticity that creates a vulnerability to injury (Johnston 2004)

Adaptive plasticity can be exploited to acquire special skills such as learning to play the piano, a new challenging sport, or a first or second language. Additional examples include the ability of children with congenital deafness to learn to hear with a cochlear implant device at less than 7 years of age or the ability of children to walk after hemispherectomy surgery for refractory epilepsy. Examples of impaired plasticity include numerous forms associated with intellectual disability, including neurofibromatosis type 1, fragile X syndrome, and Rett syndrome, which disrupt intracellular signaling cascades involved in learning and memory. Excessive plasticity is involved in the pathogenesis of temporal lobe epilepsy when abnormal neuronal circuits form in response to damage associated with mesial temporal sclerosis in the hippocampus. Excessive plasticity is also implicated in the maladaptive reorganization of somatosensory maps in the cerebral cortex. This is believed to be responsible for phantom limb pain following limb amputations or with focal dystonia associated with excessive practice in musicians.

Certain molecular mechanisms that provide a substrate for plasticity can also create an enhanced vulnerability for the developing brain. For example, synaptic mechanisms mediated by the excitatory amino acid glutamate are enhanced in the developing brain to allow greater plasticity associated with neuronal activity. However, certain insults can lead to the excessive opening of ion channels associated with these receptors, leading to the flooding of neurons and other cells with calcium, activating a cascade that leads to cell death. In these situations, molecular mechanisms designed to enable plasticity can become an 'Achilles' heel' for the immature brain. This can occur when hypoxia-ischemia or hypoglycemia causes glutamate to accumulate during hypoxic-ischemic encephalopathy, leading to receptor stimulation and excitotoxic cell death. Immature oligodendroglia in the periventricular white matter are also vulnerable to this type of injury because of enhanced activity of glutamate receptors during development. These examples of plasticity illustrate the ways in which it can influence both the healthy and disordered brain.

NEURONAL MECHANISMS FOR PLASTICITY

A variety of cellular and physiologic mechanisms contribute to plasticity in the developing brain. The most fundamental form of plasticity occurs at the level of synapses, where the strength of signaling varies according to how often and how strongly they are activated (Fig. 13.1). Two types of activity-dependent synaptic plasticity that are commonly studied in the laboratory are long-term potentiation

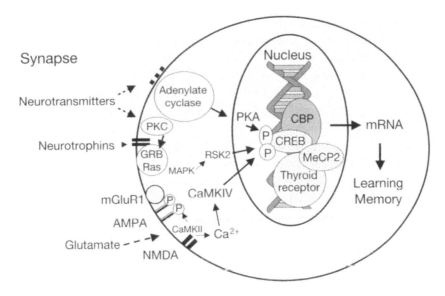

Figure 13.1 Schematic diagram of signaling pathways in neurons that are involved in activity-dependent plasticity and learning and memory. Neurotransmitters, including glutamate, gamma-aminobutyric acid (GABA), serotonin, dopamine, and norepinephrine, as well as neurotrophins such as brain-derived neurotrophic factor (BDNF), activate receptors on neuronal synapses. These receptors activate opening of ion channels and production of second messengers that signal into the nucleus. These signals in turn regulate transcription of genes by phosphorylating protein transcription factors that bind to DNA. This transcriptional activity leads to production of proteins that become integrated into synapses, leading to the storage of memories and other changes in neuronal function. CREB is a transcription factor that is important for learning and memory and is highly conserved across species, while CBP is closely linked to CREB. CBP acetylates histones, leading to unwinding of DNA and activation of transcription. MeCP2 is a transcriptional repressor that is mutated in Rett syndrome. Nuclear thyroid hormone receptor is also a transcriptional repressor unless it is occupied by thyroid hormone, which de-represses transcription of multiple genes. Abbreviations: AMPA, α-amino-3-hydroxy-5-methyliosoxazolepropionic acid; BDNF, brain-derived neurotrophic factor; CaMKIV, calcium/calmodulin kinase IV; CBP, CREB binding protein; CREB, cyclic adenosine monophosphate (cAMP) response element binding protein transcription factor; GRB: growth factor receptor bound; MAPK, mitogen activated protein kinases; MeCP2, methyl-CpG-binding protein 2; mGluR1, type I metabotropic glutamate receptor; mRNA, messenger ribonucleic acid; NMDA, N-methyl-D-aspartic acid; PKA, protein kinase A; PKC, protein kinase C; Ras, family of guanine trinucleotide binding proteins (GTPases); RSK2, ribosomal S6 kinase-2.

(LTP) and long-term depression (LTD) (Pfeiffer and Heuber 2006). LTP refers to a strengthening of activation that follows tetanic stimulation at excitatory synapses. The primary mechanism for LTP involves addition of α-amino-5-hydroxy-3-methyl-4-isoxazole propionic acid (AMPA) type glutamate receptors to the post-synaptic membrane in response to activation of N-methyl-D-aspartate

(NMDA) glutamate receptors (Fig. 13.1) (Malenka 2003). LTP is considered a physiologic correlate of acquired memory. Intracellular signaling through NMDA and AMPA receptors, as well as through receptors for other neurotransmitters and neurotrophins (e.g. metabotropic receptors for serotonin and glutamate), encodes memories and other forms of synaptic plasticity by activating the transcription of specific genes in the nucleus (Fig.13.1). For example, formation of long-term memories is thought to require gene transcription that leads to actual structural changes in synaptic networks. Further stabilization of these synaptic changes is facilitated by activation of local protein synthesis on dendritic ribosomes (Kandel 2001).

Plasticity may also involve reactivation of latent pathways in the brain. For example, rapid recovery of some language function in children after surgical excision of the left, language-dominant hemisphere (to treat intractable seizures) is attributed to recruitment of previously latent but redundant language circuits in the remaining right hemisphere (Boatman et al. 1999). Reactivation of primitive ipsilateral cortico-spinal tracts may also be responsible for recovery of proximal body and trunk movement in hemispherectomy patients (Muller et al. 1991). Persistence of neurogenesis in certain brain regions and programmed deletion of selected neurons through apoptosis may also contribute to plasticity (Raff et al. 1993, Johnston et al. 2001). Regrowth of axons may also contribute to the eventual recovery of function. Voss et al. (2006) reported evidence of aberrant subcortical white matter consistent with axonal regrowth in the brain of an adult who recovered from a minimally conscious state after many years.

Programmed overproduction and the subsequent pruning of synapses in the cerebral cortex of the immature primate brain also provides an important substrate for plasticity, allowing children to benefit from environmental influences over a prolonged postnatal period and offering an advantage for recovering from injuries. Huttenlocher (1990) reported that the number of synapses in the cerebral cortex increases rapidly in the postnatal period to a level that is approximately twice the adult level at 2 years of age. Synaptic density declines to adult levels in the late teenage years. Chugani (1998) found a similar pattern of glucose consumption in the cerebral cortex of children at different ages using positron emission tomography (PET), consistent with the observation that synaptic activity is the major consumer of glucose in the brain. Magnetic resonance imaging (MRI) has also shown similar dynamic changes in cortical thickness during development, with a thicker cortex in younger children with progressive thinning more prominent in the teenage years. Using this technique, Shaw et al. (2006) reported that a group of more intelligent children appeared to have a more plastic cortex, with an accelerated and prolonged early phase of cortical increase and vigorous thinning in early adolescence. Studies in animals indicate that the proliferation and pruning of synapses, as well as their refinement and stabilization, are strongly influenced by patterns of synaptic activity mediated by the relative balance of excitatory and inhibitory neurotransmitter receptors (Raff et al. 1993, Kandel 2001, Johnston et al. 2001, Johnston 2004).

IMPAIRED PLASTICITY IN COGNITIVE AND BEHAVIORAL SYNDROMES

Molecular lesions within the signaling pathways involved in activity-dependent plasticity are responsible for a number of developmental cognitive disorders (Table 13.1). This form of aberrant plasticity is associated with an abnormal pattern of skill acquisition and/or execution of specialized skills in the absence of discernable injury and, in most cases, a lack of gross brain malformation. However, patients with these disorders often have somatic dysmorphic features because of the ubiquitous role these signaling pathways have in other organs besides the brain.

One such disorder is fragile X syndrome (FXS), the most prevalent X-linked inherited form of mental retardation. FXS is associated with variable cognitive and language impairments as well as hyperactivity, anxiety, frequent autistic behaviors, and characteristic dysmorphic features. Brain imaging has demonstrated that the brain is larger than normal although certain areas such as the cerebellar vermis are smaller. At the microscopic level, dendritic spines appear immature suggesting a maturational arrest.

FXS is caused by an expanded trinucleotide repeat that leads to hypermethylation and inhibition of the promoter region for the fragile X mental retardation protein (FMRP). Diminished levels of FMRP, which binds to RNA within the synapses and regulates activity-dependent protein translation, is thought to impair the function and morphogenesis of excitatory synapses (Comery et al. 1997,

TABLE 13.1

Some cognitive and behavioral disorders caused by defects in neuronal signaling pathways

Fragile X syndrome
Rett syndrome
Neurofibromatosis type 1
Neurofibromatosis type 2
Tuberous sclerosis
Coffin–Lowry syndrome
Rubinstein–Taybi syndrome
Down syndrome
X-linked mental retardation with α-thalassemia
Aarskog (faciogenital dysplasia) syndrome
Non-syndromic mental retardation
Defects in Rho-GTPase signaling, mutations in PAK3, oligophrenin-1
Hypothyroidism
Lead poisoning

Huber et al. 2002, Todd and Malter 2002, Johnston 2004). These dendritic spines are implicated in the protein formation that stabilizes long-term synaptic changes (Comery et al. 1997, Huber et al. 2002, Johnston 2004). Studies conducted in mice with the gene for FMRP gene knocked out showed that activity of the group 1 glutamate metabotropic receptors (mGluR) is enhanced (Huber et al. 2002), while levels of AMPA and NMDA type glutamate receptors in the post-synaptic membrane are reduced (Snyder et al. 2001). These findings have stimulated interest in developing specific therapies for FXS using drugs that may correct these defects in signaling at the synapse.

RETT SYNDROME
Rett syndrome is a disorder in which neuronal signaling pathways are disrupted. Rett syndrome features a normal prenatal, perinatal, and early postnatal course, acquired secondary microcephaly, mental retardation, and stereotyped hand-wringing movements. Most cases are caused by mutations in the MeCP2 gene in girls. This gene codes for the MeCP2 protein transcription factor which suppresses transcription by recruiting additional transcriptional suppressors to bind to DNA (Fig. 13.1). The MeCP2 protein is predominantly expressed in neurons within the brain and has an important role in the formation and stabilization of synapses (Kaufmann et al. 2005). Data from *in vitro* neuronal cultures from mice with the MECP2 gene knockout indicate that the normal protein is phosphorylated in response to neuronal activity, causing it to be released from DNA. These data suggest that MeCP2 suppresses activity of certain genes except when neurons are depolarized and it detaches from DNA to allow transcription. One of the genes known to be controlled by MeCP2 in this way is brain-derived neurotrophic factor (BDNF) (Chen et al. 2003). This mechanism of action would allow BDNF to be transcribed in response to neuronal activity, possibly having a role in stabilizing developing synapses. Several lines of investigation suggest that Rett syndrome reflects a disorder of synaptic development and subsequently a failure of an important step in activity-dependent plasticity.

DISORDERS THAT DISRUPT SIGNALING TO CREB IN THE NUCLEUS
A number of other disorders that impair cognition and behavior are the result of disruption of the signaling cascades that connect cell-surface receptors to intra-nuclear gene transcription. Several disorders affect signaling through the transcription factor cyclic AMP response element binding protein (CREB), which has a major role in learning and memory and is highly conserved across species.

Coffin–Lowry syndrome is a sex-linked mental retardation syndrome associated with characteristic dysmorphic features caused by mutations in RSK2, the protein that phosphorylates the transcription factor CREB (Fig. 13.1). Intelligence in children with Coffin–Lowry syndrome has been correlated with the enzymatic activity of RSK2 in assays of CREB phosphorylation (Harum et al. 2001). Another modulator of CREB activity, the serine-threonine kinase DYRK1A located on chromosome 21, has been implicated in dendritic pathology associated with Down syndrome (Benavides-Piccione et al. 2004). Another related disorder is Rubinstein–Taybi syndrome (RTS), which includes severe mental retardation with a characteristic enlargement of the thumbs and great toes. It is caused by mutations in CREB binding protein (CBP), a transcriptional co-activator that is recruited by CREB. RTS and Coffin–Lowry syndrome both affect proteins that regulate the transcription of genes implicated in long-term potentiation (Petrij et al. 1995, Harum et al. 2001, Johnston 2004). A mouse model of RTS showed impairment of long-term memory and the late phase of hippocampal LTP. These deficits were correctable either by increasing the expression of CREB-dependent genes or by inhibiting histone deacetylase activity.

NEUROFIBROMATOSIS AND RELATED DISORDERS

Neurofibromatosis type 1 (NF-1) and tuberous sclerosis are neurocutaneous disorders that impair cognition and behavior. Both are caused by mutations in GTPase-activating proteins (GAP) which are linked to cell-surface receptors that regulate intracellular signaling from these receptors into the nucleus (Bernards 2003). Mutations in NF-1 and tuberous sclerosis cause these signaling pathways to become too active, leading to overgrowth (i.e. tumors) as well as cognitive impairment. In a mouse model of NF-1, impaired learning and memory has been associated with an increase in the inhibitory neurotransmitter activity mediated by GABA (Costa et al. 2002).

A similar mechanism is responsible for several non-syndromic X-linked mental retardation syndromes that result from mutations in the Rho-GTPase signaling pathways (Endris et al. 2000). The Rho-GTPases are also linked to cell-surface receptors and the axonal and dendritic cytoskeleton and these disorders are associated with abnormalities in synapse formation. Examples include mutations in oligophrenin-1, a RhoA-GAP protein and PAK3, a RhoA effector protein. Williams syndrome, which includes impaired cognition and 'cocktail party' speech without much content and excessive familiarity, may also involve a defect in Rho signaling. It is caused by a deletion on chromosome 7 in a contiguous region which includes the elastin gene, the HPC-1/syntaxin gene that codes for a protein involved in docking of synaptic vesicles and the gene for LIM kinase-1 (LIMK1). LIMK1 is linked to the Rho signaling system and may have intrinsic CREB phosphorylation activity (Yang et al. 2004).

DISORDERS OF LANGUAGE PLASTICITY

Disorders of language development in children are one of the most common problems evaluated by pediatric neurologists and developmental specialists, and language acquisition is obviously dependent on brain plasticity. The concept of language includes speech sound articulation, receptive language (i.e. comprehending information), expressive language output (which may or may not be verbal), and pragmatic language (i.e. the ability to engage in social communication with others). Language development is strongly influenced by genetic predisposition, but successful acquisition of language also depends on adaptive plasticity. For example, it is adaptive plasticity that allows infants to acquire a repertoire of sounds and gestures through imitation and learning. Infants at 6–9 months of age begin to demonstrate preferences for prosodic cues of the language that they experience in their home (Kuhl 2004, Demonet et al. 2005). Early experience and skill in the use of the phonologic features of language (e.g. rhyming) is associated with an improved acquisition of reading skill (Bradley and Bryant 1983, Rubenstein 2002, Shaywitz and Shaywitz 2005).

The experience-dependent component of learning at the behavioral level is coupled with activity-dependent plasticity at a cellular level which fine tunes the sensory cortex for use in higher level language functions. This is supported by observations in deaf children showing that exposure to speech sounds is necessary for normal speech development (Demonet et al. 2005, Harrison et al. 2005). Furthermore, deprivation of auditory sensory input is also associated with differences in higher level language function, exemplified by a greater difficulty in learning to read among deaf children (Connor and Zwolan 2004). However, the capacity of the developing brain to respond to pathologic changes in sensory input is remarkable. Although the neural input from a cochlear implant is unique and incompletely coded compared with the input from an intact peripheral auditory system, the human cortex has demonstrated the ability to learn to ascribe meaningful interpretations to this method of encoding sounds, including speech sounds (Rubinstein 2002, Demonet et al. 2005). This effect is maximal in the first 7 years of life in children. This flexibility even extends to the physical location of the cerebral cortex that processes different modalities of language. For example, Braille reading activates visual cortex in individuals born blind and communication using American Sign Language activates cortex typically associated with oral language output (Demonet et al. 2005).

PLASTICITY IN RECOVERY AFTER ACQUIRED LANGUAGE IMPAIRMENT

Beyond the fact that adaptive plasticity facilitates typical language development and is flexible enough to adapt to differences in sensory input, it is also critical for language recovery after an acquired acute brain injury. An amazing example of this

flexibility is the ability of children to recover language skills after left hemispherectomy, used to treat intractable epilepsy, even when the pre-surgical evaluation confirms
the left hemisphere as the language-dominant brain region in that individual
(Boatman et al. 1999). The mechanism for plasticity in this setting is postulated
to involve modification of synapses in redundant, probably previously latent,
neural pathways in the remaining hemisphere.

Individuals who have undergone left hemispherectomy also teach us about
laterality in neuronal plasticity. Despite extensive cortical reorganization to shift
language-dominance to the right hemisphere, there remains some subtle language
deficits (Vanlancker-Sidtis 2004). This suggests that, despite significant compensation
by the right hemisphere, there seems to be certain characteristics of the left brain
that are essential for optimal language development. One possible mechanism for
achieving left-hemisphere specificity for language could be asymmetric differences
in neurotrophic factors; an explanation that would be consistent with a recent report
of asymmetric expression of genes relevant to language development during early
brain formation (Sun et al. 2005).

LANGUAGE RECOVERY AFTER STROKE

A less dramatic example of neuronal reorganization after injury is demonstrated by
the language development of children after an early stroke (during gestation or early
infancy). Children with focal unilateral structural lesions as the result of an early
stroke typically show rapid improvement in their language skills along an unusually
steep trajectory so that eventually they 'catch up' with typically developing children (Reilly et al. 2004). Interestingly, a study comparing typically developing
children with children with lesions caused by early stroke also included a group of
children with developmental language impairment (DLI). The DLI group showed
consistently slow language improvement that did not 'catch up' to the typically
developing group (Reilly et al. 2004). This is particularly relevant to the topic of
this chapter because it suggests that a focal injury model does not account for the
clinical course of DLI and that there are some differences in the effectiveness of
neuronal plasticity in these two clinically distinct situations.

Another potential model of DLI, which has some support in the literature,
is that a diffuse, generalized brain injury better explains developmental language
impairment. A study that monitored language development in children recovering
from diffuse axonal brain injury showed that children who were younger at the
time of their injury (i.e. those who should have enhanced plasticity) actually had
slower improvement in verbal fluency than children who were older at the time of
their injury (Levin 2003). This pattern of development is more consistent with
that observed in children with DLI. Furthermore, this injury model does not
preclude the possibility that aberrant plasticity is the mechanism in both settings.
In the child with brain injury this may be an acquired problem with plasticity,

while in the case of idiopathic DLI the impaired plasticity may be genetically determined.

PLASTICITY IN SPECIFIC DEVELOPMENTAL LANGUAGE IMPAIRMENT

Although there is evidence that the group of disorders that are encompassed by the term DLI are heritable, the variability of expression within families suggests that the inheritance patterns are complex and multigenic (Bishop et al. 1995). In the past, there were no known genetic markers reliably associated with DLI that could be exploited to understand the link between the behavioral and molecular manifestations. Genetic linkage analyses have now identified associations with genes on chromosomes 2, 7, 13, 15, 16, 17, and 19 (Boyar et al. 2001, Bartlett et al. 2002, Fisher et al. 2003, SLI Consortium 2004). As expected, the phenotypes in each linkage study are different and our knowledge of the extent of these differences depends on the criteria used to measure language impairment in each study. The DLI phenotype associated with chromosome 16 was defined by poor performance on a measure of non-word repetition, while the phenotype associated with chromosome 19 was associated with poor performance on other measures of expressive language but not non-word repetition (Fisher et al. 2003). The phenotype associated with chromosome 17 is also associated with dyslexia, while the linkages to 7q31 and 13q21 appear to overlap with possible candidate genes for autistic phenotypes (Fisher et al. 2003). Partially because of the complexity of genetic expression, none of these associations is yet linked to a candidate protein that suggests a particular defect in synaptic plasticity.

AN INHERITED SPEECH DISORDER LINKED TO THE FOXP2 GENE

Recently, there has been one kindred identified with a straightforward genetic pattern of inheritance of a subtype DLI without the clear global impairment associated with the previously discussed disorders (Vargha-Khadem et al. 1995, Watkins et al. 2002a). The DLI subtype displayed in this family is characterized by expressive and receptive language weaknesses and a significant articulation deficit that persists to adulthood despite treatment. The common phenotypic feature associated in each case with abnormal FOXP2 expression is the significant articulation disorder. This symptom makes the FOXP2-associated forms of DLI unusual, because the most common forms of DLI are not associated with this degree of articulation difficulty evident clinically (Meaburn et al. 2002). This phenotype is transmitted within this kindred along an autosomal dominant inheritance pattern (Meaburn et al. 2002). Genetic testing of family members revealed a 100% correlation between being affected with the DLI subtype and an exon 14 missense mutation on chromosome region 7q31 (Lai et al. 2001). This mutation results in decreased expression of the protein FoxP2, a transcription factor that regulates gene expression in developing neural tissue (Lai et al. 2001, Shu et al. 2005). Other mutations resulting in decreased expression of the FOXP2 gene have been identified in several unrelated subjects and one case of DLI has been reported in a child with a mutation resulting in increased expression of FoxP2 (Lai et al. 2001, MacDermot et al. 2005, Somerville et al. 2005). FoxP2 belongs to the family of Forkhead box (Fox) transcription factors that bind to DNA.

Neuroimaging evaluations of this FoxP2 mutation family have also demonstrated that compared with unaffected family members, affected family members show anatomic and functional brain differences. Those affected show decreased gray matter volume in the bilateral caudate nuclei correlated with poorer performance on expressive and articulation measures of language skill (Watkins et al. 2002b, Belton et al. 2003). They also show decreased volume in cerebellar gray matter, and increased volume in the bilateral putamen, inferior frontal gyri, and planum temporale (Watkins et al. 2002b, Belton et al. 2003). Functional MRI has shown brain activation differences between affected and unaffected family members in the Broca area and the bilateral putamen on tasks contrasting silent versus articulated word generation (Liegeois et al. 2003). FoxP2 is expressed in the human thalamus, caudate, and cerebellar tissue (Lai et al. 2003). In animal studies, it has been shown to influence neuronal migration and/or maturation in the cerebellum (Lai et al. 2003).

Evidence that mutations in the FoxP2 gene disrupt neuronal plasticity in circuits required for vocal learning has also come from research on the vocal plasticity of songbirds (Scharff and Haesler 2005). It is interesting that vocal learning, which is the ability to modify innate vocalizations in relationship to a vocal model, is present in songbirds and humans but not other primates. FoxP2 expression has been shown to be increased in the basal ganglia circuits required for vocal plasticity in songbirds during periods of active learning (Teramitsu et al. 2004, Scharff and Haesler 2005). For example, zebra finches learn to sing by imitating the song of an adult tutor bird. During the critical phase of learning, the birds memorize the tutor song, but do not vocalize much. However, during the sensorimotor phase, they start singing and use auditory feedback to modify their imperfect rendition of the memorized song. FoxP2 is up-regulated both during the sensorimotor phase and the period when the final song is crystallized (Scharff and Haesler 2005). In contrast to finches, which do not modify their songs once they have been learned, adult canaries continuously modify their songs. During the spring and fall months they modify their songs, and basal ganglia circuits involved in singing behavior undergo changes in neurogenesis and other morphology (Scharff and Haesler 2005). FoxP2 expression is elevated in these neuronal circuits in both finches and canaries during periods of maximal song plasticity. FoxP2 expressing medium spiny neurons in these basal ganglia areas are the site of convergence of excitatory amino acid and dopamine circuits that are involved in plasticity (Scharff and Haesler

2005). The areas of expression of the FoxP2 gene in neuronal circuits in songbirds are analogous to the areas of the brain affected in imaging of members of the human FoxP2 family (Scharff and Haesler 2005). In addition, FoxP2 expression patterns in the human fetal brain are similar to those in the songbird (Teramitsu et al. 2004, Scharff and Haesler 2005). The linkage of FoxP2 to normal language development is further strengthened by a recent study that shows that decreased FoxP2 in mice is associated with decreased ultrasonic vocalizations which are important for pup–mother communication (Shu et al. 2005, Scharff and Haesler 2005).

This type of detailed information about one aspect of genetic factors underlying some DLI represents a significant advancement. Ongoing work toward understanding the implications of abnormal FOXP2 expression is likely to enhance our understanding of both typical and atypical language development. This area is particularly significant because it enables researchers to link cognitive, behavioral, and imaging data in humans to a molecular mechanism for developmental language plasticity in lower animals.

CONCLUSIONS

The concept of plasticity in the developing brain is one that relates to the entire spectrum of neurodevelopmental disabilities. Plasticity can be divided conveniently into adaptive plasticity, impaired plasticity, and excessive plasticity, and it is evident that plasticity can become an 'Achilles' heel' to mediate injury to the brain. Neuronal plasticity describes an alteration in neuron–neuron connectivity that occurs when synapses are modified and refined by local changes in gene and protein expression. It is expressed clinically as the brain's ability to accomplish activities such as learning, remembering, forgetting, reorganizing after changes in sensory input, and recovering function after injury.

This perspective on neurodevelopmental disabilities is valuable for the clinician because it provides a unifying underlying conceptual framework for many seemingly unrelated disorders. Recognition that many of these disorders are related to genetically based abnormalities in cell-signaling pathways is leading to the design of targeted therapies that might offer the potential for correction, especially if applied early in life. For example, abnormalities in synaptic signaling in FXS have led to a search for compounds that might provide correction which leads to improved cognitive and behavioral potential.

Recent progress in understanding the plasticity of language is particularly important, given how common language disorders are in clinical practice. Reviewing the genetics of three disorders of global development that are also associated with distinct language phenotypes (Rett, Williams, and Down syndromes), it seems unlikely that different phenotypes of DLI will be traced to a single gene defect or protein abnormality.

The genetics of DLI, uncomplicated by global cognitive impairment, has also been studied. Data from one kindred and a few other unrelated individuals have demonstrated convincing linkage between an uncommon, severe DLI subtype and the abnormal expression of the FOXP2 protein. It is anticipated that ongoing work to discover the anatomic and functional implications of abnormal FOXP2 expression will provide clues that lead us to a better understanding of the more common DLI subtypes and human language development in general.

REFERENCES

Bartlett CW, Flax JF, Logue MW, Vieland VJ, Bassett AS, Tallal P, et al. (2002) A major susceptibility locus for specific language impairment is located on 13q21. *Am J Hum Genet* 71: 45–55.

Belton E, Salmond CH, Watkins KE, Vargha-Khadem F, Gadian DG (2003) Bilateral brain abnormalities associated with dominantly inherited verbal and orofacial dyspraxia. *Hum Brain Mapp* 18: 194–200.

Benavides-Piccione R, Ballesteros-Yanez I, de Lagran MM, Elston G, Estivill X, Fillat C, et al. (2004) On dendrites in Down syndrome and DS murine models: a spiny way to learn. *Prog Neurobiol* 74: 111–126.

Bernards A (2003) GAPs galore! A survey of putative Ras superfamily GTPase activating proteins in man and *Drosophila*. *Biochim Biophys Acta* 1603: 47–82.

Bishop DV, North T, Donlan C (1995) Genetic basis of specific language impairment: evidence from a twin study. *Dev Med Child Neurol* 37: 56–71.

Boatman D, Freeman J, Vining E, Pulsifer M, Miglioretti D, Minahan R, et al. (1999) Language recovery after left hemispherectomy in children with late-onset seizures. *Ann Neurol* 46: 579–586.

Boyar FZ, Whitney MM, Lossie AC, Gray BA, Keller KL, Stalker HJ, et al. (2001) A family with a grand-maternally derived interstitial duplication of proximal 15q. *Clin Genet* 60: 421–430.

Bradley L, Bryant PE (1983) Categorizing sounds and learning to read: a causal connection. *Nature* 301: 419–421.

Buonomano DV, Merzenich MM (1998) Cortical plasticity: from synapses to maps. *Annu Rev Neurosci* 21: 149–186.

Chen R, Cohen LG, Hallett M (2002) Nervous system reorganization following injury. *Neuroscience* 111: 761–773.

Chen WG, Chang Q, Lin Y, Meissner A, West AE, Griffith EC, et al. (2003) Depression of BDNF transcription involves calcium-dependent phosphorylation of MeCP2. *Science* 302: 885–889.

Chugani HT (1998) A critical period of brain development: studies of cerebral glucose utilization with PET. *Prev Med* 27: 184–188.

Comery TA, Harris JB, Willems PJ, Oostra BA, Irwin SA, Weiler IJ, et al. (1997) Abnormal dendritic spines in fragile X knockout mice: maturation and pruning deficits. *Proc Natl Acad Sci U S A* 94: 5401–5404.

Connor CM, Zwolan TA (2004) Examining multiple sources of influence on the reading comprehension skills of children who use cochlear implants. *J Speech Lang Hear Res* 47: 509–526.

Costa RM, Federov NB, Kogan JH, Murphy GG, Stern J, Ohno M, et al. (2002) Mechanism for the learning deficits in a mouse model of neurofibromatosis type 1. *Nature* 415: 526–530.

Demonet JF, Thierry G, Cardebat D (2005) Renewal of the neurophysiology of language: functional neuroimaging. *Physiol Rev* 85: 49–95.

Endris V, Wogatzky B, Leimer U, Bartsch D, Zatyka M, Latif F, et al. (2002) The novel Rho-GTPase activating gene MEGAP/srGAP3 has a putative role in severe mental retardation. *Proc Natl Acad Sci U S A* 99: 11754–11759.

Fisher SE, Lai CS, Monaco AP (2003) Deciphering the genetic basis of speech and language disorders. *Annu Rev Neurosci* 26: 57–80.

Greenough WT, Black JE, Wallace CS (1987) Experience and brain development. *Child Dev* 58: 539–559.

Harrison RV, Gordon KA, Mount RJ (2005) Is there a critical period for cochlear implantation in congenitally deaf children? Analyses of hearing and speech perception performance after implantation. *Dev Psychobiol* 46: 252–261.

Harum KH, Alemi L, Johnston MV (2001) Cognitive impairment in Coffin–Lowry syndrome correlates with reduced RSK2 activation. *Neurology* 56: 207–214.

Huber KM, Gallagher SM, Warren ST, Bear MF (2002) Altered synaptic plasticity in a mouse model of fragile X mental retardation. *Proc Natl Acad Sci U S A* 99: 7746–7750.

Huttenlocher PR (1990) Morphometric study of human cerebral cortex development. *Neuropsychologia* 28: 517–527.

Johnson MH (1999) Cortical plasticity in normal and abnormal cognitive development: evidence and working hypotheses. *Dev Psychopathol* 11: 419–437.

Johnston MV (2003) Brain plasticity in paediatric neurology. *Eur J Paediatr Neurol* 7: 105–113.

Johnston MV (2004) Clinical disorders of brain plasticity. *Brain Dev* 26: 73–80.

Johnston MV, Nishimura A, Harum K, Pekar J, Blue ME (2001) Sculpting the developing brain. *Adv Pediatr* 48: 1–38.

Kandel ER (2001) The molecular biology of memory storage: a dialogue between genes and synapses. *Science* 294: 1030–1038.

Kaufmann WE, Johnston MV, Blue ME (2005) MeCP2 expression and function during brain development: implications for Rett syndrome's pathogenesis and clinical evolution. *Brain Dev* 27: S77–S87.

Kuhl PK (2004) Early language acquisition: cracking the speech code. *Nat Rev Neurosci* 5: 831–843.

Lai CS, Gerrelli D, Monaco AP, Fisher SE, Copp AJ (2003) FOXP2 expression during brain development coincides with adult sites of pathology in a severe speech and language disorder. *Brain* 126: 2455–2462.

Lai CS, Fisher SE, Hurst JA, Vargha-Khadem F, Monaco AP (2001) A forkhead-domain gene is mutated in a severe speech and language disorder. *Nature* 413: 519–523.

Levin HS (2003) Neuroplasticity following non-penetrating traumatic brain injury. *Brain Inj* 17: 665–674.

Liegeois F, Baldeweg T, Connelly A, Gadian DG, Mishkin M, Vargha-Khadem F (2003) Language fMRI abnormalities associated with FOXP2 gene mutation. *Nat Neurosci* 6: 1230–1237.

MacDermot KD, Bonora E, Sykes N, Coupe AM, Lai CS, Vernes SC, et al. (2005) Identification of FOXP2 truncation as a novel cause of developmental speech and language deficits. *Am J Hum Genet* 76: 1074–1080.

Malenka RC (2003) Synaptic plasticity and AMPA receptor trafficking. *Ann N Y Acad Sci* 1003: 1–11.

Meaburn E, Dale PS, Craig IW, Plomin R (2002) Language-impaired children: no sign of the FOXP2 mutation. *Neuroreport* 13: 1075–1077.

Muller F, Kunesch E, Binkofski F, Freund HJ (1991) Residual sensorimotor functions in a patient after right-sided hemispherectomy. *Neuropsychologia* 29: 125–145.

Petrij F, Giles RH, Dauwerse HG, Saris JJ, Hennekam RC, Masuno M, et al. (1995) Rubinstein–Taybi syndrome caused by mutations in the transcriptional co-activator CBP. *Nature* 376: 348–351.

Pfeiffer BE, Huber KM (2006) Current advances in local protein synthesis and synaptic plasticity. *J Neurosci* 26: 7147–7150.

Raff MC, Barres BA, Burne JF, Coles HS, Ishizaki Y, Jacobson MD (1993) Programmed cell death and the control of cell survival: lessons from the nervous system. *Science* 262: 695–700.

Reilly J, Losh M, Bellugi U, Wulfeck B (2004) 'Frog, where are you?' Narratives in children with specific language impairment, early focal brain injury, and Williams syndrome. *Brain Lang* 88: 229–247.

Rubinstein JT (2002) Paediatric cochlear implantation: prosthetic hearing and language development. *Lancet* 360: 483–485.

Scharff C, Haesler S (2005) An evolutionary perspective on FoxP2: strictly for the birds? *Curr Opin Neurobiol* 15: 694–703.

Shaw P, Greenstein D, Lerch J, Clasen L, Lenroot R, Gogtay N, et al. (2006) Intellectual ability and cortical development in children and adolescents. *Nature* 440: 676–679.

Shaywitz SE, Shaywitz BA (2005) Dyslexia (specific reading disability). *Biol Psychiatry* 57: 1301–1309.

Shu W, Cho JY, Jiang Y, Zhang M, Weisz D, Elder GA, et al. (2005) Altered ultrasonic vocalization in mice with a disruption in the Foxp2 gene. *Proc Natl Acad Sci U S A* 102: 9643–9648.

SLI Consortium (2004) Highly significant linkage to the SLI1 locus in an expanded sample of individuals affected by specific language impairment. *Am J Hum Genet* 74: 1225–1238.

Snyder EM, Philpot BD, Huber KM, Dong X, Fallon JR, Bear MF (2001) Internalization of ionotropic glutamate receptors in response to mGluR activation. *Nat Neurosci* 4: 1079–1085.

Somerville MJ, Mervis CB, Young EJ, Seo EJ, del Campo M, Bamforth S, et al. (2005) Severe expressive-language delay related to duplication of the Williams–Beuren locus. *N Engl J Med* 353: 1694–1701.

Sun T, Patoine C, Abu-Khalil A, Visvader J, Sum E, Cherry TJ, et al. (2005) Early asymmetry of gene transcription in embryonic human left and right cerebral cortex. *Science* 308: 1794–1798.

Teramitsu I, Kudo LC, London SE, Geschwind DH, White SA (2004) Parallel FoxP1 and FoxP2 expression in songbird and human brain predicts functional interaction. *J Neurosci* 24: 3152–3163.

Todd PK, Malter JS (2002) Fragile X mental retardation protein in plasticity and disease. *J Neurosci Res* 70: 623–630.

Vanlancker-Sidtis D (2004) When only the right hemisphere is left: studies in language and communication. *Brain Lang* 91: 199–211.

Vargha-Khadem F, Watkins K, Alcock K, Fletcher P, Passingham R (1995) Praxic and non-verbal cognitive deficits in a large family with a genetically transmitted speech and language disorder. *Proc Natl Acad Sci U S A* 92: 930–933.

Voss HU, Uluc AM, Dyke JP, Watts R, Kobylarz EJ, McCandliss BD, et al. (2006) Possible axonal regrowth in late recovery from the minimally conscious state. *J Clin Invest* 116: 2005–2011.

Watkins KE, Dronkers NF, Vargha-Khadem F (2002a) Behavioural analysis of an inherited speech and language disorder: comparison with acquired aphasia. *Brain* 125: 452–464.

Watkins KE, Vargha-Khadem F, Ashburner J, Passingham RE, Connelly A, Friston KJ, et al. (2002b) MRI analysis of an inherited speech and language disorder: structural brain abnormalities. *Brain* 125: 465–478.

Yang EJ, Yoon JH, Min do S, Chung KC (2004) LIM kinase 1 activates cAMP-responsive element-binding protein during the neuronal differentiation of immortalized hippocampal progenitor cells. *J Biol Chem* 279: 8903–8910.

14

CHROMOSOMAL SYNDROMES AND DEVELOPMENTAL DELAY

Sara S Cathey and Kenton R Holden

This chapter includes common chromosomal and gene abnormalities (Down syndrome, Turner syndrome, Klinefelter syndrome, and fragile X syndrome) which present with unique neurodevelopmental delays. Smith–Magenis syndrome has also been included because of its distinctive neurobehavioral phenotype. The objective of the chapter is to provide a broad overview of these disorders with an emphasis on initial historical descriptions, genetic mechanisms, neurodevelopmental and psychomotor consequences, and possible unique therapies. A general summary of therapeutic approaches to be promoted or avoided by the health care team is included.

One hurdle to overcome in an overview such as this is to decide which chromosomal/gene abnormalities to include or exclude. The present review focuses mostly on those disorders that appear frequently in children with neurodevelopmental disabilities and special needs. These disorders are a starting point for better understanding of the gene-chromosome-brain-neurodevelopment axis. Because of space limitations, important disorders such as Prader–Willi syndrome, Angelman syndrome, and Rett syndrome will not be covered and the reader is directed elsewhere for coverage of these conditions and their relationship to neurodevelopmental disabilities.

DOWN SYNDROME
Down syndrome is a multiple malformations/mental retardation syndrome caused by trisomy, of all or a large part of chromosome 21. Down syndrome is the most common genetic cause of moderate to severe intellectual disability. The majority of cases (95%) are brought about by a full trisomy 21 which is the result of meiotic non-disjunction. The single most influential factor in these cases is advanced maternal age ($\geq$35 years), since the majority of non-disjunction cases arise from maternal meiotic errors. The remaining 5% of cases arise from either Robertsonian translocations, about half of which are inherited, or from mosaicism for trisomy 21. The specific chromosome pattern does not significantly alter the pattern of learning difficulties seen in Down syndrome. Children with mosaic Down syndrome may have a less severe phenotype overall, but all children with Down syndrome have a similar profile of language and learning difficulties.

The incidence of Down syndrome is directly related to maternal age and gestational age at diagnosis. Trisomic fetuses have higher rates of spontaneous miscarriage than chromosomally normal fetuses. Prenatal screening and elective termination practices vary geographically and probably alter the incidence of Down syndrome in term neonates, typically said to be from 1 in 800 to 1 in 1000 live births (Holtzman 1996, Laws and Bishop 2004). Race does not appear to be a significant risk factor. Recurrence risk varies with the affected child's karyotype. There is no significant increased risk for parents of a child who has a *de novo* translocation. When a parent carries a balanced Robertsonian translocation, risk for recurrent Down syndrome is 3–15%, depending on which parent carries the translocation. Maternal age is the most important factor when considering possible recurrence of trisomy 21 (Hunter 2005).

John Langdon Down first recorded the easily recognized clinical characteristics of Down syndrome in 1866. The newborn with Down syndrome is hypotonic. The characteristic facial features are evident at birth, including brachycephaly, up-slanting palpebral fissures, bilateral epicanthal folds, and midface hypoplasia. The tongue is often protruding, related to the small mouth and poor tone. The ears are small and relatively square. Nuchal skin is redundant. Other physical features include small hands, short and curved fifth fingers (clinodactyly), and a high frequency of single transverse palmar creases. The feet may show a vertical plantar crease, beginning at an increased space between the first and second toes.

About half of infants with Down syndrome have a congenital heart defect. Early surgical intervention for complex congenital heart disease is now standard for children with Down syndrome. Survival in these children is comparable to children without Down syndrome who have similar heart lesions. About 10% of infants with Down syndrome also have congenital gastrointestinal malformations, with duodenal atresia the most common. Other gastrointestinal malformations include Hirschsprung disease, imperforate anus, pyloric stenosis, and tracheoesophageal fistula. Additional common gastrointestinal issues are constipation, gastroesophageal reflux, and celiac disease (Stray-Gundersen 1995, Cunniff et al. 2001, Hunter 2005).

The most potentially significant orthopedic issue for people with Down syndrom, seen in 10–15% of individuals, is atlantoaxial instability at the C1–C2 interface. A very small minority develop neurologic complications related to atlantoaxial instability (e.g. myelopathy and gait difficulty). Careful neurologic history and physical exam should be incorporated into ongoing routine evaluations (Stray-Gundersen 1995, Hunter 2005).

Thyroid disease is particularly common in Down syndrome and screening should occur at birth and yearly thereafter (Cunniff et al. 2001). The risk of leukemia in Down syndrome is 15–20 times higher than that of the general population from the ages of 1 to 10 years. Persons with Down syndrome may have a lower but still elevated risk of developing certain solid tumors, such as neuroblastoma, brain tumors, and breast cancer, but prospective studies on this issue are lacking (Satgé et al. 1998, Hunter 2005).

Vision problems, including strabismus and refractive errors, are more common in children with Down syndrome. Cataracts, although rare, are slightly more common in children with Down syndrome than in the general population. Early evaluation (by 6 months of age) for such problems can lead to early effective interventions which positively impact overall learning potential (Stray-Gundersen 1995, Cunniff et al. 2001, Hunter 2005).

Hearing loss affects approximately 60% of children with Down syndrome. Most have a conductive hearing loss related to small canals which can become easily obstructed by cerumen and skin debris, frequent otitis media with effusion, and abnormalities of the ossicular chain. Screening for hearing loss should be thorough and frequent, starting with a brainstem auditory evoked response evaluation within the first months of life. Present recommendations include audiometry evaluations semiannually until age 5 years and annually thereafter (Cunniff et al. 2001, Venail et al. 2004).

Sleep abnormalities are frequent in Down syndrome. Obstructive sleep apnea has a high incidence, but central apnea from a probable abnormal central response to hypoxia is also common and may occur in the same patient with obstructive sleep apnea. Sleep fragmentation, restless sleep, frequent arousals, and periodic leg movements are common in individuals with Down syndrome without obstructive apneas. Even in Down syndrome patients without cardiac defects, there appears to be an increased risk for pulmonary hypertension. The behavioral impact of sleep disorders is significant and includes the onset or exacerbation of attention problems, oppositional behavior, poorer academic progress than expected, and work refusal. Patients with a suspected sleep disorder require an overnight polysomnogram and an otolaryngology evaluation. Weight loss is initially indicated for obese patients with these issues. Positive airway pressure devices may help this condition and are often well tolerated (McBrien 2003).

The incidence of seizures in individuals with Down syndrome is higher than the general population, with various reports estimating rates up to approximately 15%. Seizures in Down syndrome begin either within the first two decades of life or later at age 40–50 years. An association between Down syndrome and Alzheimer disease has been recognized for decades. All Down syndrome individuals have beta-amyloid plaques and neurofibrillary tangles, the neuropathologic hallmark signs of Alzheimer disease, by 35–40 years of age (Zigman et al. 1996, Holtzman 1997, Hunter 2005). Clinical dementia appears inevitable, with an average age of onset of 51–54 years. The amyloid precursor protein is on chromosome 21, and it is theorized that overexpression of this leads to premature accumulation of the protein and eventual Alzheimer disease. The E4 allele of apolipoprotein E, on chromosome 19, has been shown to be a major risk factor for the development of Alzheimer disease. Individuals with Down syndrome who carry one or two E4 alleles develop dementia and the characteristic Alzheimer neuropathology at an earlier than expected age (Zigman et al. 1996, Holtzman 1997).

Depression is the most frequently diagnosed psychiatric disorder (i.e. dual diagnosis) in Down syndrome patients. Hallucinations commonly accompany the depression. A decline in self-care skills is common in depression arising within Down syndrome and may be incorrectly diagnosed as Alzheimer dementia. Stressor events can have a role in triggering the illness. Antidepressant medications, including selective serotonin-reuptake inhibitors (SSRIs), are often helpful and are well tolerated in individuals with Down syndrome. Although any psychiatric disorder can occur, schizophrenia (paranoid) and bipolar affective disorders have lower rates in those with Down syndrome than in the general population (Wolraich 2003).

The complications of hypotonia, lax ligaments, and decreased strength contribute to delayed early motor development in children with Down syndrome. Motor milestones are met, but at a much slower rate than in other children. Visuomotor control, balance, and agility are also areas of weakness, which have the demonstrated potential for improvement with early intervention programs. People with Down syndrome have vocal impairments including hoarseness and harshness of voice. These conditions are largely related to muscle fatigue generated by the excessive effort required to move intrinsically hypotonic laryngeal muscles (Venail et al. 2004).

Language development is the most significantly affected area of development in children with Down syndrome (Hines and Bennett 1996). Babbling is delayed in the first year of life. Expressive language development is deficient in both vocabulary and syntax. In childhood, grammar development is limited by poor verbal short-term memory (Chapman 1997, Venail et al. 2004). Children with Down syndrome have a relatively poor memory for speech sounds (i.e. phonologic memory), which is a significant barrier impeding fully normal language development. Language comprehension is less severely affected than expressive language. However, the gap between language production and comprehension continues to widen throughout childhood and adolescence. Adults with Down syndrome have a poor use of verb tense inflections, and use relatively few prepositions, pronouns, or conjunctions in speech (Laws and Bishop 2004).

Hines and Bennett (1996) systematically reviewed multiple studies exploring the impact of early intervention on the development of children with Down syndrome. Overall, positive developmental changes were seen. Specifically, levels of independence and community functioning were correlated with prior participation in early intervention programs (Hines and Bennett 1996). Language learning may continue into adulthood, making long-term speech therapy valuable (Kumin 1996, Venail et al. 2004). Children with Down syndrome can be expected to attend school, participate in extracurricular activities such as sports and community service, and later work in supported or sheltered employment positions and live semi- or fully independently in their communities.

Trisomy for chromosome 21 leads to an abnormal gene dosage. Molecular analyses of the phenotypic features associated with Down syndrome, including hypotonia, facial features, and congenital heart disease, map to 21q22.2-22.3, known as the 'Down syndrome chromosome region' (Delebar et al. 1993, Hubert et al. 1997). Many studies suggest genes outside this region are also involved epigenetically in the Down syndrome phenotype. A gene region implicated in duodenal stenosis overlaps with band 22 but extends proximally, covering a larger region of chromosome 21 (Korenberg et al. 1994). Genes within the Down syndrome chromosome region appear to make the major contributions to the intellectual disability seen in the disorder. Phenotypic mapping studies of patients with duplications of only small regions of chromosome 21 provide evidence that additional genes outside the Down syndrome chromosome region may also have a role in mental retardation/intellectual disability (Korenberg et al. 1992, 1994).

Recently, researchers have successfully created an improved mouse model of Down syndrome. This new strain of mice carries a nearly complete copy of human chromosome 21, causing trisomy for those genes, but not in every cell of the animal. These mice exhibit learning and memory deficits and heart defects like those seen in individuals with Down syndrome. Previous mouse models were trisomic for mouse chromosome 16, homologous for half of the genes on human chromosome 21. No previous mouse model exhibited congenital heart defects (Holtzman et al. 1996). The newest animal model of Down syndrome may enhance our understanding of the pathogenic mechanisms responsible for certain phenotypic features in this disorder (O'Doherty et al. 2005).

Interventions and therapies for people with Down syndrome revolve around the medical complications which vary significantly from person to person. Complicating medical factors, specifically hypotonia and cardiac defects, in addition to hearing and vision abnormalities, compromise developmental progress. As our knowledge has increased, preventive health care has become the leading advancement in optimizing the cognitive and developmental status and overall quality of life for individuals with Down syndrome.

TURNER SYNDROME

Turner syndrome, or monosomy X, is named after Henry Turner, an endocrinologist who initially described the characteristic physical features, including short stature and gonadal dysgenesis, in seven women (Turner 1938, Elsheikh et al. 2002). More than two decades later, Ford et al. (1959) demonstrated 45,X as the cause of this syndrome. Indeed, the most common chromosome constitution in Turner syndrome, seen in about half of all cases, is 45,X with complete absence of the second sex chromosome.

Monosomy X arises from non-disjunction during meiosis in a parental gamete. The single X is of maternal origin in about 70–80% of cases, consistent with paternal meiosis error rates (Nussbaum et al. 2004). If the non-disjunction occurs in the early embryonic divisions, the result is usually mosaicism in which only a proportion of cells are 45,X. Mosaicism for 45,X/46,XX confers the least severe Turner phenotype. Although these women still have short stature, they are of increased average height compared to non-mosaic individuals. Some have spontaneous puberty and menses. There is an increased risk of gonadoblastoma with the 45,X/46,XY karyotype (Elsheikh et al. 2002).

The incidence of Turner syndrome is liveborn female infants has been reported to be 1 in 2000 to 1 in 4000 (Nussbaum et al. 2004, Tyler and Edman 2004). Only about 1% of monosomy X fetuses survive to term. Why the 45,X karyotype is compatible with postnatal survival at all is unclear, given that it is nearly always lethal *in utero* (Nussbaum et al. 2004, Tyler and Edman 2004). Turner syndrome is not associated with advanced maternal age and familial recurrence of the syndrome is exceptional (Harper 1998, Gardner and Sutherland 2004).

Prenatal findings include cystic hygroma, increased nuchal thickness, coarctation of the aorta, renal anomalies, and growth retardation. No antenatal ultrasound finding is diagnostic for Turner syndrome. The diagnosis may be suspected in the newborn period in the female infant with lymphedema of the hands and feet, 'webbed' neck, and heart defects, particularly left-sided defects such as aortic valve abnormalities, coarctation of the aorta, and hypoplastic left heart. Renal and/or urologic anomalies, including horseshoe kidney and double collecting systems, are not uncommon. The incidence of thyroid disease increases with age, and nearly one-third of adults with Turner syndrome have hypothyroidism. Problems with early gross and fine motor sensory integration, delayed walking, and early language dysfunction may call attention to a problem in the preschool years. Turner syndrome may remain undiagnosed until later childhood when an evaluation for short stature and delayed sexual maturation is initiated (Tyler and Edman 2004).

Unlike other common chromosome abnormalities, Turner syndrome is not usually associated with mental retardation. The neurocognitive phenotype of Turner syndrome is consistent, regardless of the parent of origin of the deleted X chromosome (Ross et al. 2000a). Overall intelligence is normal, but the majority of these girls and women have deficits in specific areas of intellectual performance (Money 1993, Elsheikh et al. 2002). Anticipating a probable need for special educational services is prudent. Impaired visuospatial abilities, non-verbal memory, and attentional skills in these females have been well documented (Ross et al. 1995, 2000b, Mazzocco 2001, Elsheikh et al. 2002, Rourke et al. 2002). These issues are manifested in poor math skills, poor direction sense, impaired non-verbal problem-solving, difficulty with multi-tasking, and reduced attention span (Sybert and McCauley 2004). While schoolgirls with Turner syndrome work at age level in spelling, they tend to perform 2 years behind their classmates in mathematics (Rourke et al. 2002). Intelligence testing demonstrates lower performance than verbal scores (Ross et al. 1995, O'Connor et al. 2000). At least half of all girls with Turner syndrome have some degree of sensorineural hearing loss, and this frequency increases with age. It may present as early as 6 years of age and progress (Saenger et al. 2001). Monitoring for hearing loss will help avoid its possible interference with school and learning issues.

A characteristic psychosocial profile has been described in females with Turner syndrome (Elsheikh et al. 2002). Compared with healthy young girls, those with Turner syndrome have more difficulty making friends and participate in fewer social activities (Ross et al. 2000b). Anxiety and delayed social maturation, leading to feelings of isolation, are common in adolescence (Sybert and McCauley 2004, Tyler and Edman 2004). Adolescents with Turner syndrome have more peer relationship and school problems than short-statured girls without Turner syndrome (Saenger et al. 2001). Psychosocial support for these girls is an integral component of treatment in preventing low self-esteem and subsequent depressive symptoms. Obtaining a driver's license may require certain accommodations be made in order to overcome poor navigational planning and impaired spatial and directional abilities (Sybert and McCauley 2004). Dating and initiation of sexual activity may be delayed (Ross et al. 2000b). Gender identification is clearly and consistently female (Tyler and Edman 2004). Adult women with Turner syndrome tend to live with their parents longer than age-matched peers and to marry later in life. Individuals with non-verbal learning disabilities may fail to interpret social cues appropriately. Misreading facial expressions and body language contributes to awkward social interactions (Sybert and McCauley 2004).

It is difficult to quantify the true incidence of the social and behavioral problems in Turner syndrome because of confounding factors such as hormone replacement, concurrent health problems, and environmental issues contributing to learning problems and social immaturity. There is considerable variation among the population of females with Turner syndrome, and most would be considered to have only subtle social problems (McCauley et al. 2001). In surveys of adults with Turner syndrome, most indicate a reasonable satisfaction with their lifestyle and employment. Many women with Turner syndrome achieve college education and eventual vocational success. The overall incidence of psychiatric illness in women with Turner syndrome is not increased compared to the general population (Sybert 2005).

The genes thus far described as responsible for the Turner syndrome phenotype escape X-inactivation (Elsheikh et al. 2002, Nussbaum et al. 2004, Sybert 2005). Some of these genes have homologs on the Y chromosome, indicating that their presence on both sex chromosomes is needed for normal development (Elsheikh et al. 2002). Haplo-insufficiency for the short arm of the X chromosome or the homologous sequences on the Y chromosome gives a phenotype with short stature and gonadal dysgenesis.

SHOX was the first gene discovered to be involved in the Turner syndrome phenotype. Loss of the SHOX gene, located in the pseudo-autosomal region PAR1 of Xp, confers short stature and the other skeletal manifestations of Turner syndrome, including cubitus valgus and short fourth metacarpals (Kosho et al. 1999, Clement-Jones et al. 2000, Boucher et al. 2001, Sybert 2005).

It is suspected that more than one gene is responsible for the related somatic features of Turner syndrome (lymphedema, including puffy hands and feet, webbed neck, and nail dysplasia). A lymphedema critical region has been mapped to Xp11.4 (Boucher et al. 2001). The neurocognitive phenotype with visuospatial and perceptual deficits also is likely multigenic in origin. Deletion of distal Xp22.3 has been proposed to most influence the development of visuospatial perceptual abilities in Turner syndrome (Ross et al. 2000a). Both the short and the long arm of the X chromosome contain genes important for ovarian function. Candidate genes in such premature ovarian failure regions (POF1 and POF2) are currently being investigated (Sybert and McCauley 2004).

Many reviews of Turner syndrome delineate a subset of patients with mental retardation who have short stature, gonadal dysgenesis, and a ring X chromosome. Mental retardation in women with the 46,Xr(X) karyotype has been attributed to a lack of expression of the XIST gene in small rings. XIST controls X-inactivation. It is postulated that overexpression of X chromosomal material leads to mental retardation. Larger ring X that expresses XIST leads to a Turner syndrome phenotype, while the small ring that lacks XIST expression predicts mental retardation with or without other associated physical anomalies (Nussbaum et al. 2004, Sybert 2005).

Beyond early intervention, special education services, and psychosocial support, females with Turner syndrome are treated with hormonal therapy. Although Turner syndrome girls are not growth hormone deficient, treatment of short stature with growth hormone is effective and has become clinically routine. Growth hormone can accelerate growth in girls with Turner syndrome and increase final height attainment. An average gain of 10cm in final height has been reported in some studies (Elsheikh et al. 2002). The factors important in final height achieved include growth hormone regimen and years of growth hormone treatment prior to estrogenization and final closure of bone growth plates. Therapy has been initiated as early as 2 years of age. Growth hormone therapy may be carefully combined with anabolic steroid therapy in select patients who begin therapy after 8 years of age (Saenger et al. 2001).

Most girls with Turner syndrome will require estrogen therapy to induce pubertal development. Because estrogen induces closing of epiphyseal plates, limiting height growth, estrogen therapy may be delayed to maximize final height. Some studies have implicated estrogen therapy in improved psychologic function. Estrogen-treated girls self-reported improved well-being and self-esteem during the relatively awkward age of 12–16 years (Ross et al. 1996b). Improved memory function has been seen in estrogen-treated adolescents (Ross et al. 2000). Estrogen and growth hormone therapies require co-ordination and close supervision carried out by a pediatric endocrinologist as an integral member of the health care team.

KLINEFELTER SYNDROME

Klinefelter syndrome is a common chromosomal abnormality affecting approximately 1 in 600 to 1 in 800 live-born males. It was initially described in 1942 as an endocrine disorder characterized by infertility, hypogonadism with elevated gonadotropins, and gynecomastia (Klinefelter et al. 1942, Visootsak et al. 2001, Lanfranco et al. 2004). The associated 47,XXY karyotype was initially demonstrated in 1959. The supernumerary X is the result of non-disjunction during meiosis, either paternal (50–60% of cases) or maternal (40–50% of cases) in origin. Parent of origin of the extra X chromosome does not affect the specific phenotypic expression of this disorder. Mean maternal age is increased in the maternally derived cases, but paternal age is not increased, even in paternally derived cases. There appears to be no significant recurrence risk within a family (Tyler and Edman 2004, Simpson et al. 2005).

Population studies have shown that approximately 10% of cases are diagnosed prenatally, by amniocentesis, usually performed for the indication of advanced maternal age. Approximately 25% of cases are diagnosed in childhood or adulthood during evaluation for developmental delay, gynecomastia, or hypogonadism. Using incidence studies based on cytogenetic surveys of newborn infants, it is estimated that more than 60% of cases are never formally diagnosed (Ratcliffe 1999, Visootsak et al. 2001).

An X chromosome gene dosage effect is the probable mechanism for the phenotype seen in individuals with 47,XXY. Some genes on the X chromosome escape X-inactivation, leading to excess gene product formation. An increased frequency of skewed X-inactivation has been demonstrated in Klinefelter syndrome. This may be protective and explain why severe behavior and learning issues are seen in only a minority of males with Klinefelter syndrome (Simpson et al. 2005). Variants of the common 47,XXY karyotype demonstrate that the effects on physical and mental development increase with the number of extra X chromosomes present (Visootsak et al. 2001). Mosaicism for 46,XY/47,XXY imparts a less severe phenotype and these males have less developmental delay than individuals with 47,XXY. Males with 48,XXXY have severe language impairment, mild to moderate mental retardation, clinodactyly, radio-ulnar synostosis, and subtle facial dysmorphism. Males with 49,XXXXY have an even more severe phenotype (Simpson et al. 2005). These 'Klinefelter variants' are rare. The 48,XXXY karyotype is seen in approximately 1 in 50 000 male births, and 49,XXXXY in only 1 in 85 000 to 1 in 100 000 male births.

Clinical features of Klinefelter syndrome are rarely detected in infancy. Growth parameters and external genitalia are usually normal at birth. Toddlers have language delay. Motor development is usually in the normal range, although neuromotor developmental delay has been said to contribute to reduced fine and gross motor skills in some individuals with Klinefelter syndrome. Some reports have documented an increased frequency of poor muscle tone, tremor, and reduced dexterity. These issues affect writing skills and speed on timed tasks, and lead to physical awkwardness (Visootsak et al. 2001). After age 5, boys with Klinefelter syndrome demonstrate a particular growth pattern characterized by a significantly accelerated linear growth. This is mostly caused by excessive leg length, and the result is a decreased upper to lower body segment ratio. Final height is average to tall (Lanfranco et al. 2004). The body habitus of adolescents and adults is eunuchoid, with an arm span greater than height by 2–3cm, slender shoulders, and slightly widened hips (Simpson et al. 2005).

Klinefelter syndrome is the most common cause of male infertility and the diagnosis may be made as part of an infertility evaluation. Puberty occurs on time, but secondary sex characteristics fail to advance in the usual fashion. Facial, pubic, and axillary hair are sparse. Testes may initially enlarge but then involute, with a greatest final diameter typically less than 2.5cm. Prepubertal testosterone levels are within the normal range, but in adulthood these levels are low-normal to low. The gonadotropins, luteinizing hormone (LH) and follicle-stimulating hormone (FSH), begin to increase around age 12 years, and remain abnormally elevated (Tyler et al. 2004). By 13–14 years of age, most boys with Klinefelter syndrome have markedly elevated FSH and LH levels and a plateau of testosterone that is subnormal. Elevated LH leads to testicular aromatization of testosterone to estradiol. The decreased testosterone:estradiol ratio contributes to the development of gynecomastia, seen in more than 50% of adolescents with Klinefelter syndrome (Simpson et al. 2005). Klinefelter syndrome is not associated with gender identity disorders or homosexuality, but overall sexual interest may be diminished (Visootsak et al. 2001).

Although the vast majority of males with Klinefelter syndrome are azospermic, exceptional cases of paternity have been reported. These cases might be attributed to unrecognized testicular mosaicism. A karyotype analysis performed on a peripheral blood sample does not predict the chromosomal constitution of the testis cells, or the absence or presence of actual spermatogenesis (Lanfranco et al. 2004). Most adult males with Klinefelter syndrome will need to plan for adoption, artificial insemination, or use other assisted reproductive techniques. Intracytoplasmic sperm injection, using sperm recovered by testicular biopsy, has allowed some 47,XXY males to biologically father children. Pregnancies achieved by this route in this patient population have a twofold increased frequency of sex chromosome aneuploidy (Simpson et al. 2005).

There are additional medical issues associated with Klinefelter syndrome. Androgen deficiency contributes to osteoporosis, reduced muscle strength, and an increased thromboembolic risk, as a result of decreased fibrinolysis. This results in venous stasis ulcers and varicose veins, seen in 13–30% of patients (Lanfranco et al. 2004, Simpson et al. 2005). Type 2 diabetes and chronic thyroiditis are associated with Klinefelter syndrome. Other autoimmune disorders may occur with increased frequency, but adequate studies are lacking. The risk of breast cancer with Klinefelter syndrome is close to that of age-matched women. Physicians should perform annual clinical breast exams, and men should be taught self-examination. No studies support routine screening mammography. Young men with Klinefelter syndrome have an approximate risk of 1% for developing mediastinal germ cell tumors.

Although males with Klinefelter syndrome demonstrate considerable developmental variability, specific cognitive deficits in speech and language as well as executive functions are consistently noted. Secondary problems with emotional development, attention, and social interaction are also quite common. Most individuals with Klinefelter syndrome have learning problems, but still greater than 80% have IQ scores greater than 90 (Tyler et al. 2004). Verbal IQ is lower than performance IQ because of the poor vocabulary skills, limited abstract reasoning, and impaired auditory memory and processing (Graham et al. 1988, Money 1993, Radcliffe 1999). Receptive language skills are comparable for 47,XXY boys and controls except for the comprehension of complex sentence structures. Problems within the expressive language domain include difficulties with word finding and expressing an organized narrative, impaired reading and spelling, and impaired auditory memory. Auditory processing and memory, of both verbal and non-verbal material, are compromised. These deficits are manifested as reduced accuracy and rate of oral reading and an impaired comprehension of text material (Graham et al. 1988, Ratcliffe 1999). In summary, boys with Klinefelter syndrome have difficulty with word retrieval, complex grammar, and with constructing oral narratives. These deficits are similar to those seen in chromosomally intact children with dyslexia (Visootsak et al. 2001).

Care of the individual with Klinefelter syndrome requires a multidisciplinary approach. If comprehensive neurodevelopmental evaluations and early intervention therapies begin in infancy, later school difficulties appear to be reduced. Early sign language may help the child with Klinefelter syndrome communicate and decrease frustration experienced prior to the onset of speech (Simpson et al. 2005). Without early remediation, the language processing deficits of the preschooler become chronic reading and writing disabilities. These boys are more likely than peers to require special education and to fail one or more grades (Visootsak et al. 2001).

Testosterone replacement should begin when gonadotropin levels start to rise, around age 11 or 12 years. The goals are to provide age-appropriate levels of testosterone, estradiol, LH, and FSH, and to gradually induce virilization. Testosterone replacement continues for life (Tyler et al. 2004). Testosterone therapy leads to increased strength, libido, bone mineral density, body hair, and a more masculine physique. Neither gynecomastia nor fertility is improved with testosterone replacement. The testes do not respond to gonadotropin or androgen stimulation (Lanfranco et al. 2004, Simpson et al. 2005). Testosterone therapy has been promoted to enhance learning, mood, self-esteem, concentration, and energy, even when the pretreatment hormone level is in the normal range. However, some patients continue to have difficulties with language and social interactions despite years of hormone therapy. Objective long-term studies are recognized to be needed in this area (Simpson et al. 2005).

FRAGILE X SYNDROME

Fragile X syndrome (FXS) is the most common inherited cause of intellectual disability and occurs in both males and females. It is caused by an abnormal expansion of a trinucleotide repeat in the fragile X mental retardation (FMR1) gene located on the long arm of the X chromosome (Xq27.3). Unaffected individuals have approximately 5–55 tandem repetitive triplets of CGG, and this normal number of repeats is transmitted from parent to child in a stable manner. Individuals with 55–200 repeats, known as pre-mutation carriers, are not affected with the full FXS but are at risk for having children with FXS. Pre-mutations are transmitted in an inherently unstable manner, and the number of CGG repeats may expand when a female, but not a male, transmits the mutation. The probability of a mother's pre-mutation expanding to a full mutation in her offspring is increased with the mother's repeat number. Individuals with greater than 200 repeats have the full mutation and are affected with FXS (Terraciano et al. 2005, Visootsak et al. 2005). The presence of more than 200 copies of the repeat leads to methylation, and therefore inactivation, of the promoter region of the FMR1 gene.

Methylation inhibits transcription of FMR1, resulting in absence of the gene's protein product, FMR1 protein (FMRP) (Oostra and Willemsen 2003, Pandey et al. 2004). The normal function of FMRP is to transport messenger RNA from the nucleus to the ribosomes. FMRP is expressed in many tissues and is particularly abundant in neurons. There, FMRP transports specific messenger RNA along the dendrites to actively translating ribosomes near the synapses. It is the absence of FMRP that causes the mental retardation in FXS (Gantois and Kooy 2002). FXS is rarely caused by point mutations of FMR1 rather than the triplet repeat expansion.

Pre-mutation carriers do not exhibit the full FXS, but are not completely unaffected as was previously thought. An estimated 30% of male pre-mutation carriers over the age of 50 years develop the fragile X associated tremor/ataxia syndrome. Approximately 20% of female pre-mutation carriers develop premature ovarian failure (Terracciano et al. 2005). The phenotype of individuals with full mutations do not overlap with these pre-mutation phenotypes because the molecular mechanisms are distinct. Pre-mutation carriers have increased transcriptional activity of the FMR1 gene, while individuals with FXS have silenced FMR1 genes.

FXS is named for the cytogenetically visible fragile site at Xq27.3 induced by culturing cells of affected individuals in a folate-deficient media (Visootsak et al.

2005). Cytogenetic testing is negative in some affected individuals and pre-mutation carriers, but it served as the diagnostic test for FXS until the gene was cloned in 1991. DNA FMR1 analyses by Southern blot and polymerase chain reaction are now the standard methods for diagnostic testing (Hagerman 2005).

Population studies indicate the incidence of FXS is about 1 in 4000 males and 1 in 8000 females (Turner et al. 1996, Hagerman and Hagerman 2002). The pre-mutation is found in the general population at a frequency of approximately 1 in 250 females and 1 in 700 males (Hagerman 2005). All ethnic, racial, and socioeconomic backgrounds are affected.

The classic physical manifestations of FXS include particular craniofacial features (large ears, long face, prominent forehead and jaw) and macro-orchidism in most males. The facial phenotype is subtle in young children and becomes more pronounced with age, especially after puberty. Most adult males with FXS have enlarged testicles with testicular volumes of 40–60ml. The upper limit of testicular volume in normal adult males is 25–30ml (Hagerman and Hagerman 2002). Macro-orchidism does not appear to affect fertility in these individuals (Visootsak et al. 2005). Musculoskeletal findings include flat feet and hyperextensible metacarpophalangeal joints. The finger joint laxity becomes less noticeable with age. These skeletal issues, plus characteristic velvety smooth skin, suggest a connective tissue dysplasia in FXS. Abnormal elastin fibers have been demonstrated in the skin, aorta, and cardiac valves of males with FXS. Mitral valve prolapse is a common finding in affected adults, apparently developing in late adolescence or adulthood. Because of X-inactivation post-term, the phenotypic manifestations of FXS in females with full mutations are variable. About half of these women are asymptomatic. The remaining women in this category manifest variable symptoms, from learning disabilities to overt intellectual disability (Hagerman and Hagerman 2002).

FXS phenotype in full mutation individuals is characterized by global intellectual impairment and distinctive neurocognitive deficits. These specific deficits include poor attention skills, visuospatial disabilities, and difficulty processing sequential information. The degree of cognitive impairment is correlated with the deficit of FMRP (Loesch et al. 2004). The majority of males with FXS have moderate to severe mental retardation, but the entire spectrum is represented from mild to profound (Pandey et al. 2004). Females are usually less severely affected than males. Most full mutation females have IQs in the mildly retarded to low normal range (Hagerman 2005). Higher functioning individuals have incomplete methylation and therefore incomplete inactivation of FMR1. Mosaicism, where a proportion of cells have the full mutation and others have the pre-mutation, is another mechanism that allows for some production of FMRP and less severe phenotypes.

Postmortem examinations of brain tissue from individuals with FXS reveal abnormalities of neuronal dendritic spines, suggesting synaptic abnormalities. Several brain regions are enlarged, including the hippocampus, amygdala, caudate nucleus, and thalamus. The cerebellar vermis is smaller than in population norms. Seizures occur in 20% of patients and typically respond well to standard anticonvulsants (Hessl et al. 2004).

Learning problems may be the presenting feature of FXS in the young child because the physical phenotype may not be recognized until after puberty. Both males and females show a decline with age in all areas of cognitive abilities and all domains of adaptive functioning (Rittey 2003). Affected females have a more variable cognitive profile than males. Individuals with FXS have difficulty with higher level 'executive function' tasks including planning, working memory, and shifting attention. A fundamental impairment seen in FXS is weakness in inhibitory control, with an inability to regulate arousal. Males with FXS often react more strongly to environmental stimuli than individuals without FXS. This area of dysfunction is somewhat responsive to behavior modification and medications. Rapid speech, anxiety, and aggressive behaviors may be related to this underlying hyperarousal (Cornish et al. 2004).

Deficits in attention are consistently seen in FXS. Accompanying hyperactivity and impulsivity is more common in boys (80%) than girls (35%) with FXS (Hagerman 2005). Tantrums begin in the second year of life and occur commonly with excessive stimulation, such as times of transition from one environment or activity to the next. Affected children lack intrinsic self-calming skills, usually making timeouts ineffective. Anxiety is more common in individuals without hyperactivity. Social anxiety is more pronounced in females and may lead to avoidant behavior in adolescence. The hyperactivity improves with age, but aggression may worsen. Obsessive-compulsive behavior is also common in FXS.

Approximately 15–25% of individuals with FXS will meet diagnostic criteria for an autism spectrum disorder (Hagerman and Hagerman 2002, Rittey 2003). More commonly male than female, these children have severe language and social deficits and lower IQ scores than FXS children without autism. Hand flapping, hand biting, poor eye contact, shyness, and perseveration of speech are seen in most individuals with FXS. FMRP levels do not, however, correlate with the presence of autism, suggesting secondary gene effects may be additive to the FMR1 mutation (Hagerman and Hagerman 2002).

Language delays are noted in children with FXS by 2–3 years of age. Children with FXS gain expressive language skills more slowly than receptive language skills. Most research on language development has involved males with FXS, but females appear to follow a similar pattern. Males with FXS have rapid and dysrhythmic speech. They use repetitions of whole words or parts of words. Tangential language is common. They perseverate and reintroduce personally favorite topics repeatedly (Hagerman and Hagerman 2002, Visootsak et al. 2005).

Longitudinal studies emphasize the importance of early intervention to facilitate the cognitive abilities and adaptive behavioral skills in children with FXS that will enhance participation in activities of daily living. Intervention strategies should focus on strengths in receptive language and target the lower expressive language skills (Visootsak et al. 2005). Attention and behavior problems are usually the areas of greatest concern for parents of children with FXS. The majority of affected children respond well to standard therapies for attention-deficit–hyperactivity disorder. The SSRIs are useful for decreasing aggression, anxiety, and obsessive-compulsive behaviors in individuals with FXS. Occupational therapy with sensory integration techniques provides calming techniques. Families should be instructed to recognize escalating behaviors and avoid overstimulation. Counseling might help adults with FXS recognize situations that precipitate behavioral outbursts and learn self-initiated calming. Gene therapy aimed at reactivating the FMR1 gene is an area of current intense research (Rattazzi et al. 2004).

Pharmacologic specific therapy may be on the horizon. Glutamate is the neurotransmitter at most excitatory synapses in the brain. Group 1 metabotropic glutamate receptor (Gp1 mGluR) activities are increased in individuals with FXS because of absence of FMRP. The consequences of activating these receptors vary widely and may account for the delayed cognitive development and the observed neurologic and psychiatric symptoms of the disorder. Studies of Gp1 mGluR antagonists have been positive in animal models, and work in this area continues (Bear 2005).

SMITH–MAGENIS SYNDROME

Smith–Magenis syndrome (SMS) is a complex multisystem congenital anomaly/intellectual disability syndrome with striking neurobehavioral features caused by an interstitial deletion of chromosome 17p11.2 The deletions are *de novo* in the vast majority of cases, suggesting a low familial recurrence risk (Smith and Gropman 2005). Since the first report in 1982 (Smith et al. 1982), approximately 500 cases of all ages have been identified worldwide from multiple ethnic groups with a complex but distinct phenotype. Although the estimated prevalence was 1 in 25 000 in initial studies, improved cytogenetic techniques in target populations suggests that SMS is probably more common than initially suspected. Delayed diagnosis is still common because of subtle infantile and early childhood features. Lifespan does not appear to be affected by SMS, although associated co-morbid features such as epilepsy or congenital heart disease may change this prognosis for certain individuals.

SMS is considered to be a contiguous gene syndrome brought about by deletion of adjacent genes in a specific region of the short arm of chromosome 17. The size of the deletion varies from 2 to 9 megabases, but approximately 75% of affected individuals have a common deletion spanning four megabases. Most patients have cytogenetically visible deletions which can be appreciated on good quality, high resolution karyotyping. Fluorescence *in situ* hybridization with

SMS-specific probes confirms the diagnosis in the occasional equivocal case. The SMS critical region has been narrowed to a 1-megabase region that contains 25 genes. Genes responsible for the intellectual disability, craniofacial features, and behavioral and sleep disturbances are proposed to be located proximally in the critical region, while genes affecting development (physical and mental) are thought to be distally located (Smith and Gropman 2005). One gene of particular interest is the RAI1 (retinoic acid induced 1) gene. Several patients with clinically suspected SMS who lack cytogenetically detectable deletions have been found to have mutations of this gene detected with molecular sequencing (Slager et al. 2003). These patients share the characteristic facial and neurobehavioral features, but lack the short stature and structural anomalies seen in patients with deletions. The percentage of SMS cases with RAI1 mutations remains to be determined (Bi et al. 2004).

Following the initial case reports of SMS (Smith et al. 1982), subsequent reports of patients with consistent clinical findings established four major criteria for recognition of the syndrome (Stratton et al. 1986):

(1) mild to moderate brachycephaly with a broad face and nasal bridge, (2) variable midface hypoplasia, (3) short broad hands, (4) intellectual disability associated with hyperactivity and often self-destructive behaviors

Most patients have short stature and congenital malformations, for example, cleft palate, structural heart disease, or genital anomalies. Several early observed cases with typical craniofacial changes in association with short stature and obesity resembled a phenotype similar to Prader–Willi or Down syndrome. Eyes are deep-set with up-slanting palpebral fissures and heavy brows. The mouth is quite characteristic, with a fleshy tented appearance to the upper lip and open-mouth expression. As children with SMS age, the midface hypoplasia is more severe, and the forehead and jaw prominence is more striking. All patients have moderate to severe mental retardation/intellectual disability, with speech more severally affected than motor abilities. Behavior problems are very common and include hyperactivity, excessive aggression, self-stimulatory activity, and self-destructive acts. Although initially thought to be consistent with behavior commonly seen in persons with intellectually disability, this behavior profile has proven to be very typical of the SMS phenotype (Stratton et al. 1986).

Further delineation of the evolving phenotype was accomplished by a multidisciplinary clinical study of 29 patients with SMS in 1996 (Greenberg et al. 1996). This and subsequent studies found significant otolaryngologic abnormalities (conductive and sensorineural hearing loss, velopharyngeal incompetence, deep hoarse voice), ophthalmologic defects (strabismus, myopia, iris dysplasia, microcornea), scoliosis, cardiac (valvular or structural) abnormalities, renal (especially duplication of the collecting systems) anomalies, and other neurodevelopmental abnormalities. Brain imaging commonly shows ventriculomegaly. Sleep studies with electro-encephalography (EEG) are abnormal, with a predominantly reduced REM sleep dura-tion. Psychometric testing has documented intelligence quotients in individuals with SMS ranging from 20 to 78 with a mean of 47 ± 15 in 86% of the patients. Language assessments support earlier observations that expressive language is consistently more delayed than receptive language. Behaviors of SMS were previously attributed to the frustration related to the expressive language delays. Sign language is recom-mended as an adjunct to speech therapy to help improve this specific problem. The documented sleep disorder in SMS may also contribute to the behavior problems. Individuals have difficulty falling asleep and staying asleep, with frequent awakenings during the night. Half of the individuals have reduced (but not absent) REM sleep (Greenberg et al. 1996). The underlying etiology of the sleep disorder is not yet apparent.

Additional aberrant behaviors occurring in patients with SMS include self-destructive behavior with onychotillomania (pulling out fingernails and toenails), wrist biting, head banging, and polyembolokoilamania (insertion of foreign bodies into body orifices) (Greenberg et al. 1990).

Various medications have been used in attempts to modify these aberrant behaviors. The most commonly prescribed medications in a 1996 study were methylphenidate, pemoline, and thioridazine. In most cases, the medications were not effective in modifying behavior or improving attention span (Greenberg et al. 1996). Behavioral therapies remain the primary means of treating undesirable prob-lematic aberrant behaviors.

SMS has distinctive behavioral, cognitive, and neuropsychiatric abnormalities. Stereotypic and self-injurious behaviors affect 97% of individuals and distinguish SMS from many other genetic syndromes (Finucane et al. 2001). These beha-viors, in addition to erratic sleep patterns, create severe management issues. The repertoire of self-injurious behavior increases with age (self-pinching, scratching, picking). Additional behavioral abnormalities include attention seeking, hostility, impulsiveness, temper tantrums, aggression, anxiety, overactivity, destruction, and unusual motor behaviors. Two such unusual behaviors are the 'self-hug' or spas-modic upper-body squeeze, and the 'lick and flip' which is hand-licking followed by page flipping motions (Finucane et al. 1994, Smith and Gropman 2005). Also consistent are strikingly low adaptive behaviors. Adults with SMS have few skills related to activities of daily living (Shelley and Robertson 2005). Severe behavioral disturbances, especially aggression, self-injury, and impulsivity, explain the consis-tently low rates of eventual occupational attainment.

Sleep and behavioral abnormalities of SMS may be aggravated by inversion of the circadian rhythm of melatonin secretion. Tantrums in SMS correlate with a rise in serum melatonin. Melatonin rises during the day and a proposed hypothesis is that children with SMS 'struggle' against sleep. Treatment with β_1-adrenergic blockers results in significant improvement in inappropriate behaviors, increased concentration, increased hours of sleep, and delayed waking (De Leersnyder et al. 2001). Good sleep hygiene remains an important component of effective intervention.

The treatment aim is to improve the quality of life for persons with SMS and their families. Therapeutic interventions should be directed toward modifying aberrant behaviors, improving attention, treating the sleep disturbances, and providing therapies that may improve cognition and behavior (Shelley and Robertson 2005). Earlier diagnosis, and therefore earlier interventions, should be aggressively sought. Children with SMS are more alert in the early morning hours and this should be utilized to the child's advantage in educational and therapeutic settings. Teachers, special educators, nurses, caregivers, psychologists, and doctors should be well-informed about the unique aspects of this complex genetic syndrome.

SUBTELOMERIC DELETION-DUPLICATION-TRANSLOCATION SYNDROMES

Collectively, subtelomeric deletion-duplication-translocation syndromes are a frequent cause of global developmental delay/mental retardation–intellectual disability equivalent in their occurrence to Down syndrome. The subtelomeric regions are 'gene-rich' genomic regions in which DNA copy number changes (CNC) or genomic variants can be detected by a panel of subtelomeric fluorescence *in situ* hybridization (FISH) probes or by comparative genomic hybridization (CGH) microarrays (Sherr and Shevell 2006). Detection rates in the setting of moderate–severe mental retardation/intellectual disability and dysmorphology approach 10% (Wilkie 1993), while in the absence of appreciable dysmorphology diagnostic yield is 1% or less (Xu and Chen 2003). A plethora of subtelomeric CNC syndromes have been reported in the literature, and shared clinical recognizable phenotypes have been delineated (e.g. 1p36, 15q26, 22q13) through careful observation. Given ongoing advances in FISH and CGH technologies, one can expect an increase in the delineation of such syndromes in the near to intermediate future.

THERAPIES AND INTERVENTIONS

All children with chromosomal syndromes and their associated neurodevelopmental abnormalities benefit from the services of an interdisciplinary health care team. Educational, psychological, speech and language, occupational, and physical therapists, as well as social workers and other medical specialists need to be identified early for successful implementation of interventions and therapy plans. At the time of initial diagnosis of an individual, the immediate family, and possibly extended family members, should be offered genetic counseling by a certified genetic counselor or medical geneticist. Local national and international parent networks and support groups are often an invaluable resource for care providers as well as for families. The internet has facilitated these opportunities.

Beyond medical management of associated health problems, behavioral problems in many of these children require the additional efforts of an occupational therapist, early childhood educator, behavioral psychologist, or psychiatrist from an early age. Caregivers should be taught to recognize escalating behavioral problems, use positive reinforcement and calming techniques, master transition techniques, and avoid overstimulation. Behavioral issues should be addressed based on intellectual age and developmental level rather than chronologic age. Medications used acutely or chronically can often be helpful for many of these situations. Of particular interest are the SSRIs, which can be helpful in decreasing aggression and anxiety. Although SSRIs are primarily used as antidepressants in the general population, they are used more frequently for decreasing aggression, obsessive-compulsive behaviors, and anxiety in the neurodevelopmentally disabled population. Often mood stabilization is also desired and can be obtained from an atypical antipsychotic such as risperidone.

Seizures occur with increased frequency in most chromosomal or gene syndromes and usually begin in childhood. These are usually treated with standard antiepileptic drugs (AED) at normal doses. However, because some AED (carbamazepine and valproic acid) also have a beneficial effect on abnormal behaviors, consideration might be given to their use over other AED medications if other benefits–risks are equal.

Transition to adulthood may be problematic because of difficulty attaining social and financial independence from caregivers. Appropriate vocational training, apprenticeships in sheltered workshops, and committed adult supervisors help smooth the transition. Continued medical follow-up is necessary to monitor for associated medical conditions which are unique to each chromosomal or gene syndrome and to monitor medication treatments. It is important to provide early, consistent, and individualized reproductive health education to this population. Counseling on the issues of socially appropriate behavior, safety, and informed sexual choices is often a professionally daunting task which is frequently not approached with the same vigor as dealing with the medical complications of these disorders.

Alternative therapies need to be addressed. Even in the face of dissent from their long-time trusted health care provider, promised 'cures' and anecdotal evidence from the proponents of various alternative therapies drive caregivers to try these treatments. While the least that can happen is wasted time and money, more serious consequences may arise. A non-judgmental objective approach should be maintained in all discussions about the appropriateness of any therapies. Health care providers should be prepared to discuss the safety and efficacy of various proferred treatments.

There are many therapies available that have little rigorous scientific evidence to support their use. Some of these more popular treatments include:

'Nutritional' therapy (e.g. megavitamins, supplements/trace minerals, low-gluten, Feingold diet), antifungal therapy, hyperbaric oxygen, patterning, EEG biofeedback and selected drugs such as piracetam for Down syndrome, etc

There is no clear evidence that these or many other therapies benefit any child. Any future harm that may be produced has rarely been investigated. In an era when new advances in medical therapy seem like miracles, the primary care provider and other members of the health care team need to stay abreast of the latest medical information. Health care providers need to be prepared to provide accurate information to affected individuals and their families regarding both old and new proposed therapies.

CONCLUSIONS

Chromosomal and gene mutation syndromes are complex chronic conditions. Understanding the impact they can have on children, families, schools, and communities is important and necessary. Every affected individual should be given a chance to reach his/her maximum potential. Successes need to be celebrated. Many people with these conditions have learned to accentuate their talents and have become successful independent adults. Health care providers should strive to provide this opportunity to every affected individual.

REFERENCES

Bear MF (2005) Therapeutic implications of the mGluR theory of fragile X mental retardation. *Genes Brain Behav* 4: 393–398.

Bi W, Saifi GM, Shaw CJ, Walz K, Fonseca P, Wilson M, et al. (2004) Mutations in RAI1, a PHD-containing protein, in nondeletion patients with Smith–Magenis syndrome. *Hum Genet* 115: 515–524.

Boucher CA, Sargent CA, Ogata T, Affara NA (2001) Breakpoint analysis of Turner patients with partial Xp deletions: implications for the lymphoedema gene location. *J Med Genet* 38: 591–598.

Chapman RS (1997) Language development in children and adolescents with Down syndrome. *Ment Retard Dev Disabil Res Rev* 3: 307–312.

Clement-Jones M, Schiller S, Rao E, Blaschke RJ, Suniga A, Zeller R, et al. (2000) The short stature homeobox gene SHOX is involved in skeletal abnormalities in Turner syndrome. *Hum Mol Genet* 9: 695–702.

Cornish K, Sudhalter V, Turk J (2004) Attention and language in fragile X. *Ment Retard Dev Disabil Res Rev* 10: 11–16.

Cunniff C, Frias JL, Kaye C, Moeschler JB, Panny SR, Trotter TL (2001) Health supervision for children with Down syndrome. *Pediatrics* 107: 442–449.

Delabar J-M, Theophile D, Rahman Z, Chettouh Z, Blouin J-L, Prieur M, et al. (1993) Molecular mapping of twenty-four features of Down syndrome on chromosome 21. *Eur J Hum Genet* 1: 114–124.

De Leersnyder H, de Blois MC, Vekemans M, Sidi D, Villain E, Kindermans C, et al. (2001) Beta (1)-adrenergic antagonists improve sleep and behavioral disturbances in a circadian disorder, Smith–Magenis syndrome. *J Med Genet* 38: 586–590.

Elsheikh M, Dunger DB, Conway GS, Wass JAH (2002) Turner's syndrome in adulthood. *Endocr Rev* 23: 120–140.

Finucane B, Dirrigl KH, Simon EW (2001) Characterization of self-injurious behaviors in children and adults with Smith–Magenis syndrome. *Am J Ment Retard* 106: 52–58.

Finucane BM, Konar D, Haas-Givler B, Kurtz MB, Scott CI Jr (1994) The spasmodic upper-body squeeze: a characteristic behavior in Smith–Magenis syndrome. *Dev Med Child Neurol* 36: 78–83.

Ford CE, Jones KW, Polani PE, de Almeida JC, Briggs JH (1959) A sex-chromosome anomaly in a case of gonadal dysgenesis (Turner's syndrome). *Lancet* 1: 711–713.

Gantois I, Kooy RF (2002) Targeting fragile X. *Genome Biol* 3; 1014.1–1014.5.

Gardner RJM, Sutherland GR (2004) Normal parents with a chromosomally abnormal child. In: *Chromosome Abnormalities and Genetic Counseling, 3rd edn.* New York: Oxford University Press, p 258.

Graham JM Jr, Bashir AS, Stark RE, Silbert A, Walzer S (1988) Oral and written language abilities of XXY boys: implications for anticipatory guidance. *Pediatrics* 81: 795–806.

Greenberg F, Lewis RA, Potocki L, Glaze D, Parke J, Killian J, et al. (1996) Multi-disciplinary clinical study of Smith–Magenis syndrome (deletion 17p11.2). *Am J Med Genet* 62: 247–254.

Greenberg F, Smith ACM, Richter S, Magenis E, Guzzetta V, Patel PI, et al. (1990) Smith–Magenis syndrome (deletion 17p11.2) as a new contiguous gene deletion syndrome (abstract). *Am J Hum Genet* 47 (Suppl): A59.

Hagerman RJ (2005) Fragile X syndrome. In: Cassidy SB, Allanson JE (eds) *Management of Genetic Syndromes, 2nd edn.* Hoboken, New Jersey: Wiley-Liss, pp 251–263.

Hagerman RJ, Hagerman PJ (eds) (2002) *Fragile X syndrome.* Baltimore: Johns Hopkins University Press.

Harper PS (1998) Endocrine and reproductive disorders. In: *Practical Genetic Counseling, 5th edn.* Boston: Butterworth-Heinemann, p 273.

Hessl D, Rivera SM, Reiss AL (2004) The neuroanatomy and neuroendocrinology of fragile X syndrome. *Ment Retard Dev Disabil Res Rev* 10: 17–24.

Hines, S, Bennett F (1996) Effectiveness of early intervention for children with Down syndrome. *Ment Retard Dev Disabil Res Rev* 2: 96–101.

Holtzman D (1997) Alzheimer disease and Down syndrome. *Cytogenet Cell Genet* 77: 17 (Official presentations) (suppl 1).

Holtzman DM, Epstein CJ, Mobley WC (1996) The human trisomy 21 brain: insights from mouse models of Down syndrome. *Ment Retard Dev Disabil Res Rev* 2: 66–72.

Hubert RS, Mitchell S, Chen X-N, Ekemekji K, Gadomski C, Sun Z, et al. (1997) BAC and PAC contigs covering 3.5 Mb of the Down syndrome congenital heart disease region between D21S55 and MX1 on chromosome 21. *Genomics* 41: 218–226.

Hunter AGW (2005) Down syndrome. In: Cassidy SB, Allanson JE (eds) *Management of Genetic Syndromes, 2nd edn.* Hoboken, New Jersey: Wiley-Liss, pp 191–210.

Klinefelter HF, Reifenstein EC, Albright F (1942) Syndrome characterized by gynecomastia, aspermatogenesis without A-Leydigism, and increased excretion of follicle stimulating hormone. *J Clin Endocrinol* 2: 615–627.

Korenberg JR, Bradley C, Disteche CM (1992) Down syndrome: molecular mapping of the congenital heart disease and duodenal stenosis. *Am J Hum Genet* 50: 294–302.

Korenberg JR, Chen X-N, Schipper R, Sun Z, Gonsky R, Gerwehr S, et al. (1994) Down syndrome phenotypes: the consequences of chromosomal imbalance. *Proc Natl Acad Sci U S A* 91: 4997–5001.

Kosho T, Muroya K, Nagai T, Fujimoto M, Yokoya S, Sakamoto H, et al. (1999) Skeletal features and growth patterns in 14 patients with haploinsufficiency of SHOX: implications for the development of Turner syndrome. *J Clin Endocrinol Metab* 84: 4613–4621.

Kumin L (1996) Speech and language skills in children with Down syndrome. *Ment Retard Dev Disabil Res Rev* 2: 109–115.

Lanfranco F, Kamischke A, Zitzmann M, Nieschlag E (2004) Klinefelter's syndrome. *Lancet* 364: 273–283.

Laws G, Bishop DVM (2004) Verbal deficits in Down's syndrome and specific language impairment: a comparison. *Int J Lang Commun Disord* 39: 423–451.

Loesch DZ, Huggins RM, Hagerman RJ (2004) Phenotypic variation and FMRP levels in fragile X. *Ment Retard Dev Disabil Res Rev* 10: 31–41.

Mazzocco MMM (2001) Math learning disability and math LD subtypes: evidence from studies of Turner syndrome, Fragile X syndrome, and neurofibromatosis type 1. *J Learn Disabil* 34: 520–533.

McBrien DM (2003) Disorders of mental development: Down syndrome. In Wolraich ML (ed) *Disorders of Development and Learning, 3rd edn.* Hamilton, Ontario: BC Decker, pp 207–223.

McCauley E, Feuilan P, Kushner H, Ross JL (2001) Psychosocial development in adolescents with Turner syndrome. *J Dev Behav Pediatr* 22: 360–365.

Money J (1993) Specific neurocognitional impairments associated with Turner (45,X) and Klinefelter (47,XXY) syndromes: a review. *Soc Biol* 40: 147–151.

Nussbaum RL, McInnes RR, Willard HF (2004) *Thompson and Thompson Genetics in Medicine, 6th edn, Revised Reprint.* Philadelphia, Pennsylvania: Saunders.

O'Connor J, Fitzgerald M, Hoey H (2000) The relationship between karyotype and cognitive functioning in Turner syndrome. *Ir J Psychol Med* 17: 82–85.

O'Doherty A, Ruf S, Mulligan C, Hildreth V, Errington ML, Cooke S, et al. (2005) An aneuploid mouse strain carrying human chromosome 21 with Down syndrome phenotypes. *Science* 39: 2033–2037.

Oostra BA, Willemsen R (2003) A fragile balance: FMR1 expression levels. *Hum Mol Genet* 12: R249–R257.

Pandey UB, Phadke SR, Mittal B (2004) Molecular diagnosis and genetic counseling for fragile X mental retardation. *Neurol India* 52: 36–42.

Ratcliffe S (1999) Long-term outcome in children of sex chromosome abnormalities. *Arch Dis Child* 80: 192–195.

Rattazzi MC, LaFauci G, Brown WT (2004) Prospects for gene therapy in the fragile X syndrome. *Ment Retard Dev Disabil Res Rev* 10: 75–81.

Rittey CD (2003) Learning difficulties: what the neurologist needs to know. *J Neurol Neurosurg Psychiatry* 74: 30–36.

Ross JL, McCauley E, Roeltgen D, Long L, Kushner H, Feuillan P, et al. (1996) Self-concept and behavior in adolescent girls with Turner syndrome: potential estrogen effects. *J Clin Endocrinol Metab* 81: 926–931.

Ross JL, Roeltgen D, Kushner H, Wei F, Zinn AR (2000a) The Turner syndrome-associated neurocognitive phenotype maps to distal XP. *Am J Hum Genet* 67: 672–681.

Ross JL, Stefanatos G, Roeltgen D, Kushner H, Cutler GB Jr (1995) Ullrich–Turner syndrome: neurodevelopmental changes from childhood through adolescence. *Am J Med Genet* 58: 74–82.

Ross J, Zinn A, McCauley E. (2000b) Neurodevelopmental and psychosocial aspects of Turner syndrome. *Ment Retard Dev Disabil Res Rev* 6: 135–141.

Rourke BP, Ahmad SA, Collins DW, Hayman-Abello BA, Hayman-Abello SE, Warriner EM (2002) Child clinical/pediatric neuropsychology: some recent advances. *Annu Rev Psychol* 53: 309–339.

Saenger P, Albertsson Wiklnad K, Conway GS, Davenport M, Gravholt CH, Hintz R, et al. (2001) Recommendations for the diagnosis and management of Turner syndrome. *J Clin Endocrinol Metab* 86: 3061–3069.

Satgé D, Sommelet D, Geneix A, Nishi M, Malet P, Vekemans M (1998) A tumor profile in Down syndrome. *Am J Med Genet* 78: 207–216.

Shelley BP, Robertson MM (2005) The neuropsychiatry and multisystem features of the Smith–Magenis syndrome: a review. *J Neuropsychiatry Clin Neurosci* 17: 91–97.

Sherr EH, Shevell MI (2006) Mental retardation and global developmental delay. In: Swaiman KF, Ashwal S, Ferreiro DM (eds) *Pediatric Neurology: Principles & Practice, 4th edn.* Philadelphia: Mosby Elsevier, pp 799–820.

Simpson JL, Graham JM, Samango-Sprouse C, Swerdloff R (2005) Klinefelter syndrome. In: Cassidy SB, Allanson JE (eds) *Management of Genetic Syndromes, 2nd edn.* Hoboken, New Jersey: Wiley-Liss, pp 323–333.

Slager RE, Newton TL, Vlangos CN, Finucane B, Elsea SH (2003) Mutations in RAI1 associated with Smith–Magenis syndrome. *Nat Genet* 33: 466–468.

Smith ACM, Gropman AL (2005) Smith–Magenis Syndrome. In: Cassidy SB, Allanson JE (eds) *Management of Genetic Syndromes, 2nd edn.* Hoboken, New Jersey: Wiley-Liss, pp 507–525.

Smith ACM, McGavran L, Waldstein G (1982) Deletion of the 17 short arm in two patients with facial clefts. *Am J Hum Genet* 34 (Suppl): A410.

Stratton RF, Dobyns WB, Greenberg F, DeSana JB, Moore C, Fidone G, et al. (1986) Interstitial deletion of (17)(p11.2p11.2): report of six additional patients with a new chromosome deletion syndrome. *Am J Med Genet* 24: 421–432.

Stray-Gundersen K (ed) (1995) *Babies with Down Syndrome: A New Parent's Guide.* Bethesda, Maryland: Woodbine House.

Sybert VP (2005) Turner Syndrome. In: Cassidy SB, Allanson JE (eds) *Management of Genetic Syndromes, 2nd edn.* Hoboken, New Jersey: Wiley-Liss, pp 589–605.

Sybert VP, McCauley E (2004) Turner's syndrome. *N Engl J Med* 351: 1227–1238.

Terracciano A, Chiurazzi P, Neri G (2005) Fragile X syndrome. *Am J Med Genet* 137C: 32–37.

Turner G, Webb T, Wake S, Robinson H (1996) Prevalence of fragile X syndrome. *Am J Med Genet* 64: 196–197.

Turner HH (1938) A syndrome of infantilism, congenital webbed neck, and cubitus valgus. *Endocrinology* 23: 566–574.

Tyler C, Edman J (2004) Down syndrome, Turner syndrome, and Klinefelter syndrome: primary care throughout the life span. *Prim Care* 31: 627–648.

Venail F, Gardiner Q, Mondain M (2004) ENT and speech disorders in children with Down's syndrome: an overview of pathophysiology, clinical features, treatments, and current management. *Clin Pediatr* 43: 783–791.

Visootsak J, Aylstock M, Graham JM Jr (2001) Klinefelter syndrome and its variants: an update and review for the primary pediatrician. *Clin Pediatr* 40: 639–651.

Visootsak J, Warren ST, Anido A, Graham JM (2005) FragileX Syndrome: an update and review for the primary pediatrician. *Clin Pediatr* 44: 371–381.

Wilkie AO (1993) Detection of cryptic chromosomal abnormalities in unexplained mental retardation: a general strategy using hypervariable sub-telomeric DNA polymoprhisms.; *Am J Hum Genet* 53: 688.

Xu J, Chen Z (2003) Advances in molecular cytogenetics for the evaluation of mental retardation. *Am J Med Genet* 117C: 15.

Zigman W, Silverman W, Wisniewski HM (1996) Aging and Alzheimer's disease in Down syndrome: clinical and pathological changes. *Ment Retard Dev Disabil Res Rev* 2: 73–79.

15

INBORN ERRORS OF METABOLISM AND DEVELOPMENTAL DELAY

Myriam Srour and Michael Shevell

The number of metabolic conditions that cause neurodevelopmental disabilities is vast and each cannot be discussed individually because of space limitations. Rather, this chapter starts with an introductory section that discusses the features common to all metabolic disorders, followed by a general approach section, which outlines when to clinically suspect a metabolic disorder and the essential steps to take if a metabolic disorder is indeed suspected. Selected conditions in each category are then discussed as a general illustration of the most important general principles.

Metabolic disorders can be defined as a group of conditions in which there is a deficiency in production, synthesis, metabolism, storage, or transport of biochemical compounds. They can be the cause of developmental delay in 1–5% of children (Curry et al. 1997). Individually, these disorders are rare; however, collectively they constitute a large burden of morbidity and mortality. It is extremely important to identify these disorders because specific treatment may be available or acute metabolic decompensation can be avoided. In addition, prognosis and appropriate genetic counseling can be offered to the parents for whom additional pregnancies may impose a significant recurrent risk of devastating illness. Metabolic disorders pose a considerable challenge to clinicians in that they may only be faced with a small number of cases throughout their career. Additionally, each individual disorder can have a variety of different clinical presentations which may include common clinical symptomatology encountered in primary care practice.

The mechanisms by which disorders of metabolism cause disease are numerous; however, the biochemical mechanisms of brain dysfunction and resultant intellectual disability are generally poorly understood. Recent progress in understanding the mechanisms of disease in some of these disorders has provided insight into potential specific therapeutic options. However, given the small number of cases and the heterogeneity of disease severity and presentation, therapeutic trials are very difficult to carry out. Many of the therapeutic options described in this chapter have been reported only in small uncontrolled case series.

Metabolic disorders may be classified into three major groups:

1 Intoxication disorders
2 Energy production disorders
3 Storage disorders

Intoxication disorders are characterized by a symptom-free interval of variable length, which is followed by signs of either acute intoxication (i.e. vomiting, lethargy, coma, and liver failure) or chronic intoxication (i.e. progressive developmental delay, ectopia lentis, cardiomyopathy). In these disorders, an inborn error of metabolism leads to an acute or chronic accumulation of toxic compounds proximal to the metabolic block. Examples of these disorders include the aminoacidopathies (e.g. maple syrup urine disease, phenylketonuria), most organic acidemias (e.g. methymalonic acidemia, propionic acidemia), congenital urea cycle defects (e.g. ornithine transcarbamylase deficiency), and sugar intolerances (e.g. galactosemia).

Energy production disorders are caused by a deficiency in either energy production (e.g. mitochondrial disorders, disorders of carbohydrate metabolism, fatty acid oxidation disorders) or energy utilization (e.g. creatine deficiency). Symptoms tend to be multisystemic, including tissues of different embryonic origin, and developmental delay may be accompanied by hypoglycemia, hyperlacticacidemia, myopathy, and cardiomyopathy.

Storage disorders involve the abnormal synthesis or degradation of complex molecules. These include all lysosomal disorders, peroxisomal disorders, and inborn errors of cholesterol synthesis. Symptoms are progressive, permanent, and independent of food intake. Hepatosplenomegaly, white matter abnormalities, and skeletal deformities are common.

This chapter does not intend to address issues of diagnosis. Rather, it attempts to review the mechanisms by which the metabolic disorders cause developmental delay, the natural history of cognition in these disorders, and the interventions that are available that can alter or impact on cognition.

GENERAL APPROACH
When evaluating a child with developmental delay, there are several clues on history (i.e. red flags) that should prompt the search for a possible underlying metabolic disorder:

1 A history of parental consanguinity, an affected sibling or unexplained loss of a previous child – most metabolic disorders are autosomal recessive in inheritance
2 Developmental regression and the loss of previously acquired skills
3 A history of episodic bouts of acute distress such as lethargy, ataxia, or vomiting, especially in the context of an intercurrent catabolic state

4 Early refractory neonatal seizures – this may suggest biotin deficiency, pyridoxine deficiency, or a glucose transporter defect
5 Myoclonic seizures – this may suggest neuronal ceroid lipofuscinosis, sialidosis, and some of the mitochondrial disorders

On examination, there are also several findings that could suggest an underlying metabolic disorder: macrocephaly (i.e. leukodystrophies [Canavan and Alexander disease], glutaric aciduria type 1 and Tay–Sachs disease) and dysmorphic features (i.e. a long face and broad forehead in Zellweger syndrome or coarse features in the mucopolysaccharidoses), or ophthalmologic findings (cherry red spot in Tay–Sachs, GM1 gangliosidosis and Gaucher). Hepatosplenomegaly is a hallmark of storage disorders. Extrapyramidal movement abnormalities are typical of disorders affecting the basal ganglia such as Wilson disease, pantothenate kinase-associated neurodegeneration, and propionic aciduria.

The laboratory evaluation of a child with a suspected inborn error of metabolism can potentially be excessively extensive, and it is important to limit investigations to those that will be sufficiently high yield, yet the threshold for testing must be sufficiently low to avoid missing a potentially treatable case or one with an associated high familial recurrence risk. Thus, the clinician can expect a large number of negative evaluations. Most children with an inborn error of metabolism have findings other than isolated developmental delay on either history (e.g. failure to thrive, developmental regression, episodic decompensation, movement disorder, seizures) or physical examination (e.g. hepatosplenomegaly, coarse facial features). Routine non-selective screening for inborn errors of metabolism in children with developmental delay has a yield of about 1%. When suggestive clinical features are present, the yield may increase to 5–14%. A recent American Academy of Neurology practice parameter has suggested that routine metabolic testing is not indicated in the evaluation of isolated developmental delay provided that universal newborn infant screening was performed (Shevell et al. 2003).

If a metabolic disorder is suspected, core investigations include the determination of acid–base balance, glucose, ammonia, liver function, lactate, very-long-chain fatty acids (VLCFA), serum amino acid profile, urine organic acid profile, and ketones. Neuroimaging is extremely useful to identify white matter and basal ganglia abnormalities. Additional investigations should be obtained as clinical signs or symptoms suggest and include specific enzymatic and molecular analysis and electromyogram and nerve conduction studies when there is suspicion of peripheral involvement or white matter changes centrally (Fig. 15.1).

DISORDERS OF AMINO ACID AND ORGANIC ACID METABOLISM
Disorders of amino acid and organic acid metabolism are generally characterized by a toxic accumulation of a metabolite proximal to the block. An affected

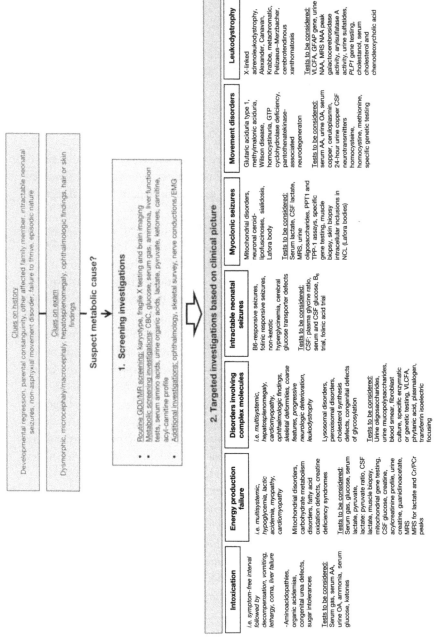

Fig. 15.1 Approach algorithm to inborn errors of metabolism causing neurodevelopmental delay. AA, aminoacids; MRS, magnetic resonance spectroscopy; NAA, N-acetyl aspartic acid; OA, organic acids; PPT1, palmitoyl protein thioesterase 1; TPP-1, tripeptidyl peptidase 1; VLCFA, very-long-chain fatty acids.

newborn infant is usually healthy at birth and for the first few days of life, and then develops an acute toxic encephalopathy with progression if unrecognized to coma. Early recognition and diagnosis improves outcome. Acidopathies can also present in older children and adolescents with progressive symptoms such as the loss of intellectual function and ataxia, or intermittently with coma related to an inter-current catabolic state. The most prominent amino acidopathies are phenylketonuria and maple syrup urine disease. The most prominent organic acidopathies are pro-prionic acidemia and methylmalonic acidemia.

Phenylketonuria

Phenylketonuria (PKU) is the best-known disorder of amino acid metabolism and was one of the first metabolic diseases to be characterized. Classic PKU results from the impaired activity of phenylalanine (PHE) hydroxylase, which converts phenylalanine to tyrosine. Hyperphenylalaninemia can also result from defects in tetrahydrofolate (BH_4) the co-cofactor of PHE hydroxylase. PKU is an autosomal recessive condition. There have been more than 400 mutations identified in the PHE hydroxylase PAH on chromosome 12q22-24.1 and most patients are compound heterozygotes, resulting in substantial phenotypic variability. Clinically, patients may present acutely in the neonatal period with an 'intoxication-type' picture charac-terized by vomiting, lethargy, and coma. If untreated, progressive symptoms such as mental retardation, microcephaly, seizures, and abnormal movements develop.

The precise mechanisms of neuronal damage are unclear, although several fac-tors are thought to have a role. Accumulation of PHE may have a direct neurotoxic effect. Magnetic resonance spectroscopy (MRS) has shown a correlation between PHE concentration and clinical outcome (Moller et al. 2003). High PHE also impairs the transport of other substances such as tyrosine and tryptophan, which may fur-ther contribute to neurotoxicity. Neuroimaging shows evidence of white matter abnor-malities, even in patients with good PHE control (Anderson et al. 2007). Myelin degradation is likely related to inhibition of oligodendrocyte-specific sulfurylase with resultant low myelin sulfatide content (Dyer et al. 1996). Additionally, recent studies have suggested that myelin formation is impaired because of reduced cholesterol synthesis (Hargreaves 2007).

Therapy of PKU involves adherence to a strict diet that is low in PHE. Early and prompt institution of the diet leads to dramatic improvement of outcome (Waisbren et al. 2007). Screening programs of newborn infants were instituted in the early 1960s with very favorable results. Because the developing brain is most vulnerable to high PHE levels, good control during childhood is most important for preventing long-term IQ loss. However, current recommendations emphasize that some form of dietary therapy should continue throughout life, because relaxa-tion of dietary restraints in school-aged children results in some loss of intelli-gence. Moreover, even with optimal treatment, there may be subtle deficits in higher cortical function (Leuzzi et al. 2004). Neuropsychologic testing demonstrates slightly higher IQ in non-affected siblings and parents (Diamond et al. 1997). Women with PKU must adhere to a strict diet before conception and throughout pregnancy to prevent devastating damage to the fetus. Unrecognized and untreated maternal PKU can result in microcephaly, severe mental retardation, and congenital heart defects in the child (Lenke and Levy 1980).

MAPLE SYRUP URINE DISEASE

Maple syrup urine disease (MSUD) is caused by the deficiency of the mitochondrial branched-chain-keto acid dehydrogenase complex which metabolizes the three branched amino acids: leucine, isoleucine, and valine. Leucine may be the most toxic of the three metabolites. As with PKU, the clinical presentation of classic MSUD is typically that of an acute intoxication, with a normal initial neonatal period (4–5 days) followed by decompensation with vomiting, lethargy, and coma. Hypertonic episodes with opisthotonus, 'boxing' and 'pedaling' movements, or slow limb elevation is often observed.

MSUD is a white-matter disease. Spongy changes in the white matter are seen on histology, and a reduction in myelin lipids (cerebrosides, proteolipids, and sulfatides) is observed. Astrocytes seem to be more sensitive to branched chain amino acids than neurons.

The disease is named for the classic burnt sugar or maple syrup odor of the urine. The diagnosis is based upon identifying abnormal metabolites, and the presence of alloleucine is diagnostic of MSUD. Enzymatic studies in cultured fibroblasts or peripheral leukocytes confirm the diagnosis.

If left untreated, MSUD results in diffuse brain edema after 1 week of age, followed by more localized edema of the deep cerebellar white matter, dorsal brainstem, cerebral peduncles, and dorsal limb of the internal capsule. Neurotoxicity may be prevented by rapid diagnosis and treatment. Acute treatment consists of rapid removal of toxic metabolites by hemodialysis or peritoneal dialysis, and the reversal of the catabolic state with total parenteral nutrition. Prevention of recurrent episodes of decompensation by dietary restriction is critical. Affected patients usually survive, but generally with significant developmental delay. However, there are patients with normal intelligence. Intellectual outcome is inversely related to the duration of metabolite elevation, and patients in whom treatment is initiated after 14 days of age rarely achieve normal intelligence (de Ogier and Saudubray 2002).

PROPIONIC ACIDEMIA

Deficiency of propionyl-CoA carboxylase, a mitochondrial biotin-dependent enzyme, results in a high level of propionate and its by-products including propionyl-carnitine, 3-hydroxypropionate, and methylcitrate. Accumulation of propionyl-CoA also results in carnitine deficiency and the synthesis of abnormal fatty acids. Patients usually present with non-specific signs in the neonatal period such as vomiting, dehydration, lethargy, and coma. Upon initial presentation, metabolic acidosis with an increased anion gap and ketonuria is seen, and hyperammonemia is always present. The clinical course is characterized by repeated relapses, usually precipitated by intercurrent infection, fever, or high protein intake. Other than developmental delay, seizures are often seen. The presence of pyramidal signs and movement disorders such as dystonia and chorea in a patient with developmental delay should prompt consideration of this underlying diagnosis.

There does not seem to be a clear correlation between enzymatic activity and clinical phenotype and there is no satisfactory explanation for why some patients have a severe life-threatening course whereas others have only mild developmental delay (Deodato et al. 2006). Differences in protein uptake, the potential contribution of gut bacteria, and activity of alternate propionate disposal mechanisms only partially explain phenotypic variability.

Treatment of acute attacks of ketosis involves the withdrawal of dietary protein, administration of sodium bicarbonate, and aggressive removal of toxin by dialysis (de Ogier and Saudubray 2002). A low-protein diet (total protein 0.5–1.5g/kg/day) or a diet selectively reduced in the content of propionate precursors such as valine appears to be the most effective treatment. Treatment helps minimize the frequency of attacks of ketosis but developmental delay still occurs. Carnitine therapy prevents carnitine depletion and helps eliminate propionic acid by formation and excretion of propionyl carnitine. Recognition of the potential contribution of gut bacteria to propionate production has led to the suggestion of chronic antimicrobial therapy. Metronidazole decreases serum and urine levels of propionate, but this is not accompanied by a definitive improvement in objective outcome (Deodato et al. 2006).

METHYMALONIC ACIDEMIA

The clinical presentation of methylmalonic acidemia is non-specific, and again is typified by an 'intoxication-type' profile. The most common form of isolated methylmalonic acidemia, the infantile/non-vitamin B_{12}-responsive form, has a catastrophic acute neonatal presentation. Investigations show severe metabolic acidosis, ketosis and ketonuria, hyperammonemia, hyperglycinemia, thrombocytopenia, and neutropenia. A less severe form, the vitamin B_{12}-responsive phenotype, occurs in the first months or years of life. Clinical signs include feeding problems, failure to thrive, hypotonia, developmental delay, and vomiting and lethargy after protein intake. In contrast to propionic acidemia, enzyme activity in this disorder correlates with clinical severity (Ledley and Rosenblatt 1997). Treatment involves dietary restriction of methylmalonic acid precursors. Also, vitamin B_{12} (cobalamin) should be given as soon as this diagnosis is suspected, as it may be beneficial even in patients with the 'vitamin B_{12} unresponsive' subtype. Carnitine and metronidazole may be used as therapeutic adjuncts with a similar rationale to that described above for propionic acidemia.

DISORDERS OF CARBOHYDRATE METABOLISM

GALACTOSEMIA

Classic galactosemia, a rare inborn error of carbohydrate metabolism, is caused by galactose-1-phosphate uridyltransferase deficiency and results in defective conversion of galactose to glucose. Galactose-1-phosphate and its metabolites such as galactitol then accumulate within cells. Galactosemia usually presents in the newborn infant fed with breast milk or a lactose-containing infant formula. Vomiting, lethargy, and signs of hepatic insufficiency are typical presenting features. Less frequently, patients may have a more chronic course with persistent poor feeding, failure to thrive, and developmental delay. Cataracts are usually seen on presentation.

Classic galactosemia is autosomal recessive and the responsible gene, *GALT*, has been localized on chromosome 9p13. Genetic heterogeneity resulting in residual galactose-1-phosphate uridyltransferase activity and environmental factors related to galactose intake are thought to be responsible for the observed phenotypic variability (Ng et al. 1994). Imaging and postpartum pathology demonstrate diffuse white matter abnormalities. Somatosensory evoked potentials are slowed. Animal studies suggest that the early increase in intracranial pressure is brought about by increased osmolality caused by high brain galactitol concentrations and concomitant alterations in glucose, adenosine triphosphate, and phosphocreatine levels. In addition, accumulated galactose and its metabolites, especially galactitol, are clearly neurotoxic (Ridel et al. 2005).

Treatment consists of withdrawal of galactose-containing formulas in the acute neonatal period and strict avoidance of galactose-containing foods. Dietary therapy helps reduce cataracts, liver failure, and sepsis, but even adequately treated patients show evidence of developmental delay. Several studies have documented a reduced IQ (mean 70–90), which does not appear to correlate to time of diagnosis, initiation of therapy, or compliance (Ridel et al. 2005). Speech delay and dyspraxia are observed in approximately 90%. A subgroup of patients develop ataxia and tremor later in their disease, which does not seem to be related to any neuroimaging findings or level of IQ. Ovarian failure is frequently seen in affected females (Bosch 2006).

UREA CYCLE DISORDERS

Inborn errors of urea synthesis are characterized by the triad of hyperammonemia, encephalopathy, and respiratory alkalosis. With the exception of arginase, patients with a complete absence of any urea cycle enzyme generally present in the newborn period with hyperammonemic coma, which, despite aggressive therapy, carries a 50% mortality. Studies of children rescued from hyperammonemic coma have shown a significant risk of mental retardation and other developmental disabilities, and neonates who remain in stage III coma for longer than 72 hours invariably have mental retardation. There is an inverse linear relationship between the duration of hyperammonemic coma and IQ. Siblings of affected patients who are treated prospectively from birth have IQs in the low normal or borderline range (Gropman and Batshaw 2004, Bachmann 2005).

Ammonia is a well-recognized neurotoxin; however, the precise mechanism of its toxicity is unclear. There may be distinct mechanisms for the effects of acute high ammonia levels and those of chronic mildly elevated levels. Acute increases in ammonia increase blood–brain barrier permeability, deplete intermediates of cell metabolism, and promote disaggregation of microtubules, whereas chronic mildly elevated levels may alter axonal development and brain amino acid and neurotransmitter levels (Cagnon and Braissant 2007). Animal studies suggest that hyperammonemia induces glutamine accumulation in astrocytes, which results in an osmotic water shift and astrocytic swelling. Indeed, pathologic examination of edematous brains reveals astrocytic swelling with normal neurons, axons, and dendrites. Finally, high glutamine levels may cause altered metabolism of neurotransmitters (Cagnon and Braissant 2007). For instance, altered serotonin metabolism has been suggested as a possible mechanism for some of the unusual behaviors (i.e. anorexia and sleeping disorders) observed in urea cycle disorders. It has been difficult to differentiate the effects of hyperammonemia from those of the hypoxia-ischemia and increased intracranial pressure that invariably accompany hyperammonemic coma (Batshaw 1984).

ORNITHINE TRANSCARBAMYLASE DEFICIENCY
Ornithine transcarbamylase deficiency is the most common urea cycle defect. This enzyme catalyzes the conversion of ornithine and carbamoyl phosphate to citrulline. Carbamoyl phosphate is necessary for the removal of ammonia from the circulation, and so its deficiency leads to hyperammonemia. It is an X-linked disorder (*OTC* gene). Males present in the neonatal period with acute hyperammonemic coma which may be lethal without treatment.

The phenotype of heterozygous female patients is very heterogeneous because of allelic heterogeneity and variable X chromosome inactivation (i.e. lyonization). Classically, approximately 85% of heterozygous females are considered to be asymptomatic, with the remaining 15% experiencing late onset symptoms (Maestri et al. 1998). These late onset symptoms are episodic, usually related to high protein loads or catabolic states, and include cyclic vomiting, headaches, lethargy, hyperventilation, ataxia, and hypotonia. Many female patients spontaneously adopt a vegetarian diet because of their natural aversion to protein. Recent studies have suggested that 'asymptomatic heterozygous females,' defined as women not demonstrating protein aversion or having episodes of hyperammonemia, show evidence of subtle cognitive deficits on detailed testing. Full scale IQ scores in these females were lower than their non-carrier sisters, with the main difference being in verbal rather than performance IQ. There is also evidence that these individuals have deficits in attention and executive functions (Gropman and Batshaw 2004).

Treatment consists of restriction of protein intake with supplemental arginine and the promotion of nitrogen removal with sodium benzoate and phenylbutarate administration. Acute hyperammonemia is treated urgently with hemodialysis. There have been reports of successful orthotopic liver transplantation with positive outcomes.

DISORDERS OF MUCOPOLYSACCHARIDE METABOLISM

The mucopolysaccharidoses (MPS) are a heterogeneous group of lysosomal storage disorders, each caused by a deficiency of an enzyme involved in the degradation of glucosaminoglycan molecules, also known as the muccopolysaccharides. The resultant accumulation of glycosaminoglycans in lysosomes causes cell dysfunction. There are 11 known enzyme deficiencies, which result in seven distinct types of MPS. All of these disorders are autosomal recessive except for MPS II (i.e. Hunter syndrome) which is X-linked. Clinically, these disorders are characterized by a multisystem involvement resulting in dysmorphic facies, organomegaly, and dysostosis multiplex. The severity of developmental delay is variable. Some MPS, such as mild forms of MPS I (Scheie syndrome), MPS IV (Morquio syndrome A and B), and MPS VI (Maroteaux–Lamy syndrome) are not known to be associated with developmental delay.

MPSI, also known as Hurler Syndrome, is the most severe of the MPS. It is a progressive multisystemic disorder that results in death in early childhood. Children appear normal at birth and diagnosis is usually made between 4 and 18 months. Facial features become progressively coarser. Various skeletal deformities, hepatosplenomegaly, and an enlarged tongue develop. Developmental delay usually appears between 12 and 24 months. Most children will only acquire limited language, because of a combination of their developmental delay, progressive hearing loss, and enlarged tongue. Other clinical features include corneal clouding, glaucoma, obstructive airway disease, and hydrocephalus secondary to a defective reabsorption of cerebrospinal fluid.

Therapy for the MPS relies on the observation that enzyme replacement is possible in cell cultures derived from MPS affected tissues. It has been estimated that only 1–2% of residual enzyme activity is needed to correct metabolic defects and alter phenotypic expression (Muenzer 2004). The currently available therapies consist of either replacing the deficient enzyme directly through the parenteral route or indirectly via hematopoietic stem cell transplantation (HSCT). A major difficulty with direct enzyme replacement therapy is that, despite high intravenous dosage, enzymes cannot effectively cross the blood–brain barrier. This effectively limits possible benefits to the central nervous system (CNS). Enzyme replacement therapy has been used for only the most severe types of MPS. HSCT relies on the observation that normal cells introduced into the patient release a small amount of the deficient enzyme into the extracellular space, which can then be taken up by the adjacent deficient cells. The new bone marrow may also produce macrophages which can clear stored material from tissues including the CNS. More than 200 children with MPS I have received HSCT (Muenzer 2004). Transplantation before the age of 24 months seems to prevent CNS involvement and reduce organomegaly. However, eye and skeletal abnormalities are not substantially improved. HSCT carries high complication rates as a result of acquired chronic immunosuppression, with a 15–20% risk of mortality.

LEUKODYSTROPHIES
The leukodystrophies form a group of diseases in which a genetically determined metabolic defect results in progressive destruction or failed development of the myelin of the CNS. Lysosomal and peroxisomal disorders are the main causes. The characteristic clinical picture is that of an initially healthy child who develops progressive neurologic deterioration with developmental delay and signs of spasticity (Table 15.1).

Metachromatic Leukodystrophy
Metachromatic leukodystrophy (MLD) arises from the deficiency of the lysosomal enzyme arylsulfatase A which results in accumulation of the sphingolipid galactosylsulfatide. This membrane lipid is found in various tissues such as the kidney and bile ducts, but particularly in the myelin of the nervous system. The accumulation of sphingolipid affects predominantly the oligodendrocytes.

Three clinical variants have been described according to age of onset: (1) late infantile, (2) juvenile, and (3) adult MLD. Late infantile MLD, the most frequent form, usually begins between the ages of 18 and 24 months. Patients develop ataxia, spastic quadriplegia, and optic atrophy. Juvenile MLD presents between the ages of 4 and 16 years, and the adult onset form presents after 16 years of age. In the juvenile and adult onset forms, psychiatric symptoms are often predominant.

The arylsulfatase gene A gene is located on chromosome 22, and over 80 different disease-causing mutations have been described. In general, severity of symptoms is related to residual enzyme activity. Homozygosity for null alleles results in zero enzyme activity and the late infantile form. Heterozygozity for a null allele or a mutation that allows some residual enzyme activity gives rise to the juvenile form. Adult forms are generally caused by mutations that allow residual enzyme activity in both alleles. Of interest, approximately 2% of the healthy population has a substantial arylsylfatase A deficiency due to a polymorphism which causes reduction of enzyme activity to only 5–10% of normal. This is termed 'pseudo-deficiency' and does not result in any evident overt clinical or metabolic abnormalities.

Currently, there is no efficient treatment available for MLD. Like MPS I, MLD is a disorder for which enzyme replacement is theoretically possible. Animal models have explored the possibility of this approach. Transduction of bone marrow with

TABLE 15.1
Selected leukodystrophies

	Age of onset	Inheritance	Defect	Main clinical features
X-linked adrenoleukodystrophy	4–10 years	X-linked	Peroxisomal membrane protein (ALDP) deficiency	Progressive impairment of cognition, vision, hearing and motor function addisonian features elevated VLCFA posterior WM changes on CT/MRI
Alexander	6 months	AD	Glial fibrillary acidic protein (GFAP) defect	Macrocephaly, seizures, spasticity, cystic white matter changes on neuroimaging, astrocytic Rosenthal fibers
Canavan	3–6 months	AR	Aspartoacylase deficiency (aminoacidopathy)	Macrocephaly, initial hypotonia then spasticity, seizures, increased NAA (urine and MRS), spongiform changes on MRI
Globoid cell leukodystrophy (Krabbe)	3–8 months	AR	Lysososmal galactosecerebrosidase deficiency	Irritability, spasticity, optic atrophy
Metachromatic leukodystrophy (late infantile form)	18–24 months	AR	Lysosomal arylsulfatase-A deficiency	Ataxia, spasticity, optic atrophy
Pelizaeus–Merzbacher	Neonatal	X-linked	Proteolipid protein 1 defect	Nystagmus, spasticity Diffusely abnormal myelin on MRI

AD, autosomal dominant; ALDP, adrenoleukodystrophy protein; AR, autosomal recessive; CT, computed tomography; MRI, magnetic resonance imaging; MRS, magnetic resonance spectroscopy; NAA, N-acetyl aspartic acid; VLCFA, very-long-chain fatty acid; WM, white matter.

a retroviral vector containing arylsulfatase A into arylsulfatase A-deficient mice successfully induced sustained expression of the enzyme in many tissues, including the brain. However, reduction of storage material was observed only in the kidney and liver, and no effect was seen on the brain (Matzner et al. 2000). Behavioral studies in treated animals did not show any benefit (Gieselmann 2003). The axonal diameter in the optic nerve and peripheral nerves which is reduced in enzyme-deficient animals is normalized with treatment, suggesting some potential therapeutic effect in the peripheral nervous system. A few cases of successful bone marrow transplantation have been reported although controlled studies have not been performed (Gorg et al. 2007).

GLOBOID CELL LEUKODYSTROPHY (KRABBE DISEASE)

Globoid cell leukodystrophy is caused by mutations in the *GALC* gene, which encodes the lysosomal enzyme galactosylceramide which degrades galactosylceremide and psychosine (galactosylsphingosine) to ceramide and galactose. The disease is characterized by progressive demyelination of the central and peripheral nervous systems. Microscopic examination of white matter demonstrates multinucleated globoid cells, near-total loss of myelin and oligodendroglia, and astrocytic gliosis. Globoid cells are macrophages that contain undigested galactosylceramide.

The great majority of patients present with severe symptoms during the first 6 months of life, but later onset forms such as juvenile and adult have also been described. Individuals with the infantile form seem healthy at birth and during the first few months of life, but then develop irritability, spasticity, and developmental delay by the age of 6 months. The peripheral nervous system is invariably involved. Patients rarely survive their second year of life. The clinical course is heterogeneous, even among individuals with the same genotype. There does not seem to be any consistent correlation between the age of onset and the residual GALC enzyme activity in leukocytes or cultured skin fibroblasts (Suzuki 2003).

In patients with advanced symptoms, there is no specific treatment besides supportive care. Individuals who are identified prior to the onset of clinical symptoms may undergo HSCT. A recent study showed that HSCT in asymptomatic newborn infants slowed the development of neurologic symptoms in a 3-year follow-up, whereas transplantation in symptomatic individuals did not significantly affect eventual neurologic outcome (Escolar et al. 2005, Boelens 2006).

X-LINKED ADRENOLEUKODYSTROPHY

X-linked adrenoleukodystrophy (X-ALD) is a peroxisomal disorder characterized by accumulation of VLCFA in the nervous system, adrenal cortex, and testes. It is caused by mutations in the *ABCD1* gene, located on chromosome Xq28, which encodes a peroxisomal membrane protein ADLP (adrenoleukodystrophy protein). The mechanism by which ADLP deficiency causes accumulation of VLCFA is still unknown.

X-ALD has two distinct forms. Adrenomyeloneuronopathy is a non-inflammatory axonopathy, which is mostly observed in adults and heterozygous female carriers and presents as a slowly progressive paraparesis. Depression or emotional disturbances are common in this setting and becomes more severe with advanced disease. The second form is an inflammatory cerebral myelinopathy and is seen almost exclusively in boys. Between the ages of 4 and 8 years, affected boys develop progressive impairment of cognition, behavior, vision, hearing, and motor function and usually become totally disabled within 2 years. The two forms often co-occur in the same family.

Recent evidence suggests that the inflammatory cerebral myelinopathy form results from the destructive autoimmune response to VLCFA-containing lipids, mediated by CD1 molecules, and CD8 cytotoxic T cells (Moser et al. 2007). There is a strong correlation between VLCFA levels and inflammatory cytokines. Treatment of X-ALD includes mandatory adrenal hormone replacement therapy for all patients with adrenal insufficiency. It is now generally accepted that bone marrow transplantation can provide long-term stabilization and occasionally reverse symptoms in the early stages of inflammatory brain disease (Shapiro et al. 2000). Lorenzo oil is a 4:1 mixture of glyceryl trioleate and glyceryl trierucate which normalizes the levels of VLCFA in the plasma of affected individuals. Lorenzo oil therapy in symptomatic boys has been disappointing, but a recent study involving asymptomatic boys less than 6 years old treated with Lorenzo oil suggests that it may reduce the probability of developing future signs (Moser et al. 2005).

DISORDERS OF TRACE METAL METABOLISM
WILSON DISEASE
Wilson disease is an autosomal recessive disorder of copper metabolism resulting in accumulation of copper in many organs and tissues. The hallmarks of the disease are liver dysfunction, neurologic symptoms, and Kayser–Fleischer corneal rings. Presentation is either with hepatic or neurologic symptoms. Initial symptoms may be very subtle, with mild tremor, speech or writing problems that are frequently diagnosed as attention-deficit–hyperactivity disorder or behavioral problems. The characteristic neurologic symptoms are those of a progressive movement disorder with dysarthria, dystonia, chorea, and, less commonly, parkinsonian. One-third of patients have psychiatric symptoms at presentation such as depression, disorganization of personality, or even overt psychosis.

The pathogenesis of liver disease is a direct result of copper accumulation in hepatocytes. Accumulated copper initially leads to mitochondrial damage, then the release of copper from necrotic hepatocytes results in oxidative stress, inflammation, and fibrogenesis. The pathogenesis of the neurologic symptoms is less clear. Copper does not accumulate in the neurons, rather it accumulates in the extracellular space and where it is believed to be a major source of free-radical production.

There is no single test for the diagnosis of Wilson disease. The diagnosis is based on typical clinical findings and laboratory anomalies (low ceruloplasmin, increased 24-hour urinary copper excretion, and high free serum copper) and can be made without further tests if two of the following findings are present: Kayser–Fleischer rings on ocular slit lamp examination, typical neurologic symptoms, and low ceruloplasmin levels. There are characteristic changes in the basal ganglia on neuroimaging. Ceruloplasmin levels are normal in 10% of cases, so proper exclusion of the diagnosis if suspected clinically requires the analysis of 24-hour urinary copper excretion.

Wilson disease results from mutations in the *ATP7B* gene, which encodes a transmembrane copper transporter that has a key role in incorporating copper into ceruloplasmin and in moving copper out of the hepatocyte and into bile. Molecular genetic testing of the *ATP7B* gene is clinically available, but the mutation detection rate varies depending on the test method and the individual's ethnicity. Complete gene sequencing detects mutations in about 98% of individuals with Wilson disease. Genetic analysis is not required for confirmation if the diagnosis can be established with the biochemical and imaging measures described above.

Wilson disease is a treatable condition, and reversal of symptoms is possible. The optimal treatment for Wilson disease is controversial. The American Association for the Study of Liver Diseases practice guidelines on Wilson disease state that initial treatment for symptomatic patients should include a chelating agent (e.g. penicillamine or trientine) which increases urinary excretion of copper. Treatment of presymptomatic patients or maintenance therapy should be accomplished with either a chelating agent or zinc. Zinc interferes with intestinal copper absorption by sharing the same carrier as copper in the enterocytes and by inducing metallothionein, an intracellular metal ligand. Penicillamine can result in an exacerbation of neurologic deficits in over 10% of individuals, and this is not always reversible. This has led to suggestions that zinc therapy alone, or therapy with tetrathiomolybdate, may be the treatment of choice in persons with only mild neurologic symptoms (Ala et al. 2007).

MITOCHONDRIAL DISORDERS
Mitochondria are the descendants of aerobic bacteria that colonized eukaryotic cells and endowed their host with aerobic metabolism. Mitochondria generate energy as adenosine triphosphate (ATP) via the electron transport chain and oxidative phosphorylation (respiratory chain). They perform other numerous tasks such as the metabolism of pyruvate, amino acids, fatty acids, and steroids.

Mitochondrial disorders are clinically diverse and are caused by either structural or functional abnormalities in the mitochondrial respiratory chain, which can arise from mutations in either the nuclear or mitochondrial DNA. These disorders have a higher prevalence than commonly believed, with estimates of 10–15 cases per 100 000 persons, which is similar to many better known neurologic diseases. Mitochondrial proteins are mainly encoded by genes located in the nuclear genome, however, 13 proteins and 24 tRNAs are encoded by mitochondrial DNA (mtDNA) (Anderson et al. 1981). The genetics of the disorders that arise from mutations in mtDNA are distinct from Mendelian genetics in several ways.

Inheritance is maternal, because all mitochondria and mtDNA in the zygote are derived from the ovum. Because mtDNA molecules are present in multiple copies (polyplasmy) in each cell and pathogenic mutations usually only affect a variable proportion of these (heteroplasmy), there exists a 'threshold' effect where a critical proportion of mtDNA must be abnormal to translate into overt clinical disease and a phenotype of interest. Heteroplasmy and the 'threshold' effect also exist at the organelle level because each mitochondrion harbors a dozen copies of mtDNA.

The pathogenesis of mitochondrial diseases involves a progressive decline in mitochondrial ATP-generating capacities, leading to energy failure and cell death in affected tissues. Mitochondrial dysfunction can affect virtually all tissues and thus the disease is most often multisystemic. However, high-energy requiring tissues such as the brain, heart, and skeletal muscle are preferentially involved.

It has become apparent that there is not a straightforward relationship between the site of mitochondrial mutations and the associated clinical phenotype. Mutations in the same gene can give rise to different symptom complexes and conversely mutations in different genes can give rise to the same clinical syndrome. For example, the A to G mutation at nucleotide 3243 of mtDNA encoding for tRNA Leu (UUR) can result in Leigh syndrome, lactic acidosis, mitochondrial encephalopathy with stroke-like episodes (MELAS), or diabetes and deafness. The great variability in clinical presentations is largely attributed to heteroplasmy and the 'threshold' effect. The main recognizable syndromes of mtDNA are summarized in Table 15.2.

Common clinical features of mitochondrial disease include ptosis, external ophthalmoplegia, proximal myopathy, pigmentary retinopathy, and diabetes mellitus. Fluctuating encephalopathy, seizures (usually myoclonic in type), migraines, and ataxia are other frequent neurologic symptoms. A mitochondrial disorder should be suspected in cases where there is progressive multisystemic involvement, especially with cardiomyopathy, diabetes, deafness, and ophthalmoplegia. Maternal inheritance of neurologic symptoms should also raise suspicion, although it is important to highlight again that many mitochondrial disorders are caused by nuclear DNA mutations and may follow a Mendelian inheritance pattern.

If the clinical picture is highly suggestive of one of the classic mitochondrial syndromes, then blood should be sent for molecular genetic analysis. Other important investigations include lactate and pyruvate in the serum and cerebrospinal fluid, plasma ketone bodies, acylcarnitine, urinary organic acid analysis, neuroimaging, and muscle biopsy. Elevated lactate with a high lactate:pyruvate ratio (>20) and positive ketone body levels are highly suggestive of a respiratory chain deficiency. In cases of Leigh syndrome or MELAS, neuroimaging may show characteristic cerebral lesions; however, in most mitochondrial disorders neuroimaging is nonspecific and may reveal cerebral atrophy with involvement of deep gray nuclei and white matter diffusely (Barkovich et al. 1993). On MRS, increases in the

TABLE 15.2
Clinical features of selected mitochondrial DNA syndromes

Kearns–Sayre–Shy syndrome
Progressive external ophthalmoplegia before age 20 years
Pigmentary retinopathy
Cerebellar ataxia
High CSF protein
Heart block

Leber hereditary optic neuropathy (LHON)
Subacute painless bilateral visual loss
Male:female 4:1

Leigh syndrome
Infantile onset
Subacute relapsing encephalopathy
Cerebellar and brainstem signs

MERRF (myoclonic epilepsy with ragged red fibers)
Progressive myoclonic epilepsy
Myopathy/ataxia
Lactic acidosis, ragged red fibers

MELAS (mitochondrial encephalopathy with lactic acidosis and stroke-like episodes)
Stroke-like episodes before age 40 years
Seizures, headaches
Ragged red fibers, lactic acidosis

NARP (neurogenic weakness with ataxia and retinitis pigmentosa)
Developmental delay, neuropathy, ataxia
Retinitis pigmentosa

---

lactate peak may be observed. Muscle biopsy may show ragged red fibers on modified Gomori stain and the absence of specific staining for succinate dehydrogenase and cytochrome oxidase. It is important to point out that normal results in any of the above tests, including the muscle biopsy, do not necessarily definitively exclude the diagnosis of a mitochondrial disorder.

The management of mitochondrial disease is primarily supportive. It includes early diagnosis and treatment of diabetes mellitus, cardiac pacing if necessary, and correction of ptosis. A variety of vitamins and co-factors have been used but clinical evidence supporting their use is lacking. Food supplements such as co-enzyme Q_{10} are well tolerated and some patients report a subjective benefit. Patients with complex I and II deficiency may benefit from oral riboflavin supplementation (vitamin B_2) (DiMauro and Mancuso 2007).

CREATINE DEFICIENCY SYNDROMES

The creatine deficiency syndromes have only been identified in the past decade. They share the common feature of absence of the creatine/phosphocreatine peak on brain MRS. Creatine and phosphocreatine are essential for normal brain function and have an important role in energy storage and transmission. Deficiencies of two key enzymes involved in creatine metabolism, L-arginine:glycine guanidinoacetate methyltransferase (GAMT), amidinotransferase (AGAT), and creatine transformer (SLCA6A8) defects can cause creatine deficiency syndromes.

The clinical presentation is heterogeneous. Most patients attract medical attention between the ages of 6 and 24 months for developmental delay. Language skills seem particularly affected.

GAMT deficiency is an autosomal recessive disorder that results in accumulation of guanidinoacetic acid (GAA), the precursor to creatine. Toxicity is likely caused by a combination of creatine deficiency and GAA toxicity. Severely affected individuals have extrapyramidal symptoms, while mildly affected individuals may only have mild developmental delay. Autistic features and seizures can be present. Diagnosis is based on an absent Creatine/Phosphocreatine peak on cerebral MRS and elevated GAA creatine and creatine in urine and plasma. Confirmation of diagnosis can be achieved through determination of GAMT activity in liver, fibroblasts, or lymphoblasts. Pharmacologic doses of oral creatine have resulted in a partial increase of brain creatine and a reduction of GAA, although levels remain significantly abnormal. There have been some reports of a partial clinical benefit with creatine supplementation, although all patients still lacked expressive language. The clinical course may reflect brain creatine levels with an initial improvement followed by a plateau in function.

Creatine transporter deficiency is an X-linked disorder. Serum and urine creatine levels are normal or elevated. The characteristic clinical feature is speech delay. Additional features include mild mental retardation and seizures. Unfortunately, oral supplementation of creatine does not result in apparent clinical improvement (Schulze 2003).

Only a handful of individuals with AGAT deficiency have been described. These individuals developed intellectual disability and severe language delay. Oral supplementation with creatine resulted in complete replenishment of creatine in the brain as measured by MRS with a rapid improvement of visual and fine motor skills and a mild improvement in verbal abilities (Schulze 2003).

CONCLUSIONS

While inborn errors of metabolism are individually rare, collectively they are an important cause of developmental delay. Their diagnosis carries a significant impact on the patient and the family. The clinician should be aware of several red flags that should trigger metabolic investigations: developmental regression, progressive neurologic deterioration, episodic neurologic symptoms, a family history of similarly affected individual, parental consanguinity, and the presence of specific dysmorphisms. Although the number of potential investigations can seem overwhelming, initial evaluation of acid–base balance, glucose, ammonia, liver function, lactate, pyruvate, serum amino acid profile, urine organic acid profile, ketones, cartinitine, acyl profile and neuroimaging will recognize – at least in a preliminary way – the majority of cases. Accurate diagnosis can allow prognostication, genetic counseling, and, in some cases, specific treatment that modifies eventual outcome.

REFERENCES

Ala A, Walker AP, Ashkan K, Dooley JS, Schilsky ML (2007) Wilson's disease. *Lancet* 369: 397–408.

Anderson S, Bankier AT, Barrell BG, et al. (1981) Sequence and organisation of the human mitochondrial genome. *Nature* 1981;290:457–65.

Anderson PJ, Wood SJ, Francis DE, Coleman L, Anderson V, Boneh A (2007) Are neuropsychological impairments in children with early-treated phenylketonuria (PKU) related to white matter abnormalities or elevated phenylalanine levels? *Dev Neuropsychol* 32: 645–668.

Bachmann C (2005) Long-term outcome of urea cycle disorders. *Acta Gastroenterol Belg* 68: 466–468.

Barkovich AJ, Good WV, Koch TK, Berg BO (1993) Mitochondrial disorders: analysis of their clinical and imaging characteristics. *Am J Neuroradiol* 14: 1119–1137.

Batshaw ML (1984) Hyperammonemia. *Curr Probl Pediatr* 14: 1–69.

Boelens JJ (2006) Trends in haematopoietic cell transplantation for inborn errors of metabolism. *J Inherit Metab Dis* 29: 413–420.

Bosch AM (2006) Classical galactosaemia revisited. *J Inherit Metab Dis* 29: 516–525.

Cagnon L, Braissant O (2007) Hyperammonemia-induced toxicity for the developing central nervous system. *Brain Res Rev* 56: 183–197.

Curry CJ, Stevenson RE, Aughton D, Byrne J, Carey JC, Cassidy S, et al. (1997) Evaluation of mental retardation: Recommendations of a Consensus Conference: American College of Medical Genetics. *Am J Med Genet* 72: 468–477.

de Ogier BH, Saudubray JM (2002) Branched-chain organic acidurias. *Semin Neonatol* 7: 65–74.

Deodato F, Boenzi S, Santorelli FM, Dionisi-Vici C (2006) Methylmalonic and propionic aciduria. *Am J Med Genet* C142: 104–112.

Diamond A, Prevor MB, Callender G, Druin DP (1997) Prefrontal cortex cognitive deficits in children treated early and continuously for PKU. *Monogr Soc Res Child Dev* 62: 1–208.

DiMauro S, Mancuso M (2007) Mitochondrial diseases: therapeutic approaches. *Biosci Rep* 27: 125–137.

Dyer CA, Kendler A, Philibotte T, Gardiner P, Cruz J, Levy HL (1996) Evidence for central nervous system glial cell plasticity in phenylketonuria. *J Neuropathol Exp Neurol* 55: 795–814.

Escolar ML, Poe MD, Provenzale JM, Richards KC, Allison J, Wood S, et al. (2005) Transplantation of umbilical-cord blood in babies with infantile Krabbe's disease. *N Engl J Med* 352: 2069–2081.

Gieselmann V (2003) Metachromatic leukodystrophy: recent research developments. *J Child Neurol* 18: 591–594.

Görg M, Wilck W, Granitzny B, Suerken A, Lukacs Z, Ding X, et al. (2007) Stabilization of juvenile metachromatic leukodystrophy after bone marrow transplantation: a 13-year follow-up. *J Child Neurol* 22: 1139–1142.

Gropman AL, Batshaw ML (2004) Cognitive outcome in urea cycle disorders. *Mol Genet Metab* 81 (Suppl 1): S58–S62.

Hargreaves IP (2007) Coenzyme Q10 in phenylketonuria and mevalonic aciduria. *Mitochondrion* (Suppl 7): S175–S180.

Ledley FD, Rosenblatt DS (1997) Mutations in mut methylmalonic acidemia: clinical and enzymatic correlations. *Hum Mutat* 9: 1–6.

Leuzzi V, Pansini M, Sechi E, Chiarotti F, Carducci C, Levi G, et al. (2004) Executive function impairment in early-treated PKU subjects with normal mental development. *J Inherit Metab Dis* 27: 115–125.

Lenke RR and Levy HL. 1980. Maternal phenylketonuria and hyperphenylalanemia: An international survey of the outcome of untreated and treated pregnancies. *NEJM* 303(21): 1202–1208.

Maestri NE, Lord C, Glynn M, Bale A, Brusilow SW (1998) The phenotype of ostensibly healthy women who are carriers for ornithine transcarbamylase deficiency. *Medicine (Baltimore)* 77: 389–397.

Matzner U, Habetha M, Gieselmann V (2000) Retrovirally expressed human arylsulfatase A corrects the metabolic defect of arylsulfatase A-deficient mouse cells. *Gene Ther* 7: 805–812.

Moller HE, Weglage J, Bick U, Wiedermann D, Feldmann R, Ullrich K (2003) Brain imaging and proton magnetic resonance spectroscopy in patients with phenylketonuria. *Pediatrics* 112: 1580–1583.

Moser HW, Mahmood A, Raymond GV (2007) X-linked adrenoleukodystrophy. *Nat Clin Pract Neurol* 3: 140–151.

Moser HW, Raymond GV, Lu SE, Muenz LR, Moser AB, Xu J, et al. (2005) Follow-up of 89 asymptomatic patients with adrenoleukodystrophy treated with Lorenzo's oil. *Arch Neurol* 62: 1073–1080.

Muenzer J (2004) The mucopolysaccharidoses: a heterogeneous group of disorders with variable pediatric presentations. *J Pediatr* 144: S27–S34.

Ng WG, Xu YK, Kaufman FR, Donnell GN, Wolff J, Allen RJ, et al. (1994) Biochemical and molecular studies of 132 patients with galactosemia. *Hum Genet* 94: 359–363.

Ridel KR, Leslie ND, Gilbert DL (2005) An updated review of the long-term neurological effects of galactosemia. *Pediatr Neurol* 33: 153–161.

Schulze A (2003) Creatine deficiency syndromes. *Mol Cell Biochem* 244: 143–150.

Shapiro E, Krivit W, Lockman L, Jambaqué I, Peters C, Cowan M, et al. (2000) Long-term effect of bone-marrow transplantation for childhood-onset cerebral X-linked adrenoleukodystrophy. *Lancet* 356: 713–718.

Shevell M, Ashwal S, Donley D, Flint J, Gingold M, Hirtz D, et al. (2003) Practice parameter: evaluation of the child with global developmental delay: report of the Quality Standards Subcommittee of the American Academy of Neurology and the Practice Committee of the Child Neurology Society. *Neurology* 60: 367–380.

Suzuki K (2003) Globoid cell leukodystrophy (Krabbe's disease): update. *J Child Neurol* 18: 595–603.

Waisbren SE, Noel K, Fahrbach K, Cella C, Frame D, Dorenbaum A, et al. (2007) Phenylalanine blood levels and clinical outcomes in phenylketonuria: a systematic literature review and meta-analysis. *Mol Genet Metab* 92: 63–70.

16

THE CEREBELLUM AND DEVELOPMENT

Catherine Limperopoulos and Adré du Plessis

Over the past decade, there has been increasing evidence supporting the complex hierarchy of genetic and cellular processes of cerebellar development in the embryonic and fetal brain. Furthermore, recent technologic and conceptual break-throughs have resulted in an improved diagnostic capability giving rise to new insights into cerebellar anomalies and cerebellar injury in the newborn infant which has led to a formal reassessment of the functional role of the cerebellum in higher order functions. Notably, our evolving understanding of the cerebellum under normal and pathologic conditions has opened a new and exciting area in contemporary pediatric neuroscience. In this chapter we provide an overview of normal cerebellar development and describe the unique susceptibility of the brain for acquired cerebellar injury in the preterm and term windows of development. Novel clinical and neuroimaging evidence describing the relationship between the cerebellum and non-motor behaviors and cognitive operations are presented and the neurodevelopmental consequences of early life cerebellar injury are summarized.

NORMAL DEVELOPMENT OF THE CEREBELLUM

Embryologically, the cerebellum is one of the first brain structures to begin development at around 4 weeks' gestation shortly after neural tube closure and perhaps paradoxically it is one of the last to reach its mature configuration. Broadly speaking, the cerebellum develops through four stages (ten Donkelaar et al. 2003). First, the cerebellar territory at the midbrain–hindbrain boundary becomes delineated. Next, two compartments for cell proliferation arise from primary and secondary neuroepithelium. From the primary neuroepithelium adjacent to the fourth ventricle, cells migrate in two directions (Fig. 16.1). Dorsal migration (8–13 weeks' gestation) leads to formation of the deep cerebellar nuclei and Purkinje cell layer. Dorsolateral migration forms the lateral rhombic lips from which tangential migration along the subpial surface of the developing cerebellum at 6–12 weeks' gestation, leads to formation of a secondary neuroepithelium, the external granular layer. This surface layer of the developing cerebellum is a site of vigorous neuronal proliferation.

The third stage, which continues well into the first postnatal year, is characterized by an inward migration of granule cells from the external granular layer

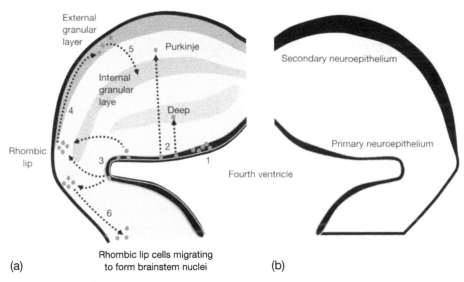

Fig. 16.1 (a) Developmental stages of cerebellar development: (1) cellular proliferation in primary neuroepithelium; (2) dorsal migration to form deep nuclei and Purkinje layer; (3) dorsolateral migration to rhombic lips; (4) tangential subpial migration to form external granular layer; (5) inward migration across Purkinje layer to form internal granular layer; (6) ventral migration to form pontine and inferior olivary nuclei. (b) Primary and secondary neuroepithelial layers forming vascular germinal matrices.

across the Purkinje layer leading to formation of the internal granular layer. Finally, the burst of proliferation in the pre-migratory cells of the external granular layer triggers the onset of cerebellar foliation, a process that continues postnatally and is completed by 7 months of age. Migration, proliferation, and arborization of the cerebellar neurons are complete by 20 months of postnatal life. This protracted development of the cerebellum renders it particularly vulnerable to a variety of developmental and acquired insults capable of derailing its normal maturational program. This review focuses specifically on acquired forms of injury during this extended period of cerebellar development.

PATHOGENESIS OF VASCULAR INJURY IN THE IMMATURE CEREBELLUM

Cerebellar hemorrhagic injury is increasingly recognized as an important lesion of the immature brain. The exact pathogenesis of cerebellar hemorrhagic injury is unclear, but is likely multifactorial, and likely includes birth trauma, preterm birth, and other factors. Furthermore, the origin and causes of cerebellar injury in the term infant are different from those in the preterm infant.

    In the term infant, cerebellar hemorrhagic injury is frequently associated with traumatic delivery such as breech presentation and prolonged labor with extensive cranial molding (Serfontein et al. 1980, Bulas et al. 1991, Huang and Lui 1995, Miall et al. 2003). Cerebellar hemorrhagic injury associated with breech or traumatic delivery and/or instrumentation is believed to be a result of severe distortion and disruption of the venous structures within the compliant neonatal skull, leading to laceration of the tentorium or falx cerebri or a traumatic cerebellar laceration along the vermis. Cerebellar hemorrhagic injury may also result from increases in venous pressure, as seen in infants on extracorporeal membrane oxygenation or earlier techniques of facemask ventilation (Serfontein et al. 1980, Miall et al. 2003). Cerebellar hemorrhagic injury in infants presenting with brainstem compression, sudden shock, and disseminated intravascular coagulation has also been described (Martin et al. 1976, Chadduck et al. 1995, Merrill et al. 1998).

In the preterm infant, previous studies suggested that cerebellar hemorrhagic injury often occured concomitantly with a supratentorial hemorrhage, and was associated with high mortality (Perlman et al. 1983, Mercuri et al. 1997). A more recently described pattern of cerebellar hemorrhagic injury in preterm infants (<1500g) may remain clinically 'silent' and is not necessarily associated with significant supratentorial bleeding (Merrill et al. 1998).

The etiology of cerebellar hemorrhagic injury in the preterm infant is likely similar to the more frequently recognized germinal matrix hemorrhage adjacent to the lateral ventricle of the immature cerebral hemisphere (Fig. 16.2). The fragile and friable nature of these transient germinal matrices makes them particularly vulnerable to ischemic or asphyxial injury. Cerebellar hemorrhagic injury may occur within the germinal matrix located in the subependymal layer of the roof of the fourth ventricle and within the subpial external granular cell layer. Subpial germinal matrix bleeding may be the source of intrahemispheric cerebellar hemorrhagic injury identified along the outer periphery of the cerebellum (Rakic and Sidman

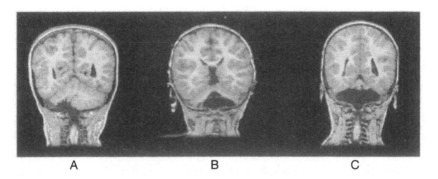

Fig. 16.2 Coronal T1-weighted magnetic resonance image of patients showing (A) right unilateral inferior cerebellar hemispheric injury; (B) bilateral inferomedial cerebellar injury; (C) extensive bilateral near-completed injury of the cerebellum.

1970, Pape et al. 1976, Merrill et al. 1998, Baumeister and Hofer 2000, Volpe 2001). Thus, cerebellar hemorrhagic injury, like the periventricular germinal matrix hemorrhages, may result from narrow range or failure of cerebral autoregulation and unstable cerebral blood flow in these fragile vascular structures (du Plessis and Volpe 2002). In addition to the effects of the initial injury, subsequent injury to the highly mitotic cerebellar precursor cells exposed to extravasated blood may further disrupt subsequent cerebellar development.

Another mechanism proposed for cerebellar injury in the preterm infant is vaso-occlusive injury in the inferior cerebellar artery distribution resulting in extensive bilateral injury to the lower cerebellar hemispheres and a 'pancake-like' appearance at follow-up (Johnsen et al. 2002, 2005). It is noteworthy that recent studies have demonstrated an important relationship between cerebellar lesions identified early in preterm life and subsequent impairment of unilateral or bilateral cerebellar growth and development (Limperopoulos et al. 2005b, 2005c, Srinivasan et al. 2006). The potential role of undetected early gestation cerebellar injury in the pathogenesis of subsequent cerebellar 'hypoplasia/aplasia' has been proposed by several investigators (Boltshauser 2004, Messerschmidt et al. 2005).

INCIDENCE OF VASCULAR INJURY IN THE IMMATURE CEREBELLUM

The exact incidence of cerebellar injury in the preterm and term born infant is unknown. In fact until recently, cerebellar hemorrhagic injury had been considered a rare condition in the neonatal period (Scotti et al. 1981, Reeder et al. 1982). Previous clinical studies estimated the incidence of cerebellar hemorrhagic injury in combined preterm and term populations at 2.5–3.6% (Reeder et al. 1982, Menezes et al. 1983, Von Gontard et al. 1988, Mercuri et al. 1997, Merrill et al. 1998). Conversely, existing neuropathologic evidence suggests that cerebellar hemorrhagic injury is more prevalent than clinically appreciated at present and is estimated to occur in 15–25% (Grunnet and Shields 1976, Donat et al. 1979) of low birth weight infants (<1500g). Recent clinical studies have corroborated these neuro-pathologic data indicating that very low birth weight infants have a particular predilection for cerebellar hemorrhagic injury (Johnsen et al. 2002, 2005, Limperopoulos et al. 2005a, Messerschmidt et al. 2005) with up to 19% of infants born under 750g developing ultrasound evidence of this injury (Limperopoulos et al. 2005a). These reports have highlighted that cerebellar hemorrhagic injury is an important but under-recognized complication of extreme preterm birth and has been under-appreciated in surviving preterm infants. Predictors of cere-bellar hemorrhagic injury include such factors as combined prenatal, intrapar-tum, and early postnatal cardiorespiratory derangements suggesting a higher degree of fetal–neonatal illness preceding the actual injury (Limperopoulos et al. 2005a).

ADVANCES IN NEUROIMAGING TECHNIQUES

The increasing availability of more sophisticated neuroimaging techniques has greatly enhanced the frequency, accuracy, and timing with which cerebellar injury is diagnosed in the newborn (Mercuri et al. 1997, Merrill et al. 1998, Miall et al. 2003, Limperopoulos et al. 2005b).

CRANIAL ULTRASOUND

Identification of cerebellar hemorrhagic injury by conventional ultrasound through the anterior fontanelle has been limited because of the highly echogenic tentorium and cerebellar vermis (Serfontein et al. 1980, Reeder et al. 1982, Di Salvo 2001). Recent use of the acoustic window provided by the mastoid fontanelle has vastly improved visualization of the posterior fossa (Baumeister and Hofer 2000, Di Salvo 2001, Correa et al. 2004). Consequently, the use of this mastoid window approach has increased the detection of acute cerebellar hemorrhagic injury at the incubator in the neonatal intensive care unit and is becoming part of the routine neonatal ultrasound protocol in many centers (Di Salvo 2001, Correa et al. 2004, Limperopoulos et al. 2005a).

MAGNETIC RESONANCE IMAGING

The widespread availability of magnetic resonance imaging (MRI) has also facilitated early and more accurate diagnosis of cerebellar injury in the newborn (Miall et al. 2003, Limperopoulos et al. 2005b). The successful application of sophisticated MRI techniques, such as 3D volumetric MRI and diffusion tensor imaging, offers the opportunity to evaluate the brain from complementary integrated perspectives to include volume and microstructure (Inder et al. 2004, Huppi and Dubois 2006). Specifically, the ability to make quantitative measurements of gray and white matter volumes in the preterm infant over the third post-conceptional trimester has advanced our understanding of normal and abnormal cerebral cortical development and myelination (Huppi and Dubois 2006). Quantitative MRI studies in preterm infants have demonstrated dramatic increases in brain growth (and its tissue subclasses) and microstructural organization of the brain after preterm birth (Huppi et al. 1998, Huppi and Dubois 2006). It has been proposed that this phase of rapid growth leaves the brain particularly vulnerable to injury and to subsequent impaired growth and microstructural developmental aberration. Recent quantitative MRI studies of the developing immature cerebellum are summarized below.

CEREBELLAR HEMORRHAGIC INJURY IN THE HIGH-RISK INFANT

To date, neuroimaging studies in preterm infants have focused largely on supratentorial injuries such as periventricular leukomalacia and intraventricular hemorrhage. However, the improved neuroimaging techniques described above, as well as the increased survival of very low birth weight infants, have allowed the delineation of different patterns of abnormal cerebellar development in ex-preterm infants following cerebellar hemorrhagic injury.

An extensive and symmetric form of cerebellar injury invariably associated with pontine hypoplasia and supratentorial parenchymal injury has been described (Martin et al. 1976, Johnsen et al. 2002, 2005, Messerschmidt et al. 2005). A broader spectrum of cerebellar injury was described in a recent retrospective 5-year case–control study (Limperopoulos et al. 2005a). In this study, 35 preterm infants with a cranial ultrasound diagnosis of cerebellar hemorrhage were studied by brain MRI. The cerebellar lesions in these infants ranged from a mild and more prevalent form (71%), which was primarily focal and unilateral, to a less common (9%) but more diffuse and extensive form of injury involving both cerebellar hemispheres and the vermis. This form of bilateral cerebellar hemorrhagic injury ranged from partial inferomedial to near-complete cerebellar destruction similar to that previously described (Messerschmidt et al. 2005). In this study, concomitant supratentorial lesions were common, but in 23% of infants injury was confined to the cerebellum (Limperopoulos et al. 2005a). Risk factors for cerebellar hemorrhagic injury included maternal (e.g. assisted conception) and intrapartum risk factors (e.g. abnormal fetal heart rate, emergent cesarean section, low Apgar scores), as well as early postnatal cardiorespiratory derangements (e.g. high-frequency ventilation, patent ductus arteriosus, lower 5-day minimum pH). Mortality and morbidity (e.g. prolonged ventilation, longer neonatal intensive care unit stay, severe retinopathy of preterm birth) was significantly higher among preterm infants who had developed cerebellar hemorrhagic injury.

THIRD TRIMESTER CEREBELLAR VULNERABILITY

Recent studies have examined the effects of preterm birth itself, as well as preterm-related brain injuries, on early postnatal cerebellar growth. Using quantitative 3D MRI techniques in preterm infants these studies have demonstrated that the growth of the immature cerebellum is particularly rapid during the third trimester of gestation. In fact, the rate of cerebellar growth during this phase far exceeded that of the cerebral hemispheres (Limperopoulos et al. 2005b). However, when compared with term infants, preterm infants show significantly smaller cerebellar volumes at term-equivalent age, indicating that cerebellar development is impeded by preterm extrauterine life even in the absence of actual demonstrable cerebral or cerebellar MRI injury (Limperopoulos et al. 2005b).

These findings raise important questions about the possibility of extrauterine factors or withdrawal of intrauterine factors operating during the early weeks of preterm life that impede cerebellar growth and development (Limperopoulos & du Plessis 2006). Moreover, cerebellar growth impairment is amplified further by associated brain injuries, even when these injuries are remote and confined to the supratentorial structures (Argyropoulou et al. 2003, Limperopoulos et al. 2005a,

Shah et al. 2006, Srinivasan et al. 2006). Together these findings suggest that the phase of rapid cerebellar development during late gestation is likely to represent a period of particular regional vulnerability in the preterm infant. Further studies are needed to determine to what extent this failure of cerebellar growth is brought about by actual cerebellar injury that is undetected by current MRI techniques, possible withdrawal of trophic influences from remote supratentorial injury, or to a paucity of trophic factors normally provided by the mother or placenta.

Advanced 3D volumetric MRI and parcellation techniques have been used to study the crossed trophic effects of cerebellar injury in preterm infants on remote cerebral projection areas and vice versa. Results showed that unilateral cerebral parenchymal injury (e.g. unilateral periventricular hemorrhagic infarction) was asso-ciated with a significantly decreased volume of the apparently uninjured contralateral cerebellar hemisphere (Limperopoulos et al. 2005c). Conversely, unilateral primary cerebellar injury was associated with a volume decrease in the contralateral cere-bral hemisphere. Of note, these effects are evident as early as term gestational age equivalent. These data provide evidence for a significant crossed trophic effect between the developing cerebral and cerebellar structures in preterm infants. These findings also provide important insights into the highly integrated anatomic and functional interactions between the cerebrum and cerebellum during normal brain development. It is postulated that crossed cerebello-cerebral diaschisis may have an important role in the long-term neurodevelopmental impairments and disabilities documented in the years following preterm birth.

These observations of an early onset failure of normal cerebellar growth may contribute to the long-term neurodevelopmental impairment described in survivors of preterm birth. Allin et al. (2001) demonstrated an association between impaired cerebellar growth in survivors of preterm birth and cognitive deficits during adoles-cence compared with those born at term. In a later report, the same investigators (Allin et al. 2005) also demonstrated that lateral cerebellar volume reductions were associated with reduced cerebral white matter volume, and impaired executive, visuospatial, and language function.

ROLE OF CEREBELLAR INJURY IN COGNITIVE–AFFECTIVE DISTURBANCES: OLD CONCEPTS REVISITED

Traditionally, the cerebellum has been known for its fundamental role in motor control and the ability to learn highly complex motor sequences (Riva and Giorgi 2000, Schmahmann 2004). In recent years, this traditional view of cerebellar func-tion as a pure motor center has been extensively challenged. Anatomic, physiologic, and functional neuroimaging studies suggest that the cerebellum participates in the organization of higher order cerebral function. Recent clinical evidence in adults has corroborated neuroanatomic and neurophysiologic findings suggesting a role for the cerebellum far beyond motor function into domains of language, thought modulation, and emotions (Schmahmann and Pandya 1991, Schmahmann and Sherman 1998, Schmahmann and Caplan 2006, Leiner et al. 1991, 1993, Fiez et al. 1992, Fiez 1996).

The clinical manifestations of the recently defined 'cerebellar cognitive affective syndrome' include core elements of executive, spatial, language, and affective disturbance (Schmahmann and Sherman 1998). Specific impairments include disturbances of executive function (e.g. planning, verbal fluency, abstract reasoning, working memory), difficulties with spatial cognition such as visuospatial organization and memory, personality change with blunting of affect or disinhibited and inappropriate behavior, and language deficits (e.g. agrammatism and dysprosodia) (Schmahmann and Pandya 1991, Schmahmann and Sherman 1998, Schmahmann 2004, Schmahmann and Caplan 2006). The constellation of deficits observed in patients with cerebellar cognitive affective syndrome suggests a disruption of the cerebellar modulation of widely distributed and divergent neural circuits that link prefrontal, posterior parietal, superior temporal, and limbic cortices with the cerebellum (Schmahmann and Sherman 1998).

The presence of these deficits in adults with cerebellar lesions can be better appreciated when considered in light of the anatomic connections linking the cerebellum with cerebral association areas and paralimbic regions. Anatomic studies have revealed direct and reciprocal connections between the cerebrum and cerebellum, and the hypothalamus and cerebellum (Dietrichs and Haines 1984). Specifically, projections to the pons arise from association areas in the dorsolateral and dorsomedial prefrontal cortex (Schmahmann and Pandya 1997), posterior parietal region (Brodal 1978, May and Andersen 1986, Schmahmann and Pandya 1989), superior temporal cortex (Schmahmann and Pandya 1991), posterior parahippocampal and dorsal prestriate regions (Fries 1990, Schmahmann and Pandya 1993) as well as from the cingulate gyrus (Vilensky and van Hoesen 1981), indicating the presence of parietal and prefrontal lobe connections with the cerebellar cortex.

In children, excision of cerebellar tumors may be followed by severe language impairments (e.g. mutism and subsequent dysarthria) and visuospatial and working memory difficulties (Levisohn et al. 2000, Beebe et al. 2005, Nagel et al. 2006, Robertson et al. 2006). Regressive personality changes, emotional lability, and poor initiation of voluntary movements have also been described (Schmahmann and Sherman 1998, Schmahmann 2004). Children with attention-deficit–hyperactivity disorder have been shown to have smaller vermian lobules VI and VII on MRI (Berquin et al. 1998), and methylphenidate significantly increased brain metabolism in these patients, most notably in the cerebellum, as well as in frontal and temporal regions (Volkow et al. 1997). It has also been demonstrated that the pathology of early infantile autism includes consistently abnormal morphologic features in the cerebellum (Bauman and Kemper 1985, 2004, Courchesne et al. 1988,

Beversdorf et al. 2005). Specifically, hypoplasia of selective vermian lobules has been described in individuals with autism, suggesting that the cerebellum may have a role in the normal development of speech-language and social skills (Courchesne et al. 1988, Courchesne 2002).

Up to 50% of survivors of very preterm birth demonstrate neuromotor and cognitive impairments (Aylward 2002, Marlow et al. 2005, Vohr and Allen 2005), reflecting the influence of early brain injury on their subsequent development. At school age, these children are more likely to be considered 'clumsy' and perform less well academically. In addition to cognitive impairments, these children manifest a constellation of neurologic signs, including dysdiadochokinesis, poor coordination of fine movements, and impaired motor sequencing (Hadders-Algra et al. 1988, Marlow et al. 1988). Based on data presented in the preceding sections, it is tempting to speculate that either direct cerebellar injury or more subtle cerebellar abnormalities resulting in cerebellar 'hypofunction' may underlie the suboptimal performance that has been widely documented of ex-preterm born individuals in learning, language, and social skills.

NEURODEVELOPMENTAL IMPACT OF EARLY LIFE CEREBELLAR INJURY

Despite recent advances in neuroimaging, the developmental and functional correlates of cerebellar hemorrhagic injury in the young infant remain poorly defined. A review of the literature indicates that the outcome of cerebellar hemorrhagic injury remains controversial. Several investigators have reported favorable outcomes (Chadduck et al. 1995, Huang and Lui 1995), while others have reported important neurodevelopmental deficits (Williamson et al. 1985, Johnsen et al. 2002, 2005, Miall et al. 2003). However, previous studies of outcome in survivors of cerebellar hemorrhagic injury have had important limitations, likely contributing to the inconsistent outcomes reported. These include small sample sizes, combined preterm and term infants, broad age distributions at follow-up testing, and a lack of standardized measures of neurodevelopmental performance as outcomes.

Very few studies have described the outcome of term infants who sustained cerebellar hemorrhagic injury in the neonatal period. Available data indicate that cerebellar hemorrhagic injury in the term infant is associated with high mortality and neurologic sequelae including microcephaly, hypotonia, truncal ataxia, intention tremor, and nystagmus. Cognitive delays ranging from mild to severe have also been described, as well as markedly disordered expressive language (Williamson et al. 1985, Miall et al. 2003). The poor outcome noted among term infants has been associated with a high frequency of serious congenital abnormalities and a high incidence of anteceding asphyxia (Miall et al. 2003). Conversely, favorable neurodevelopmental outcomes have been described in infants with cerebellar hemorrhagic injury associated with coagulopathies (Chadduck et al. 1995). It is important to note that most studies did not use standardized measures to quantify global developmental performance.

The neurodevelopmental outcome of survivors of preterm cerebellar injury has primarily focused on a selected subgroup of infants with an extensive form of cerebellar injury with associated supratentorial parenchymal injury (Johnsen et al. 2002, 2005, Bodensteiner and Johnsen 2004). These children demonstrated a high prevalence of profound neurologic impairment including microcephaly, spastic quadriplegia and diplegia, hypotonia, dystonia, ataxia, and seizures.

A recent study (Limperopoulos et al. 2007) examined the outcome of 86 preterm infants, of whom 35 with isolated cerebellar hemorrhagic injury were age-matched to 35 preterm controls, while an additional 16 had cerebellar hemorrhagic injury plus supratentorial parenchymal injury. This study used formal neurologic examinations, and a battery of standardized developmental, behavioral, and functional evaluations. Isolated cerebellar hemorrhagic injury in preterm infants was associated with a higher prevalence of global pervasive neurodevelopment disabilities and functional limitations than preterm age-matched controls. Global developmental, functional, and social–behavioral deficits (i.e. positive autism screening) were significantly more common and profound in preterm infants with injury that involved the cerebellar vermis than infants with injury confined to a single cerebellar hemisphere. Preterm infants with combined cerebellar hemorrhagic injury and supratentorial parenchymal injury were at greater risk for neuromotor impairments than those with isolated cerebellar injury, but there was no significant difference in cognitive, language, and social function at outcome assessment.

In summary, cerebellar injury in preterm infants is associated with a significant risk for adverse neurodevelopmental sequelae. The topography of cerebellar injury is correlated with different neurodevelopmental profiles, a critical factor that needs to be carefully considered when prognosticating in the clinical situation. Finally, these high rates of neurodevelopmental disabilities underscore the importance of early identification and ongoing surveillance for a broad spectrum of potential adverse outcomes.

CONCLUSIONS AND FUTURE DIRECTIONS

The rapidly increasing sophistication of neuroimaging techniques together with improved survival of seriously ill newborn infants have increased our understanding of the pathophysiologic mechanisms and consequences that underlie direct and indirect cerebellar injury in the developing infant. Early life cerebellar growth impairment, related to either direct cerebellar injury or cerebellar underdevelopment secondary to cerebral injury, has a previously under-recognized role in the long-term cognitive, behavioral, and motor deficits associated with brain injury among high-risk infants. In order to better delineate the functional relevance of early life injury to the cerebellum on cerebro-cerebellar circuitry, further quantitative volumetric, microstructural, metabolic, and functional MRI studies will need to be systematically undertaken. Furthermore, longitudinal studies on large groups of infants with discrete and well-characterized cerebellar injury will be essential in further exploring the relative contribution of cerebellar injury to the high prevalence of neurodevelopmental morbidities reported in survivors of preterm and term cerebellar injury, as well as providing new insights into lesion-deficit correlates and the potential for recovery.

REFERENCES

Allin MP, Matsumoto H, Santhouse AM, Nosarti C, AlAsady MHS, Stewart SAL, et al. (2001) Cognitive and motor function and the size of the cerebellum in adolescents born very preterm. *Brain* 124: 60–66.

Allin MP, Salaria S, Nosarti C, Wyatt J, Rifkin L, Murray RM, et al. (2005) Vermis and lateral lobes of the cerebellum in adolescents born very preterm. *Neuroreport* 7: 1821–1824.

Argyropoulou MI, Xydis V, Drougia A, Tzoufi M, Bassounas A, Andronikou S, et al. (2003) MRI measurements of the pons and cerebellum in children born preterm: associations with the severity of periventricular leukomalacia and perinatal risk factors. *Neuroradiology* 45: 730–734.

Aylward GP (2002) Cognitive and neuropsychological outcomes: more than IQ scores. *Ment Retard Dev Disabil Res Rev* 8: 234–240.

Bauman M, Kemper TL (1985) Histoanatomic observations of the brain in early infantile autism. *Neurology* 35: 866–874.

Bauman ML, Kemper TL (2005) Neuroanatomic observations of the brain in autism: a review and future directions. *Int J Dev Neurosci* 23: 183–187.

Baumeister FA, Hofer M (2000) Cerebellar hemorrhage in preterm infants with intraventricular hemorrhage: a missed diagnosis? A patient report. *Clin Pediatr* 39: 611–613.

Beebe DW, Ris MD, Armstrong FD, Fontanesi J, Mulhern R, Holmes E, et al. (2005) Cognitive and adaptive outcome in low-grade pediatric cerebellar astrocytomas: evidence of diminished cognitive and adaptive functioning in National Collaborative Research Studies (CCG 9891/POG 9130). *J Clin Oncol* 23: 5198–5204.

Berquin PC, Giedd JN, Jacobsen LK, Hamburger SD, Krain AL, Rapoport JL, et al. (1998) Cerebellum in attention-deficit hyperactivity disorder: a morphometric MRI study. *Neurology* 50: 1087–1093.

Beversdorf DQ, Manning SE, Hillier A, Anderson SL, Nordgren RE, Walters SE, et al. (2005) Timing of prenatal stressors and autism. *J Autism Dev Disord* 35: 471–478.

Bodensteiner JB, Johnsen SD (2005) Cerebellar injury in the extremely premature infant: newly recognized but relatively common outcome. *J Child Neurol* 20: 139–142.

Boltshauser E (2004) Cerebellum–small brain but large confusion: a review of selected cerebellar malformations and disruptions. *Am J Med Genet A* 1;126A: 376–385.

Brodal P (1978) The corticopontine projection in the rhesus monkey: origin and principles of organization. *Brain* 101: 251–283.

Bulas DI, Taylor GA, Fitz C, Revenis ME, Glass P, Ingram JD (1991) Posterior fossa intracranial hemorrhage in infants treated with extracorporeal membrane oxygenation: sonographic findings. *AJR Am J Roentgenol* 156: 571–575.

Chadduck WM, Duong DH, Kast JM, Donahue DJ (1995) Pediatric cerebellar hemorrhages. *Childs Nerv Syst* 11: 579–583.

Courchesne E (2002) Abnormal early brain development in autism. *Mol Psychiatry* 7: S21–23.

Courchesne E, Yeung-Courchesne R, Press GA, Hesselink JR, Jernigan TL (1988) Hypoplasia of cerebellar vermal lobules VI and VII in autism. *N Engl J Med* 318: 1349–1354.

Correa F, Enriquez G, Rossello J, Lucaya J, Piqueras J, Aso C, et al. (2004) Posterior fontanelle sonography: an acoustic window into the neonatal brain. *AJNR Am J Neuroradiol* 25: 1274–1282.

Dietrichs E, Haines DE (1984) Demonstration of hypothalamo-cerebellar and cerebello-hypothalamic fibres in a prosimian primate (*Galago crassicaudatus*). *Anat Embryol* 170: 313–318.

Di Salvo DN (2001) A new view of the neonatal brain: clinical utility of supplemental neurologic US imaging windows. *Radiographics* 21: 943–955.

Donat JF, Okazaki H, Kleinberg F (1979) Cerebellar hemorrhages in newborn infants. *Am J Dis Child* 133: 441.

du Plessis AJ, Volpe JJ (2002) Perinatal brain injury in the preterm and term newborn. *Curr Opin Neurol* 15: 151–157.

Fiez JA (1996) Cerebellar contributions to cognition. *Neuron* 16: 13–15.

Fiez JA, Petersen SE, Cheney MK, Raichle ME (1992) Impaired non-motor learning and error detection associated with cerebellar damage: a single case study. *Brain* 115: 155–178.

Fries W (1990) Pontine projection from striate and prestriate visual cortex in the macaque monkey: an anterograde study. *Vis Neurosci* 4: 205–216.

Grunnet ML, Shields WD (1976) Cerebellar hemorrhage in the premature infant. *J Pediatr Res* 88: 605–608.

Hadders-Algra M, Huisjes HJ, Touwen BC (1988) Perinatal correlates of major and minor neurological dysfunction at school age: a multivariate analysis. *Dev Med Child Neurol* 30: 472–481.

Huang LT, Lui CC (1995) Tentorial hemorrhage associated with vacuum extraction in a newborn. *Pediatr Radiol* 25 (Suppl 1): S230–231.

Huppi PS, Dubois J (2006) Diffusion tensor imaging of brain development. *Semin Fetal Neonatal Med* 11: 489–497.

Huppi PS, Warfield S, Kikinis R, Barnes PD, Zientara GP, Jolesz F, et al. (1998) Quantitative magnetic resonance imaging of brain development in premature and mature newborns. *Ann Neurol* 43: 224–235.

Inder TE, Warfield SK, Wang H, Huppi PS, Volpe JJ (2005) Abnormal cerebral structure is present at term in premature infants. *Pediatrics* 115: 286–294.

Johnsen SD, Bodensteiner JB, Lotze TE (2005) Frequency and nature of cerebellar injury in the extremely premature survivor with cerebral palsy. *J Child Neurol* 20: 60–64.

Johnsen SD, Tarby TJ, Lewis KS, Bird R, Prenger E (2002) Cerebellar infarction: an unrecognized complication of very low birthweight. *J Child Neurol* 17: 320–324.

Leiner HC, Leiner AL, Dow RS (1991) The human cerebro-cerebellar system: its computing, cognitive, and language skills. *Behav Brain Res* 44: 113–128.

Leiner HC, Leiner AL, Dow RS (1993) Cognitive and language functions of the human cerebellum. *Trends Neurosci* 16: 444–447.

Levisohn L, Cronin-Golomb A, Schmahmann JD (2000) Neuropsychological consequences of cerebellar tumour resection in children: cerebellar cognitive affective syndrome in a paediatric population. *Brain* 123: 1041–1050.

Limperopoulos C, Bassan H, Gauvreau K, Robertson RL Jr, Sullivan NR, Benson CB, et al. (2007) Does cerebellar injury in premature infants contribute to the high prevalence of long term cognitive learning and behavioral disability in survivors? *Pediatrics* 120: 584–593.

Limperopoulos C, Benson CB, Bassan H, Disalvo DN, Kinnamon DD, Moore M, et al. (2005a) Cerebellar hemorrhage in the preterm infant: ultrasonographic findings and risk factors. *Pediatrics* 116: 717–724.

Limperopoulos C, du Plessis AJ (2006) Disorders of cerebellar growth and development. *Curr Opin Pediatr* 18: 621–627.

Limperopoulos C, Soul JS, Gauvreau K, Huppi PS, Warfield SK, Bassan H, et al. (2005b) Late gestation cerebellar growth is rapid and impeded by premature birth. *Pediatrics* 115: 688–695.

Limperopoulos C, Soul JS, Haidar H, Huppi PS, Bassan H, Warfield SK, et al. (2005c) Impaired trophic interactions between the cerebellum and the cerebrum among preterm infants. *Pediatrics* 116: 844–850.

Marlow N, Hunt LP, Chiswick ML (1988) Clinical factors associated with adverse outcome for babies weighing 2000g or less at birth. *Arch Dis Child* 63 (10 Spec No): 1131–1136.

Marlow N, Wolke D, Bracewell MA, Samara M; EPICure Stugy Group (2005) Neurologic and developmental disability at six years of age after extremely preterm birth. *N Engl J Med* 352: 9–19.

Martin R, Roessmann U, Fanaroff A (1976) Massive intracerebellar hemorrhage in low-birth-weight infants. *J Pediatr* 89: 290–293.

May JG, Andersen RA (1986) Different patterns of corticopontine projections from separate cortical fields within the inferior parietal lobule and dorsal prelunate gyrus of the macaque. *Exp Brain Res* 63: 265–278.

Menezes AH, Smith DE, Bell WE (1983) Posterior fossa hemorrhage in the term neonate. *Neurosurgery* 13: 452–456.

Mercuri E, He J, Curati WL, Dubowitz LM, Cowan FM, Bydder GM (1997) Cerebellar infarction and atrophy in infants and children with a history of premature birth. *Pediatr Radiol* 27: 139–143.

Merrill JD, Piecuch RE, Fell SC, Barkovich AJ, Goldstein RB (1998) A new pattern of cerebellar hemorrhages in preterm infants. *Pediatrics* 102: e62.

Messerschmidt A, Brugger PC, Boltshauser E, Zoder G, Sterniste W, Birnbacher R, et al. (2005) Disruption of cerebellar development: potential complication of extreme prematurity. *Am J Neuroradiol* 26: 1659–1667.

Miall LS, Cornette LG, Tanner SF, Arthur RJ, Levene MI (2003) Posterior fossa abnormalities seen on magnetic resonance brain imaging in a cohort of newborn infants. *J Perinatol* 23: 396–403.

Nagel BJ, Delis DC, Palmer SL, Reeves C, Gajjar A, Mulhern RK (2006) Early patterns of verbal memory impairment in children treated for medulloblastoma. *Neuropsychology* 20: 105–112.

Pape KE, Armstrong DL, Fitzhardinge PM (1976) Central nervous system pathology associated with mask ventilation in the very low birthweight infant: a new etiology for intracerebellar hemorrhages. *Pediatrics* 58: 473–483.

Perlman JM, Nelson JS, McAlister WH, Volpe JJ (1983) Intracerebellar hemorrhage in a premature newborn: diagnosis by real-time ultrasound and correlation with autopsy findings. *Pediatrics* 71: 159–162.

Rakic P, Sidman RL (1970) Histogenesis of cortical layers in human cerebellum, particularly the lamina dissecans. *J Comp Neurol* 139: 473–500.

Reeder JD, Setzer ES, Kaude JV (1982) Ultrasonographic detection of perinatal intracerebellar hemorrhage. *Pediatrics* 70: 385–386.

Riva D, Giorgi C (2000) The cerebellum contributes to higher functions during development: evidence from a series of children surgically treated for posterior fossa tumours. *Brain* 123 (Pt 5): 1051–1061.

Robertson PL, Muraszko KM, Holmes EJ, Sposto R, Packer RJ, Gajjar A, et al. The Children's Oncology Group (2006) Incidence and severity of postoperative cerebellar mutism syndrome in children with medulloblastoma: a prospective study by the Children's Oncology Group. *J Neurosurg* 105: 444–451.

Schmahmann JD (2004) Disorders of the cerebellum: ataxia, dysmetria of thought, and the cerebellar cognitive affective syndrome. *J Neuropsychiatry Clin Neurosci* 16: 367–378.

Schmahmann JD, Caplan D (2006) Cognition, emotion and the cerebellum. *Brain* 129: 290–292.

Schmahmann JD, Pandya DN (1989) Anatomical investigation of projections to the basis pontis from posterior parietal association cortices in rhesus monkey. *J Comp Neurol* 289: 53–73.

Schmahmann JD, Pandya DN (1991) Projections to the basis pontis from the superior temporal sulcus and superior temporal region in the rhesus monkey. *J Comp Neurol* 308: 224–28.

Schmahmann JD, Pandya DN (1993) Prelunate, occipitotemporal, and arahippocampal projections to the basis pontis in rhesus monkey. *J Comp Neurol* 337: 94–112.

Schmahmann JD, Pandya DN (1997) Anatomic organization of the basilar pontine projections from prefrontal cortices in rhesus monkey. *J Neurosci* 17: 438–458.

Schmahmann JD, Sherman JC (1998) The cerebellar cognitive affective syndrome. *Brain* 121 (pt 4): 561–579.

Scotti G, Flodmark O, Harwood-Nash DC, Humphries RP (1981) Posterior fossa hemorrhages in the newborn. *J Comput Assist Tomogr* 5: 68–72.

Serfontein GL, Rom S, Stein S (1980) Posterior fossa subdural hemorrhage in the newborn. *Pediatrics* 65: 40–43.

Shah DK, Anderson PJ, Carlin JB, Pavlovic M, Howard K, Thompson DK, et al. (2006) Reduction in cerebellar volumes in preterm infants: relationship to white matter injury and neurodevelopment at two years of age. *Pediatr Res* 60: 97–102.

Srinivasan L, Allsop J, Counsell SJ, Boardman JP, Edwards AD, Rutherford M (2006) Smaller cerebellar volumes in very preterm infants at term-equivalent age are associated with the presence of supratentorial lesions. *Am J Neuroradiol* 27: 573–579.

ten Donkelaar HJ, Lammens M, Wesseling P, Thijssen HO, Renier WO (2003) Development and developmental disorders of the human cerebellum. *J Neurol* 250: 1025–1036.

Vilensky JA, van Hoesen GW (1981) Corticopontine projections from the cingulate cortex in the rhesus monkey. *Brain Res* 205: 391–395.

Vohr BR, Allen M (2005) Extreme prematurity: the continuing dilemma. *N Engl J Med* 352: 71–72.

Volkow, ND, Wang GJ, Fowler JS, et al. (1997) Topographical distribution of olivary and corticonuclear fibers in the cerebellum: a review. In: Courville E, de Montingny C, Lamarre Y (eds) *The Inferior Olivary Nucleus*. Raven Press, New York. pp 207–234.

Volpe JJ (2001) *Neurology of the Newborn*. Philadelphia, PA: WB Saunders.

von Gontard A, Arnold D, Adis B (1988) Posterior fossa hemorrhage in the newborn: diagnosis and management. *Pediatr Radiol* 18: 347–348.

Williamson WD, Percy AK, Fishman MA, Cheek WR, Desmond MM, LaFevers N, et al. (1985) Cerebellar hemorrhage in the term neonate: developmental and neurologic outcome. *Pediatr Neurol* 1: 356–360.

17
GENETIC MALFORMATIONS OF CORTICAL DEVELOPMENT

Elliott H Sherr

Understanding the mechanisms from formation of the neural tube to the full development of the human central nervous system continues to be a source of inspiration and fascination for clinicians and scientists since before the remarkable contributions of Ramón y Cajal. With the advent of modern genetics and imaging tools, astute clinician scientists have identified a number of disorders of brain development which have given us a glimpse into the mechanisms of cerebral development and also continue to humble us at the vast complexity that lies before us that remains to be understood. We are still primarily at the stage of identification with prevention and treatment yet to be effectively addressed but we can take hope from recent advances in the treatment of cancer which arose from a detailed understanding of the molecular underpinnings of neoplasms suggesting that similar progress awaits the field of neurodevelopmental disabilities. This review highlights recent advances in the genetics of human brain development, focusing on the later stages of prosencephalon development.

MICROCEPHALY

Microcephaly, or a head circumference of 3 standard deviations (SD) below the mean, is often associated with mental retardation (Dolk 1991). Microcephaly is typically divided into primary microcephaly, where the head circumference is small at birth, and secondary microcephaly, where the head does not grow adequately during postnatal development and becomes progressively smaller relative to age and sex and ethnically based standards. This latter condition will not be addressed in much detail in this review.

Seemingly, microcephaly encompasses many causes: neurodegenerative conditions such as Rett syndrome, metabolic disorders such as Glut1 haploinsufficiency, and perinatal disorders including infection (e.g. HIV) and hypoxic ischemic injury. Congenital or primary microcephaly also has many causes, which include disorders of prosencephalization (holoprosencephaly and agenesis of the corpus callosum, chromosomal disorders and disorders of cellular migration) (Table 17.1). Some of these, such as Miller–Dieker lissencephaly, are addressed in other sections.

Some primary microcephaly disorders are labeled as autosomal recessive primary microcephaly (in the past referred to as microcephaly vera). These patients have

TABLE 17.1
Causes of primary/congenital microcephaly

Intrauterine infection	*Chromosomal disorders*
Cytomegalovirus	Down syndrome
Herpes simplex	Trisomy 13 or 18
Rubella	Ring chromosomes
Varicella	Sex chromosome aneuploidy
Coxsackie B virus	
Toxoplasmosis	*Malformation disorders*
	Microcephaly vera microcephalin
Drugs and toxins	Holoprosencephaly
Alcohol	Aprosencephaly
Tobacco	Agenesis of the corpus callosum
Cocaine	Lissencephaly
Heroin	
Antiepileptics	*Other hereditary* (partial list)
Chemotherapeutics	Normal occipitofrontal circumference variant
Toluene	Smith–Lemli–Opitz syndrome
	Cornelia de Lange syndrome
Hypoxia/ischemia/stroke	Rubinstein–Taybi syndrome
Trauma	Fanconi anemia
Malnutrition	Nijmegen breakage syndrome
Endocrinopathies	
Hypoglycemia	
Hypothyroidism	
Hypopituitarism	

evidence of microcephaly by 32 weeks' gestation and are born with an occipitofrontal circumference (OFC) -4 to -12SD below the mean. Brain magnetic resonance imaging (MRI) typically shows simplification of the cerebral cortical gyral pattern with usually no evidence for a specific neuronal migrational defect (Woods et al. 2005). The patients typically have mental retardation, good motor skills, and a pleasant disposition. The incidence in northern Pakistan, where consanguinity is relatively common, is estimated to be 1 in 10 000. In England, the incidence is estimated at 1 in 1 000 000. Six genetic loci and four genes have recently been identified in these disorders, but 18/56 Pakistani families do not show linkage to any of these loci, suggesting that many additional genes will soon be identified (Woods et al. 2005). The discovery of these four genes has demonstrated the importance of cell cycle regulation in cortical development (Table 17.2). Moreover, there is now evidence to suggest that the expansion of cortex size, something that particularly links *Homo sapiens* to our immediate ancestors, may be tied to these very same genetic mechanisms.

TABLE 17.2

Genetic causes of autosomal recessive primary microcephaly

Locus name	Chromosomal region	Gene name	Function
MCPH1	8p22-pter	Microcephalin	Cell cycle entry, DNA repair
MCPH2	19q13.1-13.2	Unreported	NA
MCPH3	9q34	CDK5RAP2	Centrosomal tubulin binder
MCPH4	15q15-q21	Unreported	NA
MCPH5	1q31	ASPM	Organize MT at spindle poles
MCPH6	13q12.2	CENPJ	Found at spindle poles

The gene from the first microcephaly locus, MCPH1, or microcephalin, has been implicated in both cell cycle regulation and DNA repair. One variation of primary microcephaly was identified in a consanguineous family with a recessive 427insA mutation in microcephalin. Cells from patients showed premature chromosome condensation underlying cell cycle dysregulation (Neitzel et al. 2002, Trimborn et al. 2004). RNA interference (RNAi) experiments have shown that microcephalin regulates the transcription of Cdk1 and BRCA1, known DNA damage response genes. BRCA1 is well studied as a principal genetic risk factor for familial and non-familial breast cancer (Lee et al. 2000). MPCH1 mutant cell lines show defects in the G2-M checkpoint arrest and the normal function of MPCH1 may be to regulate phosphorylation of Cdk1 preventing premature entry into mitosis (Alderton et al. 2006). The genes involved in Seckel syndrome, another microcephaly syndrome, and ataxia telangiectasia (ataxia telangiectasia related (ATR) and ataxia telangiectasia mutated (ATM)) also participate in DNA damage repair. Both are protein kinases; ATM responds to double strand breaks in DNA and ATR is activated by single-stranded DNA. The discovery of the mechanisms of these microcephaly genes underscores the role of DNA repair in neuroblast proliferation.

A more recently described disorder, which includes microcephaly, growth retardation, and a T and B cell immunodeficiency, is caused by mutations in Cernunnos (NHEJ1 or XLF), a gene involved in the repair of double-strand DNA breaks through the non-homologous end-joining pathway (Ahnesorg et al. 2006, Buck et al. 2006). Interestingly, a recent report identified truncation of NHEJ1 in a fetus with polymicrogyria and heterotopia (Cantagrel et al. 2006). If this initial finding is confirmed, it will suggest an important mechanistic link between DNA repair and polymicrogyria as currently the causes of polymicrogyria remain mostly obscure.

The most recognized common gene cause of primary microcephaly from mutations is the gene ASPM. The role of this gene's protein product and related proteins highlight the importance of microtubule dynamics during cell division as another important cause of microcephaly. The predicted protein for ASPM contains N-terminal calponin-homology domains and up to 81 calmodulin-binding IQ domains. The *Drosophila* homolog to ASPM, Asp (abnormal spindle protein), is a microtubule-associated protein that is necessary for the aggregation of microtubules into focused spindle poles (Wakefield et al. 2001). Similarly, ASPM is localized to spindle poles during mitosis of cultured cells (Kouprina et al. 2005) as well as in mouse embryonic neuroepithelial cells (Fish et al. 2006). Moreover, RNAi reduction of ASPM causes an alteration in the orientation of the cleavage plane of these dividing neuronal precursors. This disruption of symmetric division could lead to premature termination of cell divisions in the neuroepithelium and thus microcephaly from the generation of too few neurons (Fish et al. 2006).

MCPH6 is caused by mutations in CENJP. This gene has also been found at centrosomes and spindle poles. The *Drosophila* homolog, DSas-4, appears to be essential for centriole replication (Basto et al. 2006). Flies mutated in DSas-4 lose their centrioles during development and show abnormal asymmetric cell divisions of neuroblasts. Interestingly, the flies appear to develop into morphologically normal adults. They lack flagella and cilia, and this leads to early death. In a similar mechanistic vein, MCPH3 is caused by mutation in CDK5RAP2 and, like CENJP, it is highly expressed during prenatal neurogenesis and is localized to the spindle pole of mitotic cells (Bond et al. 2005).

With the availability of the chimpanzee and human genomes, there has been considerable interest in using informatic tools to identify regions that differ significantly between humans and chimpanzees, more than would be predicted by comparison to other mammalian genomes, thus imputing a 'neutral' evolutionary rate for single nucleotide polymorphisms (SNPs). One might assume that polymorphisms that show up at a faster rate in certain genes relative to the whole genome may be under a positive evolutionary pressure to do so. This type of ongoing evolution has been seen in many of these microcephaly genes. For instance, an allele of ASPM arose in our ancestors approximately 5800 years ago and its high frequency in humans suggests that it is under a strong influence for positive selection (Mekel-Bobrov et al. 2005). Similar data have been found for microcephalin, CDK5RAP2, and CENPJ (Evans et al. 2005). This field of evolutionary analysis is still in its early phases and much more experimental testing of these hypotheses must occur before we can understand the precise implications of these observations.

In addition to primary microcephaly, there has been recent progress in the identification of other syndromic causes of microcephaly. One disorder, Feingold syndrome, results in microcephaly, esophageal and duodenal atresias, mental retardation, syndactyly, and cardiac defects. It is caused by autosomal dominant mutations (haploinsufficiency) in the MYCN gene (van Bokhoven et al. 2005). Mutations of the catalytic subunit of RAB3GAP cause the autosomal recessive Warburg micro syndrome. These patients have microcephaly, microcornea, congenital cataract, short stature, and hypogenitalism (Aligianis et al. 2005). A milder phenotype, Martsolf syndrome (congenital cataracts, hypogonadism, and mild mental retardation), was also found to be caused by mutations in RAB3GAP (Aligianis et al. 2006). A better understanding of the mechanisms underlying these mutations awaits further study.

AGENESIS OF THE CORPUS CALLOSUM

Containing over 190 million axons, the corpus callosum is the main connection between the two cerebral hemispheres. It evolved with the onset of placental mammals, as monotremes and marsupials have an anterior commissure but do not have a corpus callosum (Granger et al. 1985). Agenesis of the corpus callosum (ACC) is present in at least 1 in 4000 live births, making this the most common CNS malformation after neural tube defects (Paul et al. 2007). Normal callosal development necessitates

1 Neuronal proliferation and fate specification
2 Growth and differentiation of midline structures
3 Projection of pioneer axons across the midline
4 Guidance by these pioneer neurons for the subsequent crossing of more distant cortical projection neurons
5 Guidance of these projection neurons to contralateral (usually homotopic) target sites in the opposite (contralateral hemisphere)

In mice, many gene knockout models have been shown to result in callosal agenesis (Richards et al. 2004), but little information exists on what role these genes may have in human ACC. The genetics of human ACC is quite variable and speaks to the underlying complexity of callosal development. Current evidence suggests a combination of genetic mechanisms, including single-gene Mendelian, sporadic mutations (single-gene), and complex genetics (which may have a mixture of inherited and *de novo* mutations). Recent studies suggest that about 33% of ACC patients have an identified cause, with 10% having chromosomal anomalies and the remaining 20–25% having recognizable genetic syndromes (Bedeschi et al. 2006).

One example of a Mendelian disorder is X-linked lissencephaly with agenesis of the corpus callosum and ambiguous genitalia (XLAG), which results from a mutation in the Aristaless-related homeobox gene (ARX). First described with intractable epilepsy, profound neurodevelopmental impairment, and early lethality (Proud et al. 1992), these initial patients were all male and also had microcephaly, ACC, optic atrophy, and craniofacial dysmorphisms. Females with mutations in ARX, who were described later and who would be expected to have a wide range of clinical severity if X-inactivation was random (i.e. lyonization), ranged from completely healthy to those with spasticity, mental retardation, and seizures. MRI scans were either normal or showed isolated ACC with Probst bundles (Bonneau et al.

2002). In addition to ACC, the mouse ARX knockout mimics many of the other clinical and anatomic findings in XLAG (Sherr 2003) including a significant reduction in cortical interneurons, which likely explains the severe and uncontrollable seizures in this condition (Kitamura et al. 2002).

Another syndrome with considerable overlap between human and animal conditions is CRASH syndrome (corpus callosum agenesis, retardation, adducted thumbs, spastic paraplegia, and hydrocephalus), which is accompanied by diminutive cortico-spinal tracts within the brainstem. There is phenotypic variability, and other clinical presentations include hydrocephalus resulting from stenosis of the aqueduct of Sylvius (HSAS) and mental retardation, aphasia, shuffling gait, adducted thumbs (MASA) syndromes. CRASH is caused by mutations in the L1CAM gene that codes for a transmembrane cell adhesion protein broadly expressed in the central nervous system. L1 gene inactivation models in mice show complete or partial ACC, hydrocephalus, small cortico-spinal tracts, reduced neuron numbers, and additional abnormalities in the elaboration of apical dendrites from cortical pyramidal neurons (Demyanenko et al. 1999). Recent work suggests that inhibiting homophilic binding of the L1CAM protein can cause hydrocephalus, but that to cause ACC there must also be additional disruption of L1CAM heterophilic binding with multiple partners including integrins (Itoh et al. 2004).

Andermann syndrome, an autosomal recessive condition particularly prevalent in the Saguenay-Lac-St-Jean region of Quebec (i.e. founder effect), presents with callosal hypoplasia or ACC, cognitive impairment, episodes of psychosis, and a progressive central and peripheral neuropathy. It is caused by mutation of the potassium-chloride co-transporter KCC3 (Dupre et al. 2003). Interestingly, callosal agenesis is not present in every person with KCC3 recessive mutations and there is phenotypic variability even within the same family. This suggests a role for additional genetic or epigenetic influences. KCC3 knockout mice have similar neurodegeneration, and also have hearing loss and progressive neuropathy (Boettger et al. 2003). However, in contrast to ARX and L1 mouse mutants, these mice have a normally formed corpus callosum.

In spite of this progress on single-gene Mendelian causes of ACC, most individuals with ACC do not have a clearly inherited cause or a recognized genetic syndrome, suggesting that ACC can be caused by *de novo* genetic events. One salient example of this is Mowat–Wilson syndrome (MWS), which, in addition to ACC, presents with Hirschsprung disease, congenital heart disease, genitourinary anomalies, microcephaly, epilepsy, and severe cognitive impairment (Mowat et al. 2003). MWS is caused by inactivating heterozygous mutations in the gene ZFHX1B on chromosome 2q22, which codes for Smad interacting protein 1 (SIP1) (Zweier et al. 2005). ACC is not observed in all MWS cases, as would be expected, because haploinsufficiency or gene dosage of SIP1 likely interacts with other genetic polymorphisms to alter callosal development (Mowat et al. 2003). Gene dosage effects have been observed in mouse knockout models for the genes DCC and GAP-43 in which isolated partial ACC is observed in heterozygotes and complete ACC with additional anomalies is observed in homozygote knockout mice (Shen et al. 2002). It is likely that other cases of ACC are caused by haploinsufficiency at other genetic loci. This is exemplified by many reports of patients with ACC who have sporadic (i.e. non-inherited) chromosomal changes, with particular genomic loci identified repeatedly (Dobyns 1996).

Recent data using microarray-based comparative genomic hybridization demonstrates that patients with ACC have chromosomal deletions or duplications smaller than those that can be detected using conventional cytogenetics (Sherr et al. 2005). Indeed, in collaboration with the California Birth Defects Monitoring Program, we have demonstrated that the risk of having a child with ACC is nearly threefold higher for mothers aged 40 and above consistent with causal *de novo* chromosomal changes (unpublished observation). In addition to single-gene causes of ACC, there are likely many cases in which ACC is caused by polygenic and other complex interactions. Like many birth defects, this complex polygenic interaction will require genome-wide association studies and deep sequencing of candidate intervals containing putative genes to make progress in our understanding of these disorders.

PERIVENTRICULAR HETEROTOPIA

Periventricular nodular heterotopia (PVNH) is often seen as bilateral contiguous nodules of gray matter adjacent to the body of the lateral ventricles. The best described condition within this classification is the X-linked disorder that is primarily found in females and is associated with high rates of embryonic male lethality (Eksioglu et al. 1996). This has been explained by a cell-autonomous mosaic mechanism wherein the females will express the mutant gene in roughly half of the cortical neurons and hemizygous males will express the mutant gene in all the neurons, accounting for the high rate of male lethality. Nearly all X-linked familial cases of PVNH and 20% of the sporadic cases are caused by mutations in the filamin 1 gene (Fox et al. 1998, Sheen et al. 2001). Recently, there have also been descriptions of somatic mosaicism for FLNA mutations. This explains some of the sporadic female cases and also some of the cases in males. The FLNA gene is located at Xq28, codes for a 280kDa protein that crosslinks actin filaments into branching networks in the cytoplasm and also anchors membranes proteins to the actin cytoskeleton.

Clinically, females with FLNA-mediated PVNH usually present with epilepsy in the school aged years and can have normal intelligence. This was also evident in one male patient with 5pter trisomy (Sheen et al. 2003). Even with normal intelligence, some patients presented with deficits in reading, processing speed, and executive function on detailed psychometric testing (Chang et al. 2005). Some patients present additionally with symptoms suggestive of an Ehlers–Danlos syndrome phenotype (joint hypermobility and aortic dilatation) (Sheen et al. 2005).

FLNA mutations can also cause other syndromes. Missense mutations in patients can lead to craniofacial malformations and skeletal dysplasia syndromes such as oto-palato-digital syndromes types I and II, frontometaphseal dysplasia, and Melnick–Needles syndrome (Robertson et al. 2003). One patient has recently been reported with craniofacial dysmorphisms and PVNH who has a splice site mutation in FLNA (Hehr et al. 2006). In a mouse inactivation model, premature truncation of filamin A leads to male lethality because of incomplete septation of the cardiac outflow tract producing a severe truncus arteriosis. Ventricular septal defects and other cardiac anomalies are seen and males have midline fusion defects at the sternum and palate (Hart et al. 2006). These diverse findings underscore the diverse pleiotropic effects that disruption of the actin cytoskeleton can have on the development of multiple different organ systems of variable embryonic origin.

Other genes cause PVNH and probably more remain to be found, as demonstrated by the observation that only 20–25% of sporadic patients have FLNA mutations (Parrini et al. 2006). One rare autosomal recessive cause of PVNH is mutations in ARFGEF2 (ADP-ribosylation factor guanine nucleotide-exchange factor 2) (Sheen et al. 2004). This was identified in two consanguineous Turkish families, but has yet to be reported in sporadic cases. ARFGEF2 is expressed widely in the developing neocortex and may have an important role in vesicle trafficking in neuronal migration. There are other less common causes of PVNH such as steroid sulfatase deficiency (Ozawa et al. 2006), chromosome 5p anomalies (Sheen et al. 2003), and chromosome 1p36 deletion (Neal et al. 2006). PVNH can also be seen as part of a complex malformation syndrome (Aicardi 2005), in chromosomal disorders (Ramocki et al. 2003), or in association with other brain malformations (Wieck et al. 2005, Parrini et al. 2006).

POLYMICROGYRIA

Polymicrogyria (PMG) refers to the cortical malformation that results in abnormal lamination, a thickened cortical ribbon, and an excessive number of relatively sm ll gyral infolds. The histopathology usually shows either one single continuous layer or four layers with fusion of the molecular layer. Single-layer and four-layer anatomy can be seen in the same patient, suggesting that these findings exist within the same clinico-pathologic spectrum. The etiology of PMG is likely quite heterogeneous and in most cases the cause is currently unknown. Infection and vascular disruption have been observed as etiologic in PMG and genetic causes also contribute, including autosomal recessive, X-linked, and chromosomal disorders. PMG has been seen in association with other syndromes, but in nearly all these cases the etiology of the PMG itself remains obscure. There is some evidence of PMG-like mislayering in mouse models and this may lead to an understanding of the precise molecular pathways involved.

PMG can be focal or widespread, unilateral or bilateral. It can occur as an isolated lesion or in association with other CNS anomalies, such as PVNH, ACC, and cerebellar anomalies. The small irregular gyral pattern can be seen most readily in scans of younger patients. As the patients grow, the imaging changes to a less irregular, but more thickened cortex (Takanashi and Barkovich 2003). This is thought to be a result of the increased myelination of the subcortical white matter. The region affected by the PMG is the basis for classification. Thus, the following anatomic designations have been used: bilateral frontal polymicrogyria (BFP), bilateral frontoparietal polymicrogyria (BFPP), bilateral perisylvian poly-microgyria (BPP), bilateral parasagittal parieto-occipital polymicrogyria (BPOP), bilateral generalized polymicrogyria (BGP), and unilateral polymicrogyria.

Some of the PMG syndromes demonstrate shared clinical features, which usually correspond to the regions affected. In BPP, patients typically have pseudo-bulbar palsy with facial diplegia and weakness of the muscles of mastication. They usually also have a severe dysarthria and can have fine motor deficits. Many can have normal intelligence and some have seizures. However, patients with BFPP have global delay, esotropia, upper motor neurons signs, and epilepsy. Patients with unilateral PMG will present with hemiparesis and typically seizures. They may not have cognitive impairment, but this depends more on the underlying cause of the PMG.

One gene has recently been identified for BFPP. This is an autosomal reces-sive disorder, identified in both consanguineous and unrelated parents of Arab, European, Indian, and Pakistani origins (Piao et al. 2004). Interestingly, none of the unrelated parents were compound heterozygotes, suggesting that their parents may be consanguineous and implying that this disorder may itself be quite rare (Piao et al. 2005). This disorder is caused by mutation in the gene GPR56, which encodes an orphan G-protein-coupled receptor. This gene is highly expressed in the ventricular and subventricular zones of the developing mouse cerebral cortex, yet absent from regions where post-mitotic neurons are highest. Although earlier studies have suggested that PMG is caused by a disruption late in cortical develop-ment, after neuronal differentiation and migration, these data may be interpreted to conclude that the eventual fate of PMG is determined much earlier in develop-ment, even though it is not anatomically evident until much later.

The genetics for the remainder of PMG cases are not yet well established. A subset of patients with mutations in the AH1 gene that cause Joubert syndrome also have polymicrogyria (Dixon-Salazar et al. 2004), although many of the patients with similar mutations in AH1 do not, suggesting the existence of as yet unidentified epigenetic modifiers. Multiple patients with the deletion 22q11.2 syn-drome have polymicrogyria, suggesting that there may be an important locus for PMG in that region, although secondary vascular complications may have a role in these cases (Robin et al. 2006). The gene Cernunnos (NHEJ1), mentioned above in the discussion of microcephaly, is truncated in a single case of a patient with PMG and PVNH (Cantagrel et al. 2006). A patient has been reported with a balanced translocation that interrupts two genes: mannosidase and glutathione S-transferase genes (Leeflang et al. 2003). Multiple chromosomal loci have been associated with PMG, including 1p36 and 6q25 in patients with overlapping deletion syndromes, although the candidate genes for these regions have not yet been elucidated (WB Dobyns, personal communication). Additionally, a locus on Xq28 was putatively found in a group of BPP families. However, further progress in this region has not been reported (Villard et al. 2002). Very little is understood about cortical lamination even in animal models; thus progress in our understanding of PMG is likely to shed light on the genetic pathways directing cortical organization. One recent paper may help to make progress in developing animal models for PMG and PVNH. A forebrain specific knockout of MEKK4, one upstream member of the MAP Kinase family of serine/threonine kinases, demonstrates both periventricular heterotopia and polymicrogyria. In part, this phenotype appears to be caused by aberrant signaling through filamin (Sarkisian et al. 2006).

LISSENCEPHALY

Lissencephaly denotes a smooth-appearing cerebral cortex. This is also associated with a pathologically thickened cortical mantle that usually encompasses four cellular layers. Clinically and genetically, lissencephaly also includes pachygyria (few and broad gyri) and subcortical band heterotopia, wherein a separate layer of neurons is found below the outer cortical layer. Typically, lissencephaly has been divided into two main groups. Type I, or classic, lissencephaly encompasses syndromes caused by mutations in LIS1, DCX, ARX, RELN, and 14-3-3ε genes. This group will continue to grow, as evidenced by the recent report of alpha-tubulin mutations in patients with type I lissencephaly (Keays et al. 2007). We have also seen a similar advance in our understanding of type II lissencephaly, referred to as cobblestone lissencephaly, with the recent identification of the genes that cause Fukuyama muscular dystrophy, Walker–Warburg syndrome, and muscle–eye–brain disease and the mechanisms that link these clinically overlapping disorders together.

TYPE I LISSENCEPHALY SYNDROMES

Miller–Dieker syndrome

Patients with Miller–Dieker syndrome (MDS) are initially detected because of microcephaly, hypotonia, and poor feeding. They have a typical facial appearance and often have cardiac defects. Brain MRIs reveal severe lissencephaly throughout the cortex, typically with no antero-posterior gradient (see below). All patients have *de novo* deletions at 17p13.3 which include the LIS1 and 14-3-3ε loci.

Isolated lissencephaly

Patients with isolated lissencephaly typically have mutations in LIS1 or the X chromosome gene DCX. Patients with LIS1 mutations typically have more severe lissencephaly in the posterior aspects of the cortex, thus having a posterior> anterior imaging gradient. These patients also have profound mental retardation, seizures, and a shortened lifespan. Patients with DCX mutations usually present with two different anatomic constellations. Males with DCX mutations have an anterior>posterior gradient for their lissencephaly. They, like the LIS1 patients, are profoundly affected. Females with DCX mutations can have a subcortical neuronal layer ('double band cortex'), and this is interpreted to be caused by random X-inactivation with prescribed resulting DCX functioning in a cell-autonomous manner. There are also rare male patients with DCX who have less severe mutations and some patients with LIS1 mutations who have a double cortex, suggesting that formation of this anatomic deficit can occur through multiple mechanisms (D'Agostino et al. 2002).

Other causes of lissencephaly include mutations in the gene Reelin (Hong et al. 2000). This disorder, lissencephaly with cerebellar hypoplasia (LCH), is distinct from the aforementioned lissencephaly syndromes. These patients have globally diminished white matter volume and a very diminutive cerebellum and pons. XLAG (Kitamura et al. 2002) was addressed in the prior section on ACC.

Three lissencephaly genes (LIS1, DCX, and 14-3-3ε) have been implicated in the process of microtubule dynamics and neuronal migration. LIS1 was identified initially as a subunit for the platelet-activating factor acetyl-hydrolase, an enzyme involved in metabolism of the lipid messenger platelet activating factor (Hattori et al. 1994). However, selective knockout of the catalytic subunit of this enzyme does not affect brain development, suggesting that LIS1 might work through other mechanisms (Koizumi et al. 2003, Yan et al. 2003). In contrast, LIS1 regulates dynein function. The ortholog of LIS1 in Aspergillus, NudF, regulates nuclear movement within the cell through dynein (Xiang et al. 1995). LIS1 interacts biochemically with dynein and with dynamitin, a subunit of dynactin (Tai et al. 2002). In neurons, RNAi inhibition of LIS1 causes disruption of radial migration (Tsai et al. 2005). This disruption also occurs in radial glial precursors. There is also evidence that LIS1 participates in regulating microtubules through mitosis, which probably also accounts for the observed microcephaly together with the lissencephaly, highlighting an important mechanistic overlap between these two groups of disorders (Li et al. 2005). Deletion of 14-3-3ε results in MDS, a more severe phenotype than isolated lissencephaly. Normally, 14-3-3ε modulates LIS1 function by binding to phosphorylated NUDEL. However, if this binding does not occur or is reduced (as in MDS), then LIS1 is mislocalized and there is a downstream reduction in dynein function.

Like LIS1, DCX also has been shown to bind to microtubules (Gleeson et al. 1999) and the binding of microtububles appears to be regulated by phosphorylation of DCX (Tanaka et al. 2004). RNAi knockdown of DCX in cortical slice cultures results in migrational deficits (LoTurco and Bai 2006). Interestingly, mouse knockout models of DCX do not have these problems. All of these genes tie cell autonomous deficits in cell migration to the observed lissencephaly.

In comparison, RELN is an extracellular secreted glycoprotein that binds to α3β1 integrin, and two lipoprotein receptors, Vdlr and ApoER2. This binding leads to tyrosine phosphorylation and activation of the cytoplasmic adaptor protein disabled (Dab1). Reeler mice (i.e. mutation in reelin) and scrambler mice (i.e. mutation in disabled) have similar cortical malformations (Sheldon et al. 1997) which underscores genetically the biochemical observation that both RELN and DAB1 reside in the same signaling pathway.

As many of the causes of lissencephaly affect neuronal migration through disruption of microtubule dynamics, it is not surprising to learn that a recent publication identifies both an ENU-mutagenized mouse model and a small subset of lissencephalic patients with mutations in the alfa-tubulin gene (TUBA3) (Keays et al. 2007). The point mutation in the mice reduces GTP binding and prevents the normal heterodimerization of alfa and beta tubulin. Forty patients with cortical dysgenesis were screened for TUBA3 mutations for whom LIS1 and DCX genes had already been sequenced and hence excluded as causing lissencephaly. Two patients with *de novo* mutations in TUBA3 were identified. In both patients, agenesis of the splenium of the corpus callosum and hypoplasia of the cerebellar vermis were also noted. It will be interesting to see if other members of the microtubule network are also implicated in lissencephaly and microcephaly vera.

COBBLESTONE LISSENCEPHALY

Three clinical syndromes – Walker–Warburg syndrome (WWS), Fukuyama congenital muscular dystrophy (FCMD), and muscle–eye–brain disease (MEB) – involve these three organs: brain, muscle, and eye. Patients with one of these three syndromes each have hydrocephalus, 'cobblestone' lissencephaly, agenesis of the corpus callosum, fusion of the hemispheres, cerebellar hypoplasia, and, in some cases, occipital encephalocele. These lissencephalies have a gross 'cobblestone' appearance because there is overmigration of neurons beyond the glial limitans and subsequent clustering of these neurons beyond the molecular layer, giving a stippled appearance. Ocular abnormalities include cataracts, microphthalmia, buphthalmus, and persistent hyperplastic primary vitreous. All patients have elevated serum creatine kinase levels and a debilitating muscular dystrophy that may be overlooked clinically. Typically, patients with WWS are the most severely affected, patients with FCMD can have a quite variable outcome, and those with MEB are usually the least severely affected. Some data support phenotype–genotype correlations, but this is still early in the analysis of these patients (van Reeuwijk et al. 2005a).

The gene (fukutin) for FCMD was the first identified and at the time no clear function for the protein was known. There is a founder mutation in the gene, a retrotransposon insertion, which arose approximately 3000 years ago and is estimated to be present in 1% of the Japanese population (Colombo et al. 2000). Patients with mutations in the Fukutin related protein (FKRP) have a diverse set of clinical presentations:

1 A congenital muscular dystrophy with cerebellar cysts and mental retardation (Muntoni 2004)
2 A limb-girdle muscular dystrophy (Brockington et al. 2001)
3 A few patients with MEB disease and WWS (Beltran-Valero de Bernabe et al. 2004)

Patients with MEB usually have mutations in the O-mannose β 1,2 N acetylglu cosaminyltransferase gene (POMGnT1) (Yoshida et al. 2001). The genetics of WWS appears more complex. To date, patients have been identified with mutations in POMGnT1, POMGnT2, fukuitn, and FKRP. These genes only account for 30–40% of WWS patients, suggesting a much more complex disorder to be revealed (van Reeuwijk et al. 2005b). All of these genes share a functional role in regulating O-linked glycosylation (van Reeuwijk et al. 2005b). The myd mouse was shown to have abnormal neuronal migration and disruption of the basal lamina in addition to a muscle defect, similar to patients with cobblestone lissencephaly (Michele et al. 2002). Moreover, these defects, caused by mutation in the gene Large, could be recapitulated by a brain-specific deletion of α-dystroglycan (Moore et al. 2002). Moreover, overexpression of the glycosyltransferase encoded by the gene LARGE rescued the glycosylation defect in Large (myd) mice and in cells from individuals with other congenital muscular dystrophies, suggesting a shared mechanism and a possible strategic targeted therapeutic approach (Barresi et al. 2004).

CONCLUSIONS

The progress made to date in the genetics of deficits in brain development has come almost entirely in the last 10 years. This very rapid progress in gene identification has also led to elegant studies dissecting the molecular mechanisms of these diseases and in some cases offering insights into possible treatment modalities. In a number of categories of brain malformation, there has been a confluence of mechanisms that lead to the group of observed disorders. This has been particularly true for primary microcephaly and for cobblestone lissencephaly and, in a slightly less cohesive sense, the type I lissencephalies. This concordance may provide important insight as we look for the causes of ACC and polymicrogyria, disorders that still primarily defy precise mechanistic understanding in patients. More importantly still, the power of these genetic approaches will allow us to move beyond description and ultimately, it is hoped, to prevention and treatment.

ACKNOWLEDGMENTS

EHS is supported by grants from the NIH and the March of Dimes.

REFERENCES

Ahnesorg P, Smith P, Jackson SP (2006) XLF interacts with the XRCC4-DNA ligase IV complex to promote DNA nonhomologous end-joining. *Cell* 124: 301–313.

Aicardi J (2005) Aicardi syndrome. *Brain Dev* 27: 164–171.

Alderton GK, Galbiati L, Griffith E, Surinya KH, Neitzel H, Jackson AP, et al. (2006). Regulation of mitotic entry by microcephalin and its overlap with ATR signalling. *Nat Cell Biol* 8: 725–733.

Aligianis IA, Johnson CA, Gissen P, Chen D, Hampshire D, Hoffmann K, et al. (2005) Mutations of the catalytic subunit of RAB3GAP cause Warburg Micro syndrome. *Nat Genet* 37: 221–223.

Aligianis IA, Morgan NV, Mione M, Johnson CA, Rosser E, Hennekam RC, et al. (2006) Mutation in Rab3 GTPase-activating protein (RAB3GAP) noncatalytic subunit in a kindred with Martsolf syndrome. *Am J Hum Genet* 78: 702–707.

Barresi R, Michele DE, Kanagawa M, Harper HA, Dovico SA, Satz JS, et al. (2004) LARGE can functionally bypass alpha-dystroglycan glycosylation defects in distinct congenital muscular dystrophies. *Nat Med* 10: 696–703.

Basto R, Lau J, Vinogradova T, Gardiol A, Woods CG, Khodjakov A, et al. (2006) Flies without centrioles. *Cell* 125: 1375–1386.

Bedeschi MF, Bonaglia MC, Grasso R, Pellegri A, Garghentino RR, Battaglia MA, et al. (2006) Agenesis of the corpus callosum: clinical and genetic study in 63 young patients. *Pediatr Neurol* 34: 186–193.

Beltran-Valero de Bernabe D, Voit T, Longman D, Steinbrecher A, Straub V, Yuva Y, et al. (2004) Mutations in the FKRP gene can cause muscle–eye–brain disease and Walker–Warburg syndrome. *J Med Genet* 41: e61.

Boettger T, Rust MB, Maier H, Seidenbecher T, Schweizer M, Keating DJ, et al. (2003) Loss of K-Cl co-transporter KCC3 causes deafness, neurodegeneration and reduced seizure threshold. *EMBO J* 22: 5422–5434.

Bond J, Roberts E, Springell K, Lizarraga SB, Scott S, Higgins J, et al. (2005) A centrosomal mechanism involving CDK5RAP2 and CENPJ controls brain size. *Nat Genet* 37: 353–355.

Bonneau D, Toutain A, Laquerriere A, Marret S, Saugier-Veber P, Barthez MA, et al. (2002) X-linked lissencephaly with absent corpus callosum and ambiguous genitalia (XLAG): clinical, magnetic resonance imaging, and neuropathological findings. *Ann Neurol* 51: 340–349.

Brockington M, Yuva Y, Prandini P, Brown SC, Torelli S, Benson MA, et al. (2001) Mutations in the fukutin-related protein gene (FKRP) identify limb girdle muscular dystrophy 2I as a milder allelic variant of congenital muscular dystrophy MDC1C. *Hum Mol Genet* 10: 2851–2859.

Buck D, Malivert L, de Chasseval R, Barraud A, Fondaneche MC, Sanal O, et al. (2006) Cernunnos, a novel nonhomologous end-joining factor, is mutated in human immunodeficiency with microcephaly. *Cell* 124: 287–299.

Cantagrel V, Lossi AM, Lisgo S, Missirian C, Borges A, Philip N, et al. (2006) Truncation of NHEJ1 in a patient with polymicrogyria. *Hum Mutat* 28: 356–364.

Chang BS, Ly J, Appignani B, Bodell A, Apse KA, Ravenscroft RS, et al. (2005) Reading impairment in the neuronal migration disorder of periventricular nodular heterotopia. *Neurology* 64: 799–803.

Colombo R, Bignamini AA, Carobene A, Sasaki J, Tachikawa M, Kobayashi K, et al. (2000) Age and origin of the FCMD 3′-untranslated-region retrotransposal insertion mutation causing Fukuyama-type congenital muscular dystrophy in the Japanese population. *Hum Genet* 107: 559–567.

D'Agostino MD, Bernasconi A, Das S, Bastos A, Valerio RM, Palmini A, et al. (2002) Subcortical band heterotopia (SBH) in males: clinical, imaging and genetic findings in comparison with females. *Brain* 125: 2507–2522.

Demyanenko GP, Tsai AY, Maness PF (1999) Abnormalities in neuronal process extension, hippocampal development, and the ventricular system of L1 knockout mice. *J Neurosci* 19: 4907–4920.

Dixon-Salazar T, Silhavy JL, Marsh SE, Louie CM, Scott LC, Gururaj A, et al. (2004) Mutations in the AHI1 gene, encoding Jouberin, cause Joubert syndrome with cortical polymicrogyria. *Am J Hum Genet* 75: 979–987.

Dobyns WB (1996) Absence makes the search grow longer. *Am J Hum Genet* 58: 7–16.

Dolk H (1991) The predictive value of microcephaly during the first year of life for mental retardation at seven years. *Dev Med Child Neurol* 33: 974–983.

Dupre N, Howard HC, Mathieu J, Karpati G, Vanasse M , Bouchard JP, et al. (2003) Hereditary motor and sensory neuropathy with agenesis of the corpus callosum. *Ann Neurol* 54: 9–18.

Eksioglu YZ, Scheffer IE, Cardenas P, Knoll J, DiMario F, Ramsby G, et al. (1996) Periventricular heterotopia: an X-linked dominant epilepsy locus causing aberrant cerebral cortical development. *Neuron* 16: 77–87.

Evans PD, Gilbert SL, Mekel-Bobrov N, Vallender EJ, Anderson JR, Vaez-Azizi LM, et al. (2005) Microcephalin, a gene regulating brain size, continues to evolve adaptively in humans. *Science* 309: 1717–1720.

Fish JL, Kosodo Y, Enard W, Paabo S, Huttner WB (2006) Aspm specifically maintains symmetric proliferative divisions of neuroepithelial cells. *Proc Natl Acad Sci U S A* 103: 10438–10443.

Fox JW, Lamperti ED, Eksioglu YZ, Hong SE, Feng Y, Graham DA, et al. (1998) Mutations in filamin 1 prevent migration of cerebral cortical neurons in human periventricular heterotopia. *Neuron* 21: 1315–1325.

Gleeson JG, Lin PT, Flanagan LA, Walsh CA (1999) Doublecortin is a microtubule-associated protein and is expressed widely by migrating neurons. *Neuron* 23: 257–271.

Granger EM, Masterton RB, Glendenning KK (1985) Origin of interhemispheric fibers in acallosal opossum (with a comparison to callosal origins in rat). *J Comp Neurol* 241: 82–98.

Hart AW, Morgan JE, Schneider J, West K, McKie L, Bhattacharya S, et al. (2006) Cardiac malformations and midline skeletal defects in mice lacking filamin A. *Hum Mol Genet* 15: 2457–2467.

Hattori M, Adachi H, Tsujimoto M, Arai H, Inoue K (1994) Miller–Dieker lissencephaly gene encodes a subunit of brain platelet-activating factor acetylhydrolase [corrected]. *Nature* 370: 216–218.

Hehr U, Hehr A, Uyanik G, Phelan E, Winkler J, Reardon W (2006) A filamin A splice mutation resulting in a syndrome of facial dysmorphism, periventricular nodular heterotopia, and severe constipation reminiscent of cerebro-fronto-facial syndrome. *J Med Ge[...]* 43: 541–5[...].

Hong SE, Shugart YY, Huang DT, Shahwan SA, Grant PE, Hourihane JO, et al. (2000) Autosomal recessive lissencephaly with cerebellar hypoplasia is associated with human RELN mutations. *Nat Genet* 26: 93–96.

Itoh K, Cheng L, Kamei Y, Fushiki S, Kamiguchi H, Gutwein P, et al. (2004) Brain development in mice lacking L1-L1 homophilic adhesion. *J Cell Biol* 165: 145–154.

Keays DA, Tian G, Poirier K, Huang GJ , Siebold J, Cleak J, et al. (2007) Mutations in alpha-tubulin cause abnormal neuronal migration in mice and lissencephaly in humans. *Cell* 128: 45–57.

Kitamura K, Yanazawa M, Sugiyama N, Miura H, Iizuka-Kogo A, Kusaka M, et al. (2002) Mutation of ARX causes abnormal development of forebrain and testes in mice and X-linked lissencephaly with abnormal genitalia in humans. *Nat Genet* 32: 359–369.

Koizumi H, Yamaguchi N, Hattori M, Ishikawa TO, Aoki J, Taketo MM, et al. (2003) Targeted disruption of intracellular type I platelet activating factor-acetylhydrolase catalytic subunits causes severe impairment in spermatogenesis. *J Biol Chem* 278: 12489–12494.

Kouprina N, Pavlicek A, Collins NK, Nakano M, Noskov VN, Ohzeki J, et al. (2005) The microcephaly ASPM gene is expressed in proliferating tissues and encodes for a mitotic spindle protein. *Hum Mol Genet* 14: 2155–2165.

Lee JS, Collins K, Brown A, Lee CH, Chung JH (2000) The function of BRCA1 in DNA damage response. *Cold Spring Harb Symp Quant Biol* 65: 547–552.

Leeflang EP, Marsh SE, Parrini E, Moro F, Pilz D, Dobyns WB, et al. (2003) Patient with bilateral periventricular nodular heterotopia and polymicrogyria with apparently balanced reciprocal translocation t(1;6)(p12;p12.2) that interrupts the mannosidase alpha, class 1A, and glutathione S-transferase A2 genes. *J Med Genet* 40: e128.

Li J, Lee WL, Cooper JA (2005) NudEL targets dynein to microtubule ends through LIS1. *Nat Cell Biol* 7: 686–690.

LoTurco JJ, Bai J (2006) The multipolar stage and disruptions in neuronal migration. *Trends Neurosci* 29: 407–413.

Mekel-Bobrov N, Gilbert SL, Evans PD, Vallender EJ, Anderson JR, Hudson RR, et al. (2005) Ongoing adaptive evolution of ASPM, a brain size determinant in *Homo sapiens. Science* 309: 1720–1722.

Michele DE, Barresi R, Kanagawa M, Saito F, Cohn RD, Satz JS, et al. (2002) Post-translational disruption of dystroglycan-ligand interactions in congenital muscular dystrophies. *Nature* 418 (6896): 417–422.

Moore SA, Saito F, Chen J, Michele DE, Henry MD, Messing A, et al. (2002) Deletion of brain dystroglycan recapitulates aspects of congenital muscular dystrophy. *Nature* 418: 422–425.

Mowat DR, Wilson MJ, Goossens M (2003) Mowat–Wilson syndrome. *J Med Genet* 40: 305–310.

Muntoni F (2004) Journey into muscular dystrophies caused by abnormal glycosylation. *Acta Myol* 23: 79–84.

Neal J, Apse K, Sahin M, Walsh CA, Sheen VL (2006) Deletion of chromosome 1p36 is associated with periventricular nodular heterotopia. *Am J Med Genet A* 140: 1692–1695.

Neitzel H, Neumann LM, Schindler D, Wirges A, Tonnies H, Trimborn M, et al. (2002) Premature chromosome condensation in humans associated with microcephaly and mental retardation: a novel autosomal recessive condition. *Am J Hum Genet* 70: 1015–1022.

Ozawa H, Osawa M, Nagai T, Sakura N (2006) Steroid sulfatase deficiency with bilateral periventricular nodular heterotopia. *Pediatr Neurol* 34: 239–241.

Parrini E, Ramazzotti A, Dobyns WB, Mei D, Moro F, Veggiotti P, et al. (2006) Periventricular heterotopia: phenotypic heterogeneity and correlation with Filamin A mutations. *Brain* 129: 92–1906.

Paul LK, Brown WS, Adolphs R, Tyszka JM, Richards L, Mukherjee P, et al. (2007) Agenesis of the corpus callosum: genetic, developmental and functional aspects of connectivity. *Nat Rev Neurosci* 8: 287–299.

Piao X, Chang BS, Bodell A, Woods K, Benzeev B, Topcu M, et al. (2005) Genotype–phenotype analysis of human frontoparietal polymicrogyria syndromes. *Ann Neurol* 58: 680–687.

Piao X, Hill RS, Bodell A, Chang BS, Basel-Vanagaite L, Straussberg R, et al. (2004) G protein-coupled receptor-dependent development of human frontal cortex. *Science* 303: 2033–2036.

Proud VK, Levine C, Carpenter NJ (1992) New X-linked syndrome with seizures, acquired micrencephaly, and agenesis of the corpus callosum. *Am J Med Genet* 43: 458–466.

Ramocki MB, Dowling J, Grinberg I, Kimonis VE, Cardoso C, Gross A, et al. (2003). Reciprocal fusion transcripts of two novel Zn-finger genes in a female with absence of the corpus callosum, ocular colobomas and a balanced translocation between chromosomes 2p24 and 9q32. *Eur J Hum Genet* 11: 527–534.

Richards L, Plachez C, Ren T (2004) Mechanisms regulating the development of the corpus callosum and its agenesis in mouse and human. *Clin Genet* 66: 276–289.

Robertson SP, Twigg SR, Sutherland-Smith AJ, Biancalana V, Gorlin RJ, Horn D, et al. (2003) Localized mutations in the gene encoding the cytoskeletal protein filamin A cause diverse malformations in humans. *Nat Genet* 33: 487–491.

Robin NH, Taylor CJ, McDonald-McGinn DM, Zackai EH, Bingham P, Collins KJ, et al. (2006) Polymicrogyria and deletion 22q11.2 syndrome: window to the etiology of a commoncortical malformation. *Am J Med Genet A* 140: 2416–2425.

Sarkisian MR, Bartley CM, Chi H, Nakamura F, Hashimoto-Torii K, Torii M, et al. (2006) MEKK4 signaling regulates filamin expression and neuronal migration. *Neuron* 52: 789–801.

Sheen VL, Dixon PH, Fox JW, Hong SE, Kinton L, Sisodiya SM, et al. (2001) Mutations in the X-linked filamin 1 gene cause periventricular nodular heterotopia in males as well as in females. *Hum Mol Genet* 10: 1775–1783.

Sheen VL, Ganesh VS, Topcu M, Sebire G, Bodell A, Hill RS, et al. (2004) Mutations in ARFGEF2 implicate vesicle trafficking in neural progenitor proliferation and migration in the human cerebral cortex. *Nat Genet* 36: 69–76.

Sheen VL, Jansen A, Chen MH, Parrini E, Morgan T, Ravenscroft R, et al. (2005) Filamin A mutations cause periventricular heterotopia with Ehlers–Danlos syndrome. *Neurology* 64. 254–262.

Sheen VL, Wheless JW, Bodell A, Braverman E, Cotter PD, Rauen KA, et al. (2003) Periventricular heterotopia associated with chromosome 5p anomalies. *Neurology* 60: 1033–1036.

Sheldon M, Rice DS, D'Arcangelo G, Yoneshima H, Nakajima K, Mikoshiba K, et al. (1997) Scrambler and yotari disrupt the disabled gene and produce a reeler-like phenotype in mice. *Nature* 389: 730–733.

Shen Y, Mani S, Donovan SL, Schwob JE, Meiri KF (2002) Growth-associated protein-43 is required for commissural axon guidance in the developing vertebrate nervous system. *J Neurosci* 22: 239–247.

Sherr EH (2003) The ARX story (epilepsy, mental retardation, autism, and cerebral malformations): one gene leads to many phenotypes. *Curr Opin Pediatr* 15: 567–571.

Sherr EH, Owen R, Albertson DG, Pinkel D, Cotter PD, Slavotinek AM, et al. (2005) Genomic microarray analysis identifies candidate loci in patients with corpus callosum anomalies. *Neurology* 65: 1496–1498.

Tai CY, Dujardin DL, Faulkner NE, Vallee RB (2002) Role of dynein, dynactin, and CLIP-170 interactions in LIS1 kinetochore function. *J Cell Biol* 156: 959–968.

Takanashi J, Barkovich AJ (2003) The changing MR imaging appearance of polymicrogyria: a consequence of myelination. *AJNR Am J Neuroradiol* 24: 788–793.

Tanaka T, Serneo H, Tseng C, Kulkarni AB, Tsai LH, Gleeson JG (2004) Cdk5 phosphorylation of doublecortin ser297 regulates its effect on neuronal migration. *Neuron* 41: 215–227.

Trimborn M, Bell SM, Felix C, Rashid Y, Jafri H, Griffiths PD, et al. (2004) Mutations in microcephalin cause aberrant regulation of chromosome condensation. *Am J Hum Genet* 75: 261–266.

Tsai JW, Chen Y, Kriegstein AR, Vallee RB (2005) LIS1 RNA interference blocks neural stem cell division, morphogenesis, and motility at multiple stages. *J Cell Biol* 170: 935–945.

van Bokhoven H, Celli J, van Reeuwijk J, Rinne T, Glaudemans B, van Beusekom E, et al. (2005) MYCN haploinsufficiency is associated with reduced brain size and intestinal atresias in Feingold syndrome. *Nat Genet* 37: 465–467.

van Reeuwijk J, Brunner HG, van Bokhoven H (2005a) Glyc-O-genetics of Walker–Warburg syndrome. *Clin Genet* 67: 281–289.

van Reeuwijk J, Janssen M, van den Elzen C, Beltran-Valero de Bernabe D, Sabatelli P, Merlini L, et al. (2005b) POMT2 mutations cause alpha-dystroglycan hypoglycosylation and Walker–Warburg syndrome. *J Med Genet* 42: 907–912.

Villard L, Nguyen K, Cardoso C, Martin CL, Weiss AM, Sifry-Platt M, et al. (2002) A locus for bilateral perisylvian polymicrogyria maps to Xq28. *Am J Hum Genet* 70: 1003–1038.

Wakefield JG, Bonaccorsi S, Gatti M (2001). The drosophila protein asp is involved in microtubule organization during spindle formation and cytokinesis. *J Cell Biol* 153: 637–648.

Wieck G, Leventer RJ, Squier WM, JansenA, Andermann E, Dubeau F, et al. (2005) Periventricular nodular heterotopia with overlying polymicrogyria. *Brain* 128: 2811–2821.

Woods CG, Bond J, Enard W (2005) Autosomal recessive primary microcephaly (MCPH): a review of clinical, molecular, and evolutionary findings. *Am J Hum Genet* 76: 717–728.

Xiang X, Osmani AH, Osmani SA, Xin M, Morris NR (1995) NudF, a nuclear migration gene in Aspergillus nidulans, is similar to the human LIS-1 gene required for neuronal migration. *Mol Biol Cell* 6: 297–310.

Yan W, Assadi AH, Wynshaw-Boris A, Eichele G, Matzuk MM, Clark GD (2003) Previously uncharacterized roles of platelet-activating factor acetylhydrolase 1b complex in mouse spermatogenesis. *Proc Natl Acad Sci U S A* 100: 7189–7194.

Yoshida A, Kobayashi K, Manya H, Taniguchi K, Kano H, Mizuno M, et al. (2001) Muscular dystrophy and neuronal migration disorder caused by mutations in a glycosyltransferase, POMGnT1. *Dev Cell* 1: 717–724.

Zweier C, Thiel CT, Dufke A, Crow YJ, Meinecke P, Suri M, et al. (2005) Clinical and mutational spectrum of Mowat–Wilson syndrome. *Eur J Med Genet* 48: 97–111.

18
PERINATAL ACQUIRED BRAIN INJURY

Jerome Y Yager and Pierre Gressens

Neonatal brain injury occurs commonly and encompasses a host of disorders that include acutely acquired insults such as hypoxia-ischemia, stroke, meningitis, seizures, and metabolic disorders, as well as disorders of a more chronic and/or developmental nature such as chromosomal abnormalities, cerebral dysgenesis, and fetal exposure to environmental toxins such as alcohol, various pharmaceuticals (e.g. phenytoin), or intrauterine congenital infections. Less apparent are remote antenatal insults that occur acutely *in utero* and create injury, but allow the fetus to recover by the time of birth. Although the characterization of these insults is in many ways theoretical, as they are not observed directly, their reality is manifested in the inevitable presentation of disability. Intrauterine insults of a cerebrovascular nature such as ischemic white matter injury, a pathogenic substrate of cerebral palsy, and neonatal stroke are classic examples.

This chapter focuses on acquired perinatal brain injuries, particularly those that result from vascular compromise to the brain. Perinatal brain injury refers to that which occurs around the time of birth and, according to the definition of the World Health Organization (WHO), commences at 22 weeks' gestation and ends at day 7 of postnatal life.

Presentation of these infants is recognized by one of two clinical phenotypes. Presentation following an 'acute' insult is recognized by a constellation of clinical symptoms and signs that have become known as neonatal encephalopathy. Neonatal encephalopathy is described as a clinically defined syndrome of disturbed neurologic function in the earliest days of life in the term infant, manifested by difficulty with initiating and maintaining respiration, depression of tone and reflexes, subnormal level of consciousness, and often by coincident seizures (Nelson and Leviton 1991, Leviton and Nelson 1992). Newborn infants who experience 'remote' antepartum insults often present normally at birth, without the need for resuscitation, and do not manifest symptoms or signs of their injury until later in life. In this regard, infants may present at 6 months to 1 year of age with early handedness, seizures, cerebral palsy, and/or abnormalities of development (Bouza et al. 1994a, 1994b, Sreenan et al. 2000, Oskoui and Shevell 2005). More recent evidence links the long-term sequelae of developmental disabilities and mental health issues with perinatal events of hypoxia-ischemia and chronic placental insufficiency (Cannon and Murray 1998, Cannon et al. 2002, Badawi et al. 2006).

The consequences of perinatal injury are broad in scope, with cerebral palsy being the most frequently recognized outcome measure for perinatal brain injury. Clearly, outcomes range among a spectrum of possible disorders such as mental retardation/intellectual disability (MR/ID), cerebral palsy, epilepsy, vision and hearing loss, learning difficulties, and school failure. In general, the neurodevelopmental disabilities account for 27% of health conditions causing disability in children (National Foundation for Brain Research (US)). Among children 0–4 years of age, developmental delay is the most common disability, whereas between 5 and 14 years of age, the specific learning disabilities, including attentional difficulties and dyslexia, rank first, and chronic conditions, which include cerebral palsy and epilepsy, rank second. Almost 30% of such children have more than one type of disability (Cossette and Duclos 2002).

EPIDEMIOLOGY

Term Neonatal Hypoxia-Ischemia

Intrapartum asphyxia resulting in neonatal encephalopathy remains an important and identifiable cause of brain injury (Levene et al. 1985, Nelson and Ellenberg 1998, Badawi et al. 1998a, 2005). Badawi et al. (1998a, 1998b) found intrapartum hypoxia alone to correlate with moderate to severe neonatal encephalopathy in 4% of their series of 164 term encephalopathic infants. However, hypoxia was a compounding feature for the production of neonatal encephalopathy in an additional 25% of cases. Overall incidence rates are in the range 4.6–7.7/1000 live births (Hull and Dodd 1992).

Significant sequelae of term neonatal hypoxia-ischemia may occur in as many as 50–75% of children (Dilenge et al. 2001), and as many as 10% of cases of idiopathic mental retardation may be related to intrapartum asphyxia (Roland and Hill 1997). Most infants with mild neonatal encephalopathy appear to develop normally. Only those with moderate to severe encephalopathy appear to have significant subsequent neurologic morbidity (Finer et al. 1981, Robertson and Finer 1985, Robertson et al. 1989, Selton and Andre 1997). The Western Australian Cerebral Palsy Registry found that 13% of survivors of term neonatal encephalopathy had cerebral palsy. Among those with cerebral palsy, neonatal encephalopathy was more likely to be severe, and if severe, the children were more likely to develop spastic or dyskinetic cerebral palsy, cognitive impairment (75%), or epilepsy (53%) (Badawi et al. 2005). However, 25% of those children with mild neonatal encephalopathy, who were initially categorized as being 'non-impaired' in early testing, tested more than one school grade level below expected when entering the school system (Robertston et al. 1989). Similarly, there were significantly higher incidences of neurodevelopmental impairment and learning difficulties at adolescence among term infants born with evidence of neonatal encephalopathy at birth, but who did not develop cerebral palsy (Moster et al. 2002). Certainly, others have found that, as children reach early childhood and adolescence, cognitive and behavioral difficulties become more apparent in those infants who have experienced a mild to moderate neonatal encephalopathy, even in the absence of cerebral palsy (Gonzalez and Miller 2006).

Increasingly, there is recognition that while intrapartum asphyxia contributes to an acute neonatal encephalopathy, the latter more likely results from a combination of events that can take place during the antepartum phase and culminates in a terminal intrapartum asphyxia (Badawi et al. 1998a, 1998b). In Badawi et al.'s excellent studies, terminal intrapartum events that significantly contributed to the development of cerebral palsy were maternal pyrexia, persistent occiput posterior, and acute intrapartum events (Badawi et al. 1998b). Antepartum factors during pregnancy that contributed to a moderate or severe encephalopathy were maternal thyroid disease, severe pre-eclampsia, moderate to severe bleeding, viral infection, not having had alcohol, an abnormal placenta, and factors leading to the delivery of growth restricted baby. The latter association increased the risk of neonatal encephalopathy by 40-fold. Interestingly, the findings from this study showed that intrapartum hypoxia alone contributed to 4% of the cases with neonatal encephalopathy, and antepartum factors alone contributed to 69% of cases; however, a combination of antepartum and intrapartum factors contributed to 25% of the cases of neonatal encephalopathy. The authors concluded that the causes of newborn encephalopathy are heterogeneous and frequently follow a causal pathway that begins during the antepartum period (Badawi et al. 1998a, 1998b).

More recently, the literature suggests a strong role for chorioamnionitis as one of the most frequent causes of acquired brain damage in the perinatal period (Toti and De Felice 2001). A recent meta-analysis of chorioamnionitis and cerebral palsy indicated a positive association among preterm and term infants, with a relative risk of 4.7 for the latter group (Wu and Colford 2000). In another study, it was found that the odds ratio in term infants for the development of cerebral palsy in cases of clinical chorioamnionitis was 9.3 (Grether and Nelson 1997). Similarly, maternal fever has been linked with an increased incidence of neonatal encephalopathy (Lieberman et al. 2000, Impey et al. 2001). Several reviews of the recent epidemiologic and cytokine literature clearly support a role for inflammation and/or cytokines in perinatal brain injury (Dammann and Leviton 1997a, 2000, Shalak and Perlman 2002).

PRETERM BRAIN INJURY
Preterm birth occurs in 5–11% of all births and is responsible for 70% of neonatal deaths, with survivors accounting for 75% of neonatal morbidity (Wen et al. 2004, Joseph et al. 2007). Survivors of preterm birth have a unique distribution of brain injury that focuses on the periventricular white matter which is referred to as periventricular leukomalacia (PVL). The peak gestational age for PVL is between

24 and 32 weeks' gestation, when 25% develop consequences of motor impairment or cerebral palsy, and upwards of 50% develop cognitive and specific learning disabilities by school age (Hack et al. 2005, Litt et al. 2005, Taylor et al. 2006). Several predisposing factors have been associated with the development of PVL. In this regard, vascular development has a major role in the selective regional distribution of PVL. Vessels derived largely from the middle cerebral artery penetrate the cerebral wall from the pial surface. These long penetrators are end arteries, and do not anastomose with surrounding vessels, leaving the region they supply specifically vulnerable to a reduction in perfusion pressure. These 'watershed regions' are most prominent in the less mature infant, accounting for the prevalence of this disease in the 24–32 week gestation neonate (Miyawaki et al. 1998, Inage et al. 2000).

In combination with the above, the cerebral circulation of the immature sick newborn is largely pressure-passive (Cavazzuti and Duffy 1982, Young et al. 1982). Subcortical white matter has consistently demonstrated a more profound selective hypoperfusion than other cortical gray matter structures (Kennedy et al. 1970). During recovery from acute illness, a reduction in blood flow is seen in the white matter structures of the preterm lamb, in contrast to a normalization of cerebral blood flow to brainstem and cortical gray matter (Szymonowicz et al. 1990). Similar alterations in cerebral blood flow have been documented in the distressed human neonate (Lou et al. 1979).

In this regard, a prominent neuropathogenic correlation has been made with impaired cerebrovascular regulation, whereby the periventricular white matter is supplied by non-collateralizing end zone short penetrating arteries, making the area intrinsically topographically vulnerable to ischemia (Takashima and Tanaka 1978, Altman and Volpe 1987). The role of inflammatory-mediated brain injury through maternal–fetal infection in the preterm infant is strongly supported by the animal literature which has shown an association between inflammatory mediators and white matter injury (Duncan et al. 2002, Yoon et al. 2003). Whether this is also the case for human preterm infants is unclear at present. The exposure to intrauterine infection as an independent risk factor for cerebral palsy has been examined, yet no association was found (Grethner et al. 2003). Similarly, the blood spots of very preterm infants were examined for numerous inflammatory cytokines but the concentrations found did not distinguish between those with later cerebral palsy and controls (Nelson et al. 2003). However, recently evidence has been presented of inflammatory cells and free-radical activity in the necrotic lesions of preterm infants in human pathologic series (Billards et al. 2006, Folkerth 2006).

PATTERNS OF BRAIN INJURY

Of importance in the understanding of injury to the immature newborn brain is the recognition that developmental processes are occurring rapidly over a short time interval (Volpe 2001). Hence, brain damage is expressed in different regions of the brain in a way that is dependent on the maturational stage in which they occur, the specific region of the brain affected, and the actual severity of injury. In this regard, neuroimaging studies have shown, through single time point and serial studies, the different patterns of brain injury and their evolution over time.

Preterm infants typically express injury within the periventricular white matter regions of the brain, whereas more mature infants express their injury within gray matter structures (Fig. 18.1). Within the context of the term newborn, two patterns of brain injury have been recognized (Pasternak and Gorey 1998, Miller et al. 2005). Magnetic resonance imaging studies have distinguished those infants with basal ganglia/thalamic lesions from those with predominantly cortical watershed injuries. Further, Miller et al. (2005) were able to distinguish these forms of injury clinically in that those infants with basal ganglia and/or thalamic damage were associated with significantly more severe neonatal signs including the need

Spectrum of Neuropathologic Injury to the Immature Brain
Pre-Term   **Term**

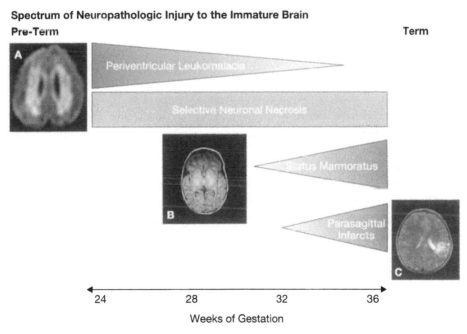

Fig. 18.1 Evolution of brain injury from 24 weeks' gestation to term. Patterns of brain injury evolve through periventricular leukomalacia (A), to injury of the basal ganglia (B), and parasagittal infarction (C). Magnetic resonance images depicting evolution of damage and change in relation to topographic sensitivity of the newborn brain to hypoxic-ischemic injury. (A) Diffusion weighted image of preterm infant depicting enhancement of white matter adjacent to lateral ventricles. (B and C) T1-weighted images of term infant indicating hyperintensity of deep gray matter nuclei (B) and peri-rolandic fissure (C), in keeping with hypoxic-ischemic injury to the more mature brain.

Photographs courtesy of Dr. Steven Miller.

for more intensive resuscitation, more severe encephalopathy, and more difficult to treat seizures. Congruent with this presentation, this latter pattern of injury was associated with a significantly more severe impairment of eventual motor and cognitive outcome.

Many of the original animal studies that had identified the pattern of perinatal brain injury to be both maturational and severity-dependent were carried out by Myers and his group in their model of ischemia in rhesus monkeys (Myers 1972a, 1972b, 1975, 1979). Although much more has been learned since these original studies, it is clear that the white matter of the preterm infant is predisposed to injury for topographic (vascular) and intrinsic (maturational) reasons. In the term infant, deep gray matter structures are more likely to be injured followed a 'near-complete pattern' or acute 'near-total' hypoxic-ischemic insult, whereas selective cortical injury occurs following a 'partial prolonged' hypoxic-ischemic pattern. These patterns follow the ontogenic sensitivity of the brain, with deeper structures being spared during incomplete ischemia.

MECHANISMS OF INJURY

The principal pathogenic mechanism underlying those patterns of brain injury described above is an impairment of cerebral blood flow, presumably resulting from an interruption of placental blood flow and gas exchange (Fig. 18.2). A curtailment of oxygen and glucose delivery results in brain cells shifting from aerobic to anaerobic patterns of glycolysis, which causes a rapid depletion of high-energy phosphate stores and an accumulation of lactic acid. The pursuant energy failure is associated with a shift in transmembrane potential, cell depolarization, and inactivation of the Na-K$^+$ ATPase pump resulting in cytotoxic edema.

Concurrent with these alterations, glutamate, the predominant excitatory amino acid, is released into the synaptic cleft and accumulates to known neurotoxic concentrations. Glutamate perpetuates neuronal swelling by enhancing the influx of sodium and chloride through voltage-gated channels and by causing a rapid elevation of intracellular Ca^{2+} (Rothman and Olney 1986, Choi 1988). In addition, glutamate induces free-radical production by depleting concentrations of glutathione, an endogenous free-radical scavenger. The increasing levels of intracellular Ca^{2+}, in concert with the accumulating 'energy debt,' promotes the initiation and facilitation of a cascade of catabolic processes culminating in eventual cell disintegration. This latter process results in the accumulation of free fatty acids secondary to membrane phospholipid turnover and the further production of excess free radicals.

There is an expanding role for the formation of oxygen free radicals in the pathogenesis of post-ischemic injury (Chan 1986, 2001). A free radical is a molecule that contains an uneven number of electrons, and is therefore inherently unstable. The major site of endogenous free-radical production is the mitochondria, where

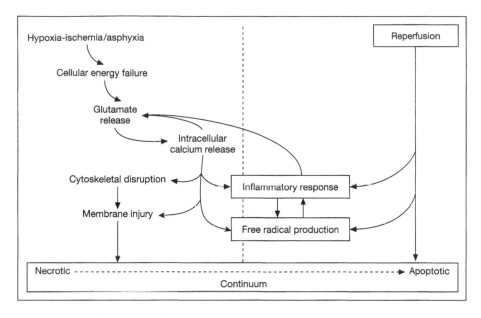

Fig. 18.2 Simplified diagram of pathophysiologic mechanisms involved in hypoxic-ischemic brain injury. Note the process of hypoxia-ischemia that triggers the cycle of events leading to cell death may take only minutes to hours, whereas reperfusion and the subsequent phase of recovery during which neuronal and glial injury continue lasts days to weeks.

Modified from Vannucci (1990) and Bona et al. (1999).

reactive intermediates arise from the oxygen used in the electron transport chain during the oxidation of substrates to form ATP and water. These intermediates interact with transition metals such as iron (Fe^{2+}), which mediate the dismutation of hydroxyl peroxide (H_2O_2) to result in the formation of the highly reactive hydroxyl radical (-OH). Pro-oxidant enzymes include (1) nitric oxide synthases, (2) cyclo-oxygenase, (3) xanthine dehydrogenase, (4) xanthine oxidase, (5) NADPH, and (6) myelo- and mono-peroxidases. Cells containing these enzymes include neurons, endothelium, astrocytes, as well as the inflammatory leukocytes and microglia/ macrophages (Chan 2001).

During ischemia and following resuscitation, reactive oxygen species (ROS) directly perpetuate brain injury by causing the disruption of cell membranes through lipid peroxidation, DNA damage, reduced glutamate reuptake, and inhibition of the sodium-potassium ATPase. Free radicals also contribute to the continued elevation of intracellular Ca^{2+}. The propagation of these events following hypoxic-ischemic insult results in the phenomenon of cell necrosis (Ginsberg et al. 1988, Fujimura et al. 1999a, 1999b, Chan 2001). Indirectly, more recent studies implicate mitochondria, apurinic/apyrimidinic endonuclease/redox factor-1 (APE/Ref-1), a DNA repair enzyme, and a transcription factor, nuclear factor κB (NF-κB), as major targets for ROS that lead to ischemic cell death through apoptosis (Fujimura et al. 1998, 1999a, 1999b, Chan 2001). In this regard, hypoxic-ischemic insults not only render the mitochondria dysfunctional, but also cause the release of cytochrome C into the cytoplasm. Here, cytochrome C activates a series of caspases leading to DNA fragmentation and apoptotic cell death (Zou et al. 1997). NF-κB and other transcription factors are regulated by the redox state of the cell (Dalton et al. 1999). Under conditions of ischemia or varying pro-inflammatory stimuli, NF-κB is activated and targets downstream inducible genes such as iNOS, COX-2, and cytokines, which are also involved in producing neuronal injury and the inflammatory response following cerebral ischemia (Yin and Juurlink 2000, Yrjanheikki et al. 2000).

Cytokines have a pivotal role in physiologic and pathologic conditions. In pathologic conditions, cytokines may be neurotoxic through their stimulation of microglia and astroglia to produce nitric oxide, ROS and excitatory amino acids. Additionally, tumor necrosis factor (TNF) may be directly toxic to neurons and glia (Merrill 1992). Cytokines, especially TNF, can also induce endothelial cells to promote the expression of adhesion molecules and enhance coagulant activity, further potentiating the cycle of ischemia, free radical production, and eventual cell death.

The inflammatory response to brain injury has been characterized by a predictable cycle of genomic responses (Bona et al. 1998, Ellison et al. 1999). Hence, in the first minutes following middle cerebral artery occlusion, c-fos, c-jun and other immediate early genes are transiently increased. This is followed by the heat-shock proteins (HSP-70, HSP-72) at 1–2 hours of recovery which lasts up to 2 days. The third wave of gene expression, peaking at about 12 hours after ischemia and lasting up to 5 days, largely comprises of the pro-inflammatory cytokines TNF-α, interleukins IL-1b and IL-6, and the anti-inflammatory cytokine IL-1ra. Chemokine expression is also elevated along with a host of various 'adhesion molecules' (ICAM-1, ELAM-1, P-selectin, CD11/CD18, and MAC-1). Not surprisingly, the noted elevation of inflammatory genes occurs in concert with the infiltration of inflammatory cells in the form of neutrophils, polymorphonuclear leukocytes, and monocytes/macrophages. In an apparent attempt to begin the process of repair, neurotrophic factors (NGF, BDNF, and p53) also appear at the site of injury. The inflammatory reaction not only contributes to lipid-membrane peroxidation, but also exacerbates the degree of tissue injury by further occluding blood flow with vascular plugging. Moreover, leukocytes enhance the generation of ROS which perpetuate the events leading to eventual necrosis or apoptosis (Blumenfeld et al. 1992, Beilharz et al. 1995, Hudome et al. 1997, Aden et al. 1999, Barone and Feuerstein 1999, Bona et al. 1999).

Cell death occurs via two separate pathways. The first, characterized by the loss of membrane integrity, signs of organelle damage, and loss of lysosomal contents, is consistent with 'necrosis.' The second, characterized by the preservation of membrane integrity, organelle structure, and lysosomal contents, but with over-all diminution of cell volume, chromatin condensation, and nuclear fragmentation, has been termed 'apoptosis.' This latter type of cell death appears to be a form of 'programmed cell death,' regulated by the Bcl-2 family of proteins which inhibit developmental cell death, and the group of Bax proteins which appear to be up-regulated in neurons destined to die. More recent evidence has also focused on the group of pro-enzymes knows as caspases, the final 'executioners' of apoptosis (MacManus and Linnik 1997, Eldadah and Faden 2000). Caspase activation occurs via both an extrinsic and an intrinsic pathway. The former is initiated by ligation of cell surface death receptors belonging to the TNF-α and Ras receptors, referred to as the death domain. Once this external complex is formed, the receptor–adapter complex binds pro-caspase 8 or 10. The intrinsic pathway is activated through the mitochondrial release of cytochrome C. As part of this regulatory process, the concentration of cellular ATP also influences the type of cell death chosen by the neuron. With complete ATP depletion necrosis occurs, whereas when ATP is only partially depleted, apoptosis is the mechanism of cell death. In that regard, it has been shown that low concentrations of glutamate caused cell death to occur within 16–24 hours, whereas high concentrations of glutamate caused death in 2–8 hours (Mattson and Furukawa 1996). These investigators found that the cell death caused by the lower concentrations of glutamate was morphologically apoptotic in nature, whereas those cells killed rapidly by the higher concentrations of glutamate were necrotic in appearance (Ferriero 2004, Perlman 2006).

Mechanisms Responsible for Maturational Sensitivities of the Newborn Infant's Brain

In addition to the predilection of deep gray matter of the term newborn infant to near-total ischemia, several animal studies have suggested that NADPH-diaphorase positive neurons are selectively spared during hypoxia-ischemia (Ferriero et al. 1988). Further studies by this same group of investigators went on to show that the concentration of NADPH-diaphorase containing neurons and hence the sparing of these neurons decreased with maturation. Thus, 7-day rat pups injected intrastriatally with quinolinic acid showed selective sparing of neurons, whereas 14-day rat pups and later ages similarly injected showed no such sparing (Ferriero et al. 1990). This line of investigation lends support for the intrinsic predisposition of the basal ganglia to injury in the term infant but not in the preterm infant, who may be protected by a higher concentration of NADPH-diaphorase positive neurons.

Significant advances have been made in the understanding of the intrinsic vulnerability of white matter to injury in the preterm infant. A series of studies have shown the maturation-dependent nature of white matter injury, suggesting that the stage of development that best coincides with vulnerability is the oligodendroglial precursors (preOLs). The decline in risk for white matter injury coincides with the onset of the mature differentiation of preOLs that initiates myelination (Back et al. 1998, 2001, 2002a, Back 2006).

At the cellular level, several investigators have shown a remarkable sensitivity of preOLs to excitotoxic injury (Oka et al. 1993, Yoshioka et al. 1996). When exposing differentiating oligodendroglia to 2mmol/l concentrations of L-glutamate a dramatic loss of cells (>90%) was observed compared with controls. Interestingly, the authors also showed that cell death was not caused by a receptor-mediated mechanism, but rather by a depletion of intracellular cysteine and a subsequent reduction in concentrations of glutathione, an important free-radical scavenger. Moreover, these investigators showed that the exquisite vulnerability of oligodendrocytes to free radical attack and cell death is maturation dependent (Yonezawa et al. 1996, Back et al. 1998). Support for the association of oxidative damage can be found in recent studies that found increased levels of isoprostanes in histopathologically confirmed cased of preterm infant with white matter injury (Back et al. 2005).

Increasingly, infectious and/or inflammatory markers are being identified as being associated with white matter disease in the newborn human. In a series of 483 singleton newborn infants, histologic chorioamnionitis was a significant predictor of periventricular echodensities (De Felice et al. 2001). In another clinical study, the relative risk of cerebral palsy in low birth weight infants was fourfold greater in those with a history of infection (Wheater and Rennie 2000). In a group of women with complicated preterm gestations, the amniotic fluid was prospectively evaluated and offspring with PVL identified on cranial ultrasound. Amniotic fluid concentrations of TNF, IL-1, and IL-6 were elevated in all infants with white matter lesions. Placental pathology also showed a higher incidence of chorioamnionitis in those with PVL than those without (Yoon et al. 1997a). Several reviews of the epidemiologic and cytokine literature clearly support a role for inflammation/cytokines in neonatal PVL (Dammann and Leviton 1997a, 1997b, 2000a, 2000b). In addition, several investigators (Yoon et al. 1997b, Kadhim et al. 2001, 2002, 2003) have identified cytokines (TNF, IL-6 and IL-1β) in the brains of autopsied infants with PVL.

ANIMAL MODELS OF BRAIN INJURY

The study of perinatal brain injury has seen tremendous recent advances. A number of different animal models have been adapted in the pursuit of enhancing our knowledge, particularly at the biochemical and molecular levels. In discussing this broad and complicated area it is not our intention to be all inclusive, but to focus on those models that have most accurately reflected the human condition of perinatal acquired brain injury in the term and preterm infant. In addition, we touch on the topic of animal models related to perinatal brain injury that have shown particular promise regarding the subsequent onset of some of the neurodevelopmental disabilities.

MONKEY

Although the primate is only infrequently utilized at the present time, the classic studies of Myers and colleagues (Myers 1972a 1972b, 1975, 1979, Brann 1975) categorized the pattern of neuronal injury into the patterns of brain injury that we see today with clinically available neuroimaging techniques. These studies further set the stage and framework for understanding the systemic and causative correlations with these injuries, allowing a more comprehensive understanding of the relationship of injury to timing and severity.

In these studies, term monkey fetuses were exposed to true asphyxia (cessation of respiratory gas exchange) by covering their heads with a rubber sac and clamping their umbilical cord at delivery. This led to an immediate rise in fetal blood pressure from an increase in peripheral vascular resistance, followed within 20 seconds by profound fetal bradycardia and an accompanying decline in arterial pressure. The blood pressure slowly falls to become pressure-passive at about 12–14 minutes post-insult. Despite this, the fetal heart rate remains at approximately 60 beats per minute for up to at least 35 minutes. In conjunction with these changes, there was a rapid decline in fetal oxygen content, a rise in carbon dioxide, and a fall in pH to approximately 6.9 during the first 12.5 minutes. At least 12 minutes of total asphyxia was required to produce *any* signs of neuropathologic injury. These results coincide with clinical studies that have looked at the duration of prolonged fetal heart rate deceleration required for neurologic morbidity, and found a period of at least 17 minutes was required before morbidity was seen (Leung et al. 1993). Neuropathologically, these monkey fetuses displayed damage predominantly within the brainstem.

In models of partial ischemia, monkey fetuses remained *in utero*, and mothers were manipulated such as to render them hypotensive. These studies indicated that the term fetus tolerated reductions in pO_2 to 30% of normal. However, when reduced to 10% of normal for periods of up to 5 hours, the fetuses became increasingly bradycardic, and hypotensive. Physiologically, they were profoundly hypoxic and acidemic with a pH <7.0. At birth they often displayed opisthotonus and decerebrate posturing as well as generalized convulsions. Pathologically, the brains showed widespread cortical tissue necrosis, and those who survived longer periods of time prior to sacrifice displayed evidence of parasagittal infarction and porencephaly.

Based on investigations over two decades, Myers and colleagues described four patterns of brain damage that related to the actual degree of hypoxia/anoxia and whether it was combined with acidemia. In addition to the cohorts described above, fetal term monkeys exposed to severe hypoxia, in the absence of acidemia, developed predominantly white matter injury, whereas those experiencing partial prolonged asphyxia combined with a terminal total asphyxial event experienced damage that focused on the basal ganglia and thalamus. Thus, both the clinical and pathologic changes produced in these term monkeys by various degrees of intrauterine asphyxia resemble closely the changes observed in perinatally damaged humans.

More recently, a model of PVL in the preterm baboon has been developed that closely resembles the pathologic substrate seen in the human preterm infant (Inder et al. 2004). In this regard, the authors found the ontogenic development of the baboon brain to be remarkably similar to that of the human, although slightly more advanced when it came to white matter development. The authors have subsequently pursued investigations involving the preterm delivery of fetal baboons at 125 days gestation (NB term 160 days), and perpetuated their survival in a 'baboon' intensive care setting for 14 days. Examination of their brains revealed white matter injury in 50% of the preterm delivered animals, with evidence of reactive astrogliosis and activated microglia. The location of the injury was predominantly in the area of the parietal and occipital lobes, often in accompaniment with ventriculomegaly. Gray matter injury was observed in 25%, with basal ganglia involvement in 6%. Overall, the findings were strikingly consistent with those recognized in the preterm human infant, indicating the strong role this model may have in future studies, particularly with respect to the investigation of potential therapeutic interventions.

SHEEP

Gray matter

The sheep has served as an effective large animal model for the study of perinatal asphyxia. Gunn and colleagues (Gunn et al. 1992, Mallard et al. 1992, 1993, Williams et al. 1992) described the neuropathologic consequences following umbilical cord occlusion in near-term fetal sheep. Brief 10-minute periods of cord occlusion resulted in transient asphyxia, accompanied by hypotension and bradycardia, together with prolonged neuronal depression on electroencephalogram (EEG). Histologically, areas of selective neuronal necrosis were found in the hippocampus. These studies were subsequently extended such that near-term sheep fetuses were exposed to repeated brief episodes of *in utero* hypoxia-ischemia for three 10-minute intervals, separated by 1 or 5 hours. The findings were compared with a single 30-minute episode of hypoxia-ischemia. Repeated episodes at 1-hour intervals resulted in a greater degree of neuronal injury; however, when separated by 5-hour intervals, the distribution of injury 'shifted' to involve the striatum almost exclusively. When episodes were repeated at much shorter intervals (every 2.5–5.0 minutes), but far more frequently (until arterial pH was 6.8), the damage was diffuse and extensive, causing infarction of the parasagittal cortex, thalamus, and cerebellum in 40% of the animals, and diffuse selective neuronal necrosis in the remainder (De Hann et al. 1997).

Experiments in which near-term fetal sheep were exposed to prolonged hypoxia-ischemia of 30, 60, or 120 minutes were carried out to correlate the duration of insult with histopathologic injury (Gunn et al. 1992). Uterine artery occlusion in this setting produced severe hypoxemia, hypercarbia, acidosis, and bradycardia. Neuronal injury in this model was inversely correlated with blood pressure during the insult, such that the lower the blood pressure the greater the damage, but interestingly no association was found with hypoxemia. Areas of greatest sensitivity included the parasagittal cortex, CA_{1-3} regions of the hippocampus, the striatum, and the thalamus, respectively.

White matter

In recent years there has been an increasing focus on models of periventricular white matter damage. In the sheep, this was first elucidated by Ting et al. (1983). These investigators developed a model whereby mid-gestational sheep fetuses (68–85 days' gestation – term 145 days) were exposed to 10% oxygen for 2 hours. Of the 38 sheep fetuses subjected to hypoxia, 29 were concomitantly rendered hypovolemic. Of the 38 fetuses, 10 died prior to delivery, and only 8 showed evidence of gross and microscopic brain injury. In that regard, hemispheric white matter was most severely damaged, with some brains showing evidence of hemorrhage and cystic degeneration. It should be noted that damage was also noted in the basal ganglia of these animals as well as the dorsolateral regions of the cortex, although to a lesser extent than the white matter damage observed. Of particular note was the finding that only those fetuses in whom the mean arterial blood pressure fell below 30mmHg showed actual brain damage, whereas none of those who maintained their blood pressure above this threshold did (irrespective of the actual degree of hypoxia experienced).

Petersson et al. (2002) detailed the neuropathologic injury to white matter in 126 day (0.85) gestation ovine fetuses following carotid artery occlusion for 30 minutes and recovery for either 48 or 72 hours. These investigators found both gray and white matter involvement; the latter was characterized by a reactive gliosis and the loss of myelin basic protein in the oligodendrocytes. The neuropathologic consequences of cerebral hypoperfusion for 30 minutes in 0.65 versus 0.9 term gestation fetal sheep was compared. These investigators confirmed the topographic specificity of white matter injury. However, both ages displayed parasagittal cortical damage and selective neuronal necrosis in the thalamus and striatum. The preterm fetuses developed subcortical infarcts with more rapidly evolving necrosis of the white matter than those closer to term (Reddy et al. 1998).

Most recently, several laboratories have developed models of white matter injury in sheep following systemic endotoxemia (Duncan et al. 2002, Mallard et al. 2003). In this regard, the use of systemic asphyxia or endotoxemia was compared for the induction of injury resembling PVL in fetal sheep that were 93–96 days of age or 0.65 of term gestation. Asphyxia was promoted by umbilical cord occlusion for 25 minutes, whereas systemic endotoxemia was caused by the IV injection of *Escherichia coli* lipoprotein polysaccharide (LPS). Interestingly, the white matter appeared particularly sensitive in both models as characterized by microglial infiltration, loss of oligodendroglia, and damage to astrocytes. In contrast, whereas systemic endotoxemia caused selective injury to white matter, umbilical cord occlusion was less specific and also resulted in neuronal necrosis in subcortical regions including the striatum and hippocampus.

A model of systemic injection of LPS over 5 days in fetal sheep at 0.65 of term gestation was also investigated. Following LPS injection, particularly over the first 2 days, there was an acute decrease in both mean arterial blood pressure and pO_2. This was accompanied by an increase in measured lactate and acidosis. Although statistically significant only over the first 2 days of injection, these data clearly show alterations to have occurred over 4 days of injection. Interestingly, these data indicate that the endotoxemia model of white matter injury is a model that combines both inflammation and ischemia as part of its pathophysiologic contribution to resulting white matter injury. It was also found that an elevation of IL-6 occurred during the first 6 hours of injection and there was a similar acute increase in TNF-α within the first 2 hours. Histopathologically, diffuse white matter injury was seen in the majority of animals with a specific periventricular involvement occurring in one-third.

The significant influence of endotoxin by administering LPS to 11 catheterized fetal sheep at 0.7 of term has been further investigated (Dalitz et al. 2003). The authors measured fetal cerebral blood flow and placental flow using microspheres. Their findings showed that while fetal cerebral blood flow did not decrease, oxygen delivery did. Specifically, both cortical and white matter oxygen delivery decreased by 36% and 28% of control at 4 and 8 hours post LPS injection, respectively. Placental blood flow decreased by 54% and 43% at 4 and 8 hours post injection. These data clearly support the role of infection in not only causing an inflammatory response, but also a hypoxic response.

Back and colleagues (Back 2006, Back et al. 2006, 2007) have elaborated on the mid-gestation (0.65 gestation) sheep as a model of PVL. In their extensive work, they have very clearly defined the maturation-dependent vulnerability of the developing oligodendroglial cell. In this regard, the sheep, at age 90–120 days (term gestation 145 days), coincides best with the 24–28 week gestation human fetus, and contains those white cells most susceptible to ischemic-induced injury. Consistent with this finding are cerebral blood flow studies indicating the selective vulnerability of the periventricular white matter to underperfusion.

RODENTS

By far the most commonly used animal for models of perinatal asphyxia is the rodent, most often the rat. In the immature animal, this model was introduced by Vannucci's group in the early 1980s and utilized the combination of unilateral common carotid artery ligation with 8% oxygen exposure in a 7-day rat pup (Rice et al. 1981). The authors described the pathologic consequences of this insult particularly within gray matter structures as columnar regions of selective neuronal necrosis through to overt infarction. Chronically, cystic infarction of the cerebral cortex may be seen within the distribution of the middle cerebral artery territory resembling the formation of a porencephalic cyst. Although the myelinogenic zones of vulnerability were discussed in this original paper, until recently these findings had largely been overlooked.

Gray matter

Perhaps one of the main advantages that the rodent model has to offer is that it has been so well characterized over the years (Vannucci 1990). In this regard, the 7-day rat pup has been variously likened to a 32–34 week human infant. The physiologic parameters of the model have shown that during the insult, the rat pup becomes hypoxic in combination with being hypocapneic as a result of hyperventilation. This results in a compensated metabolic acidosis and allows for a normal pH despite the lactic acidemia. Mean systemic blood pressure during the hypoxia-ischemic insult declines by approximately 25% (Welsh et al. 1982, Palmer et al. 1990). Regional cerebral blood flow measurements indicate a reduction of blood flow to 17–40% of control values, with those areas most vulnerable to damage displaying the lowest blood flow (Lyons et al. 1987, Vannucci et al. 1988). Cerebral metabolic correlates indicate a depletion of intracellular glucose, accompanying lactic acidosis, and a near-complete loss of high-energy phosphates within the hemisphere ipsilateral to the common carotid artery ligation (Palmer et al. 1990, Yager et al. 1991). During recovery, ATP replenishes rapidly, although this recovery is followed by a secondary decline within the first 24–48 hours of injury. The findings appear consistent with a relative lack of substrate (i.e. glucose) compared with oxygen as the underlying causative mechanism of cell death, in keeping with the findings that the contralateral hemisphere appears healthy although exposed to hypoxia in the absence of ischemia (Yager et al. 1991, 1992, 1996, Vannucci and Yager 1992, Yager and Thornhill 1997). Others have documented an increase, particularly in the striatum of excitatory amino acid release (Gordon et al. 1991), and the accumulation of intracellular calcium that arises during the terminus of the insult and into recovery phase (Vannucci et al. 2001). Pathologically, cerebral edema evolves over a period of several days, peaking at 72 hours in those animals ultimately having the most significant damage (Vannucci et al. 1993). Histologically, there is a gradation of injury observed which correlates in a linear fashion with the duration and severity of the insult (Towfighi et al. 1991, 1995, Vannucci et al. 1997). Hence, damage commences following 60 minutes of hypoxia-ischemia and progresses to produce overt infarction by 90 minutes. Neocortical damage often appears in a columnar distribution. There is also evidence of necrosis of the subcortical gray matter structures and periventricular myelinogenic zones.

Bona et al. (1999) have delineated the pro-inflammatory response that occurs during recovery in this model. In this regard, a distinctive IL-1 and TNF-α response was seen in the first 24 hours, accompanied by chemokines and macrophage inflammatory protein production. In the next phase, neutrophils transiently invade the lesion at 12–24 hours. This is followed by microglia/macrophages and astrocytes. The latter group persists for upwards of 42 days, with natural killer cells being evident from 24 hours and lymphocytes beginning to infiltrate the lesion at the end of the week following the initial insult. Cell death in this model persists for upwards of 2 weeks, particularly in the deep gray matter structures of the basal ganglia as apoptosis (Northington et al. 2001a, 2001b).

Several others have developed modifications of the Rice–Vannucci model. Renolleau et al. (1998, 1999) studied a model of transient unilateral hypoxic-ischemic injury in the 7-day rat and found that with reperfusion, the inflammatory response was much more robust and occurred in a shorter time frame, augmenting the extent of injury. Similar results were found by others (Ashwal et al. 1995, Derugin et al. 2000). Schwartz et al. (1992) utilized a model of bilateral common carotid artery ligation which they indicated produces a more uniform and severe neocortical infarction, of greater reproducibility to the unilateral model. Unfortunately, neuropathology was described at only 3 days of recovery and in our experience has an extremely high mortality rate beyond 72 hours (Yager et al., unpublished data).

White matter
As in the previously described models, recent years have seen the development of a number of rat models that focus on white matter injury. In our own laboratory, we have developed a model of transient bilateral common carotid artery ligation for periods of between 5 and 10 minutes. Assessment of the neuropathologic findings at 72 hours of recovery shows evidence of cystic infarction involving the periventricular regions of the brain reminiscent of those seen in PVL in the human neonate (Fig. 18.3) (Jelinski et al. 1999). Further elaboration of this model has shown that the cells most sensitive to the ischemic injury are O4 oligodendroglial progenitors, and in particular that they are especially sensitive to the development of ROS during reperfusion. Moreover, the white matter in this model shows particular sensitivity to cerebral blood flow in those regions that are damaged by this insult reveal abnormalities in reperfusion (suggesting pressure passivity) and a more prolonged exposure to repeated ischemia leads to abnormalities of autoregulation, despite a return to normal of cerebral blood flow, in surrounding undamaged gray matter areas.

Models of periventricular white matter injury involving a hypoxic-ischemic insult in the rat have also come from Uehara et al. (1999) who induced white matter injury following permanent bilateral common carotid artery ligation in P5 rats, and Cai et al. (2001) who studied permanent bilateral artery ligation induced

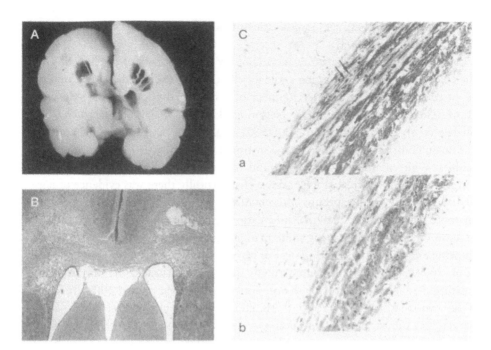

Fig. 18.3. (A) Coronal section of preterm born infant with marked evidence of cystic periventricular leukomalacia. Anterior coronal section in 10-day rat pup following bilateral common carotid artery ligation and hypoxia for 10 minutes, at 7 days of age. Note areas of cystic changes in periventricular white matter regions similar to those seen in human infant (B). Coronal section through corpus callosum stained for myelin basic protein in 7-day rat pup treated as in B. Upper section (a) is control. Note irregularity and disorganization of myelin basic protein in experimental animal (b).

in P1 rats and assessed the neuropathologic consequences on day P7 and P14 of recovery. The latter group of investigators found a reduction in the O4 staining cell, an increase in microglia and/or macrophages, and a reduction in myelin basic protein on P7, but not P14, specifically within white matter structures, again indicating the intrinsic enhanced vulnerability of the oligodendrocyte to damage from ischemia at this stage of cellular development.

Back and colleagues have led the way in the important work of delineating the rodent oligodendroglial cell lineage, and correlating this with that of the human in order to identify the correct timing for use of this model as one for human PVL. This group of investigators has identified that the window of vulnerability for white matter injury precedes myelination and coincides with a time when the late oligodendrocyte progenitor is the major target. In the human this coincides with the 24–32 week timeframe during which PVL most commonly occurs in the human, and the P2–P5 timeframe for the rat, recognizing that white matter injury does occur beyond these ages in both the human and rat (Back et al. 2001, 2002a, 2002b, Craig et al. 2003).

Infectious and inflammatory models of PVL have also been developed, given the epidemiologic data suggesting a role for clinical and subclinical chorioamnionitis as an etiologic factor in the development of cerebral palsy in children mentioned above (Grether and Nelson 1997, Nelson et al. 1998, Shalak and Perlman 2002, Shalak et al. 2002). Yoon et al. (1997) created an ascending infection and chorioamnionitis model using *E. coli* in timed pregnant (0.70 of term gestation) rabbits. White matter lesions were found in about half of those fetuses infected, but in none of those treated with saline. Histologically there was evidence of kary-orrhexis, and disorganization of white matter together with evidence of apoptosis. In more recent studies, maternal inoculation of rabbits with *E. coli* at 0.80 term gestation resulted in consistent white matter injury, with one-quarter of the brains showing evidence for the development of periventricular white matter cysts (Debillon et al. 2000, 2003a, 2003b). Interestingly, this study illustrated the importance of treating the pregnant rabbits with antibiotics as there was almost 100% mortality if no treatment was provided. In this model, focal white matter cysts, accom-panied by a robust inflammatory response and diffuse cell death, which mimic the white matter damage seen in very and extremely preterm infants, occur in the absence of a detectable neocortical inflammatory response.

The effects of ibotenate, a potent glutamate agonist, during various periods of gestation has been studied in both mouse and hamster models (Gressens et al. 1996). Newborn hamsters intracerebrally injected on P0 displayed neuronal migration dis-orders graded from nodular to extensive heterotopias which resembled the human dysgenetic features of lissencephaly and the double-cortex syndrome. Mice injected on P0 exhibited features of microgyria, and when injected on P5, after completion of neuronal migration of the cortical plate, ibotenate caused extensive neuronal loss in all cortical layers and the formation of porencephalic cysts resembling white mat-ter injury in the newborn human. These authors have subsequently utilized this model in the investigation of the underlying pathophysiology of perinatal brain injury and the application of numerous potential therapeutic interventions (Dommergues et al. 2003, Husson et al. 2005, Keller et al. 2006, Rangon et al. 2006).

This body of work by has been further illuminated by examining the effects of fetal growth restriction (FGR) on white matter injury in the preterm brain. In a first model, pregnant dams were exposed to chronic intrauterine hypoxia (10% O_2) from E5 to E20 (Baud et al. 2004). The FGR rat pups displayed typical white matter lesions that were consistent with those seen in PVL. In addition, there was an evolution of changes that were age-dependent, such that rat pups examined as early as E19 showed inflammatory changes in the white matter, with lesions developing most prominently at P3, and a delay in myelination being seen by P14 and tapering off by P21 (Table 18.1).

TABLE 18.1
Percentage and type of hypoxic injury in rat pups exposed to intrauterine chronic hypoxia.

Gestational age	White matter inflammation (%)	Focal white matter lesions (%)	Astrogliosis (%)	Myelination delay (%)
E19	80	0	Nd	Nd
P0	100	79	Nd	Nd
P3	100	94	0	Nd
P7	20	20	67	95
P14	0	0	100	100
P21	Nd	0	83	17

Nd, not determined.
Source: Modified from Baud et al. (2004) with permission.

Subsequent investigations utilized a model in unilateral uterine artery ligation to induce FGR (Olivier et al. 2005, 2007). Again, this model of FGR displayed white matter injury associated with an inflammatory response and increased apoptotic cell death. In addition, myelination remained defective even into adulthood. When the effects of unilateral uterine artery ligation on E17 was combined with an excitotoxic lesion on P5, investigators found that the white matter injury was found to be decreased in rat pups who were determined to have 'moderate FGR', but increased in those with severe FGR. The investigators concluded that this 'double-hit' model of white matter injury provides neuroprotection under conditions of moderate FGR as a result of a hypoxic preconditioning effect. However, the lack of protection in the rat pups with severe FGR suggests that there is a threshold beyond which damage may be too severe to recover. This substantiates at a basic level the role of multiple events in the causation of perinatal brain injury that has been evident in clinically oriented studies (Badawi et al. 1998b).

CLINICAL MANIFESTATIONS OF PERINATAL BRAIN INJURY AND OUTCOME
TERM INFANTS
Perinatal brain injuries may manifest themselves acutely, around the time of birth, or not be evident for weeks and months subsequently. Substantiating this latter statement are studies that showed that non-disabled survivors of neonatal encephalopathy at 8 years of age were significantly more likely to be a school grade below their peers (Robertson et al. 1989). In the Western Australian Cohort of children with moderate or severe neonatal encephalopathy, only 10% of patients had cerebral palsy, although a total of 39% had poor outcomes, suggesting that the majority of children had abnormalities of development in the absence of

cerebral palsy (Dixon et al. 2002). In this regard, the hypothesis has been put forward that while many infants may experience their initial insult antepartum, a considerable number have contributory events around the time of birth during the intrapartum delivery (Badawi et al. 1998b). This latter conceptual model also suggests that many cases of neonatal encephalopathy may result from a 'double-hit' phenomenon, in that the newborn may experience an antepartum vascular, infectious, or toxic exposure, leading to initial physiologic compromise that 'primes the pump' for further instability and additional exposure to insults during the birth and delivery process (Badawi et al. 1998b, Gressens 2000, Baud et al. 2004).

Asphyxial events that significantly compromise the fetus around the time of birth present themselves as a neonatal encephalopathy. Neonatal encephalopathy has been described as 'a clinically defined syndrome of disturbed neurologic function in the earliest days of life in the term infant, manifested by difficulty with initiating and maintaining respiration, depression of tone and reflexes, subnormal level of consciousness, and often by seizures' (Nelson and Leviton 1991). The appearance and grouping of this constellation of symptoms are used to categorize the grading of Stages I, II, and III, which correspond to 'mild,' 'moderate,' and 'severe' encephalopathy. Evidence would suggest that the current classification of neonatal encephalopathy has important prognostic validity. Specifically, neonates classified as 'mild' are very (indeed, highly) likely to have a favorable outcome, whereas evidence of 'severe' encephalopathy in the first week is associated with a high rate of later severe disability or death. In the National Collaborative Perinatal Study, only 31% of those infants with an Apgar score of 3 or less at 20 minutes survived to 7 years of age. However, among the survivors, 80% were free of major disability (Nelson and Ellenberg 1981).

Longitudinal studies to school age by Robertson et al. (1989) and Robertson and Grace (1992) in Canada and recent studies in Australia (Badawi et al. 1998b, 2001, 2005) have provided compelling evidence for this association between the extremes of neonatal encephalopathy and outcome. However, those with 'moderate' encephalopathy (i.e. the majority of infants) may or may not have long-term developmental sequelae, posing a significant prognostic difficulty in the clinical situation. In this regard, 21% of infants with moderate hypoxic-ischemic encephalopathy were found to be disabled at 3.5 years of age, with decreased motor and cognitive skills and lower IQs (Robertson et al. 1989). By 8 years of age, the mortality rate of infants born with hypoxic-ischemic encephalopathy was 13%. Of the 75% who survived, 16% had impairments which included cerebral palsy, blindness, cognitive delay, epilepsy, and hearing loss. Children with a history of moderate encephalopathy were significantly more impaired in intellect, visuomotor integration, and receptive language, as well as school readiness areas of reading, spelling, and mathematics. Interestingly, even those children who were free of motor impairment were twice as likely to be more than one grade level below their peer group (Robertson and Finer 1985, Robertson et al. 1989).

In children with perinatal or remote stroke, very little information currently exists on outcome. In a review of cases of cerebral infarction detected at term, 46 children had been followed for a mean of 3.5 years. One-third of the children were normal. Cerebral palsy was present in 22 of the 46, with cognitive impairment compromising 19 of the children. Only 8 of the 31 who were impaired had a single disability, with 23 having multiple impairments. Predictors of abnormal outcome were the presence of an abnormal neurologic examination at discharge, and the presence of neonatal seizures (Sreenan et al. 2000). An excellent recent review of perinatal stroke indicates a greater likelihood of hemiplegic cerebral palsy in those children with presumed or remote perinatal stroke compared to those with acute infarction (Glomb et al. 2001, Kirton and deVeber 2006).

Neonatal seizures are the most common expression of underlying acute neurologic compromise presenting in the newborn period. It is part of the symptom complex that makes up moderate or severe grades of neonatal encephalopathy. One of the outstanding current controversies relates to whether or not these seizures, in conjunction with hypoxic-ischemic encephalopathy, actually contributes to brain injury. Increasingly, it is becoming clear through animal experimentation and clinical research that seizures in the newborn period, which complicate an underlying hypoxic-ischemic encephalopathy, contribute to the brain damaging effects of the latter (Ben-Ari and Holmes 2006). In a series of experiments utilizing the Rice–Vannucci model of hypoxia-ischemia in the 7-day rat pup, an experimental induction of prolonged clinical and electrographically documented seizures was performed. Our studies revealed a marked increase, particularly in hippocampal cell death, in those animals in whom hypoxia-ischemia was complicated by seizures, compared with those who did not have seizures (Wirrell et al. 2001). Further examination of the model revealed that in those pups in whom damage was exacerbated, energy reserves did not recover to the same extent between hypoxia-ischemia and seizure onset as it did in controls. Furthermore, extracellular concentrations of glutamate levels were elevated significantly above both control values and those in whom damage was not worsened (Yager et al. 2002). Exacerbation of brain injury by seizures complicating hypoxia-ischemia in the newborn has been substantiated in humans (Miller et al. 2002). Utilizing magnetic resonance spectroscopy investigators have shown that in newborn infants experiencing seizures there was an independently associated increase in lactate:choline ratio as a function of anaerobic metabolism, and NAA:choline ratio as a function of cell compromise in both the basal ganglia and intervascular zone of babies experiencing seizures compared to those who did not.

Although cerebral palsy has been the sine quo non outcome measure for perinatal asphyxia, it is now increasingly evident that with longer follow-up, other deficits may arise in children who do not express cerebral palsy as a phenotype. In a recent review of the animal and human literature, substantiating findings in both were noted which clearly indicate that not all perinatal asphyxia results in cerebral palsy, but rather a complex and evolving host of outcomes that spans both cognitive and motor aspects of development (Gonzalez and Miller 2006). Certainly, additional literature further suggests a role for perinatal asphyxia in such mental health disorders including autism and schizophrenia. In a review of 239 surviving infants who had experienced term moderate or severe neonatal encephalopathy, 12 (5%) were given a diagnosis of autism spectrum disorder by 5 years of age, compared with only 5 of 563 controls (0.08%). According to these data, newborn infants who had experienced neonatal encephalopathy at birth were 5.9 times more likely to have autism than the general population (Badawi et al. 2006). Others have found a strong association between fetal growth restriction, which strongly predisposes to perinatal hypoxia, and later onset schizophrenia (Nilsson et al. 2005).

PRETERM INFANTS

The most commonly quoted neurologic sequela of preterm birth is cerebral palsy. It is more common as gestational age decreases and has a higher prevalence amongst boys than girls. The overall reported incidence is approximately 10% of preterm born infants and is most often either of the spastic or dyskinetic type. However, as in the term infant, developmental delay takes on an increasingly important role, particularly as children move towards their school years (Marlow et al. 2005). In a study of 308 surviving preterm infants born before 26 weeks' gestation, 241 were assessed at a median age of 6 years, and compared with 160 term born classmates. The rates of severe, moderate, and mild disability were 22%, 24%, and 34%, respectively. Disabling cerebral palsy was present in 12% of children. Among children who were diagnosed with severe disability at 30 months of age, abnormalities persisted to 6 years of age in 86% (Marlow et al. 2005). Adverse outcomes were consistently noted more often in boys (Wood et al. 2005). A meta-analysis of preterm outcomes revealed significantly lower cognitive scores than the term born comparison group, and that these scores were directly proportional to declining gestational age. Moreover, these infants had higher rates of attention-deficit disorder, and internalizing and externalizing behaviors (Bhutta et al. 2002). European studies show that upwards of 20% of very low birth weight infants are behind 1 year in school, and an additional 25% require special education intervention by the time they are 8–9 years of age (Hille et al. 1994). Interestingly, one-third of infants born between 32 and 36 weeks' gestation (near term) also require special educational needs (Huddy et al. 2001). Although few studies exist on adult survivors, 242 such survivors of very low birth weight were found to have significantly lower IQs, were less likely to be enrolled in post-secondary education, and were less likely to finish high school than their peers (Hack et al. 2002, Hack and Klein 2006).

Finally, a recent study reviewed the outcomes of those preterm infants with unilateral cerebral lesions, as assessed by ultrasound in the neonatal period. In this cohort of patients, verbal function was preserved over non-verbal function irrespective of the lateralization of the lesion. Furthermore, children with left-sided lesions did more poorly than those children with right-sided lesions at 8 years of age (Vollmer et al. 2006).

THERAPEUTIC INTERVENTIONS (NOW AND IN THE FUTURE)
Neuroprotection of the neonatal brain continues to be a health care priority given the lifelong emotional and economic repercussions of perinatal brain injury. In this regard, early childhood costs for each child born preterm has been estimated at a cumulative expense of approximately $26 000 for the first 3–5 years of life (Clements et al. 2007). Recent advances in our understanding of the mechanisms involved in both term and preterm brain injury has provided tremendous opportunities to identify potential targets in the biologic substrate for neuroprotection that may ameliorate long-term outcome (Saliba et al. 2007).

Several neuroprotective approaches are currently being tested in animal models of perinatal brain damage, including drugs targeting glutamate receptors, inflammation, cytokines, macrophage activation, antioxidant molecules, and strategies such as growth factors and stem cell replacement therapy, all aimed at improving post-lesional plasticity and tissue repair (Gressens et al. 2005, Bouslama et al. 2006, Keller et al. 2006, Gressens 2007, Saliba et al. 2007, Sizonenko et al. 2007, Welin et al. 2007). Certainly the most promising of these approaches currently available has been the introduction of post-ischemic hypothermia. In this regard, a National Institutes of Health sponsored trial of post-ischemic hypothermia randomized term infants diagnosed with perinatal asphxia to receive whole-body cooling at 33.5°C for 72 hours. At follow-up of 18–22 months, 102 and 106 infants had been enrolled in the experimental and control groups, respectively. Death or moderate or severe disability occurred in 44% of the hypothermic group compared to 62% of controls and the rate of cerebral palsy was also significantly reduced to 19% in hypothermics compared to 30% of controls (Shankaran et al. 2005). The CoolCap Study Group reported on their group of 218 patients, 110 of whom received head cooling to a rectal temperature of 34–35°C for 72 hours within 6 hours of asphyxia. This group did not find a significant difference in death or severe disability at 18 months follow-up between the hypothermic and control groups (Gluckman et al. 2005). The smaller clinical trial of Eicher et al. (2005) examined the effect of whole-body cooling to 33°C for 48 hours within 6 hours of asphyxia. Patient data were analyzed at 12 months. In this study, severely abnormal motor scores were recorded in 64% of normothermic controls compared to 24% of the hypothermic group. Combined outcome of death or severe disability revealed significantly fewer adverse outcomes in the hypothermic group (52%) than the normothermic controls (Eicher et al. 2005).

Numerous therapeutic agents have been shown to be neuroprotective in animal models of neonatal stroke and hypoxia-ischemia (Ferriero 2005). However, translating these agents to the clinical setting is challenging, given that many of the agents utilized in the treatment of hypoxia-ischemia or stroke may be detrimental to the developing nervous system. In this regard, several studies have shown the detrimental effects of therapeutically developed pharmaceuticals on the maturing nervous system (Ikonomidou et al. 2001, Gressens et al. 2002, Ikonomidou and Turski 2002, Olney et al. 2002, 2004a, 2004b, Bittigau et al. 2003). Olney and colleagues used MK801, a well-known N-methyl-D-aspartate (NMDA) antagonist, to protect the 7-day rat pup brain from traumatic injury. Surprisingly, these investigators found that not only did this potentially therapeutic drug not protect the brain, but it actually increased the amount of damage observed (Ikonomidou et al. 1999, Pohl et al. 1999). The same has held true for a host of other pharmaceutical agents that have routinely been used in the care of newborn infants. Fredriksson et al. (2004) found profound neurodegeneration of cells in the cortex of 10-day-old mice (equivalent to term newborn infants) following exposure to ketamine, a frequently used anesthetic agent. When tested 2 months later, these mice showed severe deficits of learning, memory retention, and habituation, the latter being a good indication of 'anxiety.'

CONCLUSIONS

Perinatal brain injury continues to be common and contributes to lifelong emotional and economic hardship for numerous children and families. The last two decades have seen an explosion of knowledge regarding the underlying etiology of this disorder and this has provided the theoretical underpinning and rational for potential targeted interventions. Post-ischemic hypothermia is the first step in this direction, although much work still needs to be done and there remains as yet no effective intervention for those most severely affected. Given the sensitivity of the developing brain to the toxic effect of medications currently used in the treatment of hypoxia-ischemia and stroke, new approaches will clearly need to take into account their safety and efficacy, not only for the developing human brain but perhaps for the pregnant mother as well. In the long run, it is very likely that we will witness the development of multifaceted interventions that pinpoint various aspects of the complex and interdigital pathophysiologic cycle leading to cell death. In this regard, interventions that provide benefit to preterm babies will likely be preventive in nature, and as such require the treatment of mother as well as baby. Clearly, these will be numerous challenges to biologically modifying outcomes for the next decade.

REFERENCES

Aden U, Bona E, Hagberg H, Fredholm BB (1999) Changes in c-fos mRNA in the neonatal rat brain following hypoxic ischemia. *Neurosci Lett* 180: 91–95.

Altman DI, Volpe JJ (1987) Cerebral blood flow in the newborn infant: measurement and role in the pathogenesis of periventricular and intraventricular hemorrhage. *Adv Pediatr* 34: 111–138.

Ashwal S, Cole DJ, Osborne S, Osborne TN, Pearce WJ (1995) A new model of neonatal stroke: reversible middle cerebral artery occlusion in the rat pup. *Pediatr Neurol* 12: 191–196.

Back SA, (2006) Perinatal white matter injury: the changing spectrum of pathology and emerging insights into pathogenetic mechanisms. *Ment Retard Dev Disabil Res Rev* 12: 129–140.

Back SA, Gan X, Li Y, Rosenberg PA, Volpe JJ (1998) Maturation-dependent vulnerability of oligodendrocytes to oxidative stress-induced death caused by glutathione depletion. *J Neurosci* 18: 6241–6253.

Back SA, Han BH, Luo NL, Chricton CA, Xanthoudakis S, Tam J, et al. (2002a) Selective vulnerability of late oligodendrocyte progenitors to hypoxia-ischemia. *J Neurosci* 22: 455–463.

Back SA, Luo NL, Borenstein NS, Levine JM, Volpe JJ, Kinney HC (2001) Late oligodendrocyte progenitors coincide with the developmental window of vulnerability for human perinatal white matter injury. *J Neurosci* 21: 1302–1312.

Back SA, Luo NL, Borenstein NS, Volpe JJ, Kinney HC (2002b) Arrested oligodendrocyte lineage progression during human cerebral white matter development: dissociation between the timing of progenitor differentiation and myelinogenesis. *J Neuropathol Exp Neurol* 61: 197–211.

Back SA, Luo NL, Mallinson RA, O'Malley JP, Wallen LD, Frei B, et al. (2005) Selective vulnerability of preterm white matter to oxidative damage defined by F2-isoprostanes. *Ann Neurol* 58: 108–120.

Back SA, Riddle A, Hohimer AR (2006) Role of instrumented fetal sheep preparations in defining the pathogenesis of human periventricular white-matter injury. *J Child Neurol* 21: 582–589.

Back SA, Riddle A, McClure MM (2007) Maturation-dependent vulnerability of perinatal white matter in premature birth. *Stroke* 38: 724–730.

Badawi N, Dixon G, Felix JF, Keogh JM, Petterson B, Stanley FJ, et al. (2006) Autism following a history of newborn encephalopathy: more than a coincidence? *Dev Med Child Neurol* 48: 85–89.

Badawi N, Felix JF, Kurinczuk JJ, et al. (2005) Cerebral palsy following term newborn encephalopathy: a population-based study. *Dev Med Child Neurol* 47: 293–298.

Badawi N, Keogh JM, Dixon G, Kurinczuk JJ (2001) Developmental outcomes of newborn encephalopathy in the term infant. *Indian J Pediatr* 68: 527–530.

Badawi N, Kurinczuk JJ, Keogh JM, Alessandri LM, O'Sullivan F, Burton PR, et al. (1998a) Antepartum risk factors for newborn encephalopathy: the Western Australian case–control study. *BMJ* 317: 1549–1553.

Badawi N, Kurinczuk JJ, Keogh JM, Alessandri LM, O'Sullivan F, Burton PR, et al. (1998b) Intrapartum risk factors for newborn encephalopathy: the Western Australian case–control study. *BMJ* 317: 1554–1558.

Badawi N, Watson L, Petterson B, Blair E, Slee J, Haan E, et al. (1998c) What constitutes cerebral palsy? *Dev Med Child Neurol* 40: 520–527.

Barone FC, Feuerstein GZ (1999) Inflammatory mediators and stroke: new opportunities for novel therapeutics. *J Cereb Blood Flow Metab* 19: 819–834.

Baud O, Daire JL, Dalmaz Y, Fontaine RH, Krueger RC, Sebag G, et al. (2004) Gestational hypoxia induces white matter damage in neonatal rats: a new model of periventricular leukomalacia. *Brain Pathol* 14: 1–10.

Beilharz EJ, Williams CE, Dragunow M, Sirimanne ES, Gluckman PD (1995) Mechanisms of delayed cell death following hypoxic-ischemic injury in the immature rat: evidence for apoptosis during selective neuronal loss. *Brain Res Mol Brain Res* 29: 1–14.

Ben-Ari Y, Holmes GL (2006) Effects of seizures on developmental processes in the immature brain. *Lancet Neurol* 5: 1055–63.

Benjelloun N, Renolleau S, Represa A, Ben-Ari Y, Charriaut-Marlangue C (1999) Inflammatory responses in the cerebral cortex after ischemia in the P7 neonatal rat. *Stroke* 30: 1916–1924.

Bhutta AT, Cleves MA, Casey PH, Cradock MM, Anand KJ (2002) Cognitive and behavioral outcomes of school-aged children who were born preterm: a meta-analysis. *JAMA* 288: 728–737.

Billiards SS, Haynes RL, Folkerth RD, Trachtenberg FL, Liu LG, Volpe JJ, et al. (2006) Development of microglia in the cerebral white matter of the human fetus and infant. *J Comp Neurol* 497: 199–208.

Bittigau P, Sifringer M, Ikonomidou C (2003) Antiepileptic drugs and apoptosis in the developing brain. *Ann N Y Acad Sci* 993: 103–114.

Blumenfeld KS, Welsh FA, Harris VA, Pesenson MA (1992) Regional expression of c-fos and heat shock protein-70 mRNA following hypoxia-ischemia in immature rat brain. *J Cereb Blood Flow Metab* 12: 987–995.

Bona E, Andersson AL, Blomgren K, Gilland E, Puka-Sundvall M, Gustafson K, et al. (1999) Chemokine and inflammatory cell response to hypoxia-ischemia in immature rats. *Pediatr Res* 45: 500–509.

Bona E, Hagberg H, Løberg EM, Bågenholm R, Thoresen M (1998) Protective effects of moderate hypothermia after neonatal hypoxia-ischemic: short and long term outcome. *Pediatr Res* 43: 738–745.

Bouslama M, Chauvière L, Fontaine RH, Matrot B, Gressens P, Gallego J (2006) Treatment-induced prevention of learning deficits in newborn mice with brain lesions. *Neuroscience* 141: 795–801.

Bouza H, Dubowitz LM, Rutherford M, Pennock JM (1994a) Prediction of outcome in children with congenital hemiplegia: a magnetic resonance imaging study. *Neuropediatrics* 25: 60–66.

Bouza H, Rutherford M, Acolet D, Pennock JM, Dubowitz LM (1994b) Evolution of early hemiplegic signs in full-term infants with unilateral brain lesions in the neonatal period: a prospective study. *Neuropediatrics* 25: 201–207.

Brann AW (1975) Central nervous system findings in the newborn monkey following severe *in utero* partial asphyxia. *Neurology* 25: 327–338.

Cai Z, Pang Y, Xiao F, Rhodes PG (2001) Chronic ischemia preferentially causes white matter injury in the neonatal rat brain. *Brain Res* 898: 126–135.

Cannon M, Murray RM (1998) Neonatal origins of schizophrenia. *Arch Dis Child* 78: 1–3.

Cannon TD, van Erp TG, Rosso IM, Huttunen M, Lönnqvist J, Pirkola T, et al. (2002) Fetal hypoxia and structural brain abnormalities in schizophrenic patients, their siblings, and controls. *Arch Gen Psychiatry* 59: 35–41.

Cavazzuti M, Duffy TE (1982) Regulation of local cerebral blood flow in normal and hypoxic newborn dogs. *Ann Neurol* 11: 247–257.

Chan PH (1996) Role of oxidants in ischemic brain damage. *Stroke* 27: 1124–1129.

Chan PH (2001) Reactive oxygen radicals in signaling and damage in the ischemic brain. *J Cereb Blood Flow Metab* 21: 2–14.

Choi DW (1988) Glutamate neurotoxicity and diseases of the nervous system. *Neuron* 1: 623–634.

Clements KM, Barfield WD, Ayadi MF, Wilber N (2007) Preterm birth-associated cost of early intervention services: an analysis by gestational age. *Pediatrics* 119: e866–874.

Cossette L, Duclos E (2002) *A Profile of Disability in Canada, 2001.* Ottawa: Statistics Canada, Housing, Family and Social Statistics Division December, 2002.

Craig A, Ling Luo N, Beardsley DJ, Wingate-Peatse N, Walker DW, Hohimer AR, et al. (2003) Quantitative analysis of perinatal rodent oligodendrocyte lineage progression and its correlation with human. *Exp Neurol* 181: 231–240.

Dalitz P, Harding R, Rees SM, Cock ML (2003) Prolonged reductions in placental blood flow and cerebral oxygen delivery in preterm fetal sheep exposed to endotoxin: possible factors in white matter injury after acute infection. *J Soc Gynecol Investig* 10: 283–290.

Dalton TP, Shertzer HG, Puga A (1999) Regulation of gene expression by reactive oxygen. *Annu Rev Pharmacol Toxicol* 39: 67–101.

Dammann O, Leviton A (1997a) Maternal intrauterine infection, cytokines, and brain damage in the preterm newborn. *Pediatr Res* 42: 1–8.

Dammann O, Leviton A (1997b) Does prepregnancy bacterial vaginosis increase a mother's risk of having a preterm infant with cerebral palsy? *Dev Med Child Neurol* 39: 836–840.

Dammann D, Leviton, A (2000a) Placental cytokine expression in preterm labor and the fetal inflammatory response. *Cytokine* 12: 176–7.

Dammann O, Leviton A (2000b) Role of the fetus in perinatal infection and neonatal brain damage. *Curr Opin Pediatr* 12: 9–104.

De Felice C, Toti P, Laurini RN, Stumpo M, Picciolini E, Todros T, et al. (2001) Early neonatal brain injury in histologic chorioamnionitis. *J Pediatr* 138: 101–104.

De Haan HH, Gunn AJ, Williams CE, Gluckman PD (1997) Brief repeated umbilical cord occlusions cause sustained cytotoxic cerebral edema and focal infarcts in near-term fetal lambs. *Pediatr Res* 41: 96–104.

Debillon T, Gras-Leguen C, Leroy S, Caillon J, Rozé JC, Gressens P (2003a) Patterns of cerebral inflammatory response in a rabbit model of intrauterine infection-mediated brain lesion. *Brain Res Dev Brain Res* 145: 39–48.

Debillon T, Gras-Leguen C, Verielle V, Caillon J, Rozé JC, Gressens P (2003b) Effect of maternal antibiotic treatment on fetal periventricular white matter cell death in a rabbit intrauterine infection model. *Acta Paediatr* 92: 81–86.

Debillon T, Gras-Leguen C, Verielle V, Winer N, Caillon J, Rozé JC, et al. (2000) Intrauterine infection induces programmed cell death in rabbit periventricular white matter. *Pediatr Res* 47: 736–742.

Derugin N, Wendland M, Muramatsu K, Roberts TP, Gregory G, Ferriero DM, et al. (2000) Evolution of brain injury after transient middle cerebral artery occlusion in neonatal rats. *Stroke* 31: 1752–1761.

Dilenge M-E, Majnemer A, Shevell MI (2001) Long-term developmental outcome of asphyxiated term neonates. *J Child Neurol* 16: 781–792.

Dixon G, Badawi N, Kurinczuk JJ, Keogh JM, Silburn SR, Zubrick SR, et al. (2002) Early developmental outcomes after newborn encephalopathy. *Pediatrics* 109: 26–33.

Dommergues MA, Plaisant F, Verney C, Gressens P (2003) Early microglial activation following neonatal excitotoxic brain damage in mice: a potential target for neuroprotection. *Neuroscience* 121: 619–628.

Duncan JR, Cock ML, Scheerlinck JP, Westcott KT, McLean C, Harding R, et al. (2002) White matter injury after repeated endotoxin exposure in the preterm ovine fetus. *Pediatr Res* 52: 941–949.

Eicher DJ, Wagner CL, Katikaneni LP, Hulsey TC, Bass WT, Kaufman DA, et al. (2005) Moderate hypothermia in neonatal encephalopathy: efficacy outcomes. *Pediatr Neurol* 32: 11–17.

Eldadah Y, Faden AI (2000) Caspase pathways, neuronal apoptosis, and CNS injury. *J Neurotrauma* 17: 811–829.

Ellison JA, Barone FC, Feuerstein GZ (1999) Matrix remodeling after stroke: de novo expression of matrix proteins and integrin receptors. *Ann N Y Acad Sci* 890: 204–222.

Ferriero DM (2004) Neonatal brain injury. *N Engl J Med* 351: 1985–1995.

Ferriero DM (2005) Protecting neurons. *Epilepsia* 46: 45–51.

Ferriero DM, Arcavi LJ, Sagar SM, McIntosh TK, Simon RP (1988) Selective sparing of NADPH-diaphorase neurons in neonatal hypoxia-ischemia. *Ann Neurol* 24: 670–676.

Ferriero DM, Arcavi LJ, Simon RP (1990) Ontogeny of excitotoxic injury to nicotinamide adenine dinucleotide phosphate diaphorase reactive neurons in the neonatal rat striatum. *Neuroscience* 36: 417–424.

Finer NN, Robertson CM, Richards RT, Pinnell LE, Petters KL (1981) Hypoxic-ischemic encephalopathy in terms neonates: perinatal factors and outcome. *J Pediatr* 98: 112–117.

Folkerth RD (2006) Periventricular leukomalacia: overview and recent findings. *Pediatr Dev Pathol* 9: 3–13.

Fredriksson A, Archer T, Alm H, Gordh T, Eriksson P (2004) Neurofunctional deficits and potentiated apoptosis by neonatal NMDA antagonist administration. *Behav Brain Res* 153: 367–376.

Fujimura M, Morita-Fujimura Y, Kawase M, Chan PH (1999a) Early decrease of apurinic/apyrimidinic endonuclease expression after transient focal cerebral ischemia in mice. *J Cereb Blood Flow Metab* 19: 495–501.

Fujimura M, Morita-Fujimura Y, Murakami K, Kawase M, Chan PH (1998) Cytosolic redistribution of cytochrome c after transient focal cerebral ischemia in rats. *J Cereb Blood Flow Metab* 18: 1239–1247.

Fujimura M, Morita-Fujimura Y, Narasimhan P, Copin JC, Kawase M, Chan PH (1999b) Copper-zinc superoxide dismutase prevents the early decrease of apurinic/apyrimidinic endonuclease and subsequent DNA fragmentation after transient focal cerebral ischemia in mice. *Stroke* 30: 2408–2415.

Ginsberg MD, Watson BD, Busto R, Yoshida S, Prado R, Nakayama H, et al. (1988) Peroxidative damage to cell membranes following cerebral ischemia: a cause of ischemic brain injury? *Neurochem Pathol* 9: 171–193.

Gluckman PD, Wyatt JS, Azzopardi D, Ballard R, Edwards AD, Ferriero DM, et al. (2005) Selective head cooling with mild systemic hypothermia after neonatal encephalopathy: multicentre randomised trial. *Lancet* 365: 663–670.

Golomb MR, MacGregor DL, Domi T, Armstrong DC, McCrindle BW, Mayank S, et al. (2001) Presumed pre- or perinatal arterial ischemic stroke: risk factors and outcomes. *Ann Neurol* 50: 163–168.

Gonzalez FF, Miller SP (2006) Does perinatal asphyxia impair cognitive function without cerebral palsy? *Arch Dis Child Fetal Neonatal Ed* 91: F454–459.

Gordon KE, Simpson J, Statman D, Silverstein FS (1991) Effects of perinatal stroke on striatal amino acid efflux in rats studied with *in vivo* microdialysis. *Stroke* 22: 928–932.

Gressens P (2000) Mechanisms and disturbances of neuronal migration. *Pediatr Res* 48: 725–730.

Gressens P (2007) Drug companies and neuroprotection of the newborn: any hope for a love story? *Acta Paediatr* 96: 485–486.

Gressens P, Marret S, Evrard P (1996) Developmental spectrum of the excitotoxic cascade induced by ibotenate: a model of hypoxic insults in fetuses and neonates. *Neuropathol Appl Neurobiol* 22: 498–502.

Gressens P, Rogido M, Paindaveine B, Sola A (2002) The impact of neonatal intensive care practices on the developing brain. *J Pediatr* 140: 646–53.

Gressens P, Spedding M, Gigler G, Kertesz S, Villa P, Medja F, et al. (2005) The effects of AMPA receptor antagonists in models of stroke and neurodegeneration. *Eur J Pharmacol* 519: 58–67.

Grether JK, Nelson KB (1997) Maternal infection and cerebral palsy in infants of normal birth weight. *JAMA* 278: 207–211.

Grether JK, Nelson KB, Walsh E, Willoughby RE, Redline RW (2003) Intrauterine exposure to infection and risk of cerebral palsy in very preterm infants. *Arch Pediatr Adolesc Med* 157: 26–32.

Gunn AJ, Parer JT, Mallard EC, Williams CE, Gluckman PD (1992) Cerebral histologic and electrocorticographic changes after asphyxia in fetal sheep. *Pediatr Res* 31: 486–491.

Hack M, Flannery DJ, Schluchter M, Cartar L, Borawski E, Klein N (2002) Outcomes in young adulthood for very-low-birth-weight infants. *N Engl J Med* 346: 149–157.

Hack M, Klein N (2006) Young adult attainments of preterm infants. *JAMA* 295: 695–696.

Hack M, Taylor HG, Drotar D, Schluchter M, Cartar L, Andreias L, et al. (2005) Chronic conditions, functional limitations, and special health care needs of school-aged children born with extremely low-birth-weight in the 1990s. *JAMA* 294: 318–325.

Hille ET, den Ouden AL, Bauer L, van den Oudenrijn C, Brand R, Verloove-Vanhorick SP (1994) School performance at nine years of age in very premature and very low birth weight infants: perinatal risk factors and predictors at five years of age. Collaborative Project on Preterm and Small for Gestational Age (POPS) Infants in The Netherlands. *J Pediatr* 125: 426–434.

Huddy CL, Johnson A, Hope PL (2001) Educational and behavioural problems in babies of 32–35 weeks gestation. *Arch Dis Child Fetal Neonatal Ed* 85: F23–28.

Hudome S, Palmer C, Roberts RL, Mauger D, Housman C, Towfighi J (1997) The role of neutrophils in the production of hypoxic-ischemic brain injury in the neonatal rat. *Pediatr Res* 41: 607–616.

Hull J, Dodd KI (1992) Falling incidence of hypoxic-ischaemic encephalopathy in term infants. *Br J Obstet Gynaecol* 99: 386–391.

Husson I, Rangon CM, Lelievre V, Bemelmans AP, Sachs P, Mallet J, et al. (2005) BDNF-induced white matter neuroprotection and stage-dependent neuronal survival following a neonatal excitotoxic challenge. *Cereb Cortex* 15: 250–261.

Ikonomidou C, Bittigau P, Koch C, Genz K, Hoerster F, Felderhoff-Mueser U, et al. (2001) Neurotransmitters and apoptosis in the developing brain. *Biochem Pharmacol* 62: 401–405.

Ikonomidou C, Bosch F, Miksa M, Bittigau P, Vöckler J, Dikranian K, et al. (1999) Blockade of NMDA receptors and apoptotic neurodegeneration in the developing brain. *Science* 283: 70–74.

Ikonomidou C, Turski L (2002) Why did NMDA receptor antagonists fail clinical trials for stroke and traumatic brain injury? *Lancet Neurol* 1: 383–386.

Impey L, Greenwood C, Sheil O, MacQuillan K, Reynolds M, Redman C (2001) The relation between pre-eclampsia at term and neonatal encephalopathy. *Arch Dis Child Fetal Neonatal Ed* 85: F170–172.

Inage YW, Itoh M, Takashima S (2000) Correlation between cerebrovascular maturity and periventricular leukomalacia. *Pediatr Neurol* 22: 204–208.

Inder T, Neil J, Yoder B, Rees S (2004) Non-human primate models of neonatal brain injury. *Semin Perinatol* 28: 396–404.

Jelinski SE, Yager JY, Juurlink BHJ (1999) Preferential injury of oligodendroblasts by a short hypoxic-ischemic insult results in long-term effects on myelination. *Brain Res* 815: 150–153.

Joseph KS, Huang L, Liu S, Ananth CV, Allen AC, Sauve R, et al. (2007) Reconciling the high rates of preterm and postterm birth in the United States. *Obstet Gynecol* 109: 813–822.

Kadhim H, Tabarki B, De Prez C, Rona AM, Sebire G (2002) Interleukin-2 in the pathogenesis of perinatal white matter damage. *Neurology* 58: 1125–1128.

Kadhim H, Tabarki B, De Prez C, Sebire G (2003) Cytokine immunoreactivity in cortical and subcortical neurons in periventricular leukomalacia: are cytokines implicated in neuronal dysfunction in cerebral palsy? *Acta Neuropathol (Berl)* 105: 209–216.

Kadhim H, Tabarki B, Verellen G, De Prez C, Rona AM, Sebire G (2001) Inflammatory cytokines in the pathogenesis of periventricular leukomalacia. *Neurology* 56: 1278–1284.

Keller M, Yang J, Griesmaier E, Gorna A, Sarkozy G, Urbanek M, et al. (2006) Erythropoietin is neuroprotective against NMDA-receptor-mediated excitotoxic brain injury in newborn mice. *Neurobiol Dis* 24: 357–366.

Kennedy C, Grave GD, Jehle JW, Sokoloff L (1970) Blood flow to white matter during maturation of the brain. *Neurology* 20: 613–618.

Kirton A, deVeber G (2006) Cerebral palsy secondary to perinatal ischemic stroke. *Clin Perinatol* 33: 367–386.

Leung AS, Leung EK, Paul RH (1993) Uterine rupture after previous cesarean delivery: maternal and fetal consequences. *Am J Obstet Gynecol* 169: 945–950.

Levene ML, Kornberg J, Williams THC (1985) The incidence and severity of post-asphyxial encephalopathy in full-term infants. *Early Hum Dev* 11: 21–26.

Leviton A, Nelson KB (1992) Problems with definitions and classifications of newborn encephalopathy. *Pediatr Neurol* 8: 85–90.

Lieberman E, Lang J, Richardson DK, Frigoletto FD, Heffner HJ, Cohen A (2000) Intrapartum maternal fever and neonatal outcome. *Pediatrics* 105: 8–13.

Litt J, Taylor HG, Klein N, Hack M (2005) Learning disabilities in children with very low birthweight: prevalence, neuropsychological correlates, and educational interventions. *J Learn Disabil* 38: 130–141.

Lou HC, Lassen NA, Friis-Hansen B (1979) Impaired autoregulation of cerebral blood flow in the distressed newborn infant. *J Pediatr* 94: 118–121.

Lyons DT, Vasta F, Vannucci RC (1987) Autoradiographic determination of regional cerebral blood flow in the immature rat. *Pediatr Res* 21: 471–476.

MacManus JP, Linnik MD (1997) Gene expression induced by cerebral ischemia: and apoptotic perspective. *J Cereb Blood Flow Metab* 17: 815–832.

Mallard C, Welin AK, Peebles D, Hagberg H, Kjellmer I (2003) White matter injury following systemic endotoxemia or asphyxia in the fetal sheep. *Neurochem Res* 28: 215–223.

Mallard EC, Gunn AJ, Williams CE, Johnston BM, Gluckman PD (1992) Transient umbilical cord occlusion causes hippocampal damage in the fetal sheep. *Am J Obstet Gynecol* 167: 1423–1430.

Mallard EC, Williams CE, Gunn AJ, Gunning MI, Gluckman PD (1993) Frequent episodes of brief ischemia sensitize the fetal sheep brain to neuronal loss and induce striatal injury. *Pediatr Res* 33: 61–65.

Marlow N, Wolke D, Bracewell MA, Samara M (2005) Neurologic and developmental disability at six years of age after extremely preterm birth. *N Engl J Med* 352: 9–19.

Mattson MP, Furukawa K (1996) Programmed cell life: anti-apoptotic signaling and therapeutic strategies for neurodegenerative disorders. *Restor Neurol Neurosci* 9: 191–205.

Merrill JE (1992) Tumor necrosis factor alpha, interleukin 1 and related cytokines in brain development: normal and pathological. *Dev Neurosci* 14: 1–10.

Miller SP, Ramaswamy V, Michelson D, Barkovich AJ, Holshouser B, Wycliffe N, et al. (2005) Patterns of brain injury in term neonatal encephalopathy. *J Pediatr* 146: 453–460.

Miller SP, Weiss J, Barnwell A, Ferriero DM, Latol-Hajnal B, Ferrer-Rogers A, et al. (2002) Seizure-associated brain injury in term newborns with perinatal asphyxia. *Neurology* 58: 542–548.

Miyawaki T, Matsui K, Takashima S (1998) Developmental characteristics of vessel density in the human fetal and infant brains. *Early Hum Dev* 53: 65–72.

Moster D, Lie RT, Markestad T (2002) Joint association of Apgar scored and early neonatal symptoms with minor disabilities at school age. *Arch Dis Child Fetal Neonatal Ed* 86: F16–21.

Myers RE (1972a) Brain damage induced by umbilical cord compression at different gestational ages in monkeys. In: Goldsmith EI, Moor-Jankowski J (eds) *Second Conference on Experimental Medicine and Surgery in Primates*. New York: S. Karger, pp 394–425.

Myers RE (1972b) Two patterns of perinatal brain damage and their conditions of occurrence. *Am J Obstet Gynecol* 112: 246–276.

Myers RE (1975) Four patterns of perinatal brain damage and their conditions of occurence in primates. *Adv Neurol* 10: 223–234.

Myers RE (1979) A unitary theory of causation of anoxic and hypoxic brain pathology. *Adv Neurol* 26: 195–213.

Nelson KB, Dambrosia JM, Grether JK, Phillips TM (1998) Neonatal cytokines and coagulation factors in children with cerebral palsy. *Ann Neurol* 44: 665–675.

Nelson KB, Ellenberg JH (1981) Apgar scores as predictors of chronic neurologic disability. *Pediatrics* 68: 36–44.

Nelson KB, Ellenberg JH (1998) Antecedents of cerebral palsy: multivariate analysis of risk. *N Eng J Med* 315: 81–86.

Nelson KB, Grether JK, Dambrosia JM, Walsh E, Kohler S, Satyanarayana G, et al. (2003) Neonatal cytokines and cerebral palsy in very preterm infants. *Pediatr Res* 53: 600–607.

Nelson KB, Leviton A (1991) How much of neonatal encephalopathy is due to birth asphyxia? *Am J Dis Child* 145: 1325–1331.

Nilsson E, Stalberg G, Lichtenstein P, Cnattingius S, Olausson PO, Hultman CM (2005) Fetal growth restriction and schizophrenia: a Swedish twin study. *Twin Res Hum Genet* 8: 402–408.

Northington FJ, Ferriero DM, Flock DL, Martin LJ (2001) Delayed neurodegeneration in neonatal rat. thalamus after hypoxia-ischemia is apoptosis. *J Neurosci* 21: 1931–1938.

Northington FJ, Ferriero DM, Graham EM, Traystman RJ, Martin LJ (2001) Early neurodegeneration after hypoxia-ischemia in neonatal rat Is necrosis while delayed neuronal death is apoptosis. *Neurobiol Dis* 8: 207–219.

Oka A, Belliveau MJ, Rosenberg PA, Volpe JJ (1993) Vulnerability of oligodendroglia to glutamate: pharmacology, mechanisms, and prevention. *J Neurosci* 13: 1441–53.

Olivier P, Baud O, Bouslama M, Evrard P, Gressens P, Verney C (2007) Moderate growth restriction: deleterious and protective effects on white matter damage. *Neurobiol Dis* 26: 253–263.

Olivier P, Baud O, Evrard P, Gressens P, Verney C (2005) Prenatal ischemia and white matter damage in rats. *J Neuropathol Exp Neurol* 64: 998–1006.

Olney JW, Wozniak DF, Jevtovic-Todorovic V, Farber NB, Bittigau P, Ikonomidou C (2002) Drug-induced apoptotic neurodegeneration in the developing brain. *Brain Pathol* 12: 488–498.

Olney JW, Young C, Wozniak DF, Ikonomidou C, Jevtovic-Todorovic V (2004a) Anesthesia-induced developmental neuroapoptosis. Does it happen in humans? *Anesthesiology* 101: 273–275.

Olney JW, Young C, Wozniak DF, Jevtovic-Todorovic V, Ikonomidou C (2004b) Do pediatric drugs cause developing neurons to commit suicide? *Trends Pharmacol Sci* 25: 135–139.

Oskoui M, Shevell MI (2005) Profile of pediatric hemiparesis. *J Child Neurol* 20: 471–476.

Palmer C, Brucklacher RM, Christensen MA, Vannucci RC (1990) Carbohydrate and energy metabolism during the evolution of hypoxic-ischemic brain damage in the immature rat. *J Cereb Blood Flow Metab* 10: 227–235.

Pasternak JF, Gorey MT (1998) The syndrome of acute near-total intrauterine asphyxia in the term infant. *Pediatr Neurol* 18: 391–398.

Perlman JM (2006) Summary proceedings from the neurology group on hypoxic-ischemic encephalopathy. *Pediatrics* 17: S28–33.

Petersson KH, Stopa EG, Faris RA, Sadowska GB, Hanumar RC, Stonestreet BS (2002) White matter injury after cerebral ischemia in ovine fetuses. *Pediatr Res* 51: 68–76.

Pohl D, Bittigau P, Ishimaru MJ, Stadthaus D, Hubner C, Olney JW, et al. (1999) N-methyl-D-aspartate antagonists and apoptotic cell death triggered by head trauma in developing rat brain. *Proc Natl Acad Sci U S A* 96: 2508–2513.

Rangon CM, Dicou E, Goursaud S, Mounien L, Jégou S, Janet T, et al. (2006) Mechanisms of VIP-induced neuroprotection against neonatal excitotoxicity. *Ann N Y Acad Sci* 1070: 512–517.

Reddy K, Guan J, Marks K, Bennet L, Gunning M, Gunn A, et al. (1998) Maturational change in the cortical response to hypoperfusion injury in the fetal sheep. *Pediatr Res* 43: 674–682.

Renolleau S, Aggoun-Zouaoui D, Ben-Ari Y, Charriaut-Marlangue C (1998) A model of transient unilateral focal ischemia with reperfusion in the P7 neonatal rat: morphological changes indicative of apoptosis. *Stroke* 29: 1454–1460; discussion 61.

Rice JE, Vannucci RC, Brierley JB (1981) The influence of immaturity on hypoxic-ischemic brain damage in the rat. *Ann Neurol* 9: 131–41.

Robertson C, Finer N (1985) Term infants with hypoxic-ischemic encephalopathy: outcome at 3.5 years. *Dev Med Child Neurol* 27: 473–484.

Robertson CM, Finer NN, Grace MG (1989) School performance of survivors of neonatal encephalopathy associated with birth asphyxia at term. *J Pediatr* 114: 753–760.

Robertson CM, Grace MG (1992) Validation of prediction of kindergarten-age school-readiness scores of nondisabled survivors of moderate neonatal encephalopathy in term infants. *Can J Public Health* 83: S51–57.

Roland EH, Hill A (1997) How important is perinatal asphyxia in the causation of brain injury? *Ment Retard Dev Disabil Res Rev* 3: 22–27.

Rothman SM, Olney JW (1986) Glutamate and the pathophysiology of hypoxic-ischemic brain damage. *Ann Neurol* 19: 105–111.

Saliba E, Favrais G, Gressens P (2007) Neuroprotection of the newborn: from bench to cribside. *Semin Fetal Neonatal Med* 12: 239–240.

Schwartz PH, Massarweh WF, Vinters HV, Wasterlain CG (1992) A rat model of severe neonatal hypoxic-ischemic brain injury. *Stroke* 23: 539–546.

Selton D, Andre M (1997) Prognosis of hypoxic-ischaemic encephalopathy in full-term newborns: value of neonatal electroencephalopathy. *Neuropediatrics* 28: 276–280.

Shalak LF, Laptook AR, Jafri HS, Ramilo O, Perlman JM (2002) Clinical chorioamnionitis, elevated cytokines, and brain injury in term infants. *Pediatrics* 110: 673–680.

Shalak LF, Perlman JM (2002) Infection markers and early signs of neonatal encephalopathy in the term infant. *Ment Retard Dev Disabil Red Rev* 8: 4–9.

Shankaran S, Laptook AR, Ehrenkranz RA, Tyson JE, McDonald SA, Donovan EF, et al. (2005) Whole-body hypothermia for neonates with hypoxic-ischemic encephalopathy. *N Engl J Med* 353: 1574–1584.

Sizonenko SV, Bednarek N, Gressens P (2007) Growth factors and plasticity. *Semin Fetal Neonatal Med* 12: 241–249.

Sreenan C, Bhargava R, Robertson CM (2000) Cerebral infarction in the term newborn: clinical presentation and long-term outcome. *J Pediatr* 137: 351–355.

Szymonowicz W, Walker AM, Yu VY, Stewart ML, Cannata J, Cussen L (1990) Regional cerebral blood flow after hemorrhagic hypotension in the preterm, near-term, and newborn lamb. *Pediatr Res* 28: 361–366.

Takashima S, Tanaka K (1978) Development of cerebrovascular architecture and its relationship to periventricular leukomalacia. *Arch Neurol* 35: 11–16.

Taylor HG, Klein N, Drotar D, Schluchter M, Hack M (2006) Consequences and risks of <1000-g birth weight for neuropsychological skills, achievement, and adaptive functioning. *J Dev Behav Pediatr* 27: 459–469.

Ting P, Yamaguchi S, Bacher JD, Killens RH, Myers RE (1983) Hypoxic-ischemic cerebral necrosis in mid-gestational sheep fetuses: physiopathologic correlations. *Exp Neurol* 80: 227–245.

Toti P, De Felice C (2001) Chorioamnionitis and fetal/neonatal injury. *Biol Neonate* 79: 201–204.

Towfighi J, Yager JY, Housman C, Vannucci RC (1991) Neuropathology of remote hypoxic-ischemic damage in the immature rat. *Acta Neuropathol* 81: 578–587.

Towfighi J, Zec N, Yager J, Housman C, Vannucci RC (1995) Temporal evolution of neuropathological changes in an immature rat model of cerebral hypoxia-ischemia (HI): A light microscopic study. *Acta Neuropathol* 90: 375–386.

Uehara H, Yoshioka H, Kawase S, Nagai H, Ohmae T, Hasegawa K, et al. (1999) A new model of white matter injury in neonatal rats with bilateral carotid artery occlusion. *Brain Res* 837: 213–220.

Vannucci RC (1990) Experimental biology of cerebral hypoxia-ischemia: relation to perinatal brain damage. *Pediatr Res* 27: 317–326.

Vannucci RC, Brucklacher RM, Vannucci SJ (2001) Intracellular calcium accumulation during the evolution of hypoxic-ischemic brain damage in the immature rat. *Brain Res Brain Res Rev* 126: 117–120.

Vannucci RC, Christensen MA, Yager JY (1993) Nature, time-course, and extent of cerebral edema in perinatal hypoxic-ischemic brain damage. *Pediatr Neurol* 9: 29–34.

Vannucci RC, Lyons DT, Vasta F (1988) Regional cerebral blood flow during hypoxia-ischemia in immature rats. *Stroke* 19: 245–250.

Vannucci RC, Rossini A, Towfighi J, Vannucci SJ (1997) Measuring the accentuation of the brain damage that arises from perinatal cerebral hypoxia-ischemia. *Biol Neonate* 72: 187–191.

Vannucci RC, Yager JY (1992) Glucose, lactic acid, and perinatal hypoxic-ischemic brain damage. *Pediatr Neurol* 8: 3–12.

Vollmer B, Roth S, Riley K, O'Brien F, Baudin J, De Haan M, et al. (2006) Long-term neurodevelopmental outcome of preterm children with unilateral cerebral lesions diagnosed by neonatal ultrasound. *Early Hum Dev* 82: 655–661.

Volpe JJ (2001) *Neurology of the Newborn, 4th edn.* Philadelphia: WB Saunders.

Welin AK, Svedin P, Lapatto R, Sultan B, Hagberg H, Gressens P, et al. (2007) Melatonin reduces inflammation and cell death in white matter in the mid-gestation fetal sheep following umbilical cord occlusion. *Pediatr Res* 61: 153–158.

Welsh FA, Vannucci RC, Brierley JB (1982) Columnar alterations of NADH florescence during hypoxia-ischemia in immature rat brain. *J Cereb Blood Flow Metab* 2: 221–228.

Wen SW, Smith G, Yang Q, Walker M (2004) Epidemiology of preterm birth and neonatal outcome. *Semin Fetal Neonatal Med* 9: 429–435.

Wheater M, Rennie JM (2000) Perinatal infection is an important risk factor for cerebral palsy in very-low-birth weight infants. *Dev Med Child Neurol* 42: 364–367.

Williams CE, Gunn AJ, Mallard C, Gluckman PD (1992) Outcome after ischemia in the developing sheep brain: an electroencephalographic and histological study. *Ann Neurol* 31: 14–21.

Wirrell EC, Armstrong EA, Osman LD, Yager JY (2001) Prolonged seizures exacerbate perinatal hypoxic-ischemic brain damage. *Pediatr Res* 50: 445–454.

Wood NS, Costeloe K, Gibson AT, Hennessy EM, Marlow N, Wilkinson AR (2005) The EPICure study: associations and antecedents of neurological and developmental disability at 30 months of age following extremely preterm birth. *Arch Dis Child Fetal Neonatal Ed* 90: F134–140.

Wu YW, Colford JM (2000) Chorioamnionitis as a risk factor for cerebral palsy. *JAMA* 284: 1417–1424.

Yager JY, Armstrong EA, Miyashita H, Wirrell EC (2002) Prolonged neonatal seizures exacerbate hypoxic-ischemic brain damage: correlation with cerebral energy metabolism and excitatory amino acid release. *Dev Neurosci* 24: 367–381.

Yager JY, Brucklacher RM, Vannucci RC (1991) Cerebral oxidative metabolism and redox state during hypoxia-ischemia and early recovery in the immature rat. *Am J Physiol* 262: H1102–1108.

Yager JY, Brucklacher RM, Vannucci RC (1992) Cerebral energy metabolism during hypoxia-ischemia and early recovery in immature rats. *Am J Physiol* 262: H672–677.

Yager JY, Brucklacher RM, Vannucci RC (1996) Paradoxical mitochondrial oxidation in perinatal hypoxic-ischemic brain damage. *Brain Res* 712: 230–238.

Yager JY, Thornhill J (1997) The effect of age on susceptibility to hypoxic-ischemic brain damage. *Neurosci Biobehav Rev* 21: 167–175.

Yin K, Juurlink BH (2000) Regulation of expression of nuclear factor kappa B RelA in oligodendrocytes: effect of hypoxia. *Neuroreport* 11: 1877–1881.

Yonezawa M, Back SA, Gan X, Rosenberg PA, Volpe JJ (1996) Cystine deprivation induces oligodendroglial death: rescue by free radical scavengers and by a diffusible glial factor. *J Neurochem* 67: 566–573.

Yoon BH, Kim CJ, Romero R, Jun JK, Park KH, Choi ST, et al. (1997a) Experimentally induced intrauterine infection causes fetal brain white matter lesions in rabbits. *Am J Obstet Gynecol* 177: 797–802.

Yoon BH, Romero R, Kim CJ, Koo JN, Choe G, Syn HC, et al. (1997b) High expression of tumor necrosis factor-alpha and interleukin-6 in periventricular leukomalacia. *Am J Obstet Gynecol* 177: 406–411.

Yoon BH, Romero R, Lim JH, Shim SS, Hong JS, Shim JY, et al. (2003) The clinical significance of detecting Ureaplasma urealyticum by the polymerase chain reaction in the amniotic fluid of patients with preterm labor. *Am J Obstet Gynecol* 189: 919–924.

Yoshioka A, Bacskai B, Pleasure D (1996) Pathophysiology of oligodendroglial excitotoxicity. *J Neurosci Res* 46: 427–437.

Young RS, Hernandez MJ, Yagel SK (1982) Selective reduction of blood flow to white matter during hypotension in newborn dogs: a possible mechanism of periventricular leukomalacia. *Ann Neurol* 12: 445–448.

Yrjanheikki J, Koistinaho J, Copin JC, de Crespigny A, Moseley ME, Chan PH (2000) Spreading depression-induced expression of c-fos and cyclooxygenase-2 in transgenic mice that overexpress human copper/zinc-superoxide dismutase. *J Neurotrauma* 17: 713–718.

Zou H, Henzel WJ, Liu X, Lutschg A, Wang X (1997) Apaf-1, a human protein homologous to *C. elegans* CED-4, participates in cytochrome c-dependent activation of caspase-3. *Cell* 90: 405–413.

19

NON-PERINATAL ACQUIRED BRAIN INJURY

David J Michelson and Stephen Ashwal

Brain injury is a common cause of death and permanent disability in children worldwide. Detailed study of the causes of brain injury in childhood, as well as of its developmental and economic consequences, seeks to improve the focus of the preventative and intervention efforts of public health, medical, and rehabilitation communities. Laboratory research into the molecular and cellular mechanisms underlying brain injury continues to suggest novel therapeutic strategies that may improve eventual clinical outcomes. This research is also uncovering many important ways in which the developing brain differs from the adult brain in its response to both acquired injury and therapeutic intervention.

EPIDEMIOLOGY

While injury to the brain can occur in the context of any number of primary illnesses and injuries, with a wide array of presentations, the proximate causes of neuronal loss and permanent disability fall largely within the categories of hypoxia-ischemia and trauma.

HYPOXIC-ISCHEMIC BRAIN INJURY

Cerebral blood flow can be compromised in the distribution of a single artery, as in an acute ischemic stroke (AIS), or to the entire brain at once, as in global ischemia from cardiopulmonary arrest. The incidence of AIS in children has varied widely by report and population studied, ranging from 0.6 to 8 per 100 000 (Lynch and Han 2005), but appears to be increasingly recognized over time with advances in diagnostic medical technology, particularly neuroimaging. The causes of AIS also vary widely by report, but bacterial meningitis, congenital structural cardiac disorders, coagulopathies, vasculopathies, and viral infections account for most identified causes. Some risk factors, such as sickle cell disease, moyamoya, and genetic coagulation disorders, vary in prevalence by ethnic background. Half of the children who present with symptoms of AIS have no past medical history and about one-third have no identified risk factors on detailed medical evaluation (Ganesan et al. 2003). Arterial dissection can occur after seemingly trivial trauma in patients without any underlying risk factors and is a more common cause of AIS in children and adolescents than in older adults.

Cardiac disorders are the most commonly identified risk factor for childhood AIS, accounting for 25–50% of hospitalized cases in the United States and Canada, with congenital heart defects (CHD) making up the majority of such cases. Ischemia related to CHD can be caused by spontaneous embolism of an intra-cardiac thrombus, capillary sludging from polycythemia brought about by chronic cyanosis, or from complications of necessary diagnostic and surgical procedures. Children undergoing the Fontan procedure with pulmonary banding have a par-ticularly high rate of ischemic complications (Chun et al. 2004).

Hematologic and coagulation disorders are more commonly associated with AIS in children than in adults. Sickle cell disease, anemia, and genetic and acquired thrombophilias are found in more than half of the children studied in the United States and the United Kingdom, often either in combination with one another or with additional risk factors also evident (Chan and deVeber 2000). Children with sickle cell disease have an over 200-fold increased risk of AIS related to large and small vessel arteriopathy, with 10% experiencing a clinically symptomatic event before adolescence and more than twice as many found to have had clinically silent events on neuroimaging and detailed cognitive testing (White et al. 2006). The genetic and acquired coagulation disorders most commonly identified in children with AIS include protein C deficiency, protein S deficiency, factor V G1691A (Leiden) mutation, methylenetetrahydrofolate reductase C677T thermolabile mutation, pro-thrombin G20210A (Poort) mutation, and elevations in plasma homocystine, antiphosholipid antibodies, and lipoprotein (Haywood et al. 2005).

Arteriopathies causing AIS include both infectious and inflammatory vas-culitides, and non-inflammatory disorders such as arterial dissection, moyamoya syndrome, fibromuscular dysplasia, transient cerebral vasculopathy, and congenitally hypoplastic vessels. Infection contributes to the risk of AIS through the direct invasion of blood vessels, endothelial damage which leads to clot induction, ele-vation of prothrombotic inflammatory cytokines and factors, and consumption of antithrombotic proteins. AIS has been found to complicate systemic infection, sepsis, meningitis, encephalitis, and brain abscess, with a prevalence of 27% in one study of bacterial meningitis (Snyder et al. 1981). Viral infections with varicella, human immunodeficiency virus, parvovirus B19, and influenza A have been linked to AIS. Varicella infection can also cause a transient angiopathy and stenosis of the distal internal carotid and proximal middle cerebral and anterior cerebral arteries. The incidence of AIS appears to be increased by as much as threefold after nat-ural varicella infection and has also been reported following vaccination (Wirrell et al. 2004).

The most common clinical signs of AIS are acute hemiplegia, seizures, dys-phasia, and an altered level of consciousness. The subtlety with which these signs may present in infancy can in some cases so delay diagnosis that it is difficult to assign the onset of injury confidently to the postnatal period.

TABLE 19.1
Causes of cardiopulmonary arrest in children

Upper airway disease	Central nervous system infection
Foreign body aspiration	Intoxications
Croup and supraglottitis	Botulism
Airway trauma (blunt and penetrating)	Increased intracranial pressure
Abscess and airway infection	Status epilepticus
Angioedema	
	Cardiovascular disease
Lower airway disease	Hypovolemic, septic, or cardiogenic shock
Asthma and bronchopulmonary dysplasia	Congenital heart defect
Pneumonia and pneumonitis	Dysrhythmia
Foreign body aspiration	Coronary artery disease
Drowning	Myocarditis or pericarditis
Chest trauma	
	Other
Neurologic disease	Sudden infant death syndrome
Head or cervical spine trauma	Metabolic disorders

Children can develop hypoxic-ischemic injury from primary cardiac dysfunction and arrest but, unlike adults, in whom cardiac causes predominate, the most common causes of cardiopulmonary arrest in children are disorders in which there is initially primary airway compromise, such as drowning, choking (i.e. airway obstruction), and trauma with loss of airway patency (Table 19.1). This often leads to asphyxia-hypoxia and ischemia further complicated by combined respiratory and metabolic acidosis (Young et al. 2004). The causes of out-of-hospital cardiac arrest found in one large prospective population-based study are listed in Table 19.2.

Children who experience primary respiratory failure initially demonstrate hypertension and tachycardia followed eventually by hypotension and bradycardia, and finally by pulseless electrical activity and asystole. This differs significantly from sudden cardiac arrest in that there is in this context a gradual decrease in the delivery of substrates to the brain, rather than an abrupt termination. This has negative consequences for the progression of cellular injury. Persistent, but severely compromised, blood flow prolongs the delivery of glucose under anaerobic conditions, worsening eventual tissue acidosis, and prolongs the delivery of platelets and procoagulant factors under inflammatory conditions, worsening microvascular plugging and the prospects for reperfusion when blood flow is restored (Bittigau et al. 1999). These consequences are seen in experimental asphyxia, which causes more scattered microinfarction and hemorrhage and greater basal ganglia injury than does sudden cardiac arrest from ventricular fibrillation (Vaagenes et al. 1997).

TABLE 19.2
Causes of out-of-hospital cardiac arrest in children

Cause of arrest	N	%
Sudden infant death syndrome	136	23
Trauma	118	20
Respiratory	96	16
Submersion	73	12
Cardiac	48	8
Central nervous system	35	6
Burn	6	1
Poisoning	6	1
Other	63	10
Unknown	20	3

Source: Young et al. (2004).

TRAUMATIC BRAIN INJURY

Traumatic brain injury (TBI) is consistently among the leading causes of death and neurodevelopmental disability in childhood. Among children aged 1–14 years in the United States, accidental head injury is responsible for more deaths than all other childhood illnesses combined, with approximately 475 000 cases per year resulting in 37 000 hospitalizations and 2685 deaths (Langlois et al. 2004). Among children under 1 year of age, homicide is the leading cause of death. The available data are difficult to analyze for mechanisms of injury, but particular etiologies do clearly vary considerably with age, with a higher incidence of non-accidental injuries in infants, falls and vehicle-vs-pedestrian accidents in toddlers, sports-related injuries and bicycle crashes in juveniles, and motor vehicle accidents in adolescents.

CLASSIFICATION

The Glasgow Coma Scale (GCS), which was initially designed to describe trauma patients, has gained wide acceptance as a shorthand method for describing the level of responsiveness of patients with an acute encephalopathy of any cause. The total GCS score, ranging from 3 to 15, is determined by the addition of the patient's highest score for responses in ocular, verbal, and motor categories. Scales for use in preverbal children have been adapted from the GCS, as shown in Table 19.3, although their implementation has been modest and they still await validation in large studies. Alternatives for use in patients of all ages have been proposed that would eliminate verbal response ratings altogether in favor of scoring the more diagnostic and prognostically valuable brainstem reflexes and respiratory drive (Wijdicks 2006).

TABLE 19.3
Comparison of Glasgow Coma Score (GCS) and Modified GCS

Score		Glasgow Coma Scale	Children's Coma Scale
Eye opening	4	Spontaneous	Spontaneous
	3	To command	To sound
	2	To pain	To pain
	1	None	None
Verbal response	5	Oriented	Age-appropriate vocalization, smile, or orientation to sound
	4	Confused, disoriented	Irritable, consolable, uncooperative, aware of the environment
	3	Inappropriate words	Irritable, inconsistently consolable
	2	Incomprehensible sounds	Inconsolable, unaware of the environment, restless, agitated
	1	None	None
Motor response	6	Obeys commands	Obeys commands, spontaneous movements
	5	Localizes pain	Localizes pain
	4	Withdraws	Withdraws
	3	Abnormal flexion to pain	Abnormal flexion to pain
	2	Abnormal extension to pain	Abnormal extension to pain
	1	None	None
Best Total Score	15		

Source: Modified from Reilly et al. (1988).

TBI severity has traditionally been classified by the GCS score on presentation, with mild TBI defined as scores of 13–15, moderate as scores 9–12, and severe as scores of 8 or less (scores that also roughly indicate that a patient is comatose). However, the GCS score on presentation is not a particularly accurate predictor of the eventual outcome, even with modification (Lieh-Lai et al. 1992). The vast majority of pediatric TBI is initially categorized as mild, with 90% of children who are brought to an emergency room for evaluation being seen and released after assessment. Still, persistent cognitive and behavioral impairment can be found in some of these children when full evaluations are later performed.

PATHOPHYSIOLOGY
HYPOXIC-ISCHEMIC BRAIN INJURY
Neurons subjected to hypoxia, ischemia, or hypoglycemia suffer injury from cellular energy failure. With abrupt interruption of all substrate delivery, as with sudden cardiac arrest, brain oxygen stores and consciousness are lost within seconds and

glucose and adenosine triphosphate (ATP) stores are depleted within 5 minutes (Hoxworth et al. 1999). There are immediate and delayed phases to the further progression of injury, each with a distinct histopathologic appearance and biochemical processes. The principal cause of immediate cell death, excitotoxicity, results in a pattern of cell necrosis. Delayed death results from the activation of apoptotic pathways, promoted by multiple factors, including both ischemia and subsequent reperfusion, which cause oxidative injury and inflammation.

Early injury
Cellular energy failure leads to the loss of ion homeostasis and depolarization of neuronal membranes, accumulation of the excitatory neurotransmitter glutamate within synapses, and subsequent unregulated activation of ionotropic glutamate receptors, allowing the influx of toxic concentrations of Ca^{2+} and Na^+ into neurons (Fig. 19.1).

Ionotropic glutamate receptors are classified based on their *in vitro* responsiveness to N-methyl-D-aspartate (NMDA), alpha amino-3-hydroxy-5-methyl-4-isoxazolepropionic acid (AMPA), or kainic acid. The heteromeric NMDA receptor is composed of structural NMDAR1 and modulatory NMDAR2A–2D subunits. The NMDA receptor is normally inhibited by a Mg^{2+} ion that blocks its ion channel but under conditions of membrane depolarization and Ca^{2+} influx, this inhibition can be lost, allowing influx of Ca^{2+}, Na^+, and K^+. Sustained activation

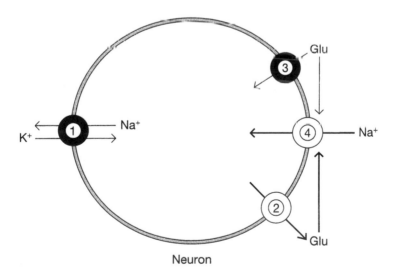

Neuron

Fig. 19.1 Energy failure causes (1) Na^+/K^+-ATPase dysfunction, intracellular Na^+ accumulation and neuronal membrane depolarization, (2) voltage-mediated release of glutamate (Glu), and (3) decreased ATP-dependent neuronal and glial glutamate reuptake. Glutamate stimulates ionotropic receptors (4) that allow further Na^+ influx and depolarization.

of NMDA channels for more than 3 minutes permitting ion influx has been shown to be sufficient to cause necrotic cell death (Benveniste et al. 1984, Takagi et al. 1993).

AMPA receptors are composed of subunits GluR1–GluR5, allow influx of Na^+ and K^+ ions with activation, and are usually impermeable to Ca^{2+} because of the expression of inhibitory GluR2 subunits. Kainic acid receptors, composed of GluR5–7 and KA1–2 subunits, are also permeable only to Na^+ and K^+. Prolonged activation of AMPA or kainic acid receptors for more than 60 minutes can lead to oncotic cell death because of the influx of Na^+ and water. Some neurons in the cortex and striatum express AMPA receptors made with fewer GluR2 subunits, thus making them more Ca^{2+} permeable and intrinsically prone to excitotoxic injury (Weiss et al. 1994, Kim et al. 2001).

Neurons normally have a steep gradient between their intracellular concentration of free Ca^{2+}, approximately 100nmol/l, and the extracellular concentration which is in the range 1–2mmol/l. This gradient is maintained through multiple pathways for Ca^{2+}, including influx through plasma membrane voltage-gated and ligand-gated channels, efflux through the plasma membrane Na^+/Ca^{2+} exchangers and Ca^{2+}-ATPases, release from the endoplasmic reticulum through inositol triphosphate (IP3) gated channels and from mitochondria through Na^+/Ca^{2+} exchangers, efflux into the endoplasmic reticulum through Ca^{2+}-ATPases and into mitochondria through electrophoretic uniport mechanisms, and binding to target proteins (Gunter and Pfeiffer 1990, Carafoli 1991). Energy failure leads to an accumulation of intracellular Ca^{2+} by changing the flux through many of these pathways (Fig. 19.2), although activation of NMDA receptors appears to have the major role (Greenberg et al. 1990).

Persistent intracellular Ca^{2+} overload activates a number of enzymes that contribute to cell death. The calpains and cathepsins are proteases that are activated by Ca^{2+} to cleave a number of specific target proteins, including spectrin, fodrin, and the nuclear factor κB (NF-κB), which leads to a remodeling of dendrites, disruption of membrane and cytoplasmic transportation, and changes in gene expression (Wang 2000). Cytosolic phospholipase A_2 is activated by Ca^{2+} to relocate to the plasma membrane and catalyze the breakdown of glycerophospholipids to lysophospholipids and free fatty acids (FFA), including arachidonic acid, which is then further metabolized to produce prostaglandins, leukotrienes, reactive oxygen species, and platelet-activating factors (Sapirstein and Bonventre 2000). Metabotropic glutamate receptors use G-protein-coupled second messenger pathways to activate phospholipase C which hydrolyzes plasma membrane phosphatidylinositol to diacylglycerol (DAG) and IP3. DAG is further hydrolyzed to additional arachidonic acid and other FFA which contribute directly to cytotoxic injury by increasing membrane fluidity neurotransmitter release, facilitating brain edema, and by inhibiting oxidative phosphorylation and ATPases (Perkin and Ashwal 2006).

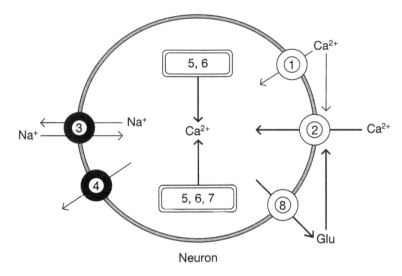

Fig. 19.2 Intracellular Na^+ accumulation and membrane depolarization from energy failure leads to intracellular Ca^{2+} overload through open (1) voltage-gated Ca^{2+} channels and (2) Ca^{2+} permeable NMDA- and AMPA-type glutamate receptors on the plasma membrane, failure of plasma membrane (3) Na^+/Ca^{2+} exchange and (4) ATP-dependent Ca^{2+} efflux, release of sequestered Ca^{2+} from the endoplasmic reticulum and mitochondria through (5) Na^+/Ca^{2+} exchange and failure of (6) ATP-dependent Ca^{2+} transporters and (7) mitochondrial electrophoretic uniports. Ca^{2+} accumulation increases release of glutamate (8), promoting further Ca^{2+} influx through ligand-gated channels.

Many of the major families of protein kinases are also affected by the elevation in Ca^{2+}. The mitogen-activated protein kinases (MAPK), the p42/p44 extracellular-signal-regulated kinases (ERK), the c-Jun N-terminal kinases (JNK), the stress-activated protein kinases (SAPK), and p38 are activated by Ca^{2+} and calcium/calmodulin protein kinase II (CaMKII) is inhibited (Fukunaga et al. 1992, Xia et al. 1996, Kawasaki et al. 1997, Ko et al. 1998, Schwarzschild et al. 1999, Vanhoutte et al. 1999). Increased activity of Ca^{2+}/Mg^{2+}-activated endonucleases and DNAseII leads to the cleavage of DNA between nucleosomes leaving fragments of multiples of 200 base pairs called DNA ladders (Robertson et al. 2000). Finally, energy failure and intracellular Ca^{2+} accumulation lead to an increase in the concentration of Ca^{2+} within mitochondria which contributes to a further reduction in oxidative phosphorylation, the production of reactive oxygen species, and the release of cytotoxic compounds, such as cytochrome C, through a disrupted mitochondrial membrane (Wang et al. 1994, Luetjens et al. 2000, Rego et al. 2000, Ward et al. 2000).

There are a number of mechanisms through which energy failure promotes the generation of free radicals, highly reactive molecules with one or more unpaired electrons in their outer orbits that are capable of causing substantial unregulated damage to cellular macromolecues through oxidation. Activated calpain converts xanthine dehydrogenase to xanthine oxidase, which catalyzes the conversion of xanthine and hypoxanthine, in abundance in the ATP deprived cell, to uric acid producing a superoxide O_2-radical in the process (McCord et al. 1985). Superoxide is also normally formed in mitochondria through the reaction of oxygen with electrons that have escaped from the electron transport chain. Accumulation of Ca^{2+} within the mitochondria during energy failure diverts the flow of electrons from the electron transport chain and depolarizes the mitochondrial membrane leading to an increased production of free radicals (Rego et al. 2000). Free radical production is greatly increased by the delivery of oxygen to ischemic tissue during the reperfusion process (Piantadosi and Zhang 1996).

Cellular defenses against endogenous free radicals involve the superoxide dismutases (SOD), which convert superoxide to hydrogen peroxide (H_2O_2), and catalase and glutathione peroxidase, which convert hydrogen peroxide to water (H_2O) and oxygen (O_2). Within neurons, Cu^{2+}/Zn^{2+}-SOD is found mainly in the cytosol and Mn^{2+}-SOD is found mainly within the mitochondrial matrix. Other naturally occurring antioxidants include vitamin C (ascorbate), vitamin E (alpha-tocopherol), glutathione, and co-enzyme Q.

Reaction of superoxide with nitric oxide (NO) produces the more freely diffusing peroxynitrite radical ($ONOO^-$) which carries out destructive oxidation and nitration of lipids, proteins, and DNA through its two by-products: the hydroxyl radical (OH^-) and nitrogen dioxide radical (NO_2^-) (Beckman 1996). Production of NO is increased in the context of energy failure. Neuronal nitric oxide synthase (nNOS) is activated by increased intracellular Ca^{2+} concentrations through CAMKII phosphorylation (Knowles and Moncada 1994, Samdani et al. 1997). Elevated intracellular NO exacerbates energy failure by activating the DNA repair enzyme poly ADP-ribose polymerase (PARP), depleting both ATP and the pool of beta-nicotinamide adenine dinucleotide (NAD^+) available for accepting electrons in mitochondrial ATP synthesis (Brookes et al. 1999).

Transition metals also contribute to free radical formation. Iron-binding proteins release Fe^{3+} during ischemia allowing it (along with other reduced transition metals) to catalyze hydroxyl radical formation through the Haber–Weiss/Fenton reaction between hydrogen peroxide and superoxide (White et al. 1985). Release of Zn^{2+} from presynaptic vesicles (along with glutamate in excitatory neurons), entry through Ca^{2+} and Zn^{2+} channels (Colvin et al. 2000), and participation in free radical production, possibly through the cyclooxygenase, 5-lipooxygenase, and protein kinase C (PKC) activation are all possible mechanisms that contribute to excitotoxic cell injury (Sensi et al. 1999, Im et al. 2004).

Excitotoxicity proceeds through this cascade of intracellular Na^+ and Ca^{2+} overload, secondary influx of Cl^- and H_2O, direct signal transduction and enzyme activation, free radical injury, and organelle injury to lead to cell death by swelling (oncosis) and plasma membrane destruction (Choi 1987). Cells dying in this way further release glutamate and other compounds into the extracellular space where they contribute to the additional excitotoxic mediated deaths of neighboring cells.

Late injury

Cells that manage to survive the immediate injuries mediated through excitotoxicity, because of only transient or partial energy failure, with restoration of energy metabolism prior to irreversible injury, may still be lost through programmed cell death or apoptosis. The apoptotic cascade is a highly regulated process with key mechanisms that are energy dependent, including novel gene transcription and protein synthesis (Martin et al. 1998).

Whereas necrotic cells undergo oncotic cytosolic expansion, irregular DNA fragmentation, and plasma membrane lysis, apoptotic cells become smaller and rounder as (1) their cytoskeleton is broken down by activated proteases, (2) their DNA is condensed and fragmented by endonucleases, (3) their nucleus is broken into dense chromatin bodies, and (4) the cell is broken into plasma membrane wrapped vesicles called apoptotic bodies. These remnants are phagocytosed by activated microglia and macrophages which recognize the exposed phosphatidyl-seriene on the apoptotic cell surface (Borisenko et al. 2003). The histopathologic and biochemical differences between necrosis and apoptosis are summarized in Table 19.4.

Apoptosis can be triggered by extracellular or intracellular processes. Binding of tumor necrosis factor (TNF) to plasma membrane TNF receptors induces receptor trimerization and coupling to the TNF receptor associated death domain

TABLE 19.4
Comparison of necrosis and apoptosis

Finding	Necrosis	Apoptosis
Histopathology		
Pattern	Ischemic core	Scattered within penumbra
Cell volume	Swollen	Shrunken
Cell membrane	Disrupted	Intact
Chromatin	Clumped	Condensed
Response	Inflammation	Phagocytosis
Biochemistry		
Timing after injury	Early (4 hours)	Delayed (24 hours)
Energy	Depleted	Required
Enzyme pathway	Truncated	Complete
Protein synthesis	Independent	Dependent
DNA	Degraded	Fragmented

protein. Binding of the Fas ligand causes Fas receptor coupling with Fas associated protein with death domain. These receptor complexes catalyze autocleavage and activation of two pro-enzymes, procaspase 8 and 10. These cysteine proteases are considered initiators of the apoptotic cascade in that they in turn activate the effectors of the family, caspase 3, 6, and 7, which cleave essential structural, signaling, DNA repair, and cell-cycle proteins (Jin et al. 2001a).

Intracellular stresses, including Ca^{2+} overload and free radical injury, can increase the permability of the inner mitochondrial membrane, cause swelling of the mitochondrial matrix, and lead to depolarization and disruption of the outer mitochondrial membrane. During this process, a mitochondrial permeability transition pore (MTP) is formed, through which mitochondrial proteins such as cytochrome C are released into the cytosol. Cytochrome C interacts with the apoptosis protease activating factor 1 (apaf-1), ATP, and another initiator caspase, procaspase 9, to form a complex referred to as an apoptosome (Zou et al. 1997). Within this complex, procaspase 9 cleaves itself to form active caspase 9, which then activates procaspase 3 to effect subsequent steps in the apoptotic cascade. Caspase 3 also cleaves and activates more procaspase 9 in a possible feed-forward cycle that helps to ensure that the apoptotic cascade, once initiated, progresses to completion. Cytosolic cytochrome C also blocks the IP3-gated channels of the endoplasmic reticulum, amplifying cytosolic Ca^{2+} overload and magnifying the apoptotic cascade (Boehning et al. 2003).

Mitochondrial depolarization can also lead to apoptosis through caspase-independent mechanisms. Formation of the MTP also allows release of apoptosis inducing factor (AIF), a mitochondrial flavoprotein, which translocates to the nucleus and causes the DNA to undergo fragmentation (Susin et al. 1999). Other mitochondrial proteins that promote apoptosis when released into the cytosol include endonuclease G, Htr2A/Omi, and Smac/Diablo (Chai et al. 2000, Li et al. 2001, Suzuki et al. 2001).

Mitochondrial permeability and MTP formation is regulated by the B-cell lymphoma 2 (Bcl-2) family of proteins. The members of this family that promote apoptosis include Bax, Bid, and Bad, which facilitate mitochondrial protein release. Other Bcl-2 family members, including Bcl-2 and Bcl-xl, inhibit apoptosis by inhibiting the pro-apoptotic members of the family (Antonsson et al. 1997). P53 activation by cell injury leads to Bax up-regulation (Isenmann et al. 1998). Activation of intracellular signaling pathways, such as JNK and p38 MAPK, promote Bax activity through phosphorylation and inactivation of Bcl-2 and Bcl-xl (Srivastava et al. 1999, Ghatan et al. 2000, Kharbanda et al. 2000, Tournier et al. 2000). Translocation of Bax and Bad to the mitochondria is increased under conditions of cellular acidosis and Ca^{2+} overload (Khaled et al. 1999, Khaled and Durham 2001). Growth factor induced protein kinase B activation protects cells by phosphorylating and inactivating Bad and caspase 8 and 9 (Jenkins et al. 2001).

Some of the same processes that are involved in the early necrosis of severely injured cells contribute to the late apoptotic death of stressed cells. PARP activation, with consequent NAD^+ and ATP depletion, contributes to apoptosis by exacerbating energy failure and plasma and mitochondrial membrane depolarization (Du et al. 2003). Acidosis caused by anaerobic metabolism and lactic acid and CO_2 build-up further promotes activation of cytochrome C dependent caspases and acidic endonucleases (Matsuyama et al. 2000). Elevated intracellular Ca^{2+} concentration may also indirectly promote apoptosis through blocking of neurotrophic factors and activation of calpains, caspases, PLA2, and endonucleases (Rordorf et al. 1991, Neumar et al. 1996, Namura et al. 1998, Rosenbaum et al. 1998, Gwag et al. 1999).

Restoration of cerebral blood flow after a period of ischemia paradoxically delivers the substrates to injured cells that are necessary for the energy dependent mechanisms of apoptosis to occur. Delivery of oxygen to these cells also allows greater production of injurious free radicals. Reperfusion also allows elements of the immune system to contribute to brain injury through the production of IL-1 and TNF-α, NO and free radicals, and cytokines which disrupt the blood–brain barrier (BBB), worsening cerebral edema and hemorrhage (Danton and Dietrich 2003).

TRAUMATIC BRAIN INJURY

Early injury

The purely mechanical traumatic injuries arising from deformation and deceleration forces acting on the cranial tissues during impact consist of skull fractures, epidural and subdural hemorrhages, subarachnoid hemorrhages, cortical contusions, and diffuse axonal injury (DAI). Secondary hypoxic-ischemic injury often arises from associated blood loss, cardiopulmonary arrest, intracranial pressure effects on cererebral blood flow, and the mass effect of intracranial hemorrhages that may cause cerebral herniation with compression of the brainstem or small or large blood vessels. The pathology of trauma is heterogeneous, with mixed areas of contusional necrosis, excitotoxicity, axonal injury, and inflammation.

In experiments with primates, DAI within the subcortical white matter, corpus callosum, and brainstem accounted for 35% of the morbidity and mortality when there was no large hematoma (Gennarelli et al. 1982). The classic conception of DAI as caused entirely by shearing forces at the time of injury has been modified by recent research showing that there is a complex pathophysiology through which all but the most severe primary axonal injury progresses toward disconnection. Shearing and tensile forces increase axolemmal permeability (microporation) and increase intracellular concentrations of Ca^{2+}, which activates calpain and caspase proteases leading to the digestion of microtubules and neurofilaments of the axonal cytoskeleton and transaxonal transport system. Accumulation of untransported vesicles and organelles promotes axonal swelling, detachment, and formation of the 'retraction ball' that is the classic histopathology description brought about by continued anterograde transport from the soma to the end of the proximal segment. These classic findings may be absent in severe axonal injury as Ca^{2+} overload can reverse anterograde transport, preventing eventual axon swelling and retraction ball formation (Marmarou et al. 2005).

Increased Ca^{2+} permeability results directly from axonal deformation, but increased Na^+ permeability also leads to membrane depolarization and entry of Ca^{2+} through voltage-gated channels (Wolf et al. 2001). Ca^{2+} mediated calpain and calmodulin activation leads to proteolysis and compaction of cytoskeletal neurofilaments such as the alpha chain of tetrameric spectrin (Buki et al. 1999, Okonkwo et al. 1998). Intracellular accumulation of Na^+ and Ca^{2+} leads to swelling and membrane disruption of axonal mitochondria, through direct effects or via calpain mediated neurofilament proteolysis (Buki and Povlishock 2006). Membrane damage causes opening of the MTP, release of cytochrome C and AIF, and activation of caspases. Caspase 3 degrades the remaining beta chains of spectrin, completely undermining cytoskeletal stability and causing plasma membrane disruption and disconnection (Wang et al. 1998).

While physical transection of an axon close to its soma leads rapidly to cell necrosis, traumatic axonal injury does not, a result attributed to a slower loss of ion homeostasis (Stone et al. 2001). Many neurons that suffer traumatic axotomy appear capable of both survival and repair. The downstream segment of the injured axon undergoes Wallerian degeneration over weeks to months with a gradual breakdown of the myelin sheath and axon cylinder, disconnection and loss of distal nerve terminals, and deafferentation of target neurons. Concomitant hypoxic-ischemic injury adds to the severity of the axonal changes caused by trauma as common cytotoxic pathways are involved (Bartus 1997).

Widespread neuronal microporation and depolarization also leads to a dramatic, but brief, increase in glutamate release which precipitates the death of some cells by excitotoxic mechanisms (Tolias and Bullock 2004). In the first weeks after injury, some regions of the brain, especially those around the actual contusion sites, show impaired mitochondrial oxidative metabolism as reflected by an increased glucose utilization and lactate production (Vespa et al. 2004). Thereafter, glucose utilization falls below normal levels in dysfunctional areas and remains suppressed until there is actual clinical recovery (Nakayama et al. 2006). Pericontusional areas have also been shown to suffer late apoptosis of neurons and oligodendrocytes (Zhang et al. 2003). Increased cerebrospinal fluid (CSF) concentrations of the apoptosis regulating Bcl-2 family of proteins have been found to be correlated with TBI severity and outcome in infants and children (Clark et al. 2000). Higher CSF Bcl-2 concentrations are correlated with survival after severe TBI (Ng et al. 2000).

Brain that is in contact with a hemorrhage appears to be at the highest risk of apoptosis. The occurrence of traumatic subarachnoid hemorrhage (SAH) is associated with more severe brain injury and less favorable outcome although controversy remains as to whether this is simply because the SAH is induced by more intense trauma or because the SAH itself induces additional irreversible brain injury through vasospasm and ischemia (Armin et al. 2006). The consequences of even isolated SAH are potentially severe.

In the early phase, there is a dramatic rise in intracranial pressure (ICP), a loss of cerebral autoregulation, a drop in cerebral blood flow, disruption of the BBB, development of cerebral edema, and acute arterial vasopasm. Profound global ischemia results initiating the complex excitotoxic and apoptotic cascades discussed above (Ostrowski et al. 2006). The ischemia is different than that which occurs with cardiac arrest or vascular occlusion, in that the extravasated blood and increased ICP cause sustained hypoperfusion, enhanced local inflammation, and greater oxidative injury (Ostrowski et al. 2005).

Oxyhemoglobin from lysed red blood cells and endothelin-1 from ruptured blood vessels are released into the subarachnoid space and depress neuronal and glial Na^+/K^+-ATPase activity, resulting in a wave of depolarization and excitatory neurotransmitter release that spreads across the surface of the brain (Petzold et al. 2003). Levels of serotonin and 20-hydroxyeiscosatetraenoic acid (20-HETE) increase in the CSF after SAH, causing profound vasoconstriction and a reduction in cerebral blood flow to 30% below that of baseline. Serotonin is likely to derive from activated platelets and to induce the production of 20-HETE through stimulation of $5\text{-}HT_{1B}$ receptors and activation of phospholipase A_2 (Cambj-Sapunar et al. 2003). Oxyhemoglobin also contributes to vasoconstriction by scavenging and metabolizing the NO produced by endothelial cells that would normally induce vascular smooth muscle relaxation (Schwartz et al. 2000).

Late injury

Late injury from SAH procedes through mechanisms similar to those seen in global ischemia. After TBI there is an up-regulated transcription of HIF-1α (Yu et al. 2001), a protein which binds with the tumor suppressor p53 to increase the transcription of other pro-apoptotic proteins, such as BNIP3, which heterodimerizes with and then inactivates the apoptosis repressors Bcl-2 and Bcl-xL (Vande Velde et al. 2000). The inflammatory response to ischemia is magnified by the presence of extravasated blood and its breakdown products within the subarachnoid space. Factors that are increased within brain tissue and blood vessels include ICAM-1, IL-1β, IL-6, and TNF-α (Prunell et al. 2005).

Cerebral edema after SAH is caused by a combination of (1) cytotoxic edema from Na^+/K^+ ATPase inhibition and excitotoxicity, and (2) vasogenic edema from BBB breakdown. Blood breakdown products compromise the BBB by increasing the permeability of interendothelial tight junctions (i.e. paracellular flux) and by increasing endothelial transcytosis (i.e. transcellular flux). SAH induced HIF-1α

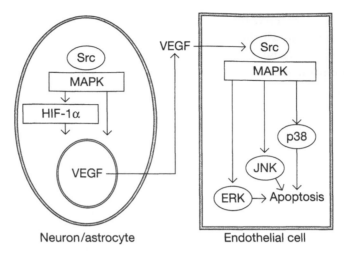

Fig. 19.3 Subarachnoid hemorrhage leads to neuronal and glial activation of Scr-MAPK and induction of HIF-1α, both of which increase transcription of vascular endothelial growth factor (VEGF), which acts on neighboring endothelial cells through Src-MAPK and downstream pathways, including ERK1/2, JNK, and p38, to promote apoptosis and vascular permeability.

Source: Modified from Ostrowski et al. (2006).

activity and Src-MAPK activity promotes the increased transcription of vascular endothelial growth factor (VEGF) in neurons and astrocytes near the cerebral arteries (Irving and Bamford 2002). This paracrine hormone in turn activates endothelial Src-MAPK, leading to BBB disruption and endothelial apoptosis through p38, JNK, and ERK pathways (Fig. 19.3). Cerebral edema increases ICP and lowers overall cerebral persusion pressure. Vasogenic edema, increased ICP, and cerebral hypoperfusion are exacerbated by the decreases in plasma osmolarity and volume caused by the increases in brain natriuretic factor (BNF) and atrial natriuretic factor (ANF) seen after SAH (Wijdicks et al. 1997).

Apoptosis occurs in endothelial cells exposed to a number of factors present after SAH, including oxyhemoglobin, natriuretic factors, TNF-α, and thromboxane A₂ (TXA2). Cells proceed through plasma membrane breakdown to an increased production of intracellular TXA2, which inhibits the phosphorylation of Akt, impairing cell survival (Gao et al. 2000). Detachment of damaged endothelial cells from the basement membrane allows contact between ATP and the vascular smooth muscle layer, promoting vasoconstriction, and between the collagen of the internal lamina and platelets and clotting factors, promoting intravascular thrombosis (Clower et al. 1994). Ischemia activates endothelial matrix metalothionine proteases 2 and 9, which also contribute to breakdown of the BBB and especially to hemorrhagic transformation of an area of infarction (Dijkhuizen et al. 2002).

Subarachnoid blood, by releasing reduced iron, produces reactive oxygen species, including the potent hydroxyl (OH⁻) radical. Oxyhemoglobin also inhibits smooth muscle $Na^+/K^+ATPase$, promoting muscle contraction through cell depolarization and Ca^{2+} influx (Zhang and Cook 1994). Finally, free oxyhemoglobin inhibits the normal vasodilatory effect of adenosine (Kajita et al. 1996).

SECONDARY BRAIN INJURY

Physiologic derangements, including hypotension, hypoxia, hyperglycemia, and hyperthermia, occur during and after the acute resuscitation of a brain injured patient and can worsen injuries and outcomes (Kochanek et al. 2001). Interventions to ameliorate the metabolic processes involved in cell death, other than induced hypothermia, have not yet translated from laboratory success in animal models to observable benefits in clinical trials or practice, but physiologic monitoring to maintain adequate cerebral blood flow, delivery of normal concentrations of oxygen and glucose, and normal temperature has been shown to be of significant value. Improvements in morbidity and mortality incurred by children who are transferred to a pediatric trauma center may in part reflect the importance of this ongoing physiologic monitoring (Densmore et al. 2006).

In most such centers, treatment of TBI is oriented toward monitoring ICP and taking steps to avoid intracranial hypertension, including head elevation, sedation, CSF drainage, osmotherapy, paralysis, hypothermia, barbiturate coma, and decompressive craniectomy. While multiple studies have shown these therapies to effectively lower ICP, it has been more difficult to show that they indeed have a long-term clinical benefit (Adamides et al. 2006). Whether efforts to minimize secondary brain injury should focus on avoiding intracranial hypertension or on maintaining optimal mean arterial blood pressure, cerebral perfusion pressure, or tissue oxygenation is currently an area of ongoing controversy in the management of head trauma patients (Kochanek 2006).

The influence of systemic blood pressure on traumatic injury has been demonstrated by animal studies showing that contusive injuries are larger with either inadequate or excessive pressures (Kroppenstedt et al. 1999) and by retrospective studies in children that show that higher blood pressures are strongly associated with survival (White et al. 2001). After global ischemic injury, cerebral perfusion to many areas remains impaired despite adequate system blood pressure. The mechanisms for this 'no reflow' phenomenon include mechanical blockage of capillaries by red blood cell sludging, white blood cell chemotaxis, disseminated intravascular coagulation, and endothelial cell swelling (Ginsberg and Myers 1972). Further flow restriction is likely to result from imbalances in such vasoactive factors as NO, adenosine, endothelin, and prostaglandins in the microvascular environment.

Hyperventilation is particularly to be avoided early in resuscitation efforts, when cerebral blood flow is already compromised. Hypocarbia causes vasoconstriction of cerebral arterioles, respiratory alkalosis reduces the dissociation of oxygen from hemoglobin, and the increased intrathoracic pressures generated by hyperventilation reduce cardiac filling, mean arterial pressures, and cerebral perfusion (Skippen et al. 1997).

Patients with severe brain injury may undergo a period of early spontaneous hypothermia followed by subsequent fever (Hickey et al. 2000). Numerous animal studies have shown the beneficial effects of hypothermia and the deleterious effects of hyperthermia on the ultimate extent of brain injury from various causes. Several mechanisms have been proposed to explain the protective effects of hypothermia, including reduction of overall metabolic demand, decreased synthesis and release of glutamate and free radicals, stabilization of lipid membranes, and decreased activity of destructive enzymes, including proteases, lipases, and endonucleases. Hypothermia rescues hippocampal CA1 neurons from ischemic injury at least in part by attenuating the down-regulation of AMPA GluR2 subunits (Colbourne et al. 2003). Clinical trials have established the benefit of induced hypothermia for adults with out-of-hospital cardiac arrest (Nolan et al. 2003) and for newborn infants experiencing perinatal asphyxia (Gluckman et al. 2005). It has been recommended that rewarming be avoided, fever treated aggressively, and induced hypothermia considered for all patients with brain injury (Hickey and Calloway 2005).

INCREASED VULNERABILITY OF CHILDREN
There are a number of physiologic characteristics that place the neurons of young children at greater risk of injury. The immature nervous system is engaged in active synapse formation, pruning, and myelination. Synaptogenesis peaks in different regions of the brain at different ages, but generally is maximal at around 6 years of age. The number of excitatory neurotransmitter receptors seen in the brain consequently also peaks in early childhood. Immature NMDA receptors are made up of subunits that make them more permeable to Ca^{2+} with normal activation and thus the neurons more prone to excitotoxic injury under conditions of excessive activation. Immature AMPA receptors also gate more Ca^{2+} and desensitize more slowly (Erecinska et al. 2004). $GABA_A$ receptor activation in very young animals causes depolarization, because of high intracellular Cl^- concentrations, and only shifts toward causing an inhibitory hyperpolarization as chloride gradients change with time (Khazipov et al. 2004).

Immature neurons and glia are particularly sensitive to signals promoting apoptosis, as apoptosis has a role in normal pruning, which occurs between the ages of 8 months and 11 years and decreases the number of neurons by more than half in some regions (Raff et al. 1993). A second wave of exuberant synaptogenesis and pruning also occurs during adolescence, especially within the frontal lobes (Giedd et al. 1999). Many of the proteins involved in regulating apoptosis, such as caspase 3, Apaf-1, Bcl-2, and Bax, are up-regulated in immature neurons (Ota et al. 2002). Immature neurons have also been found to have higher concentrations of free iron and to be intrinsically predisposed to greater free radical production, mitochondrial injury, and release of pro-apoptotic factors.

Immature neurons have 5–40% lower expression and activity of endogenous antioxidants, including Cu^{2+}/Zn^{2+}-SOD, Mn^{2+}-SOD, glutathione peroxidase, glutathione, and ascorbate, predisposing them to greater injury from free radical production (Bayir et al. 2006). They also have lower expression of the metallothionein enzymes that help to regulate transition metals and effectively limit their availability to participate in free radical production (Natale et al. 2004). The breakdown of free hemoglobin to biliverdin, which has antioxidant properties, depends on the expression of heme oxygenase (HO) in neurons and glia. The lower levels of neuronal HO found in the immature brain may contribute to greater neurodegeneration after hemorrhagic injury (Sun et al. 1990). Calcium-sensitive mitochondrial NOS has a higher expression in immature neurons, leading to greater peroxynitrite production under conditions of oxidative stress.

The high cellular activity of the developing brain translates into a greater energy demand and usage. Measurement by ^{31}phosphate magnetic resonance spectroscopy shows metabolic rates in children aged 3–8 years that are double those seen in adults (Hanaoka et al. 1998). This may contribute further to a greater susceptibility to injury from compromised energy cellular production.

In clinical practice, diffuse cerebral edema is more commonly seen in infants and children than in adults after severe TBI. The mechanical compliance of the developing skull and its membranous sutures may allow greater cranial deformation and more diffuse injury after an impact trauma (Margulies and Thibault 2000). In animal models, immaturity also results in (1) enhanced diffusion through the extracellular space of excitotoxic neurotransmitters (Van Lookeren Campagne et al. 1994), (2) a more intense inflammation in response to injury (Adelson et al. 1998), and (3) greater breakdown of the BBB (Schleien et al. 1991). Diffuse edema is not seen in animal models of trauma unless there is a superimposition of hypotension or hypoxia (Adelson et al. 1996), suggesting that these factors frequently contribute to pediatric TBI, as is recognized in infants subjected to inflicted (i.e. non-accidental) trauma (Berger et al. 2006). Pediatric victims of inflicted trauma may also develop more delayed apoptotic injury as CSF studies have been shown higher levels of cytochrome C, lower levels of Bcl-2, and greater delayed elevation of neuron specific enolase (Berger et al. 2002, Satchell et al. 2005).

There are also some physiologic characteristics of immature neurons that are protective against injury. For example, immature mitochondria appear to be better able to maintain normal function in the presence of elevated cytoplasmic Ca^{2+} (Robertson et al. 2004).

RECOVERY

Recovery of neurologic function advances in concert with several distinct processes, including repair and metabolic normalization of injured neurons, changes in existing synaptic connections, and the development of new synaptic connections (Weiloch and Nicolich 2006). The metabolic derangement seen in injured neurons, sometimes referred to as diaschesis, includes hypometabolism, neurovascular uncoupling, and aberrant neurotransmitter release (Kim et al. 2005). Ischemic neurons suffer a collapse of their dendritic spines with beading of actin aggregates that impairs connectivity even after recovery to normal metabolism (Zhang et al. 2005c). New spines are formed with time, but often in new locations and with different histologic features.

The mechanisms by which synaptic connections are modified are no different from those involved in normal learning, but they are enhanced early in recovery by the activation and release of survival, growth, and repair promoting proteins including activity regulated cytoskeletal associated protein (arc), nerve growth factor induced gene A (NGFI-A), homer, brain-derived neurotrophic factor (BDNF), and growth-associated protein-43 (GAP-43). Beyond the first week after injury, these growth factors are balanced by an up-regulated production of chondroitin sulfate proteoglycans which hamper axonal growth (Carmichael et al. 2000). Glia release factors that promote and inhibit axonal outgrowth as well as lipids that enhance myelination and glial–neuronal interactions (Badan et al. 2003). Myelin-associated proteins, such as Nogo-A, oligodendrocyte-myelin glycoprotein (OMgp), and myelin-associated glycoprotein (MAG), inhibit axonal growth cone extension through stimulation of Nogo-66 receptors (Buchli and Schwab 2005).

Excitatory neurotransmission is enhanced by the up-regulation of NMDA receptors and down-regulation of $GABA_B$ receptors, creating the conditions for enhanced axonal sprouting and long-term potentiation (LTP) similar to those seen in early development. The waves of synchronous depolarization seen during development are also seen in areas of brain recovery (Butz et al. 2004). After a severe unilateral injury, more axonal sprouting, dendritic arborization, and sp· ᵓ remodeling are seen in the contralateral hemisphere (Johansson 2004), unmasking dormant but pre-existing connections that allow very early recovery of function (Metz et al. 2005).

New neuronal progenitor cells are created in the subventricular zone for several months after injury, but it is unclear whether these cells become incorporated into the brain as mature neurons or merely contribute to the recovery of existing neurons and networks through the production of growth factors (Zhang et al. 2005b, Thored et al. 2006).

PROGNOSIS

OUTCOME CLASSIFICATION

One of the most commonly used measures of clinical outcome in adults is the Glasgow Outcome Scale (GOS), which includes the broad categories of good recovery, moderate disability, severe disability, vegetative state, and death. Use of the GOS in children with moderate to severe TBI fails to identify those within the 'good outome' category who have significant and persistent neuropsychologic impairments. The King's Outcome Scale for Childhood Head Injury (KOSCHI) and Pediatric Cerebral Performance Category Scale (PCPCS) are modifications of the GOS that take into account the developmental immaturity of young children (Fiser 1992, Crouchman et al. 2001). Table 19.5 compares these basic outcome measures.

The Rancho Los Amigos scale is a commonly used measure of cognitive recovery that was originally developed for use in adults by Hagen Malkmus and Durham in 1972. Its eight functional categories are as follow:

1 No response
2 Generalized response
3 Localized response
4 Confused and agitated
5 Confused and inappropriate but non-agitated
6 Confused but appropriate
7 Automatic and appropriate
8 Purposeful and appropriate

The Functional Inventory Measure for Children (WeeFIM) and Pediatric Evaluation of Developmental Independence (PEDI) are detailed measures adapted for use in children that quantify independence in a number of domains (Ziviani et al. 2001). The WeeFIM is one of the most popular functional outcome measures for use in pediatric studies, but it is still limited in its ability to describe the capabilities of very young children. The Kries Outcome Scale (KOS) is a functional measure specifically adapted for use in adolescents (Haley et al. 2004).

HYPOXIC-ISCHEMIC BRAIN INJURY

The outcome of focal stroke depends on the location and extent of injury but also on the underlying cause. Children presenting with a decreased level of consciousness, seizures, involvement of the complete middle cerebral artery territory, or greater than 10% of their intracranial volume tend to have poorer outcomes (Ganesan et al. 1999). A review of over 1300 published cases of AIS in childhood found that, on average, 30% (5–78%) have good neurologic outcomes, 60% (9–90%) are left with significant functional deficits, and 10% (0–16%) succumb to their injury or

TABLE 19.5
Comparison of outcome measures

Outcome	GOS	KOSCHI	PCPCS
Good recovery	5) Resumption of normal activities despite any minor neurologic or psychologic deficits	5a) Changes from baseline have no impact on well-being or function 5b) Complete recovery	1) at age appropriate level School age child attends regular school classroom
Mild disability	Not defined	Not defined	2) conscious, alert, and able to interact at an age appropriate level School age child attends regular school classroom but grade may not be age appropriate May have a mild neurologic deficit
Moderate disability	4) Disabled but independent in daily life, with varying degrees of dysphasia, hemiparesis, ataxia, intellectual and memory deficits, and personality changes	4a) Mostly independent but in need of supervision or help for physical or behavioral problems 4b) Age appropriately independent with learning and behavior problems or neurologic sequelae affecting function	3) Conscious, performs age-appropriate independent activities of daily life School age child attends special education classroom May have learning deficit
Severe disability	3) Conscious but disabled, dependent upon others for daily support due to mental and/or physical limitations	3a) Able to move to command or make purposeful spontaneous movements 3b) Incapable of self-care but fully conscious and able to communicate 3c) Highly dependent but fully conscious and able to assist in daily activities	4) Conscious but dependent on others for daily support because of impaired brain function
Vegetative state	2) Exhibits no obvious cortical function	2) No evidence of ability to communicate or to respond to commands	5) Any degree of unawareness, including coma
Death	1	1	6

GOS, Glasgow Outcome Scale; KOSCHI, King's Outcome Scale for Childhood Head Injury; PCPCS, Pediatric Cerebral Performance Category Scale.

underlying disease (Lynch and Han 2005). In one study of 90 patients with at least 2 years of follow-up, motor deficits were absent in 31%, mild in 18%, moderate in 28%, and severe in 23%. The same study found expressive or receptive language disorders in 29% of survivors although, unlike stroke in adults, the side of the lesion did not influence neuropsychologic performance (deVeber et al. 2000). Psychiatric and behavioral problems, especially attention-deficit–hyperactivity disorder (ADHD) and anxiety disorders, are found in as many as 59% of patients after childhood stroke (Max et al. 2002).

The morbidity and mortality of global hypoxic-ischemic injury tends to be greater than that of AIS, although the pattern and extent of injury depends on the severity and duration of substrate deprivation. Those regions of the brain that lie in watershed vascular territories, or whose neurons are particularly susceptible to ischemia, because of their relatively high metabolic demands or low antioxidant defenses, suffer more extensive injury after relatively short periods of ischemia. The hippocampal CA1 pyramidal neurons, cerebellar Purkinje cells, thalamic reticular neurons, medium sized striatal neurons, and the pyramidal neurons of layers III, V, and VI of the neocortex are the most sensitive to ischemia, leading survivors to develop prominent disturbances in memory, balance and gait, level of consciousness, emotion, and cognition. Prolonged ischemia causes more pronounced cell loss within the arterial watershed regions. Carbon monoxide poisoning results in particular injury to the hippocampus and globus pallidus, with consequent parkinsonian-like features and cognitive dysfunction. Mild to moderate asphyxia, with compromised oxygen and glucose delivery and significant tissue acidosis, has been shown to cause preferential injury of the subcortical white matter (Meng et al. 2006). Purely hypoxic events not associated with ischemia, even when prolonged and severe, appear to cause little neuronal injury other than synaptic dysfunction. Myoclonus and seizures are common during recovery because of neuronal excitability from selective GABA depletion; however, neurologic outcome is generally good after synaptic regeneration (Miyamoto and Auer 2000).

Reports related to predicting outcomes in brain injury in children are often limited by their small sample size and the retrospective nature of their data collection. In one prospective study of 42 children who had a persistently impaired level of consciousness 24 hours after a hypoxic-ischemic injury, 16 had a good outcome, with 4 of these having mild to moderate disability (Mandel et al. 2002). Of the 26 children with a poor outcome, 7 had severe disability or survived in a persistent vegetative state and 19 died (8 after withdrawal of therapy). Poor outcome occurred in 91% of those with initial cardiopulmonary resuscitation exceeding 10 minutes and in all of those with (1) GCS less than 5, (2) no spontaneous respirations, (3) absent pupillary reflexes at 24 hours, (4) discontinuous electroencephalographic (EEG) activity, (5) epileptiform EEG activity, or (6) bilaterally absent N20 latencies on somatosensory evoked potential testing. Other studies have found a similarly strong predictive value to these clinical and electrophysiologic parameters (Jacinto et al. 2001).

Magnetic resonance proton spectroscopy (MRS) has been shown to have considerable predictive power in the context of global hypoxic-ischemic and traumatic brain injury, with severely diminished N-acetyl aspartate and elevations of lactate correlating strongly with poor outcomes in children with asphyxia (Kreis et al. 1996), cardiac arrest (Berek et al. 1995), and severe trauma (Ashwal et al. 2006). Advances in neuroimaging may allow prediction of the specific cognitive and performance deficits of survivors. Among the promising technologies currently in development is magnetic resonance diffusion tensor imaging (DTI), which reflects the myelination and spatial orientation of axons. Early reports have shown that DTI accurately reflects *in vivo* axonal disruption after ischemia (Sotak 2002) and traumatic brain injury (Wilde et al. 2006).

TRAUMATIC BRAIN INJURY

Prognosis for recovery after TBI relates to the location of focal injuries and to the overall severity of injury. The limbic and heteromodal association areas on the undersurface of the anterior frontal and temporal lobes are those areas most often injured by a high velocity impact with the petrous bones, sphenoid wings, and cribriform plate of the skull. Patients with contusions thus frequently develop impaired executive functioning, working memory, memory encoding and retrieval, attention and behavior modulation.

In children with mild TBI, the most commonly reported symptoms include headache, dizziness, fatigue and decreased memory, concentration, and tolerance for frustration. These symptoms generally resolve rapidly, but one study found that of children with mild TBI, nearly 5.7% remained symptomatic at 1 month and 1.7% remained symptomatic at 10 months after TBI (Hooper et al. 2004). While the long-term prognosis for recovery is excellent, parents and teachers need to be prepared for the possibility that older children will have difficulty returning to school and that subtle deficits in attention, memory, and learning may not be initially apparent in preschool age children (Barlow et al. 2005). Delayed cognitive decline also results from late cortical and subcortical neurodegeneration. This is more pronounced during development and has been attributed to ongoing apoptosis, inflammation, and denervation atrophy (Pullela et al. 2006). Following TBI in childhood, hippocampal volume can continue to decrease even into adulthood (Tasker et al. 2005).

Children who have a more severe TBI are much more likely to have lasting impairments in consciousness, cognition and behavior. Post-traumatic epilepsy, often refractory to medical management, develops in up to 20% of children after TBI, with the incidence higher with more severe initial trauma and with younger age (Ratan et al. 1999). In the absence of significant focal injuries, the length of coma and of post-traumatic amnesia correlate well to injury severity and eventual outcome. In an analysis of outcomes after severe TBI, children between the ages of 5 and 10 years did better than adolescents and adults. However, children under 4 years old had the worst outcomes and were more likely to develop secondary hypotension and subdural hematoma (Levin et al. 1992). The relative contributions of age and of the unique pathophysiology of inflicted trauma could not be determined in this study.

Inflicted non-accidental trauma is associated with a number of factors that could potentially contribute to the poorer outcomes relative to accidental trauma, including the occurrence of multiple insults (Raghupathi et al. 2004), secondary hypotension and hypoxemia (Parizel et al. 2003), delays in presentation (Gilliland 1998), seizures (King et al. 2003), and cervical spinal cord injury (Gattan and Ellenbogen 2002). Genetic and socioeconomic factors may also predispose these children to poorer long-term recovery (Gleckman et al. 1999).

Even those children whose academic skills return to normal are at risk for school failure because of subsequent behavioral problems. The severity of observed behavior problems is correlated with the severity of the injury, but is even more strongly predicted by the premorbid function of the child and his family (Rivara et al. 1992, Schwartz et al. 2003). A prior diagnosis of ADHD is associated with even more behavioral problems after TBI. Children with ADHD also develop more head trauma because of their relative impulsivity than their peers, making it somewhat difficult to attribute causality and effect accurately (Brehaut et al. 2003). Family socioeconomic status and coping ability has repeatedly been shown to significantly influence recovery (Yeates and Taylor 2005) and efforts to improve family function may be important to a child's ultimate success.

Of the large number of genes that could potentially influence an individual's response and ultimate prognosis after injury, two have been studied extensively. Approximately 15% of the population carry at least one apolipoprotein E epsilon-4 (APOE4) allele and thus are at an increased risk for more severe cognitive impairment after even mild TBI. The effect seems especially robust in children and young adults and appears to be brought about by the lack of the other APOE alleles, APOE2 or APOE3. These protective alleles are associated with improved endogenous antioxidant activity and attenuated reactive gliosis. Carriers of one APOE4 have an odds ratio of a poor outcome ranging from 3.6 (Teasdale et al. 2005) to 13.9 (Friedman et al. 1999). Inheritance of the IL-1 RN allele 2 has also been associated with complications of head trauma, especially contusions and subarachnoid hemorrhages after severe TBI, with an odds ratio of 4.6 for heterozygotes (Hadjigeorgiou et al. 2005).

PLASTICITY

Children are at once at an advantage and at a disadvantage relative to adults in their capacity for rehabilitation from severe brain injury. Kennard carried out studies in the 1930s in which she found that infant monkeys experienced less behavioral impairment than adult monkeys after identical experimental cortical lesioning. Subsequent observations have largely confirmed this age-related resiliency, known as the Kennard principle, to be generally true in humans. Children undergoing early hemispherectomy for medically intractable epilepsy have relatively good outcomes, demonstrating the remarkable capacity of the still developing brain to relocate cortical function to homologous regions in the contralateral hemisphere (Bittar et al. 2002). Children between 1 and 2 years of age recover particularly well from brain injury, possibly because this is the age at which dendritic and synaptic growth is at its peak (Kolb et al. 2000). However, the capacity for this type of plasticity depends greatly on injury location and age at time of injury even during childhood. Lesions of the motor cortex are the most amenable to compensation by ipsilateral and contralateral reorganization (Chapman and McKinnon 2000), but there is a gradually worsening of prognosis for language recovery after resection of the dominant hemisphere after age 8 years (Vining et al. 1997).

Young children who have global and bilateral injuries may not only be less able to recover prior function, but they frequently acquire cognitive, attentional, and perceptual deficits that impair their ability to recover and advance developmentally. Some of these deficits may not be apparent in children injured at an early age until they enter school and have higher real demands placed upon their abilities. In long-term studies, children with severe traumatic brain injury, especially the youngest of those studied, show a deceleration in their rate of recovery several years after injury (Ewing-Cobbs et al. 2004a). Infants who have moderate to severe traumatic brain injury have greater impairments in learning, memory, and inhibition than school age children (Ewing-Cobbs et al. 2004b).

IMPLICATIONS FOR TREATMENT AND RESEARCH

Further understanding of the patterns and particular physiologic characteristics of injury in the developing brain promises to improve our ability to prevent, ameliorate, and rehabilitate brain injury in children.

PREVENTION

Most causes of severe brain injury have been shown to be amenable to prevention, but widespread implementation often suffers from a lack of either public awareness or acceptance. For example, despite intensive educational and enforcement efforts, the vast majority of 4- to 8-year-old children who die as passengers in motor vehicle accidents are unrestrained or wear adult seat belts not adapted for their development. Primary care providers, government public heath institutions, and advocacy organizations must continue to expand their efforts to prevent child abuse, pedestrian collisions, alcohol-related motor vehicle accidents, exposure to choking hazards, and inadequate and improper use of car seats, helmets, and child-proof barriers.

Secondary prevention of AIS is effective in children with some known risk factors. The Stroke Prevention in Sickle Cell Study Project (STOP) showed that serial blood transfusions produced a dramatic 92% reduction in the incidence of first clinical stroke in children with sickle cell disease and intracranial stenosis documented by transcranial Doppler ultrasound (Adams et al. 1998). Current recommendations are to use transfusion to maintain a hemoglobin S concentration below 30% in this particular at-risk population. The risk of AIS in children with CHD is reduced by earlier surgical treatment and shorter intraoperative time periods for cardiac arrest and bypass. Retrospective studies also suggest a role for aspirin in reducing the incidence of AIS in children with CHD (Barker et al. 2005). Antiplatelet agents and anticoagulation have not yet been shown to be effective for prevention of AIS in other populations at risk, although their use, at least for some period of time, is recommended by most specialists as tertiary prevention after an initial first stroke. Large multicenter clinical trials of these therapies are currently being organized and their results are eagerly anticipated (Sofronas et al. 2006).

NEUROPROTECTION

Translating successful pharmacologic interventions from animal models to humans has been frustratingly difficult, but there continues to be great promise for strategies to rescue cells from Ca^{2+} influx and excitotoxicity, block the biochemical pathways leading to apoptosis, and reduce injury from free radicals and inflammation.

NMDA-receptor antagonists such as dextromethorphan and dizocilpine (MK801) provide significant neuroprotection in animal models of cerebral ischemia (Li et al. 1999), but their use in humans is complicated by significant side effects such as delirium and psychosis (Rossberg et al. 2002). Furthermore, their use in models of childhood brain injury reduces necrosis, but greatly increases apoptosis (Pohl et al. 1999). Calcium-channel blockers would seem to be attractive candidates for reducing excitotoxic injury, but their use in animal experiments and clinical trials have generally failed to show benefit, possibly because of deleterious hypotensive effects (Lazarewicz et al. 1990, Roine et al. 1990, Calle et al. 1993). Anticonvulsants that block voltage-gated Na^+ channels and reduce membrane depolarization have shown modest promise in animal models with phenytoin (Artru and Michenfelder 1981) and lamotrigine (Imaizumi et al. 1995) producing reductions in extracellular glutamate, lactate, cerebral edema, and cell death. Barbiturates hyperpolarize membranes and decrease cerebral metabolism but have shown no benefit in animals or patients with global ischemic injury (Steen et al. 1979, Rossberg et al. 2002).

The cyclooxygenase inhibitor nimesulide has only been tested in animals but improves survival of hippocampal neurons (Candelario-Jalil et al. 2002). Magnesium infusion reduces hippocampal injury in animal models of ischemia (Miles et al. 2001, Zhu et al. 2005), possibly through NMDA channel blockade, competitive inhibition of Ca^{2+} binding sites, and vasodilation of arterioles, but large clinical trials in the setting of cardiac arrest and trauma have shown no benefit (Muir et al. 2004, Temkin et al. 2007).

Selective kappa-type opioid receptor agonists, such as the experimental agent BRL 52537, have been shown to have a neuroprotective effect in models of ischemia (Boutin et al. 1999), although only in male animals, possibly through an attenuation of Ca^{2+} influx and of neuronal NO production (Zeynalov et al. 2005). Sigma-1 receptor agonists, such as 4-phenyl-1-(4-phenylbutyl) piperadine (PPBP), seem to confer potent neuroprotection in ischemic models through reduction in Ca^{2+} influx, neuronal NO production, and glutamate release (Goyagi et al. 2001).

Other pharmacologic agents that have been considered promising for thera- peutic trials in ischemia include (1) anesthetics such as etomidate, ketamine, and propofol, (2) sodium-channel blockers such as mexiletine and lidocaine, (3) cata- cholamine receptor agonists such as dexmedetomidine, and (4) xanthine oxidase inhibitors such as allopurinol (Weigl et al. 2005).

Excitotoxic injury and necrosis progress within the first minutes to hours after injury, presenting a narrow possible window for therapeutic intervention. The more slowly progressing pathways involved in apoptosis offer a window of hours to days for therapeutic benefit. Theoretically feasable approaches include (1) inhibit- ing initiation with soluble TNF receptors, antiexcitotoxic agents, or antioxidants, (2) attenuating the apoptotic cascade with hypothermia, Bcl-2 mimetics, or with caspase, protease, endonuclease, and PARP inhibitors, and (3) promoting survival with the up-regulation of stress proteins and activation of PKB (Zhang et al. 2005d). Systemic administration of the pan-caspase inhibitor Boc-aspartyl fluoromethyl- ketone reduces injury in animal models of ischemia (Morita-Fujimura et al. 1999). Inhibitors of PARP, such as 5-iodo-6-amino-1,2-benzopyrone, improve functional outcomes in animal models of TBI when given at moderate doses but impair memory performance when given at higher doses (Satchell et al. 2003).

The pathophysiology of DAI suggests several targets for intervention to ame- liorate injury severity. Hypothermia has been shown to lessen experimental axonal disconnection through inhibition of calpain proteolysis of alpha spectrin (Maxwell et al. 1999). Large clinical trials of controlled hypothermia for TBI have thus far shown ICP reduction but no evident outcome improvement (Seppelt 2005). More recent small clinical trials, using moderate selective head cooling for severe TBI, suggest that the idea still has merit but requires refinement of technique (Liu et al. 2006).

Cyclosporine is thought to target and block the MTP. In animal models of DAI, therapeutic doses have been shown to decrease the swelling and rupture of axonal mitochondria, calpain-associated proteolysis and neurofilament compaction, and axon disconnection (Okonkwo et al. 2003). Preliminary clinical trials in humans have shown that cyclosporine is safe and possibly effective, encouraging further study in larger trials. Another immunomodulatory agent, FK506, also attenuates axonal injury after trauma, in this case through inhibition of both calcineurin and of neurofilament compaction (Marmarou and Povlishock 2006). Despite microdialysis studies in humans with TBI correlating the duration and degree of extracellular glutamate elevations with eventual outcomes, clinical trials with NMDA antagonists have thus far shown no evident benefit (Povlishock 2000).

Given the popularity of adult models of stroke and of neonatal models of asphyxia, it is likely that most neuroprotective therapies will be studied in clinical trials involving patients at the extremes of the lifespan. It is clear, however, that therapeutic responses may be significantly better or worse in preschool age and school age children. In the near future, trials of hypothermia for brain injury are needed to determine the role this should play in the resuscitation and intensive care of children.

REHABILITATION

Opportunities to enhance the recovery of children may exist during acute hospitalization, during formal rehabilitation and long after hospital discharge. Animal models show a clear benefit from a variety of therapies, including rearing in an enriched environment, infusion of growth factors, and the introduction of stem cells. Clinical trials are needed to show whether the benefits of these approaches would accrue to brain injured children.

Forced training of a paretic limb and indirect electrical or magnetic stimulation of injured cortex improves functional recovery (Hummel and Cohen 2005). Providing brain injured rodents with an enriched environment – putting them into large cages with toys, tools, and other animals, or training them in new skills – enhances their overall functional recovery. The effects are again primarily seen in the contralateral hemisphere, with increased transcription of growth-promoting genes and increased dendritic arborization and spine density of pyramidal neurons. Environmental enhancement promotes the generation of neuronal stem cells and precursor cells within the subventricular zone and striatum, but these are most likely contributing to the growth and recovery of existing networks (Matsumori et al. 2006). A blunted response to enrichment has been seen in P17 rats, associated with the earlier post-injury expression of the inhibitory NMDA receptor NR21 subunit, suggesting at least one mechanism by which plasticity decreases with age (Giza et al. 2006).

A number of pharmacologic therapies show promise for stimulating recovery in animal models. Erythropoietin given after ischemic injury increases the production of VEGF and BDNF and promotes neurogenesis, angiogenesis, and improved functional outcome (Wang et al. 2004). Granulocyte colony-stimulating factor, which is up-regulated in brain tissue after injury, can be given exogenously to improve functional outcomes, probably through decreased apoptosis and enhanced neurogenesis (Schneider et al. 2005). Other therapies that benefit recovery processes in animal models include heparin binding epidermal growth factor-like growth factor (Sugiura et al. 2005), hydroxyl-methyl-guanine Co-A reductase inhibitors (statins) (Chen et al. 2003), phosphodiesterase-5 inhibitors (Zhang et al. 2005a), sigma-1 receptor agonists, and inosine (Chen et al. 2002). Inhibition of axonal Nogo-66 receptors, either with an antigen (Lee et al. 2004) or an antibody (Seymour et al. 2005), leads to the dramatic improvement in axonal growth and functional recovery, even when initiated as late as a week after injury.

Bone marrow derived stem cells or progenitor cells, either transplanted directly into the injured area or delivered systemically, have shown an encouraging ability to boost recuperation, through much the same mechanisms as those pluripotent cells endogenously generated in the subventricular zone (Shen et al. 2006). Fetal embryonic stem cells, however, appear capable of fully differentiating into mature neurons and integrating themselves into both the cortical and striatal neural networks (Hayashi et al. 2006).

The timing of these interventions appears to be crucial to their success. Environmental stimulation of animals in the first 2 days after injury can be detrimental and the benefits of enrichment are lost if it is initiated more than 30 days after injury (Nygren and Wieloch 2005). Some pharmacologic agents both provide neuroprotection immediately after injury and enhance later recovery, including EPO, G-CSF, sigma-1 agonists, and fibroblast growth factor. Other agents have opposite effects on neuroprotection and regeneration. GABA receptor agonists, NMDA receptor antagonists, MMP inhibitors, and some anti-inflammatory agents are neuroprotective when given early after injury, but can impair rehabilitation if given later (Zhao et al. 2006). Caspases and other elements of the apoptotic cascade appear to have an important role in synaptic remodeling, suggesting that prolonged inhibition can negatively affect repair and recovery (Gillman and Mattson 2002).

CONCLUSIONS

While much has been learned regarding the basic processes by which acquired brain injury proceeds and results in disability, much remains to be learned regarding effective medical and rehabilitation interventions. A further challenge exists on a level of community and social policy to modify behavior to exert an effect of primary prevention.

REFERENCES

Adamides AA, Winter CD, Lewis PM, Cooper DJ, Kossmann T, Rosenfeld JV (2006) Current controversies in the management of patients with severe traumatic brain injury. *ANZ J Surg* 76: 163–174.

Adams RJ, McKie VC, Hsu L (1998) Prevention of a first stroke by transfusions in children with sickle cell anemia and abnormal results on transcranial Doppler ultrasonography. *N Engl J Med* 339: 5–11.

Adelson PD, Robichaud P, Hamilton RL, Kochanek PM (1996) A model of diffuse traumatic brain injury in the immature rat. *J Neurosurg* 85: 877–884.

Adelson PD, Whalen M, Robichaud P, Carlos T, Kochanek P (1998) Blood–brain barrier permeability and acute inflammation in two models of TBI in the immature rat: a preliminary report. *Acta Neurochir Suppl* 71: 104–106.

Antonsson B, Conti F, Ciavatta AM, Montessuit S, Lewis S, Martinou I, et al. (1997) Inhibition of Bax channel-forming activity by Bcl-2. *Science* 277: 370–372.

Armin SS, Colohan AR, Zhang JH (2006) Traumatic subarachnoid hemorrhage: our current understanding and its evolution over the past half century. *Neurol Res* 28: 445–452.

Artru AA, Michenfelder JD (1981) Anoxic cerebral potassium accumulation reduced by phenytoin: mechanism of cerebral protection? *Anesth Analg* 60: 41–45.

Ashwal S, Holshouser BA, Tong KA (2006) Use of advanced neuroimaging techniques in the evaluation of pediatric traumatic brain injury. *Dev Neurosci* 28: 309–326.

Badan I, Buchhold B, Hamm A, Gratz M, Walker LC, Platt D, et al. (2003) Accelerated glial reactivity to stroke in aged rats correlates with reduced functional recovery. *J Cereb Blood Flow Metab* 23: 845–854.

Barker PC, Nowak C, King K, Mosca RS, Bove EL, Goldberg CS (2005) Risk factors for cerebrovascular events following Fontan palliation in patients with a functional single ventricle. *Am J Cardiol* 96: 587–591.

Barlow KM, Thomson E, Johnson D, Minnus RA (2005) Late neurologic and cognitive sequelae of inflicted traumatic brain injury in infancy. *Pediatrics* 116: e174–e185.

Bartus R (1997) The calpain hypothesis of neurodegeneration: evidence for a common cytotoxic pathway. *Neuroscientist* 3: 314–327.

Bayir H, Kochanek PM, Kagan VE (2006) Oxidative stress in immature brain after traumatic brain injury. *Dev Neurosci* 28: 420–431.

Beckman JS (1996) Oxidative damage and tyrosine nitration from peroxynitrite. *Chem Res Toxicol* 9: 836–844.

Benveniste H, Drejer J, Schousboe A, Diemer NH (1984) Elevation of the extracellular concentrations of glutamate and aspartate in rat hippocampus during transient cerebral ischemia monitored by intracerebral microdialysis. *J Neurochem* 43: 1369–1374.

Berek K, Lechleitner P, Luef G, Felber S, Saltuari L, Schinnerl A, et al. (1995) Early determination of neurological outcome after prehospital cardiopulmonary resuscitation. *Stroke* 26: 543–549.

Berger RP, Adelson PD, Richichi R, Kochanek PM (2006) Serum biomarkers after traumatic and hypoxemic brain injuries: insight into the biochemical response of the pediatric brain to inflicted brain injury. *Dev Neurosci* 28: 327–335.

Berger RP, Janesko KL, Wisniewski SR, Adelson PD, Clark RSB, Ruppel R, et al. (2002) Neuron-specific enolase and S100B in cerebrospinal fluid after severe traumatic brain injury in infants and children. *Pediatrics* 109: E31.

Bittar RG, Rosenfeld JV, Klug GL, Hopkins IJ, Simon Harvey A (2002) Resective surgery in infants and young children with intractable epilepsy. *J Clin Neurosci* 9: 142–146.

Bittigau P, Sifringer M, Pohl D, Stadthaus D, Ishimaru M, Shimizu H, et al. (1999) Apoptotic neurodegeneration following trauma is markedly enhanced in the immature brain. *Ann Neurol* 45: 724–735.

Boehning D, Patterson RL, Sedaghat L, Glebova NO, Kurosaki T, Snyder SH (2003) Cytochrome c binds to inositol (1,4,5) triphosphate receptors amplifying calcium dependent apoptosis. *Nat Cell Biol* 5: 1051–1061.

Borisenko GG, Matsura T, Liu SX, Tyurin VA, Jianfei J, Serinkan FB, et al. (2003) Macrophage recognition of externalized phosphatidylserine and phagocytosis of apoptotic Jurkat cells: existence of a threshold. *Arch Biochem Biophys* 413: 41–52.

Boutin H, Dauphin F, MacKenzie ET, Jauzac P (1999) Differential time-course decreases in nonselective mu-, delta-, and kappa-opioid receptors after focal cerebral ischemia in mice. *Stroke* 30: 1271–1277.

Brehaut JC, Miller A, Raina P, McGrail KM (2003) Childhood behavior disorders and injuries among children and youth: a population based study. *Pediatrics* 111: 262–269.

Brookes PS, Bolanos JP, Heales SJ (1999) The assumption that nitric oxide inhibits mitochondrial ATP synthesis is correct. *FEBS Lett* 446: 261–263.

Buchli AD, Schwab ME (2005) Inhibition of nogo: a key strategy to increase regeneration, plasticity and functional recovery of the lesioned central nervous system. *Ann Med* 37: 556–567.

Buki A, Povlishock JT (2006) All roads lead to disconnection? Traumatic axonal injury revisited. *Acta Neurochir (Wien)* 148: 181–193.

Buki A, Siman R, Trojanowski JQ, Povlishock JT (1999) The role of calpain-mediated spectrin proteolysis in traumatically induced axonal injury. *J Neuropathol Exp Neurol* 58: 365–375.

Butz M, Gross J, Timmermann L, Moll M, Freund HJ, Witte OW, et al. (2004) Perilesional pathological oscillatory activity in the magnetoencephalogram of patients with cortical brain lesions. *Neurosci Lett* 355: 93–96.

Calle PA, Paridaens K, De Ridder LI, Buylaert WA (1993) Failure of nimodipine to prevent brain damage in a global brain ischemia model in the rat. *Resuscitation* 25: 59–71.

Cambj-Sapunar L, Yu M, Harder DR, Roman RJ (2003) Contribution of 5-hydroxytryptamine$_{1B}$ receptors and 20-hydroxyeiscosatetraenoic acid to fall in cerebral blood flow after subarachnoid hemorrhage. *Stroke* 34: 1269–1275.

Candelario-Jalil E, Alvarez D, Gonzalez-Falcon A, Garcia-Cabrera M, Martinez-Sanchez G, Merino N, et al. (2002) Neuroprotective efficacy of nimesulide against hippocampal neuronal damage following transient forebrain ischemia. *Eur J Pharmacol* 453: 189–195.

Carafoli E (1991) Calcium pump of the plasma membrane. *Physiol Rev* 71: 129–153.

Carmichael ST, Archibeque I, Luke L, Nolan T, Momiy J, Li S (2005) Growth-associated gene expression after stroke: evidence for a growth-promoting region in peri-infarct cortex. *Exp Neurol* 193: 291–311.

Chai J, Du C, Wu JW, Kyin S, Wang X, Shi Y (2000) Structural and biochemical basis of apoptotic activation by Smac/DIABLO. *Nature* 406: 855–862.

Chan AK, deVeber G (2000) Prothrombotic disorders and ischemic stroke in children. *Semin Pediatr Neurol* 7: 301–308.

Chapman SB, McKinnon L (2000) Discussion of developmental plasticity: factors affecting cognitive outcome after pediatric traumatic brain injury. *J Commun Disord* 33: 333–344.

Chen J, Zhang ZG, Li Y, Wang Y, Wang L, Jiang H, et al. (2003) Statins induce angiogenesis, neurogenesis, and synaptogenesis after stroke. *Ann Neurol* 53: 743–751.

Chen P, Goldberg DE, Kolb B, Lanser M, Benowitz LI (2002) Inosine induces axonal rewiring and improves behavioral outcome after stroke. *Proc Natl Acad Sci U S A* 99: 9031–9036.

Choi DW (1987) Ionic dependence of glutamate neurotoxicity. *J Neurosci* 7: 369–379.

Chun DS, Schamberger MS, Flaspohler T (2004) Incidence, outcome, and risk factors for stroke after the Fontan procedure. *Am J Cardiol* 93: 117–119.

Clark RS, Kochanek PM, Adelson PD, Bell MJ, Carcillo JA, Chen M, et al. (2000) Increases in bcl-2 protein in cerebrospinal fluid and evidence for programmed cell death in infants and children after severe traumatic brain injury. *J Pediatr* 137: 197–204.

Clower BR, Yamamoto Y, Cain L, Haines DE, Smith RR (1994) Endothelial injury following experimental subarachnoid hemorrhage in rats: effects on brain blood flow. *Anat Rec* 240: 104–114.

Colbourne F, Grooms SY, Zukin RS, Buchan AM, Bennett MV (2003) Hypothermia rescues hippocampal CA1 neurons and attenuates downregulation of the AMPA receptor GluR2 subunit after forebrain ischemia. *Proc Natl Acad Sci U S A* 100: 2906–2910.

Colvin RA, Davis N, Nipper RW, Carter PA (2000) Zinc transport in the brain: routes of zinc influx and efflux in neurons. *J Nutr* 130: 1484S–1487S.

Crouchman M, Rossiter L, Colaco T, Forsyth R (2001) A practical outcome scale for paediatric head injury. *Arch Dis Child* 84: 120–124.

Danton GH, Dietrich WD (2003) Inflammatory mechanisms after ischemia and stroke. *J Neuropathol Exp Neurol* 62: 127–136.

Densmore JC, Lim HJ, Oldham KT, Guice KS (2006) Outcomes and delivery of care in pediatric injury. *J Pediatr Surg* 41: 92–98.

DeVeber G, MacGregor D, Curtis R, Mayank S (2000) Neurologic outcome in survivors of childhood arterial ischemic stroke and sinovenous thrombosis. *J Child Neurol* 15: 316–324.

Dijkhuizen RM, Asahi M, Wu O, Rosen BR, Lo EH (2002) Rapid breakdown of microvascular barriers and subsequent hemorrhagic transformation after delayed recombinant tissue plasminogen activator treatment in a rat embolic stroke model. *Stroke* 33: 2100–2104.

Du L, Zhang X, Han YY, Burke NA, Kochanek PM, Watkins SC, et al. (2003) Intramitochondrial poly-ADP ribosylation contributes to NAD$^+$ depletion and cell death induced by oxidative stress. *J Biol Chem* 278: 18426–18433.

Erecinska M, Cherian S, Silver IA (2004) Energy metabolism in mammalian brain during development. *Prog Neurobiol* 73: 397–445.

Ewing Cobbs L, Barnes M, Fletcher JM, Levin HS, Swank PR, Song J (2004a) Modeling of longitudinal academic achievement scores after pediatric traumatic brain injury. *Dev Neuropsychol* 25: 107–133.

Ewing-Cobbs L, Prasad MR, Landry SH, Kramer L, DeLeon R (2004b) Executive functions following traumatic brain injury in young children: a preliminary analysis. *Dev Neuropsychol* 26: 487–512.

Fiser DH (1992) Assessing the outcome of pediatric intensive care. *J Pediatr* 121: 68–74.

Friedman G, Froom P, Sazbon L, Grinblatt I, Shochina M, Tsenter J, et al. (1999) Apolipoprotein E-epsilon4 genotype predicts a poor outcome in survivors of traumatic brain injury. *Neurology* 52: 244–248.

Fukunaga K, Soderling TR, Miyamoto E (1992) Activation of Ca^{2+}/calmodulin-dependent protein kinase II and protein kinase C by glutamate in cultured rat hippocampal neurons. *J Biol Chem* 267: 22527–22533.

Ganesan V, Ng V, Chong WK, Kirkham FJ, Connelly A (1999) Lesion volume, lesion location, and outcome after middle cerebral artery territory stroke. *Arch Dis Child* 81: 295–300.

Ganesan V, Prengler M, McShane MA, Wade AM, Kirkham FJ (2003) Investigation of risk factors in children with arterial ischemic stroke. *Ann Neurol* 53: 167–173.

Gao Y, Yokota R, Tang S, Ashton AW, Ware JA (2000) Reversal of angiogenesis *in vitro*, induction of apoptosis, and inhibition of AKT phosphorylation in endothelial cells by thromboxane A(2). *Circ Res* 87: 739–745.

Gennarelli TA, Thibault LE, Adams JH, Graham DI, Thompson CJ, Marcincin RP (1982) Diffuse axonal injury and traumatic coma in the primate. *Ann Neurol* 12: 564–574.

Ghatan S, Ellenbogen RG (2002) Pediatric spine and spinal cord injury after inflicted trauma. *Neurosurg Clin N Am* 13: 227–233.

Ghatan S, Larner S, Kinoshita Y, Hetman M, Patel L, Xia Z, et al. (2000) p38 MAP kinase mediates bax translocation in nitric oxide-induced apoptosis in neurons. *J Cell Biol* 150: 335–347.

Giedd JN, Blumenthal J, Jeffries NO, Castellanos FX, Liu H, Zijdenbos A, et al. (1999) Brain development during childhood and adolescence: a longitudinal MRI study. *Nat Neurosci* 2: 861–863.

Gilliland MG (1998) Interval duration between injury and severe symptoms in nonaccidental head trauma in infants and young children. *J Forensic Sci* 43: 723–725.

Gilman CP, Mattson MP (2002) Do apoptotic mechanisms regulate synaptic plasticity and growth-cone motility? *Neuromolecular Med* 2: 197–214.

Ginsberg MD, Myers RE (1972) The topography of impaired microvascular perfusion in the primate brain following total circulatory arrest. *Neurology* 22: 998–1011.

Giza CC, Maria NS, Hovda DA (2006) N-methyl-D-aspartate receptor subunit changes after traumatic injury to the developing brain. *J Neurotrauma* 23: 950–961.

Gleckman AM, Bell MD, Evans RJ, Smith TW (1999) Diffuse axonal injury in infants with nonaccidental craniocerebral trauma: enhanced detection by beta-amyloid precursor protein immunohistochemical staining. *Arch Pathol Lab Med* 123: 146–151.

Gluckman PD, Wyatt JS, Azzopardi D, Ballard R, Edwards AD, Ferriero DM, et al. (2005) Selective head cooling with mild systemic hypothermia after neonatal encephalopathy: multicentre randomised trial. *Lancet* 365: 663–670.

Goyagi T, Goto S, Bhardwaj A, Dawson VL, Hurn PD, Kirsch JR (2001) Neuroprotective effect of σ1-receptor ligand, 4-phenyl-1-(4-phenylbutyl) piperidine (PPBP) is linked to reduced neuronal nitric oxide production. *Stroke* 32: 1613–1620.

Greenberg JH, Uematsu D, Araki N, Hickey WF, Reivich M (1990) Cytosolic free calcium during focal cerebral ischemia and the effects of nimodipine on calcium and histologic damage. *Stroke* 21: IV72–IV77.

Gunter TE, Pfeiffer DR (1990) Mechanisms by which mitochondria transport calcium. *Am J Physiol* 258: 755–C786.

Gwag BJ, Canzoniero LM, Sensi SL, DeMaro JA, Koh JY, Goldberg MP, et al. (1999) Calcium ionophores can induce either apoptosis or necrosis in cultured cortical neurons. *Neuroscience* 90: 1339–1348.

Hadjigeorgiou GM, Paterakis K, Dardiotis E, Dardioti M, Aggelakis K, Tasiou A, et al. (2005) IL-1RN and IL-1B gene polymorphisms and cerebral hemorrhagic events after traumatic brain injury. *Neurology* 2005 65: 1077–1082.

Haley SM, Graham RJ, Dumas HM (2004) Outcome rating scales for pediatric head injury. *J Intensive Care Med* 19: 205–219.

Hanaoka S, Takashima S, Morooka K (1998) Study of the maturation of the child's brain using 31P-MRS. *Pediatr Neurol* 18: 305–310.

Hayashi J, Takagi Y, Fukuda H, Imazato T, Nishimura M, Fujimoto M, et al. (2006) Primate embryonic stem cell-derived neuronal progenitors transplanted into ischemic brain. *J Cereb Blood Flow Metab* 26: 906–914.

Haywood S, Liesner R, Pindora S, Ganesan V (2005) Thrombophilia and first arterial ischaemic stroke: a systematic review. *Arch Dis Child* 90: 402–405.

Hickey RW, Callaway CW (2005) Asphyxia. In: Tisherman SA, Sterz F (eds) *Therapeutic Hypothermia.* New York: Springer, pp 119–134.

Hickey RW, Kochanek PM, Ferimer H, Graham SH, Safar P (2000) Hypothermia and hyper-thermia in children after resuscitation from cardiac arrest. *Pediatrics* 106: 118–122.

Hooper SR, Alexander J, Moore D, Sasser HC, Laurent S, King J, et al. (2004) Caregiver reports of common symptoms in children following a traumatic brain injury. *NeuroRehabilitation* 19: 175–189.

Hoxworth JM, Xu K, Zhou Y, Lust WD, LaManna JC (1999) Cerebral metabolic profile, selective neuron loss, and survival of acute and chronic hyperglycemic rats following cardiac arrest and resuscitation. *Brain Res* 821: 467–479.

Hummel FC, Cohen LG (2005) Drivers of brain plasticity. *Curr Opin Neurol* 18: 667–674.

Im JY, Kim D, Lee KW, Kim JB, Lee JK, Kim DS, et al. (2004) COX-2 Regulates the insulin-like growth factor I-induced potentiation of $Zn^{(2+)}$-toxicity in primary cortical culture. *Mol Pharmacol* 66: 368–376.

Imaizumi S, Kurosawa K, Kinouchi H, Yoshimoto T (1995) Effect of phenytoin on cortical Na^+-K^+-ATPase activity in global ischemic rat brain. *J Neurotrauma* 12: 231–234.

Irving EA, Bamford M (2002) Role of mitogen- and stress-activated kinases in ischemic injury. *J Cereb Blood Flow Metab* 22: 631–647.

Isenmann S, Stoll G, Schroeter M, Krajewski S, Reed JC, Bahr M (1998) Differential regulation of Bax, Bcl-2, and Bcl-X proteins in focal cortical ischemia in the rat. *Brain Pathol* 8: 49–62.

Jacinto SJ, Gieron-Korthals M, Ferreira JA (2001) Predicting outcome in hypoxic-ischemic brain injury. *Pediatr Clin North Am* 48: 647–660.

Jenkins LW, Dixon CE, Peters G, Gao WM, Zhang X, Adelson PD, et al. (2001) Cell signaling: serine/threonine protein kinases and traumatic brain injury. In: Clark RS, Kochanek PM (eds) *Brain Injury*. Boston: Kluwer Academic Publishers, pp 163–180.

Jin K, Graham SH, Mao X, Nagayama T, Simon RP, Greenberg DA (2001a) Fas (CD95) may mediate delayed cell death in hippocampal CA1 sector after global cerebral ischemia. *J Cereb Blood Flow Metab* 21: 1411–1421.

Jin K, Graham SH, Nagayama T, Goldsmith PC, Greenberg DA, Zhou A, Simon RP (2001b) Altered expression of the neuropeptide-processing enzyme carboxypeptidase E in the rat brain after global ischemia. *J Cereb Blood Flow Metab* 21: 1422–1429.

Johansson BB (2004) Functional and cellular effects of environmental enrichment after experimental brain infarcts. *Restor Neurol Neurosci* 22: 163–174.

Kajita Y, Dietrich HH, Dacey RG Jr (1996) Effects of oxyhemoglobin on local and propagated vasodilatory responses induced by adenosine, adenosine diphosphate, and adenosine triphosphate in rat cerebral arterioles. *J Neurosurg* 85: 908–916.

Kawasaki H, Morooka T, Shimohama S, Kimura J, Hirano T, Gotoh Y, et al. (1997) Activation and involvement of p38 mitogen-activated protein kinase in glutamate-induced apoptosis in rat cerebellar granule cells. *J Biol Chem* 272: 18518–18521.

Khaled AR, Durum SK (2001) From cytosol to mitochondria: the Bax translocation story. *J Biochem Mol Biol* 34: 391–394.

Khaled AR, Kim K, Hofmeister R, Muegge K, Durum SK (1999) Withdrawal of IL-7 induces Bax translocation from cytosol to mitochondria through a rise in intracellular pH. *Proc Natl Acad Sci U S A* 96: 14476–14481.

Kharbanda S, Saxena S, Yoshida K, Pandey P, Kaneki M, Wang Q, et al. (2000) Translocation of SAPK/JNK to mitochondria and interaction with Bcl-x(L) in response to DNA damage. *J Biol Chem* 275: 322–327.

Khazipov R, Khalilov I, Tyzio R, Morozova E, Ben-Ari Y, Holmes GL (2004) Developmental changes in GABAergic actions and seizure susceptibility in the rat hippocampus. *Eur J Neurosci* 19: 590–600.

Kim DY, Kim SH, Choi HB, Min C, Gwag BJ (2001) High abundance of GluR1 mRNA and reduced Q/R editing of GluR2 mRNA in individual NADPH-diaphorase neurons. *Mol Cell Neurosci* 17: 1025–1033.

Kim YR, Huang IJ, Lee SR, Tejima E, Mandeville JB, van Meer MP, et al. (2005) Measurements of BOLD/CBV ratio show altered fMRI hemodynamics during stroke recovery in rats. *J Cereb Blood Flow Metab* 25: 820–829.

King WJ, MacKay M, Sirnick A (2003) Canadian Shaken Baby Study Group. Shaken baby syndrome in Canada: clinical characteristics and outcomes of hospital cases. *CMAJ* 168: 155–159.

Knowles RG, Moncada S (1994) Nitric oxide syntheses in mammals. *Biochem J* 298: 249–258.

Ko HW, Park KY, Kim H, Han PL, Kim YU, Gwag BJ, et al. (1998) Ca^{2+}-mediated activation of c-Jun N-terminal kinase and nuclear factor kappa B by NMDA in cortical cell cultures. *J Neurochem* 71: 1390–1395.

Kochanek PM (2006) Pediatric traumatic injury: quo vadis? *Dev Neurosci* 28: 244–255.

Kochanek PM, Clark RS, Ruppel RA, Dixon CE (2001) Cerebral resuscitation after traumatic brain injury and cardiopulmonary arrest in infants and children in the new millennium. *Pediatr Clin North Am* 48: 661–681.

Kolb B, Gibb R, Gorny G (2000) Cortical plasticity and the development of behavior after early frontal cortical injury. *Dev Neuropsychol* 18: 423–444.

Kreis R, Arcinue E, Ernst T, Shonk TK, Flores R, Ross BD (1996) Hypoxic encephalopathy after near-drowning studied by quantitative 1H-magnetic resonance spectroscopy. *J Clin Invest* 97: 1142–1154.

Kroppenstedt SN, Kern M, Thomale UW, Schneider GH, Lanksch WR, Unterberg AW (1999) Effect of cerebral perfusion pressure on contusion volume following impact injury. *J Neurosurg* 90: 520–526.

Langlois J, Rutland-Brown W, Thomas K (2004) *Traumatic Brain Injury in the United States: Emergency Department Visits, Hospitalizations, and Deaths.* Atlanta, Georgia: Centers for Disease Control and Prevention, National Center for Injury Prevention and Control.

Lazarewicz JW, Pluta R, Puka M, Salinska E (1990) Diverse mechanisms of neuronal protection by nimodipine in experimental rabbit brain ischemia. *Stroke* 21: 108–110.

Lee JK, Kim JE, Sivula M, Strittmatter SM (2004) Nogo receptor antagonism promotes stroke recovery by enhancing axonal plasticity. *J Neurosci* 24: 6209–6217.

Levin HS, Aldrich EF, Saydjari C, Eisenberg HM, Foulkes MA, Bellefleur M, et al. (1992) Severe head injury in children: experience of the Traumatic Coma Data Bank. *Neurosurgery* 31: 435–443.

Li LY, Luo X, Wang X (2001) Endonuclease G is an apoptotic DNase when released from mitochondria. *Nature* 412: 95–99.

Li MM, Payne RS, Reid KH, Tseng MT, Rigor BM, Schurr A (1999) Correlates of delayed neuronal damage and neuroprotection in a rat model of cardiac-arrest-induced cerebral ischemia. *Brain Res* 826: 44–52.

Lieh-Lai MW, Theodorou AA, Sarnaik AP, Meert KL, Moylan PM, Canady AI (1992) Limitations of the Glasgow Coma Scale in predicting outcome in children with traumatic brain injury. *J Pediatr* 120: 195–199.

Liu WG, Qiu WS, Zhang Y, Wang WM, Lu F, Yang XF (2006) Effects of selective brain cooling in patients with severe traumatic brain injury: a preliminary study. *J Int Med Res* 34: 58–64.

Luetjens CM, Bui NT, Sengpiel B, Munstermann G, Poppe M, Krohn AJ, et al. (2000) Delayed mitochondrial dysfunction in excitotoxic neuron death: cytochrome c release and a secondary increase in superoxide production. *J Neurosci* 20: 5715–5723.

Lynch JK, Han CJ (2005) Pediatric stroke: what do we know and what do we need to know? *Semin Neurol* 25: 410–423.

Mandel R, Martinot A, Delepoulle F, Lamblin MD, Laureau E, Vallee L, et al. (2002) Prediction of outcome after hypoxic-ischemic encephalopathy: a prospective clinical and electrophysiologic study. *J Pediatr* 141: 45–50.

Margulies SS, Thibault KL (2000) Infant skull and suture properties: measurements and implications for mechanisms of pediatric brain injury. *J Biomech Eng* 122: 364–371.

Marmarou CR, Povlishock JT (2006) Administration of the immunophilin ligand FK506 differentially attenuates neurofilament compaction and impaired axonal transport in injured axons following diffuse traumatic brain injury. *Exp Neurol* 197: 353–362.

Marmarou CR, Walker SA, Davis CL, Povlishock JT (2005) Quantitative analysis of the relationship between intra-axonal neurofilament compaction and impaired axonal transport following diffuse traumatic brain injury. *J Neurotrauma* 22: 1066–1080.

Martin DP, Schmidt RE, DiStefano PS, Lowry OH, Carter JG, Johnson EM (1988) Inhibitors of protein synthesis and RNA synthesis prevent neuronal death caused by nerve growth factor deprivation. *J Cell Biol* 106: 829–844.

Matsumori Y, Hong SM, Fan Y, Kayama T, Hsu CY, Weinstein PR, et al. (2006) Enriched environment and spatial learning enhance hippocampal neurogenesis and salvages ischemic penumbra after focal cerebral ischemia. *Neurobiol Dis* 22: 187–198.

Matsuyama S, Llopis J, Deveraux QL, Tsien RY, Reed JC (2000) Changes in intramitochon-drial and cytosolic pH: early events that modulate caspase activation during apoptosis. *Nat Cell Biol* 2: 318–325.

Max JE, Mathews K, Lansing AE (2002) Psychiatric disorders after childhood stroke. *J Am Acad Child Adolesc Psychiatry* 41: 555–562.

Maxwell WL, Donnelly S, Sun X, Fenton T, Puri N, Graham DI (1999) Axonal cytoskeletal responses to nondisruptive axonal injury and the short-term effects of posttraumatic hypothermia. *J Neurotrauma* 16: 1225–1234.

McCord JM, Roy RS, Schaffer SW (1985) Free radicals and myocardial ischemia: the role of xanthine oxidase. *Adv Myocardiol* 5: 183–189.

Meng S, Qiao M, Scobie K, Tomanek B, Tuor UI (2006) Evolution of magnetic resonance imaging changes associated with cerebral hypoxia-ischemia and a relatively selective white matter injury in neonatal rats. *Pediatr Res* 59: 554–559.

Metz GA, Antonow-Schlorke I, Witte OW (2005) Motor improvements after focal cortical ischemia in adult rats are mediated by compensatory mechanisms. *Behav Brain Res* 162: 71–82.

Miles AN, Majda BT, Meloni BP, Knuckey NW (2001) Post-ischemic intravenous administra-tion of magnesium sulfate inhibits hippocampal CA1 neuronal death after transient global ischemia in rats. *Neurosurgery* 49: 1443–1450.

Miyamoto O, Auer RN (2000) Hypoxia, hyperoxia, ischemia, and brain necrosis. *Neurology* 54: 362–371.

Morita-Fujimura Y, Fujimura M, Kawase M, Murakami K, Kim GW, Chan PH (1999) Inhibition of interleukin-1b converting enzyme family proteases (caspases) reduces cold injury-induced brain trauma and DNA fragmentation in mice. *J Cereb Blood Flow Metab* 19: 634–642.

Muir KW, Lees KR, Ford I, Davis S; Intravenous Magnesium Efficacy in Stroke (IMAGES) Study Investigators (2004) Magnesium for acute stroke (Intravenous Magnesium Efficacy in Stroke trial): randomised controlled trial. *Lancet* 363: 439–445.

Nakayama N, Okumura A, Shinoda J, Nakashima T, Iwama T (2006) Relationship between regional cerebral metabolism and consciousness disturbance in traumatic diffuse brain injury without large focal lesions: an FDG-PET study with statistical parametric mapping analysis. *J Neurol Neurosurg Psychiatry* 77: 856–862.

Namura S, Zhu J, Fink K, Endres M, Srinivasan A, Tomaselli KJ, et al. (1998) Activation and cleavage of caspase-3 in apoptosis induced by experimental cerebral ischemia. *J Neurosci* 18: 3659–3668.

Natale JE, Knight JB, Cheng Y, Rome JE, Gallo V (2004) Metallothionein I and II mitigate age dependent secondary brain injury. *J Neurosci Res* 78: 303–314.

Neumar RW, Hagle SM, DeGracia DJ, Krause GS, White BC (1996) Brain mu-calpain autolysis during global cerebral ischemia. *J Neurochem* 66: 421–424.

Ng I, Yeo TT, Tang WY, Soong R, Ng PY, Smith DR (2000) Apoptosis occurs after cerebral contusions in humans. *Neurosurgery* 46: 949–956.

Nolan JP, Morley PT, Hoek TL, Hickey RW (2003) Therapeutic hypothermia after cardiac arrest. An advisory statement by the Advancement Life Support Task Force of the International Liaison Committee on Resuscitation. *Resuscitation* 57: 231–235.

Nygren J, Wieloch T (2005) Enriched environment enhances recovery of motor function after focal ischemia in mice, and downregulates the transcription factor NGFI-A. *J Cereb Blood Flow Metab* 25: 1625–1633.

Okonkwo DO, Melon DE, Pellicane AJ, Mutlu LK, Rubin DG, Stone JR, et al. (2003) Dose-response of cyclosporin A in attenuating traumatic axonal injury in rat. *Neuroreport* 3: 463–466.

Okonkwo DO, Pettus EH, Moroi J, Povlishock JT (1998) Alteration of the neurofilament sidearm and its relation to neurofilament compaction occurring with traumatic axonal injury. *Brain Res* 784: 1–6.

Ostrowski RP, Colohan AR, Zhang JH (2005) Mechanisms of hyperbaric oxygen-induced neuroprotection in a rat model of subarachnoid hemorrhage. *J Cereb Blood Flow Metab* 25: 554–571.

Ostrowski RP, Colohan AR, Zhang JH (2006) Molecular mechanisms of early brain injury after subarachnoid hemorrhage. *Neurol Res* 28: 399–414.

Ota K, Yakovlev AG, Itaya A, Kameoka M, Tanaka Y, Yoshihara K (2002) Alteration of apoptotic protease-activating factor-1 (APAF-1)-dependent apoptotic pathway during development of rat brain and liver. *J Biochem (Tokyo)* 131: 131–135.

Parizel PM, Ceulemans B, Laridon A, Ozsarlak O, Van Goethem JW, Jorens PG (2003) Cortical hypoxic-ischemic brain damage in shaken baby (shaken impact) syndrome: value of diffusion-weighted MRI. *Pediatr Radiol* 33: 868–871.

Perkin RM, Ashwal S (2006) Hypoxic-ischemic encephalopathy in infants and older children. In: Swaiman KF, Ashwal S, Ferriero DM (eds) *Pediatric Neurology: Principles and Practice*, 4th edn. Philadelphia: Mosby, pp 1471–1512.

Petzold GC, Einhaupl KM, Dirnagl U, Dreier JP (2003) Ischemia triggered by spreading neuronal activation is induced by endothelin-1 and hemoglobin in the subarachnoid space. *Ann Neurol* 54: 591–598.

Piantadosi CA, Zhang J (1996) Mitochondrial generation of reactive oxygen species after brain ischemia in the rat. *Stroke* 27: 327–332.

Pohl D, Bittigau P, Ishimaru MJ, Stadthaus D, Hubner C, Olney JW, et al. (1999) N-methyl-D-aspartate antagonists and apoptotic cell death triggered by head-trauma in developing rat brain. *Proc Natl Acad Sci U S A* 96: 2508–2513.

Povlishock JT (2000) Pathophysiology of neural injury: therapeutic opportunities and challenges. *Clin Neurosurg* 46: 113–126.

Prunell GF, Svendgaard NA, Alkass K, Mathiesen T (2005) Inflammation in the brain after experimental subarachnoid hemorrhage. *Neurosurgery* 56: 1082–1092.

Pullela R, Raber J, Pfankuch T, Ferriero DM, Claus CP, Koh SE, et al. (2006) Traumatic injury to the immature brain results in progressive neuronal loss, hyperactivity and delayed cognitive impairments. *Dev Neurosci* 28: 396–409.

Raff MC, Barres BA, Burne JF, Coles HS, Ishizaki Y, Jacobson MD (1993) Programmed cell death and the control of cell survival: lessons from the nervous system. *Science* 262: 695–700.

Raghupathi R, Mehr MF, Helfaer MA, Margulies SS (2004) Traumatic axonal injury is exacerbated following repetitive closed head injury in the neonatal pig. *J Neurotrauma* 21: 307–316.

Ratan SK, Kulshreshtha R, Pandey RM (1999) Predictors of posttraumatic convulsions in head-injured children. *Pediatr Neurosurg* 30: 127–131.

Rego AC, Santos MS, Oliveira CR (2000) Glutamate mediated inhibition of oxidative phosphorylation in cultured retinal cells. *Neurochem Int* 36: 159–166.

Reilly PL, Simpson DA, Sprod R, et al. (1988) Assessing the conscious level in infants and young children: a pediatric version of the Glasgow Coma Scale. *Childs Nerv Syst* 4: 30–33.

Rivara JB, Fay GC, Jaffe KM, Polissar NL, Shurtleff HA, Martin KM (1992) Predictors of family functioning one year following traumatic brain injury in children. *Arch Phys Med Rehabil* 73: 899–910.

Robertson CL, Bucci CJ, Fiskum G (2004) Mitochondrial response to calcium in the developing brain. *Brain Res Dev Brain Res* 151: 141–148.

Robertson JD, Orrenius S, Zhivotovsky B (2000) Review: nuclear events in apoptosis. *J Struct Biol* 129: 346–358.

Roine RO, Kaste M, Kinnunen A, Nikki P, Sarna S, Kajaste S (1990) Nimodipine after resuscitation from out-of-hospital ventricular fibrillation: a placebo-controlled, double-blind, randomized trial. *JAMA* 264: 3171–3177.

Rordorf G, Uemura Y, Bonventre JV (1991) Characterization of phospholipase A2 (PLA2) activity in gerbil brain: enhanced activities of cytosolic, mitochondrial, and microsomal forms after ischemia and reperfusion. *J Neurosci* 11: 1829–1836.

Rosenbaum DM, D'Amore J, Llena J, Rybak S, Balkany A, Kessler JA (1998) Pretreatment with intraventricular aurintricarboxylic acid decreases infarct size by inhibiting apoptosis following transient global ischemia in gerbils. *Ann Neurol* 43: 654–660.

Rossberg MI, Bhardwaj A, Hurn PD, Kirsch JR (2002) Principles of cerebroprotection. In: Murray MJ, Coursin DB, Pearl RG, Prough GS (eds) *Critical Care Medicine: Perioperative Management*. Philadelphia: Lippincott Williams & Williams, pp 225–235.

Samdani AF, Dawson TM, Dawson VL (1997) Nitric oxide synthase in models of focal ischemia. *Stroke* 28: 1283–1288.

Sapirstein A, Bonventre JV (2000) Phospholipases A2 in ischemic and toxic brain injury. *Neurochem Res* 25: 745–753.

Satchell MA, Lai Y, Kochanek PM, Wisniewski SR, Fink EL, Siedberg NA, et al. (2005) Cytochrome c, a biomarker of apoptosis, is increased in cerebrospinal fluid from infants with inflicted brain injury from child abuse. *J Cereb Blood Flow Metab* 25: 919–927.

Satchell MA, Zhang X, Kochanek PM, Dixon CE, Jenkins LW, Melick JA, et al. (2003) A dual role for poly-ADP-ribosylation in spatial memory acquisition after traumatic brain injury in mice involving NAD$^+$ depletion and ribosylation of 14-3-3 gamma. *J Neurochem* 85: 697–708.

Schleien CL, Koehler RC, Shaffner DH, Eberle B, Traystman RJ (1991) Blood–brain barrier disruption after cardiopulmonary resuscitation in immature swine. *Stroke* 22: 477–483.

Schneider A, Kruger C, Steigleder T, Weber D, Pitzer C, Laage R, et al. (2005) The hematopoietic factor G-CSF is a neuronal ligand that counteracts programmed cell death and drives neurogenesis. *J Clin Invest* 115: 2083–2098.

Schwartz AY, Sehba FA, Bederson JB (2000) Decreased nitric oxide availability contributes to acute cerebral ischemia after subarachnoid hemorrhage. *Neurosurgery* 47: 208–214.

Schwartz L, Taylor HG, Drotar D, Yeates KO, Wade SL, Stancin T (2003) Long-term behavior problems following pediatric traumatic brain injury: prevalence, predictors, and correlates. *J Pediatr Psychol* 28: 251–263.

Schwarzschild MA, Cole RL, Meyers MA, Hyman SE (1999) Contrasting calcium dependencies of SAPK and ERK activations by glutamate in cultured striatal neurons. *J Neurochem* 72: 2248–2255.

Sensi SL, Yin HZ, Carriedo SG, Rao SS, Weiss JH (1999) Preferential Zn^{2+} influx through Ca^{2+}-permeable AMPA/kainate channels triggers prolonged mitochondrial superoxide production. *Proc Natl Acad Sci U S A* 96: 2414–2419.

Seppelt I (2005) Hypothermia does not improve outcome from traumatic brain injury. *Crit Care Resusc* 7: 233–237.

Seymour AB, Andrews EM, Tsai SY, Markus TM, Bollnow MR, Brenneman MM, et al. (2005) Delayed treatment with monoclonal antibody IN-1 1 week after stroke results in recovery of function and corticorubral plasticity in adult rats. *J Cereb Blood Flow Metab* 25: 1366–1375.

Shen LH, Li Y, Chen J, Zhang J, Vanguri P, Borneman J, et al. (2006) Intracarotid transplantation of bone marrow stromal cells increases axon-myelin remodeling after stroke. *Neuroscience* 137: 393–399.

Skippen P, Seear M, Poskitt K, Kestle J, Cochrane D, Annich G, et al. (1997) Effect of hyperventilation on regional cerebral blood flow in head-injured children. *Crit Care Med* 25: 1402–1409.

Snyder RD, Stovring J, Cushing AH, Davis LE, Hardy TL (1981) Cerebral infarction in childhood bacterial meningitis. *J Neurol Neurosurg Psychiatry* 44: 581–585.

Sofronas M, Ichord RN, Fullerton HJ, Lynch JK, Massicotte MP, Willan AR, et al. (2006) Pediatric stroke initiatives and preliminary studies: what is known and what is needed? *Pediatr Neurol* 34: 439–445.

Sotak CH (2002) The role of diffusion tensor imaging in the evaluation of ischemic brain injury: a review. *NMR Biomed* 15: 561–569.

Srivastava RK, Sollott SJ, Khan L, Hansford R, Lakatta EG, Longo DL (1999) Bcl-2 and Bcl-X(L) block thapsigargin-induced nitric oxide generation, c-Jun NH(2)-terminal kinase activity, and apoptosis. *Mol Cell Biol* 19: 5659–5674.

Steen PA, Milde JH, Michenfelder JD (1979) No barbiturate protection in a dog model of complete cerebral ischemia. *Ann Neurol* 5: 343–349.

Stone JR, Singleton RH, Povlishock JT (2001) Intra-axonal neurofilament compaction does not evoke local axonal swelling in all traumatically injured axons. *Exp Neurol* 172: 320–331.

Sugiura S, Kitagawa K, Tanaka S, Todo K, Omura-Matsuoka E, Sasaki T, et al. (2005) Adenovirus-mediated gene transfer of heparin-binding epidermal growth factor-like growth factor enhances neurogenesis and angiogenesis after focal cerebral ischemia in rats. *Stroke* 36: 859–864.

Sun Y, Rotenberg MO, Maines MD (1990) Developmental expression of heme oxygenase isozymes in rat brain: two HO-2 mRNAs are detected. *J Biol Chem* 265: 8212–8217.

Susin SA, Lorenzo HK, Zamzami N, Marzo I, Snow BE, Brothers GM, et al. (1999) Molecular characterization of mitochondrial apoptosis-inducing factor. *Nature* 397: 441–446.

Suzuki Y, Imai Y, Nakayama H, Takahashi K, Takio K, Takahashi R (2001) A serine protease, HtrA2, is released from the mitochondria and interacts with XIAP, inducing cell death. *Mol Cell* 8: 613–621.

Takagi K, Ginsberg MD, Globus MY, Dietrich WD, Martinez E, Kraydieh S, et al. (1993) Changes in amino acid neurotransmitters and cerebral blood flow in the ischemic penumbral region following middle cerebral artery occlusion in the rat: correlation with histopathology. *J Cereb Blood Flow Metab* 13: 575–585.

Tasker RC, Salmond CH, Westland AG, Pena A, Gillard JH, Sahakian BJ, et al. (2005) Head circumference and brain and hippocampal volume after severe traumatic brain injury in childhood. *Pediatr Res* 58: 302–308.

Teasdale GM, Murray GD, Nicoll JA (2005) The association between APOE epsilon4, age and outcome after head injury: a prospective cohort study. *Brain* 128: 2556–2561.

Temkin NR, Anderson GD, Winn HR, Ellenbogen RG, Britz GW, Schuster J, et al. (2007) Magnesium sulfate for neuroprotection after traumatic brain injury: a randomised controlled trial. *Lancet Neurol* 6: 29–38.

Thored P, Arvidsson A, Cacci E, Ahlenius H, Kallur T, Darsalia V, et al. (2006) Persistent production of neurons from adult brain stem cells during recovery after stroke. *Stem Cells* 24: 739–744.

Tolias CM, Bullock MR (2004) Critical appraisal of neuroprotection trials in head injury: what have we learned? *NeuroRx* 1: 71–79.

Tournier C, Hess P, Yang DD, Xu J, Turner TK, Nimnual A, et al. (2000) Requirement of JNK for stress-induced activation of the cytochrome c-mediated death pathway. *Science* 288: 870–874.

Vaagenes P, Safar P, Moossy J, Rao G, Diven W, Ravi C, et al. (1997) Asphyxiation versus ventricular fibrillation cardiac arrest in dogs. Differences in cerebral resuscitation effects: a preliminary study. *Resuscitation* 35: 41–52.

Van Lookeren Campagne M, Verheul JB, Nicolay K, Balazs R (1994) Early evolution and recovery from excitotoxic injury in the neonatal rat brain: a study combining magnetic resonance imaging, electrical impedance, and histology. *J Cereb Blood Flow Metab* 14: 1011–1023.

Vande Velde C, Cizeau J, Dubik D, Alimonti J, Brown T, Israels S, et al. (2000) BNIP3 and genetic control of necrosis-like cell death through the mitochondrial permeability transition pore. *Mol Cell Biol* 20: 5454–5468.

Vanhoutte P, Barnier JV, Guibert B, Pages C, Besson MJ, Hipskind RA, et al. (1999) Glutamate induces phosphorylation of Elk-1 and CREB, along with c-fos activation, via an extracellular signal-regulated kinase-dependent pathway in brain slices. *Mol Cell Biol* 19: 136–146.

Vespa P, McArthur DL, Alger J, O'Phelan K, Hattori N, Wu C, et al. (2004) Regional heterogeneity of post-traumatic brain metabolism as studied by microdialysis, magnetic resonance spectroscopy and positron emission tomography. *Brain Pathol* 14: 210–214.

Vining EP, Freeman JM, Pillas DJ, Pyzik PL, Avellino AM, Carson BS, Freeman JM (1997) Why would you remove half a brain? The outcome of 58 children after hemispherectomy: the Johns Hopkins experience: 1968 to 1996. *Pediatrics* 100: 163–171.

Wang GJ, Randall RD, Thayer SA (1994) Glutamate-induced intracellular acidification of cultured hippocampal neurons demonstrates altered energy metabolism resulting from Ca^{2+} loads. *J Neurophysiol* 72: 2563–2569.

Wang KK (2000) Calpain and caspase: can you tell the difference? *Trends Neurosci* 23: 20–26.

Wang KK, Posmantur R, Nath R, McGinnis K, Whitton M, Talanian RV, et al. (1998) Simultaneous degradation of alpha II- and beta II-spectrin by caspase 3 (CPP32) in apoptotic cells. *J Biol Chem* 273: 22490–22497.

Wang L, Zhang Z, Wang Y, Zhang R, Chopp M (2004) Treatment of stroke with erythropoietin enhances neurogenesis and angiogenesis and improves neurological function in rats. *Stroke* 35: 1732–1737.

Ward MW, Rego AC, Frenguelli BG, Nicholls DG (2000) Mitochondrial membrane potential and glutamate excitotoxicity in cultured cerebellar granule cells. *J Neurosci* 20: 7208–7219.

Weigl M, Tenze G, Steinlechner B, Skhirtladze K, Reining G, Bernardo M, et al. (2005) A systematic review of currently available pharmacological neuroprotective agents as a sole intervention before anticipated or induced cardiac arrest. *Resuscitation* 65: 21–39.

Weiloch W, Nicolich K (2006) Mechanisms of neural plasticity following brain injury. *Curr Opin Neurobiol* 16: 258–264.

Weiss JH, Turetsky D, Wilke G, Choi DW (1994) AMPA/kainate receptor-mediated damage to NADPH diaphorase-containing neurons is Ca^{2+} dependent. *Neurosci Lett* 167: 93–96.

White BC, Krause GS, Aust SD, Eyster GE (1985) Postischemic tissue injury by iron-mediated free radical lipid peroxidation. *Ann Emerg Med* 14: 804–809.

White DA, Moinuddin A, McKinstry RC, Noetzel M, Armstrong M, DeBaun M (2006) Cognitive screening for silent cerebral infarction in children with sickle cell disease. *J Pediatr Hematol Oncol* 28: 166–169.

White JR, Farukhi Z, Bull C, Christensen J, Gordon T, Paidas C, et al. (2001) Predictors of outcome in severely head-injured children. *Crit Care Med* 29: 534–540.

Wijdicks EF (2006) Clinical Scales for Comatose Patients: The Glasgow Coma Scale in Historical Context and the New FOUR Score. *Rev Neurol Dis* 3: 109–117.

Wijdicks EF, Schievink WI, Burnett JC Jr (1997) Natriuretic peptide system and endothelin in aneurysmal subarachnoid hemorrhage. *J Neurosurg* 87: 275–280.

Wilde EA, Chu Z, Bigler ED, Hunter JV, Fearing MA, Hanten G, et al. (2006) Diffusion tensor imaging in the corpus callosum in children after moderate to severe traumatic brain injury. *J Neurotrauma* 23: 1412–1426.

Wirrell E, Hill MD, Jadavji T, Kirton A, Barlow K (2004) Stroke after varicella vaccination. *J Pediatr* 145: 845–847.

Wolf JA, Stys PK, Lusardi T, Meaney D, Smith DH (2001) Traumatic axonal injury induces calcium influx modulated by tetrodotoxin-sensitive sodium channels. *J Neurosci* 21: 1923–1930.

Xia Z, Dudek H, Miranti CK, Greenberg ME (1996) Calcium influx via the NMDA receptor induces immediate early gene transcription by a MAP kinase/ERK-dependent mechanism. *J Neurosci* 16: 5425–5436.

Yeates KO, Taylor HG (2005) Neurobehavioural outcomes of mild head injury in children and adolescents. *Pediatr Rehabil* 8: 5–16.

Young KD, Gausche-Hill M, McClung CD, Lewis RJ (2004) A prospective, population-based study of the epidemiology and outcome of out-of-hospital pediatric cardiopulmonary arrest. *Pediatrics* 114: 157–164.

Yu R, Gao L, Jiang S, Guan P, Mao B (2001) Association of HIF-1alpha expression and cell apoptosis after traumatic brain injury in the rat. *Chin J Traumatol* 4: 218–221.

Zeynalov E, Nemoto M, Hurn PD, Kohler RC, Bhardwaj A (2005) Neuroprotective effect of selective kappa receptor agonist is gender specific and linked to reduced neuronal nitric oxide. *J Cereb Blood Flow Metab* 26: 414–420.

Zhang H, Cook D (1994) Cerebral vascular smooth muscle potassium channels and their possible role in the management of vasospasm. *Pharmacol Toxicol* 75: 327–336.

Zhang L, Zhang RL, Wang Y, Zhang C, Zhang ZG, Meng H, et al. (2005a) Functional recovery in aged and young rats after embolic stroke: treatment with a phosphodiesterase type 5 inhibitor. *Stroke* 36: 847–852.

Zhang RL, Zhang ZG, Chopp M (2005b) Neurogenesis in the adult ischemic brain: generation, migration, survival, and restorative therapy. *Neuroscientist* 11: 408–416.

Zhang S, Boyd J, Delaney K, Murphy TH (2005c) Rapid reversible changes in dendritic spine structure in vivo gated by the degree of ischemia. *J Neurosci* 25: 5333–5338.

Zhang X, Chen Y, Jenkins LW, Kochanek PM, Clark RS (2005d) Bench-to-bedside review: apoptosis/programmed cell death triggered by traumatic brain injury. *Critical Care* 9: 66–75.

Zhang X, Graham SH, Kochanek PM, Marion DW, Nathaniel PD, Watkins SC, et al. (2003) Caspase-8 expression and proteolysis in human brain after severe head injury. *FASEB J* 17: 1367–1369.

Zhao BQ, Wang S, Kim HY, Storrie H, Rosen BR, Mooney DJ, et al. (2006) Role of matrix metalloproteinases in delayed cortical responses after stroke. *Nat Med* 12: 441–445.

Zhu H, Meloni BP, Bojarski C, Knuckey MW, Knuckey NW (2005) Post-ischemic modest hypothermia (35°C) combined with intravenous magnesium is more effective at reducing CA1 neuronal death than either treatment used alone following global cerebral ischemia in rats. *Exp Neurol* 193: 361–368.

Ziviani J, Ottenbacher KJ, Shephard K, Foreman S, Astbury W, Ireland P (2001) Concurrent validity of the Functional Independence Measure for Children (WeeFIM) and the Pediatric Evaluation of Disabilities Inventory in children with developmental disabilities and acquired brain injuries. *Phys Occup Ther Pediatr* 21: 91–101.

Zou H, Henzel WJ, Liu X, Lutschg A, Wang X (1997) Apaf-1, a human protein homologous to *C. elegans* CED-4, participates in cytochrome c-dependent activation of caspase-3. *Cell* 90: 405–413.

20

NEW CONCEPTS IN THE REHABILITATION OF CHILDREN WITH DEVELOPMENTAL DISABILITIES: OCCUPATIONAL THERAPY AND PHYSICAL THERAPY PERSPECTIVES

Annette Majnemer and Johanna Darrah

THE ART AND SCIENCE OF REHABILITATION

Rehabilitation (from Latin; 'to equip' or 'to make fit') focuses on restoring or enhancing an individual's abilities and capacities to perform and participate in meaningful everyday activities through the use of remediation and training (to improve or acquire skills), compensation and adaptation (to modify tasks or environment to enhance function) (Seelman 2000, Majnemer et al. 2009). Rehabilitation of children with developmental disabilities occurs against a background of ongoing growth and development, whereby the child is faced with new challenges and demands on an ongoing basis. Pediatric rehabilitation efforts are aimed at facilitating functional successes with respect to the child's attainment of meaningful tasks and activities that are desired for the stage of development and associated cultural expectations. This is achieved with family members as integral partners in the rehabilitation process (Helders et al. 2003, Majnemer et al. 2009).

There has been an important shift in the *art* of rehabilitation. Initially, therapeutic approaches adopted a medical model, focusing on diminishing the identified impairments associated with the medical condition. Evidence overall does not strongly support the effectiveness of interventions aimed at decreasing or 'fixing' deficits with the expectation that functional performance will also improve (Butler and Darrah 2001, Case Smith 2005). Increasingly, a biopsychosocial view is being advocated which broadens the scope of rehabilitation strategies, placing equal importance on both the intrinsic characteristics of the individual (e.g. aspects of the medical condition, personal characteristics) and the extrinsic factors within that person's environment that may either facilitate or pose barriers to full functioning and participation (Helders et al. 2003). This biopsychosocial model provides a framework not only for practice, but also for rehabilitation research and health policy decisions. Rehabilitation specialists increasingly appreciate that disability is the product of the interaction between attributes of the individual (i.e. impairments, functional status, personal and social qualities) and the environment (i.e. physical, social, attitudinal) that they live in (Seelman 2000). As a result, the goals of intervention are more holistic, and include enhancing personal autonomy, productivity, and life satisfaction (Majnemer et al. 2009). Therapeutic interventions increasingly address the psychosocial processes, as well as the medical factors, that collectively influence overall functioning (Johnston et al. 2006). Furthermore, recognition of the importance of the environmental context of the individual has spurred greater interest in developing disease prevention and health promotion initiatives by rehabilitation specialists in the general community. Examples of these initiatives include developmental screening and stimulation programs for young children at risk for disability, fitness and other recreational programs for children and youth with disabilities, and family support groups.

Most biomedical disciplines concentrate on an organ system or a technology; however, rehabilitation has an overarching and integrative perspective with respect to how a person functions in the context of the surrounding environment (Whyte 2005). Rehabilitation as a *science* is a study of function or the process by which disability occurs and the factors that influence this process. Scientific discovery is aimed at improving our understanding of the impairments and activity limitations that underlie a health condition, coupled with identification of those related factors that modify or mediate functional performance. These factors may have a positive effect (i.e. enable) or a negative effect (i.e. disable) on functioning.

Rehabilitation science requires expertise from many disciplines, to include specific rehabilitation and medical specialties, but also now broadening to include biomedical engineering, epidemiology, basic science disciplines, sociology, architecture, and economics. The Institute of Medicine has endorsed that rehabilitation should be recognized as a scientific field of study and recommended that the intrinsic science should be strengthened with an increasing emphasis placed on the enabling–disabling process (Seelman 2000). The rehabilitation peer-reviewed literature has grown exponentially with descriptions of the extent and nature of disability in target populations, identification of factors associated with disablement or recovery, and more refined intervention strategies and assessment methods for children with developmental disabilities. However, there is a need for more 'science' as many aspects of childhood disability (causes, outcomes, and interventions) remain unclear along the continuum extending from the underlying pathology to a fulfilling and satisfying life for these children and their families (Majnemer and Limperopoulos 2002, Johnston et al. 2006). This chapter specifically focuses on the recent scientific and educational advances that have influenced the disciplines of occupational therapy and physical therapy.

Concurrent with novel theoretical frameworks and scientific evidence that support rehabilitation practice has been an upgrading in the minimum educational requirements for occupational therapy and physical therapy professional degrees.

All US and most Canadian programs now have Master's degree professional programs, with many US programs moving from a Master's level to a Clinical Doctorate designation. In addition, many rehabilitation specialists with Bachelor's level training are returning for post-professional graduate degrees in rehabilitation science or related fields. These higher degree programs ensure that therapists gain critical appraisal and research methodology skills, thus facilitating greater participation in clinical research and enhanced awareness, understanding, and utilization of evidence in their practice (www.caot.ca, www.physiotherapy.ca, www.aota.org, www.apta.org, Mayston 2005). Graduate level education is more likely to stimulate reflective practice, and a greater commitment to self-directed lifelong learning. The movement to graduate-level training (professional and post-professional) is an important vehicle for transmitting new scientific discoveries in rehabilitation science to the practice arena.

A second important educational development has been the pursuit of doctoral and postdoctoral research training by a subset of rehabilitation specialists. This growing pool of qualified academic researchers in rehabilitation are contributing to a growing scientific knowledge base to support and guide practice decisions. Given the wide scope of the field, researchers typically work collaboratively with investigators from other disciplines who bring complementary expertise to complex research questions (Seelman 2000, Whyte 2005, Johnston et al. 2006). The scientific caliber and rigor of the research methodology has steadily improved, further contributing to important advances in rehabilitation as a science.

Evidence-based practice involves clinical decision-making that integrates information from three primary sources: (1) the best available research evidence, (2) clinical expertise and professional judgment, and (3) the client's/patient's values and preferences (www.physiotherapy.ca, Sackett 2000, Johnston et al. 2006, Manns and Darrah 2006). High quality research can be used as a basis to develop practice guidelines, systematic reviews, and web-based research materials that clinicians can use as additional information sources for clinical decision-making. Formal and informal learning opportunities need to be promoted and supported by clinical managers, so as to continually integrate evidence-based knowledge and skills into the practice arena (CAOT position statement on Continuing Professional Education 2006). Furthermore, clinicians should be encouraged to reflect and learn from past personal experience, and apply clinical reasoning and problem-solving skills in collaboration with the child and their families, to ensure best practice (Manns and Darrah 2006).

In summary, the art and science of rehabilitation is enriched by contributions from the physical, biologic, psychologic, and social sciences (Frontera et al. 2005). Theoretical concepts and the evidence that underlie rehabilitation science are slowly catching up to the art of rehabilitation practice; however, strong evidence is still lacking in many specific practice areas (Whyte 2005, Johnston et al. 2006). Building research capacity in rehabilitation science is therefore a priority, by increasing the pool of well-qualified researchers, and providing appropriate infrastructure, funding opportunities, and a supportive environment for enabling interdisciplinary collaborations (Frontera et al. 2005, Whyte 2005). Concurrent with new developments in the art and science of rehabilitation, there is a greater emphasis being placed on a more holistic and integrated view of developmental disability (Whyte 1998, Seelman 2000). In the next section, key concepts that have contributed to changes in occupational therapy and physical therapy practice are described.

NEW CONCEPTS IN REHABILITATION THAT ARE INFLUENCING PRACTICE
International Classification of Functioning, Disability and Health
The World Health Organization has recently endorsed the International Classification of Functioning, Disability and Health (ICF) (WHO 2001), a conceptual framework for classifying and describing a person's health status. It represents a major revision of the former International Classification of Impairment, Disability and Handicap, a model of disablement (Bornman 2004). The ICF adopts a biopsychosocial view which recognizes that a person's health status and functional abilities are not only related to attributes of the health condition (e.g. severity, type of impairments), but are also in part a socially created phenomenon (e.g. architectural barriers, societal attitudes) (Fougeyrollas et al. 1998, WHO 2001, Majnemer and Limperopoulos 2002). The ICF components are interactive, with no presupposed a priori hierarchical relationship. The first part of the classification scheme describes two components of functioning and disability: (1) body function and structure representing physiologic, psychologic (body function), and anatomic (body structure) characteristics of the individual, and (2) activity and participation, representing tasks at the individual level (activity) and involvement in life roles (participation). Each component can be described in both positive and negative terms. Deficits in these components are described as impairments (body structure and function), activity limitations, or participation restrictions. The second part of the classification describes contextual factors that may serve to either facilitate or hinder functional potential. These contextual factors may be personal attributes not specifically related to the health condition (e.g. demographic characteristics, lifestyle preferences) or environmental characteristics (e.g. physical, social and attitudinal) (WHO 2001, Majnemer 2006).

Wide endorsement of this multilevel conceptual model has helped promote broader perspectives in the assessment and treatment of children with developmental disability. A variety of new measures are being developed for infants, children, and youth, designed to evaluate the different components of the ICF, including participation and contextual factors. For example, there are new measures of activity and participation such as the Children's Assessment of Participation and Enjoyment (CAPE) and the Life-Habits (LIFE-H) assessment (Fougeyrollas et al. 2001, King et al. 2004). The School Function Assessment (Coster et al. 1998) evaluates a child's abilities in the specific contextual framework of the school setting. Traditionally, the majority of occupational and physical therapy measures for children with disabilities focused on assessing characteristics solely at the level of body function and structure such as muscle tone (e.g. Ashworth scale), primitive reflexes (e.g. Fiorentino), sensorimotor skills (e.g. Miller Assessment for Preschoolers), and isolated hierarchical developmental skills (e.g. Griffiths Developmental Scale). New measures such as the Pediatric Evaluation of Disability Inventory and the WeeFIM (functional independence measure for children) emphasize functional abilities in a holistic manner, by documenting modifications to the task (i.e. adaptations needed) and environment (i.e. level of assistance required) that enable the child to accomplish expected everyday activities successfully.

The ICF also differentiates a child's capacity (what the child is *capable* of doing) versus performance (what the child actually *does* in their everyday life), which is important to consider in clinical practice. It serves to remind therapists that rehabilitation interventions need to identify and minimize any obstacles that undermine performance in the child's usual environment (Manns and Darrah 2006). It cannot be routinely assumed that changes at one component necessarily result in changes of skills represented by the other components. The ICF framework specifically cautions against the traditional assumption of a linear causal relationship between skills or functions represented under different components. For example, an improvement in attention span (body function component) will not necessarily result in a similar level of improvement in reading, writing, and mathematic skills (activities component) in the classroom, or in enhanced social integration (participation component) in the schoolyard. Similarly, changes in muscle strength (body function component) may not necessarily result in changes in the child's ability to kick a ball or play soccer with peers (activity and participation components). Furthermore, the ICF model has influenced intervention strategies and program goals such that they are more multidimensional, incorporating different components of the ICF classification to achieve the desired goals of intervention. For example, in order to achieve independence in securing fastenings on clothing, the therapist may simultaneously work on remediation and training at the level of body function (e.g. improving upper extremity bilateral coordination and sequencing, breaking down the task into components and practicing parts of the task using feedback), while also temporarily applying aids and adaptations such as Velcro or elasticized clothing, so that the child can very quickly achieve success at the functional activity. As such, the child achieves independence in self-care, while continuing to work on the component skills that would allow the child to do the activity in another manner.

A more holistic approach to the ongoing evaluation and treatment of children with developmental disabilities, as framed by the ICF, ensures that function is achieved as soon as possible, even while skill development is still being addressed. Rehabilitation interventions should support a child's mastery of activities that are meaningful to that child and that support participation and social integration (Goldstein et al. 2004). Furthermore, contextual factors such as environmental supports and a child's intrinsic motivation are potentially modifiable and therefore should be carefully considered as part of a package of rehabilitation interventions (Majnemer 2006). Increasingly, health promotion initiatives that encourage and maintain health and well-being in spite of disability are being planned by rehabilitation specialists.

NEW TRANSACTIVE THEORIES IN REHABILITATION
Recent theoretical concepts in rehabilitation emphasize the complex transactional relationships between the person with a disability, the tasks or occupations and roles they fulfill in everyday life, and the environments in which they live in. For example, the Person–Environment–Occupation Model (PEO) (Law et al. 1996) of occupational performance builds on concepts such as client-centered practice and environment–behavior theories. This model recognizes the important influence of environment on behavior, and encourages the therapist to pursue multiple avenues at the levels of the person, the environment or the task to elicit functional change. Similarly, the dynamic systems theory stipulates that developmental acquisitions occur as a result of the dynamic ongoing interactions of subsystems within the child, influenced by the characteristics of the task and the environment. The child's behaviors or developmental acquisitions are the end product of multiple intrinsic (i.e. child's characteristics) and extrinsic (i.e. task-specific, environmental) components (Shumway-Cook and Woollacott 1995). The child's intrinsic factors (e.g. neurologic, biomechanical, anthropometric measures, temperament, cognition) provide the possibilities or preliminary blueprint of the child; however, the environmental contextual factors influence the timing, sequence, and quality of eventual developmental achievements that are realized and their timing. Through trial and error, interactions with the environment foster the selection and refinement of behavioral repertoires (Shumway-Cook and Woollacott 1995, Hadders-Algra 2000, Helders et al. 2003).

Greater appreciation of the importance of the task and the environment, in addition to the intrinsic abilities and disabilities of the child, has prompted new emerging therapeutic approaches that go beyond restoring or acquiring skills as framed by 'normal' or typical development, to solving functional challenges by considering varying context-specific adaptive strategies that ensure success of the developmental skill needed. The therapist acts as a facilitator, identifying both factors that limit functional performance and strengths within the child and the environment that will contribute to functional success of an activity or goal (Darrah and Bartlett 1995, Burton and Davis 1996, Darrah et al. 2001, Helders et al. 2003). For example, a child with poor eye–hand co-ordination and manual dexterity may have difficulty learning to write legibly, which may negatively impact on academic performance and self-esteem (McHale and Cermak 1992, Mather and Roberts 1995). The therapist may choose to work on improving specific sensorimotor precursors to handwriting legibility such as tactile sensitivity, in-hand manipulation, grasp pattern, and perceptual-motor skills, while simultaneously introducing a laptop computer to ensure adequate functioning and participation in the classroom. At the same time, other adaptive strategies such as modified pencil grips, a clipboard to stabilize the paper, and visual cues on the paper may be explored to enhance immediate writing performance. This is essential for everyday tasks that require legible handwriting such as completing forms, making lists, and taking notes in class.

Transactive theories such as the PEO and dynamic systems have encouraged therapists to broaden their approach and imagination to consider an array of solutions to functional challenges, and to realize that different environments may require different solutions. For example, an adolescent with a diagnosis of cerebral palsy may crawl to get around at home, use a walker in the school setting, and use a power chair to hang out at the mall with their friends. The best solution results from the interaction of the child's abilities, task requirements, and contextual factors.

FAMILY-CENTERED CARE

Family-centered care involves a partnership between parents and service providers so that families are active participants in their child's rehabilitation process. Family-centered service principles clearly articulate that parents know their children best. Family-centered service acknowledges that families are different and each is unique, and that optimal child functioning occurs within a supportive family and community context (Rosenbaum et al. 1998). Families identify the extent of their involvement, which may change depending on their comfort level and the rehabilitation goals identified. Goals of treatment are identified collaboratively with input from the family, child, and therapist. Within this framework, the therapist is viewed as a collaborator, not an expert. This change in service delivery has created an environment more conducive to the identification of functional goals at the components of activity and participation rather than focusing exclusively at the component of impairment. Care is respectful, supportive, and addresses family needs and concerns. Close communication with families ensures that they have realistic expectations about their child's outcome. Research evidence indicates that family-centered service leads to more positive outcomes for the child, parent, and family (Rosenbaum et al. 1998). The desired outcomes from a family-centered approach include developmental gains for the child, improved psychologic adjustment, enhanced parental knowledge about child development, reductions in parents' psychologic distress, and increased parental satisfaction with service (Hostler 1991, Rosenbaum et al. 1998, Law et al. 2003).

Family-centered services ensure that the rehabilitation process is individualized and goals are meaningful to the child and family. This collaborative approach enables parents to become more effective and participating caregivers (Rosenbaum et al. 1998, Helders et al. 2003, Law et al. 2003, Majnemer et al. 2009).

DISABILITY STUDIES

Traditionally, disability was viewed as a problem within the person and the goal was to fix, heal, or prevent the problem (Rioux 1994). Persons with disabilities advocated for a change in this perspective, suggesting that disability is a 'socio-political' rather than a 'medical' issue. The social construction model of disability put forward that society's values and beliefs partition persons into 'disabled' and 'able-bodied' members of society, and prevent the full participation of persons with disabilities in the broader community (Law and Dunn 1993). Condeluci (1995), in his interdependent model, suggests that an individual with a disability is a 'consumer' with special needs and it is the responsibility of society to meet those needs. For persons with disabilities, issues such as living independently, finding meaningful work, and accessible physical and social environments are more important than looking 'normal.' As therapists enter into dialogue with adults with disabilities and read the disability studies literature, they realize that what is most important to persons with disabilities is not perceptual concepts, sequencing skills, or a correct pencil grasp, but rather fuller involvement in desired life roles and community activities. Therapists are beginning to rethink therapy goals with young children to reinforce the concept of functional success with less emphasis on typical development as the expected outcome or 'criterion standard' of successful rehabilitation efforts. The net result is more emphasis on community integration and participation in activities that are most important to the child and family.

LIFESPAN APPROACH TO REHABILITATION

Traditionally, the focus of intervention for children with developmental disabilities has been on intensive direct intervention, predominantly during the infant and preschool years. This approach evolved from two concepts. First, the concept of neural plasticity suggested that neurologic systems are more amenable to remediation at young ages. From a remediation model, a child was more likely to exhibit improvements in development if he/she received intensive treatment early in development. Secondly, historically the perception was that when a child entered school, academic learning took precedence over rehabilitation services such as occupational therapy and physical therapy. As a result, the intensity and frequency of occupational and physical therapy services often decreased dramatically when a child became school age.

With the adoption of a biopsychosocial model, therapists now realize that families of children with developmental disabilities need support, consultation, and often intervention throughout the lifespan as new challenges emerge. Short intense periods of therapy at critical transition points are often recommended to ensure functional success during key developmental or social transitions such as entering or leaving school, preparing to live independently, and seeking employment. Youth with disabilities go through the same transition processes and challenges as their peers without disabilities (Wehman 1996, Stewart et al. 2001). Families report that dealing with service issues of older children and adolescents can be frustrating and exhausting (Darrah et al. 2002). Therapy approaches are gradually changing to embrace a lifespan approach to intervention for persons with disabilities (Barnhart 2001), with a growing awareness that the child and family will need ongoing support, consultation and intervention. New intervention strategies such as short periods of intensive therapy, new 'transitions' programs, periodic assessments at key points, consultation, and collaborative goal-setting with families collectively reflect the adaptation lifespan approach to therapy.

INFLUENCE OF NEW ADVANCES ON OCCUPATIONAL AND PHYSICAL THERAPY PRACTICE

A more integrated approach to therapeutic assessment and intervention strategies for children with developmental disabilities has resulted in a greater emphasis on functional goals, an awareness of the prime importance of the family in the child's rehabilitation journey, an appreciation that there may be more than one solution to a child's attainment of optimum functional independence, and a lifespan approach to the management of children with developmental disabilities. The assumption that the desired outcome for children with developmental disabilities is always to approximate typical developmental patterns and expectations has received less and less emphasis, replaced instead with the goals of functional success and broader social participation. These changes in approach to intervention are evident across different diagnoses including, for example, children with physical impairments (Burton and Davis 1992), cerebral palsy (Law et al. 1998, Ketelaar et al. 2001), developmental coordination disorder (Missiuna et al. 2001), and autism (Bodf h 2004).

The curricula of educational programs for occupational and physical therapy students (Darrah et al. 2006) and practice guidelines for therapists (American Physical Therapy Association 2001) also reflect these changing concepts. Client-centered services, models of health status, a lifespan perspective, and functional goals are all emphasized in the new curricula. Because these changes have appeared in theory, practice, and education, they will undoubtedly become increasingly adopted over time in general clinical practice. The next important step in rehabilitation will be the rigorous and systematic evaluation of intervention approaches implemented based on these new concepts.

REHABILITATION RESEARCH – NEW DIRECTIONS

Rehabilitation science is a burgeoning science, and the clinical research emphasis during the last two decades has been primarily directed at the development of reliable and valid outcome measures in order to evaluate the outcomes of rehabilitation interventions (Finch et al. 2002, Majnemer and Mazer 2004). The emphasis on developing outcome measures represents an important first step of a research agenda. Clinical research in pediatric rehabilitation is now changing focus to the systematic evaluation of intervention strategies. Research evaluating the effects of different intervention approaches is sparse and the methodologic rigor of most available studies has unfortunately been less than ideal, with a preponderance of case studies and quantitative descriptive studies and low-power small-sample efforts (Ottenbacher 1995). Concomitant with this new emphasis on intervention studies, approaches to research are changing in four important ways:

1 An increased methodologic rigor
2 A broader scope of outcomes examined
3 An increased emphasis on an interdisciplinary approach
4 The explicit recognition of the importance of personal and environmental factors as mediators of interventions

Clinical researchers are applying more rigorous research methods in their clinical studies. Randomized clinical trials are appearing in the literature, often using multisite data collection to increase the sample size of conditions with low prevalence. However, given the highly complex and individualized nature of many interventions provided to children with developmental disabilities and the ethical dilemma of withholding treatment, randomized clinical trials are not always possible. Researchers using non-randomized methods still try to strengthen their research design by including a power analysis, recruiting more homogeneous samples to control for various possible confounding variables such as age and severity, standardizing both the intervention and outcome measures, and using independent blinded raters to measure outcome.

Traditionally, clinical research outcomes in this area have focused on documenting changes in the intrinsic abilities of the child represented by the ICF component of body function and structure (e.g. developmental deficits or abnormalities). Outcomes such as range of motion, cognitive functioning, attention span, co-ordination, articulation, and sensory processing have been studied with the assumption that improvement of these deficits or impairments would necessarily and likely result in overall functional improvement. Functional outcomes that focus on everyday activities (e.g. putting on a coat, walking up stairs, listening to a story) have been less evident in research studies. These functional abilities representing the ICF component of activity are now routinely measured in outcome research.

In addition to functional abilities, researchers are also beginning to evaluate outcomes which include the child's participation in social and recreational activities (Sloper et al. 1990, Simeonsson et al. 2001, Law et al. 2006). More recently, measures of a child's functioning and participation are complemented with assessments of extrinsic factors that may possibly influence outcome. In particular, family attributes such as coping, stress, and adaptability are recognized as having a powerful influence on a child's functioning and well-being (Magill-Evans et al. 2001, Majnemer and Limperopoulos 2002, Majnemer et al. 2006). As a result of the shift from biomedically oriented child-focused outcomes to more psychosocial family-focused outcomes, current research will yield information not only about the child's functional abilities, but also about the challenges faced across various domains by families of children with developmental disabilities.

This change in focus from a medically oriented approach to a biopsychosocial approach has resulted in more complex interactive models of determinants of outcome, which examine the dynamic effects of child, family, and environmental influences on a child's outcome (King et al. 2002). Research concepts and models that address the complex interplay between the child's intrinsic capabilities and environmental influences (social, attitudinal, and physical) are appearing more frequently in the literature (Colver 2005). Although studies that examine the effects of an intervention to minimize impairments are still important, the new multidimensional studies contribute to clinicians' appreciation of factors that influence the effectiveness of interventions, and to their increasing understanding of the potential influence of an intervention on many levels of functioning, both at the level of the child, and in the context of their family unit.

The emphasis on interdisciplinary research has resulted in new collaborations between basic and clinical researchers. As a result, research is emerging that attempts to link form (basic science) and function to understand the direct relationship between genes and brain anomalies with behavior and development (Als et al. 2004, Crnic and Hagerman 2004). Increased research collaborations across the rehabilitation disciplines of occupational therapy, physical therapy, and speech-language pathology are appearing that evaluate relationships among the different skill domains in children (Darrah et al. 2003). As clinicians become more sophisticated consumers of research, their role as research collaborators is also increasing. Clinicians are experts at the identification and refinement of relevant clinical research questions that have an immediate impact on families and children with disabilities. All of these factors are moving research towards a more rigorous and thorough evaluation of intervention effectiveness with multidimensional outcomes that are meaningful both to families and to clinicians (Table 20.1).

TABLE 20.1

Examples of conceptual shifts in focus at the theoretical, clinical, research and educational levels of rehabilitation practice for children with disabilities

	Traditional focus	Contemporary focus
Theory	Neuromaturational approach with emphasis on neurologic maturation of central nervous system as the primary determinant of typical developmental skills	Transactive theories such as dynamic systems, ecological task analysis, person–environment–occupation that consider the interaction of person, task and environment in the acquisition of developmental abilities
	Assumption that changes in physiologic components (e.g. muscle strength, tactile sensitivity, attention span, memory) would automatically result in improved functional skills (e.g. walking, dressing, reading)	Relationship between physiologic–anatomic parameters and functional abilities cannot be assumed and must be systematically evaluated
	Deficit model of disability that emphasizes impairments within the person – internalizes the challenges of disability	Social action model of disability that emphasizes that a person with a disability has different needs that need to be addressed in a social context – externalizes the challenges of disability as a socially created process
Clinical	Child focused	Interactive approach that considers child, task and the environment
	Remediation approach with typical development as the gold standard	Adaptive approach with success of functional skills as the gold standard
	One preconceived ideal developmental skill solution transferred to different environments	Different solutions expected in different environments
	Therapists as 'expert' providing advice to parents and identifying goals of treatment	Parents as the most important member of the team that work collaboratively to identify meaningful goals and intervention strategies
Research	Development of reliable and valid outcome measures that are developmentally appropriate	Systematic evaluation of intervention approaches and determinants of participation and well-being
	Small heterogeneous samples	Larger, often multisite homogeneous samples
	Research questions focusing primarily at components of body function and structure	Research questions focusing on components of body function and structure, activity and participation and the interaction among the components
	Discipline-specific research teams	Interdisciplinary research teams that include basic and clinician scientists, service providers and families
Professional education	Undergraduate training	Graduate training at master's and doctoral level
	Emphasis on acquisition of clinical skills	Emphasis on acquisition of clinical skills and evidence-based research evaluative skills

CONCLUSIONS

Clinical practice is greatly enriched by an expanding repertoire of approaches to intervention that may be offered to children with developmental disabilities, influenced by recent advances in the explosion of new knowledge and theories of rehabilitation. Key driving forces are listed below:

1 The ICF framework promotes a more holistic view of the child's functioning and health. This model assists the therapist in deciding what to do (which areas need to be considered), but not how to do it.

2 There is increased appreciation of the importance of a transactive approach to the therapeutic process, recognizing the dynamic interplay between the child's abilities, the expectations and constraints of the task, and the different environments the child interacts with. Developmental acquisitions are experience and context-dependent; therefore therapists more readily accept compensatory adaptive patterns, and help the child and family to find functional solutions, by capitalizing on intrinsic strengths and by modifying the task or environment.

3 Working in partnership with families ensures that goals are meaningful (i.e. individually relevant) and that child and family needs and concerns are appropriately addressed.

4 Therapists are placing a greater emphasis on community integration and social participation, because of its importance to overall health and well-being.

5 There is greater recognition of the need for periodic injections of rehabilitation throughout childhood and adolescence (i.e. lifespan approach), so as to address new challenges and life roles.

Integration and adoption of these new concepts in the rehabilitation of children with developmental disabilities are fueled by several mechanisms. First, educational curricula for rehabilitation programs are now actively promoting these new concepts into course content. Secondly, current research is increasingly moving from tool development to the evaluation of interventions, with a greater interest in the interaction of a multitude of factors that likely influence outcome, both intrinsic and extrinsic to the child. Collectively, ongoing educational and research advances will ensure that rehabilitation practice is increasingly evidence-based and aimed at promoting and enhancing the health and well-being of children and youth with disabilities and their families.

REFERENCES

American Occupational Therapy Association (AOTA) website: www.aota.org (accessed June 2006).
Als H, Duffy FH, McAnulty GB, Rivkin MJ, Vajapeyam S, Mulkern RV, et al. (2004) Early experience alters brain function and structure. *Pediatrics* 113: 846–857.
American Physical Therapy Association (2001) *Guide to Physical Therapist Practice, 2nd edn.* American Physical Therapy Association.

Barnhart RC (2001) Aging adult children with developmental disabilities and their families: challenges for occupational therapists and physical therapists. *Phys Occup Ther Pediatr* 21: 69–82.

Bodfish JW (2004) Treating the core features of autism: are we there yet? *Ment Retard Dev Disabil Res Rev* 10: 318–326.

Bornman J (2004) The World Health Organisation's terminology and classification: application to severe disability. *Disabil Rehabil* 26: 182–188.

Burton AW, Davis WE (1992) Optimizing the involvement and performance of children with physical impairments. *Pediatr Exerc Sci* 4: 236–246.

Burton AW, Davis WE (1996) Ecological task analysis: utilizing intrinsic measures in research and practice. *Hum Mov Sci* 15: 285–314.

Butler C, Darrah J (2001) Effects of neurodevelopment treatment (NDT) for cerebral palsy: an AACPDM evidence report. *Dev Med Child Neurol* 43: 778–790.

Canadian Occupational Therapy Association (CAOT) website; www.caot.ca.

Canadian Physiotherapy Association (CPA) website; www.physiotherapy.ca.

CAOT Position Statement: Continuing Professional Education, www.caot.ca, 2006.

Case-Smith J (2005) Efficacy of interventions to enhance hand function. In: Henderson A, Pehoski C (eds) *Hand Function in the Child: Foundations for Remediation 2nd edn.* St. Louis: Mosby.

Colver A (2005) A shared framework and language for childhood disability. *Dev Med Child Neurol* 47: 780–784.

Condeluci A (1995) *Interdependence: The Route to Community, 2nd edn.* Winter Park, FL: CRC Press.

Coster W, Deeney TA, Haltiwanger JT, Haley SM (1998) *School Function Assessment: User's Manual.* San Antonio, TX: Therapy Skill Builders.

Crnic LS, Hagerman R (2004) Fragile X syndrome: frontiers of understanding gene–brain–behavior relationships. *Ment Retard Dev Disabil Res Rev* 10: 1–2.

Darrah J, Bartlett D (1995) Dynamic systems theory and management of children with cerebral palsy: unresolved issues. *Infants Young Child* 8: 52–59.

Darrah J, Law M, Pollock, N (2001) Innovations in practice. Family-centered functional therapy: a choice for children with motor dysfunction. *Infants Young Child* 13: 79–87.

Darrah J, Magill-Evans JE, Adkins R (2002) How well are we doing? Families of adolescents or young adults with cerebral palsy share their perceptions of service delivery. *Disabil Rehabil* 24: 542–549.

Darrah J, Hodge M, Magill-Evans J, Kembhavi G (2003) Stability of serial assessments of motor and communication abilities in typically developing infants: implications for screening. *Early Hum Dev* 72: 97–110.

Darrah J, Loomis J, Manns T, Norton B, May L (2006) Role of conceptual models in a physical therapy curriculum: application of an integrated model of theory, research, and clinical practice. *Physiother Theory Pract* 22: 239–250.

Finch E, Brooks D, Stratford P, Mayo, N (2002) *Physical Rehabilitation Outcome Measures, a Guide to Enhanced Clinical Decision Making, 2nd edn.* Toronto: Canadian Physiotherapy Association.

Fougeyrollas P, Noreau L, Bereron H, Cloutier R, Dion SA, St-Michel G (1998) Social consequences of long term impairments and disabilities: conceptual approach and assessment of handicap. *Int J Rehabil Res* 21: 127–141.

Fougeyrollas P, Noreau L, St-Michel G (2001) *Life Habits Measure: shortened version (LIFE-H 3.0).* Lac St-Charles, Quebec, Canada: CQIDIH.

Frontera WR, Fuhrer MJ, Jette AM, Chan L, Cooper RA, Duncan PW, et al. (2005) Rehabilitation medicine summit: building research capacity. *Am J Phys Med Rehabil* 84: 913–917.

Goldstein DNE, Cohn E, Coster W (2004) Enhancing participation for children with disabilities: application of the ICF enablement framework to pediatric physical therapy practice. *Pediatr Phys Ther* 16: 114–120.

Hadders-Algra M (2000) The neuronal group selection theory: an attractive framework to explain variation in normal motor development. *Dev Med Child Neurol* 42: 707–715.

Helders PJM, Engelbert RHH, Custers JWH, Gorter JW, Takken T, Van Der Net J (2003) Creating and being created: the changing panorama of paediatric rehabilitation. *Pediatr Rehabil* 6: 5–12.

Hostler SL (1991) Family-centered care (review). *Pediatr Clin North Am* 38: 1545–1560.

International Classification of Functioning, Disability and Health (ICF) website; www.who.int/classification/icf, 2001 (accessed May 2006).

Johnston MV, Sherer M, Whyte J (2006) Applying evidence standards to rehabilitation research. *Am J Med Rehabil* 8a5: 292–309.

Ketelaar M, Vermeer A, 't Hart H, van Petegem-van Beek E, Helders PJM (2001) Effects of a functional therapy program on motor abilities of children with cerebral palsy. *Phys Ther* 81: 1534–1545.

King G, Tucker MA, Baldwin P, Lowry K, LaPorta J, Martens L (2002) A life needs model of pediatric service delivery: services to support community participation and quality of life for children and youth with disabilities. *Phys Occup Ther Pediatr* 22: 53–77.

King G, Law M, King S, Hurley P, Hanna S, Kertoy M, et al. (2004) *Children's Assessment of Participation and Enjoyment (CAPE) and Preferences for Activities of Children (PAC)*. San Antonio, TX: Harcourt Assessment.

Law M, Cooper BA, Strong S, Stewart D, Rigby P, Letts L (1996) The person–environment–occupation model: a transactive approach to occupational performance. *Can J Occup Ther* 63: 9–23.

Law M, Darrah J, Pollock N, King G, Rosenbaum P, Russell D, et al. (1998) Family-centered functional therapy for children with cerebral palsy: an emerging practice model. *Phys Occup Ther Pediatr* 18: 83–102.

Law M, Dunn W (1993) Perspectives on understanding and changing the environments of children with disabilities. *Phys Occup Ther Pediatr* 13: 1–17.

Law M, Hanna S, King G, Hurley P, King S, Kertoy M, et al. (2003) Factors affecting family-centered service delivery for children with disabilities. *Child Care Health Dev* 29: 357–366.

Law M, King G, King S, Kertoy M, Hurley P, Rosenbaum P, et al. (2006) Patterns of participation in recreational and leisure activities among children with complex physical disabilities. *Dev Med Child Neurol* 48: 337–342.

Magill-Evans J, Darrah J, Pain K, Adkins R, Kratochvil M (2001) Are families with adolescents and young adults with cerebral palsy the same as other families? *Dev Med Child Neurol* 43: 466–472.

Majnemer A (2006) Assessment tools for cerebral palsy: new directions. *Future Neurol* 1: 755–763.

Majnemer A, Birnbaum R, Kennedy E. (2009) Rehabilitation: the role of occupational therapy and physical therapy. In: Maria BL (ed) *Current Management in Child Neurology, 4th edn.* Hamilton: BC Decker, pp 407–412.

Majnemer A, Limperopoulos C (2002) The importance of outcome determination in pediatric rehabilitation (annotation). *Dev Med Child Neurol* 44: 773–777.

Majnemer A, Limperopoulos C, Shevell M, Rohlicek C, Tchervenkov C, Rosenblatt B (2006) Health and well-being of children with congenital cardiac malformation, and their families, following open-heart surgery. *Cardiol Young* 16: 157–164.

Majnemer A, Mazer B (2004) New directions in the outcome evaluation of children with cerebral palsy. *Semin Pediatr Neurol* 11: 11–17.

Manns PJ, Darrah J (2006) Linking research and clinical practice in physical therapy: strategies for integration. *Physiotherapy* 92: 88–94.

Mather N, Roberts R (1995) *Informal assessment and instruction in written language: a practitioner's guide for students with learning disabilities*. Brandon, VT: Clinical Psychology Publishing.

Mayston M (2005) Evidence-based physical therapy for the management of children with cerebral palsy (Editorial). *Dev Med Child Neurol* 47: 795.

McHale K, Cermak SA (1992) Fine motor activities in elementary school: preliminary findings and provisional implications for children with fine motor problems. *Am J Occup Ther* 46: 898–903.

Missiuna C, Mandich AD, Polatajko H, Malloy-Miller T (2001) Cognitive orientation to daily occupational performance (CO-OP): Part 1. Theoretical foundations. *Phys Occup Ther Pediatr* 20: 69–82.

Ottenbacher KJ (1995) Why rehabilitation research does not work (as well as we think it should). *Arch Phys Med Rehabil* 76: 123–129.

Rioux MH (1994) New research directions and paradigms: disability is not measles. In: Rioux M, Bach M (eds) *Disability is not Measles: New Research Paradigms in Disability*. North York, Ontario: Roeher Institute, pp 1–7.

Rosenbaum P, King S, Law M, King G, Evans J (1998) Family-centered service: a conceptual framework and research review. *Phys Occup Ther Pediatr* 18: 1–20.

Sackett DL, Straus SE, Richardson WS, Rosenberg W, Haynes RB (2000) *Evidence-Based Medicine How to Practice and Teach EBM, 2nd edn*. Toronto: Churchill Livingstone.

Seelman KD (2000) Rehabilitation science. *Technol Disabil* 12: 77–83.

Shumway-Cook A, Woollacott MJ (eds) (1995) *Motor Control: Theory and Practical Applications*. Baltimore: Williams & Wilkins.

Simeonsson RJ, Carlson D, Huntington GS, McMillen JS, Brent JL (2001) Students with disabilities: a national survey of participation in school activities. *Disabil Rehabil* 23: 49–63.

Sloper P, Turner S, Knussen C, Cunningham C (1990) Social life of school children with Down's syndrome. *Child Care Health Dev* 16: 235–251.

Stewart D, Law M, Rosenbaum P, Willms DG (2001) A qualitative study of the transition to adulthood for youth with physical disabilities. *Phys Occup Ther Pediatr* 21: 3–21.

Wehman P (ed) (1996) *Life beyond the classroom. Transition strategies for young people with disabilities, 2nd edn*. Baltimore: Paul H Brookes.

Whyte J (1998) Enabling America: a report from the Institute of Medicine on rehabilitation science and engineering. *Arch Phys Med Rehabil* 79: 1477–1480.

Whyte J (2005) Training and retention of rehabilitation researchers. *Am J Phys Med Rehabil* 84: 969–975.

World Health Organization (2001) *International Classification of Functioning, Disability and Health*. World Health Organization, Geneva.

21

EARLY INTERVENTION IN DEVELOPMENTAL DISABILITIES

David A Kube and Frederick B Palmer

Early intervention for infants and children is a system of services designed to prevent or ameliorate developmental delay or other symptoms in children with, or at risk for, disability or delay. Early intervention programs may be public or private, formal or informal, home- or center-based, and usually involve active ongoing parent participation. Services may be provided by professionals from a wide variety of disciplines working alone or as part of interdisciplinary teams. Trained non-professionals, including family members, may be an important part of these programs and service delivery. The focus is usually on children with, or at risk for, neurodevelopmental disabilities and is generally thought to include infants from birth to 3–5 years.

Prevalence data for global developmental mental retardation/intellectual disability, speech and language impairment, and other neurodevelopmental disabilities in children from birth to 3 years of age are incomplete for many reasons. There is difficulty in making accurate developmental diagnoses at these early ages. Common diagnostic criteria are not universally and systematically applied. Eligibility for most intervention programs is not based on diagnosis but on an identification of delay (which may or may not be confirmed) or certain indicators of risk for later eventual delay or disability. Available prevalence figures are usually based on data from older children. Nevertheless, available data are instructive.

In developed countries, the prevalence of intellectual disability (i.e. mental retardation) is generally felt to be in the range 1–2%, with most falling into mild ranges of delay (Petterson et al. 2005, Bhasin et al. 2006). Cerebral palsy has a birth prevalence of about 2 per 1000 live births (Odding et al. 2006). Speech and language impairment occurs in 3–7% of preschool children (Catts et al. 2002) and autism spectrum disorders are now reported in as many as 6 per 1000 children (Rutter 2005, Rice et al. 2007). In the United States, in 2004 there were 282 733 children aged from birth to 3 years receiving early intervention services through federally mandated and funded programs. This represents 2.3% of the United States' birth to 3 years population (Office of Special Education Programs 2005). Limited but similar data are available from other developed countries. For example, in Bavaria, 4% of children up to the age of 3 years need early intervention services, about one-third of them recognized as having severe cognitive or physical disabilities (European Agency for Development in Special Needs Education 2005).

NEUROPLASTICITY AND EARLY INTERVENTION

The rationale for early intervention in children with developmental disabilities is usually tied to the concept of neuroplasticity (Johnston et al. 2001). While the basic structure and function of the developing brain is genetically programmed, experience-dependent changes throughout infancy, childhood, adolescence, and adulthood individualize and shape development. These mechanisms are ongoing, not only serving to establish learning and memory, but also to fine-tune and shape cognition, language, and behavior over time, the overt manifestations of neuro-development (Post and Weiss 1997). As experiences vary, learning, memory and thus cognition, language and behavior vary. Synapses that fire repeatedly or persistently undergo changes that result in potentiation and preservation, rather than depression, pruning and loss. Thus, the complex arrays of neural interconnections, which are the substrate of neurodevelopment, are formed. An emerging understanding of the scientific underpinnings of neuroplasticity has helped support the long-standing logical, but not always verified or accepted, contention that *early* stimulation in typically developing children – and early treatments and interventions for children with neurodevelopmental disabilities – will be of greatest potential benefit.

Although links between basic studies of neuroplasticity and the clinical effects of early interventions have yet to be established, there are several clinical examples in disability, which readily support the concept but illustrate different aspects. Children develop amblyopia after prolonged abnormal visual input in early childhood. Recent studies suggest calcarine cortical loss occurs in such children (Mendola et al. 2005). Loss of NMDA R1 expression (Murphy et al. 2004) and metabolic activity (Wong et al. 2005) has been shown in visual cortex in animals after mono-cular deprivation. Patching the non-impaired eye well before age 6 years reduces the likelihood and severity of amblyopia in the impaired eye, presumably through experienced-based cortical changes, although attenuation of cortical loss has not yet been demonstrated. In amblyopic children younger than 7 years of age, improved visual evoked potentials have been demonstrated after stimulation of the amblyopic eye by patching the better eye (Weiss and Kelly 2004). Interestingly, some adults with amblyopia who lose vision in their better eye do recover some function in their amblyopic eye, indicating a potential for reversibility lasting even into adult-hood (El Mallah et al. 2000).

Constraint-induced therapy for individuals with hemiplegia has recently been shown to offer considerable benefit in young children. In constraint-induced therapy, the child's better arm is restrained 6 hours per day to force the use of the hemiplegic arm, and presumably improve function through underlying neuroplasticity mechanisms. For children with hemiplegia, constraint-induced therapy for only 21 days has resulted in an improved amount and quality of movement of the hemiplegic arm compared with a randomly assigned control group receiving traditional therapy (Taub et al. 2004). These changes were functionally meaningful for the child and were sustained at 6 months' follow-up. Research suggests that the age of treatment is not the critical factor and that older children can have the same positive benefits as younger ones from constraint-induced practice (Gordon et al. 2006).

Earlier but similar studies in adults 6 months to 17 years following stroke also showed substantial sustained improvement in arm and hand function following constraint of the uninvolved arm. Cortical mapping demonstrated enlarged and shifted motor output areas (Liepert et al. 2000). Similar cortical changes have been seen in adults following stroke who received early intensive speech therapy to enhance language skills (Blasi et al. 2002), suggesting that such changes may be widespread phenomena.

A third example supporting a neuroplasticity model for early intervention is the treatment of severe congenital hearing loss. In a case–controlled study, Yoshinaga-Itano et al. (1998) demonstrated that children with severe congenital hearing loss identified and intervened upon (language stimulation, amplification) before 6 months of age had consistently better language outcomes than did infants with severe hearing loss identified after 6 months of age. Children identified between 6 and 12 months had no better outcomes than those identified after 12, 18, 24 or 36 months. These findings suggest a sensitive (or in this case critical) time period (i.e. 'window of opportunity') exists for early intervention in these children in the first year of life.

A similar study (Moeller 2000) supports Yoshinaga-Itano et al.'s findings that later onset intervention is associated with poorer language development outcomes at 5 years of age. However, the poor language outcomes associated with later onset intervention were partially ameliorated by high levels of family participation in the intervention, compliance with recommended treatment sessions, communication with the child, and advocacy for the child.

CONTEXTUAL MODEL OF EARLY INTERVENTION

Family involvement as a factor interacting with intervention in determining neurodevelopmental outcome suggests a broader contextual model of early intervention espoused by Guralnick (1997). Family characteristics, family stressors, and culture interact to create specific and individual 'family profiles' of parent–child interaction, parent-directed child experience (necessary for experience-dependent learning), and general health and safety for the child with or at risk for a disability. These profiles influence child development and eventual functional outcomes. Broad-based intervention programs, according to this model, should address multiple variables affecting development; social and financial supports, parent information, child rearing, and direct interventions or therapy services. Targets include the child, parent, and family. Efforts targeting the community and policy-makers are also important because they influence the broader context of the individual child's learning experience.

EVIDENCE-BASED APPROACH TO EARLY INTERVENTION: CHILDREN AT RISK

When evaluating intervention studies, it is useful to consider children at risk for disability separately from those with actual diagnosed disabilities. While risk may be biologic, environmental, or both, many studies do not distinguish between sources of risk. Indeed, given the interplay between nature and nurture that underpins our conceptualization of early neurodevelopment, separation of environmental and biologic risk may indeed be arbitrary and meaningless. In prominent intervention studies of children at risk, subjects are children whose mothers had mental retardation, children who already showed evidence of early developmental delay, children from families in poverty with additional social risk factors, or premature and low birth weight infants from socially at risk families (Ramey and Ramey 1999). Risk may also be related to family variables that may affect the child's development later in life such as maternal IQ, maternal education level, age of the mother (especially if she is a teenager), single parent status, and lack of extended family support (Bailey et al. 1999). Children from households with parents with poor coping skills, mental health disorders, or substance abuse may also be at risk and could benefit from intervention programs. Other medical risk factors may need to be taken into account such as children exposed to alcohol or other toxins *in utero*, malnutrition, iron deficiency anemia, genetic disorders, and known structural brain abnormalities. It is not feasible to study the effects of early interventions in all high-risk settings, and indeed, legislative mandates for treatment may preclude such systematic study.

Studies of children at risk for disability, particularly cognitive delay, offer the largest body of evidence of treatment effect. These studies illustrate the wide range of outcome domains that need to be considered in thoroughly evaluating early interventions. Cognitive, language and related academic development are important outcomes frequently addressed. Several early intervention programs that provided intensive early educational services reduced the incidence of borderline intellectual functioning and mental retardation in children, particularly those from impoverished families or those with parents with documented low intellectual functioning or mental retardation (Martin et al. 1990, Ramey and Ramey 1999). Findings from the Infant Health and Development Program (1990) show that children born with low birth weight who received early intervention services had higher IQ levels than the control group. Developmental interventions starting in the nursery and continuing for the first year of life in a group of high risk premature infants had a positive and significant effect on their cognitive development as measured by the Bayley Scales of Infant Development (Resnick et al. 1988). More recent studies such as Project CARE, the Portage Program in the Gaza Strip, and the Home Visiting Study in Jamaica have all shown measurable improvement in cognitive skills following participation in early intervention programs (Bryant and Maxwell 1997). Challenges include identifying those children and families most likely to benefit. Low maternal IQ and poor family educational attainment are interrelated factors worthy of focus. Programs that serve a heterogeneous group of children, provide a structured curriculum, and target their efforts on parents and children together and collectively appear to be the most effective (Shonkoff and Hauser-Cram 1987).

DURATION OF FOLLOW-UP

While short-term changes in cognition are often reported, these changes are not consistently seen after long-term follow-up. In a number of intense long-term research projects providing early intervention services to preschoolers at risk for mental retardation/intellectual disability (e.g. Milwaukee, Carolina, Ypsilanti, and Syracuse), initial short-term goals noted were improved academic (i.e. readiness) scores and IQ. However, early IQ gains made in certain preschool programs dissipated over time (Westinghouse Learning Corporation 1969).

In other programs, children from low income and under-educated families or those whose mothers had low IQs showed improved intellectual ability and a reduction in mental retardation/intellectual disability (Ramey and Ramey 1999). These effects were maintained into adolescence, but only when interventions were provided in preschool, but not when initiated after preschool (Campbell and Ramey 1995, Campbell et al. 2001). As the subjects of these studies have been followed long term, other beneficial long-term outcomes have become apparent. These positive 'sleeper effects' occurred in the areas of reduced grade retention, need for special education services, better achievement test scores, and more positive attitudes and values (Lazar and Darlington 1979, Bryant and Maxwell 1997).

In the Perry Preschool Project, children who received preschool interventions, and now followed to 40 years of age, show many positive outcomes in the area of academic, social, family, and occupational functioning. The overall economic benefits to participants and their communities are striking. At age 40, the return on investment was over $17 for every dollar invested (in constant 2000 dollars) (Schweinhart and Weikart 1980, Schweinhart et al. 1993, 2005). Children from low income families who participated in a Chicago public school preschool program also showed better educational and social outcomes at 20 years (Reynolds et al. 2001). Large public early intervention programs such as Head Start show less prominent but still important reduction in delays as measured by grade retention and special education placement rates (Anderson et al. 2003). Measurement of intervention outcomes after short-term follow-up may overestimate immediate cognitive benefits, but will underestimate or not recognize important and perhaps more meaningful long-term benefits. As in other interventions, subjects need to be followed for extended periods of time, a difficult methodologic challenge, if full effects are to be demonstrated.

EDUCATIONAL OUTCOMES

Early intervention programs have had a positive impact on educational outcomes including less grade retention, better math scores, and increased high school graduation rates (Lazar and Darlington 1979, Schweinhart and Weikart 1980). Intense early educational intervention in children at socioeconomic risk can reduce the rate of failing a grade during elementary school (Ramey and Ramey 1994). Other long-term follow-up studies have found that early intervention participants completed more years of school, had a lower drop-out rate, and lower rates of grade retention. They also spent more time in school and were more likely to graduate from high school (Reynolds et al. 2001, Hawkins et al. 2005). Furthermore, a decreased rate of special education was noted among participants and they were less likely to utilize special education services in middle school (Lazar and Darlington 1979, Reynolds et al. 2001). At 18 years of age, participants in the early intervention arm of the Infant Health and Development Program who weighed 2001–2499g at birth had better mathematics performance and better receptive vocabulary skills than those of similar birth weight in the contrast group. Interestingly, and consistent with findings at ages 5 and 8 years, these sustained benefits were not seen in infants with birth weights less than 2000g. This may reflect a greater risk for neurologic injury in these lower birth weight children or other complex factors yet to be clarified (McCormick et al. 2006).

BEHAVIORAL HEALTH OUTCOMES

Certainly, some of the cognitive, academic, family, and occupational outcomes may be associated with behavioral changes, including those captured by behavioral health measures. Early intervention services implemented at various ages have shown behavioral health benefits. In a study of high risk preterm infants and their caregivers, behavior problems were significantly reduced, while the quality of caregiver interaction was improved when intervention services were started in the newborn nursery (Resnick et al. 1988).

The Brookline Early Education Project, a non-randomized, matched cohort, controlled study developed for both urban and suburban children, used family-centered early health and developmental interventions starting 3 months *before* birth and lasting through kindergarten to promote eventual school readiness. As adults, participants who had received early intervention had less depression and reported higher self-confidence. They also reported overall more positive healthy behaviors and more confidence in their abilities to manage their own health than controls. These effects were seen primarily in urban, but not suburban, participants. Thus, infants from lower socioeconomic backgrounds had the greatest benefits. That is, the intervention was associated with partial amelioration of the negative behavioral health effects of lower socioeconomic status (Palfrey et al. 2005).

In the Seattle Social Development Project, intervention services were implemented in early elementary school and consisted of teacher training in instruction and classroom management, child social and emotional skill development, parent training in behavior management and academic support, and parenting/modeling skills to reduce drug use. As adults, participants had better regulation of emotions and less depression. Those participating in the program for longer periods showed more favorable outcomes. The benefits did not appear to fade with time (Hawkins et al. 2005).

IMPROVED FAMILY AND SOCIETAL OUTCOMES
Improvements are also seen as a by-product of early intervention in family and social dynamics. In the Perry Preschool study, adults were more likely to own their own home, less likely to be on welfare, and more likely to be married, lending stability to their own lives and those of their families. There was a decreased incidence of teenage pregnancy (Schweinhart and Weikart 1980). Significantly more males participated in raising their own children (Schweinhart and Weikart 1993, Schweinhart et al. 1993, 2005). Better social functioning was seen in adults who received early intervention in the Brookline Early Education Project. They had a higher level of eventual educational attainment, were less likely to have a low income status, and were more likely to have private health insurance coverage (Palfrey et al. 2005).

Only long-term follow-up can assess effects of interventions on juvenile and adult crime. Follow-up from the Perry Preschool Project and the Chicago Child–Parent Center project showed that participants had fewer arrests as adults, lower rates of juvenile arrests, lower rates of arrest for violence, and fewer drug arrests (Schweinhart and Weikart 1980, Reynolds et al. 2001, Schweinhart et al. 2005). Timing of intervention services may be an important factor in the area of crime reduction, with earlier intervention being most important, as seen in the Seattle Social Project (Hawkins et al. 2005).

As adults, children participating in the early intervention programs showed overall increased levels of employment, including more hours worked on a weekly or annual basis (Schweinhart and Weikart 1980, Hawkins et al. 2005).

EVIDENCE-BASED APPROACH TO EARLY INTERVENTION: CHILDREN WITH DISABILITIES
In children with diagnosed neurodevelopmental disabilities, the studied and evaluated effects of early intervention are less clear. Disabilities are diverse, complex, and frequently co-occurring: (1) study samples are thus far unacceptably small or,

if sufficiently large, unacceptably heterogeneous, (2) treatments are not well stand-ardized or must be individualized, (3) long-term outcomes are not measured, and (4) broad or family-centered approaches are intrinsically difficult to study. Because of these barriers, the simple question 'Does early intervention work?' may be even more simplistic when asked about children with neurodevelopmental disabilities than those found to be at risk. Nevertheless, certain conclusions can be drawn and opportunities for research are many.

SPECIFIC LANGUAGE IMPAIRMENT

Interventions in children with speech and language impairments have seen con-siderable study. Six to eight percent of preschool children have language delay, most of them developmental language disorders. While outcomes are variable, preschool age children with speech and language delays or disorders have poorer academic outcomes as older children (Catts et al. 2002), more behavior problems (Cohen et al. 1998a, 1998b, 2000, Vallance et al. 1999) and have less skilled occupations as adults (Felsenfeld et al. 1994).

A meta-analysis of speech and language therapy interventions identified 25 randomized controlled trials of speech and language interventions in children with primary speech or language disorders. Results suggested positive short-term treat-ment effects for phonologic, expressive vocabulary, and possibly expressive syntax outcomes. Receptive language outcomes were not affected for those with receptive language delays. The meta-analysis allowed evaluation of the effects of type of treatment, but found no particular advantage for group vs. individual therapy or professional vs. trained parent implementation of treatment (Law et al. 2003).

A more recent meta-analysis reached similar conclusions and highlighted the limited range of outcomes studied. In this meta-analysis, only six of the 25 reviewed trials assessed non-language health or daily function outcomes. Most studies were short term in nature. Long-term outcomes including important academic outcomes in elementary school or later childhood were typically not assessed or part of the evaluation paradigm (Nelson et al. 2006). The effects of early intervention in autism spectrum disorders are beyond the scope of this chapter, but offer some support for early intervention in language disorders and highlight the need for the early detection of these common disabilities (Dumont-Mathieu and Fein 2005, Francis 2005).

MOTOR DISORDERS

Motor disorders, particularly cerebral palsy, have been subject to trials evaluating interventions, including early intervention. Cerebral palsy trials are all compromised by an inherent emphasis on short-term outcomes emphasizing objective measures of motor impairment only. A meta-analysis of the effects of neurodevelopmental therapy (NDT) performed under the auspices of the American Academy of

Cerebral Palsy and Developmental Medicine identified 21 studies involving 416 individual children of varying age, type and severity of cerebral palsy, and associated disabilities. Most of the 101 outcomes assessed showed no advantage from therapy and only four of the 16 favorable results were rated as 'clinically significant' (Butler and Darrah 2001). However, one randomized controlled trial of NDT in infants with spastic diplegia found motor and cognitive benefits from the contrast group (a broad infant stimulation curriculum) compared to NDT (Palmer et al. 1988, 1990). The advantage of the broader based intervention is consistent with the contextual model of early intervention and is consistent with the short-term positive outcomes in children at risk for disability demonstrated in the Infant Health and Development Program (1990) and the other studies summarized above. In another review of the effects of early intervention on motor development, some developmental programs where parents were actively involved and engaged produced a positive effect on motor development (Blauw-Hospers and Hadders-Algra 2005).

INTELLECTUAL DISABILITIES

Studies of early intervention in intellectual disability (mental retardation) are few. Randomized controlled trials with adequate power have simply not been performed and likely will not, given ethical restraints. Rather, 'second generation' (Guralnick 1997) research focusing on indications for specific interventions, the timing of such interventions, varying combinations of interventions, and the integration of interventions into co-ordinated systems of care seems to be more indicated. The literature on Down syndrome early intervention is summarized in a concise review by Spiker and Hopmann (1997). Early studies suggesting evident developmental benefits helped solidify support for mandated early intervention services in the United States and elsewhere. For example, Connolly et al. (1980) in a non-randomized follow-up study of 20 infants with Down syndrome compared with 53 children with Down syndrome living in the community but not exposed to early intervention, showed improved motor, self-help, and cognitive outcomes at 3–6 years of age in the group receiving early intervention. Subsequent follow-up of a subsample during adolescence showed sustained advantages in intellectual and adaptive domains in the early intervention group with no evident decline in adaptive skills that is often noted in Down syndrome (Connolly et al. 1993).

Gibson and Harris (1988), in a qualitative review of 21 Down syndrome early intervention studies, noted short-term gains in social, self-help, and some developmental skills, but a lack of comparable gains in either cognition or language skills. Further, these short-term gains were not sustained over the long term, although the studies and their follow-up were limited.

In a study of motor development in children with Down syndrome receiving NDT, there was no advantage in eventual developmental outcome over children receiving a developmental skills curriculum. The most powerful predictor of outcome after 1 year of treatment was the a priori level of development upon enrollment or entry into the study. The authors concluded there was no evidence to suggest that motor intervention accelerated development or improved the quality of movement beyond what could be expected on the basis of maturation alone (Mahoney et al. 2001).

Dunst et al. (1988) have been strong proponents of the contextual model for intervention effects, and therefore the importance of providing social supports for families as an important component of early intervention. Social support includes: (1) formal supports from professionals, social agencies, early intervention programs, and (2) informal supports from family, friends, social groups, and other resources. Evidence suggests that social supports have direct, mediating, and moderating contextual influences on development in children with disabilities and their families. Dunst et al. (1997) also suggest that it is the informal supports that have the greatest effect on actual observable behavioral functioning when compared to formal (professional) supports. Further, the greater the breadth of social supports, the larger contribution it has to eventual outcome. In a time of increasing health and educational costs, it is easy to see the potential of informal, but defined, social supports as an essential component of comprehensive early intervention strategies.

FUTURE DIRECTIONS AND CHALLENGES
SYSTEMATIC EVALUATION OF THE RIGHT OUTCOMES
'Is early intervention effective?' is a hopelessly general question. Any review of the effectiveness of early intervention finds evidence that *certain* interventions delivered in *certain* ways and with *certain* timing and intensity show benefit for *certain* children with *certain* risks or *certain* disabilities, when *certain* outcomes are measured.

The research challenge is to identify these 'certain' determinants of treatment effectiveness and explore the individual differences that influence treatment response (Blair and Ramey 1997). Certain general conclusions seem justified. Children from environmentally deprived backgrounds often benefit most from early intervention programs (Parry 1992). Long-term studies are required to identify what may be very important long-term benefits to children and to communities (Schweinhart et al. 2005). Broad-based infant intervention programs have shown advantage over focused particular programs, possibly because of the diverse nature of disability and risk. When biologic risk factors such as low birth weight are present, the effects of early intervention may be attenuated, or alternatively interventions may need to be modified to address the specific neurodevelopmental needs of the child at heightened biologic risk (Olds 2006). Speech and language therapy appears to be effective for phonologic and expressive language disorders, specifically for expressive vocabulary in preschoolers. There is mixed evidence for its effectiveness in expressive syntax difficulties and little evidence for its effectiveness in receptive language delay (Law 2004).

A comprehensive approach to outcome measurement is necessary. It has become clear that functional outcomes must be assessed in any evaluation of program effectiveness (Msall 2005). A systematic approach to evaluating early interventions services should address many of the following domains.

TIMING, INTENSITY, AND QUALITY OF INTERVENTIONS

Timing of intervention services is important. A review of intervention programs from birth to 3 years showed that better outcomes are associated with earlier implementation of services (Shonkoff and Hauser-Cram 1987). The intensity of the program and the breadth of involvement with the family have direct positive effects on outcomes in the areas of IQ, development, and behavior (US Department of Health and Human Services 1985). Positive effects are also obtained if interventions are started early in preschool and elementary school (Reynolds et al. 2001). Permanent effects may be produced if interventions are started as late as elementary school depending on the type of eventual outcome assessed (Hawkins et al. 2005). The greatest cognitive benefits have been seen in high risk children who actively participated in intensive high-quality center-based early intervention programs (Martin et al. 1990, Ramey and Ramey 1994). Program intensity, not unexpectedly, varies widely. Published intervention programs vary in (1) duration (from 1 to 5 years), (2) content (child curriculum only vs. additional health care, infant nutrition, and parenting/family supports), and (3) time (2.5 hours per day, to full-day programs or home-based programs with visits once or twice weekly) (Ramey and Ramey 1999). The quality of interventions is also variable and may include a wide range of therapeutic, education, prevention, and support services targeted to the child, parent, and family, either individually or collectively.

FAMILY, COMMUNITY, AND CULTURAL VARIABLES

Listening to and learning from parents is crucial in the development of appropriate interventions (i.e. family-centered approach). Individual programs should ideally be developed based on specific identification of the family's needs and from an understanding of the family's cultural background and expectations. In a study of low income, predominantly African-American, pregnant women and their families participating in an Early Head Start program, important outcomes for parents were not limited to their child's cognitive ability. Parents were also concerned whether their children were ready for school and socially and emotionally healthy (McAllister et al. 2005). When evaluating intervention services for preterm infants, investigators found that it was necessary to work together with the family when providing service in a setting outside the home in order to obtain positive sustainable benefits (Resnick et al. 1988). Families often report that they desired more intervention services than they were actually receiving (Mahoney and Filer 1996).

EARLY INTERVENTION, COMMUNITY OUTCOMES, AND SYSTEMS OF CARE

It may be necessary to rethink the concept of early interventions. Not just focusing on a specific age or high-risk group, but on ways that early intervention can have a much broader impact on the community as a whole. When comprehensive intervention, education, family, and health services were provided through the Chicago public school system to preschoolers and early elementary school children, social and educational outcomes for all were improved (Reynolds et al. 2001). In addition to cognitive and physical outcomes, other outcomes not limited to social/emotional adaptability, independence, criminal involvement, and employment of individuals should be assessed. Counseling, support, parent empowerment, and skills transference to families may be important services to incorporate in early intervention. Cross-agency efforts requiring much collaboration are necessary to accomplish this. Indicators for quality services should include the extent to which services are co-ordinated across providers and agencies, the appropriateness of services based on the specific needs of the individual child and family, and the extent to which a partnership is established between parents and professionals (Bailey et al. 1999). Ancillary complex community issues such as housing problems, neighborhood violence, or the presence of environmental toxins may presumably affect intervention outcomes. Program costs need to be analyzed in the context of long-term effects of potential benefits which may be difficult to quantify across the entire range of important outcome variables, including the potential long-range benefits for communities (Lynch 2005).

CONCLUSIONS

Effects of early intervention for children with neurodevelopmental disabilities and those at risk can be seen as overt measurable manifestations of neuroplasticity in the developing organism. Modifying factors include age of treatment, type, intensity, and duration of interventions offered, and a wide variety of possible contextual factors including family, socioeconomic, and community environment. Evidence for intervention effectiveness varies by treatment provided and the actual outcome measured. Short-term benefits, such as cognitive differences in preschoolers, are often seen but may diminish or even disappear with time, especially when interventions are not sustained. However, certain benefits may be sustained, such as upper extremity functioning in children with hemiplegia who receive intensive practice associated with constraint-induced therapy. Long-term effects may not be initially apparent, but may actually offer the greatest long-term benefits such as decreased crime and improved academic, social and family outcomes seen decades after preschool interventions in children at socioeconomic risk.

REFERENCES

Anderson LM, Shinn C, Fullilove MT, Scrimshaw SC, Fielding JE, Normand J, et al. (2003) The effectiveness of early childhood development programs: a systematic review. *Am J Prev Med* 24 (3 Suppl): 32–46.

Bailey DB, Aytch LS, Odom SL, Symons F, Wolery M (1999) Early intervention as we know it. *Ment Retard Dev Disabil Res Rev* 5: 11–20.

Bhasin TK, Brocksen S, Avchen RN, Van Naarden Braun K (2006) Prevalence of four developmental disabilities among children aged 8 years: Metropolitan Atlanta Developmental Disabilities Surveillance Program, 1996 and 2000. *MMWR Surveill Summ* 55: 1–9.

Blair C, Ramey CT (1997) Early intervention for low-birth-weight infants and the path to second-generation research. In: Guralnick MJ (ed) *The Effectiveness of Early Intervention.* Baltimore: Paul H. Brookes, pp 77–97.

Blasi V, Young AC, Tansy AP, Petersen SE, Snyder AZ, Corbetta M (2002) Word retrieval learning modulates right frontal cortex in patients with left frontal damage. *Neuron* 36: 159–170.

Blauw-Hospers CH, Hadders-Algra M (2005) A systematic review of the effects of early intervention on motor development. *Dev Med Child Neurol* 47: 421–432.

Bryant D, Maxwell K (1997) The effectiveness of early intervention for disadvantaged children. In: Guralnick MJ (ed) *The Effectiveness of Early Intervention.* Baltimore: Paul H. Brooks, pp 23–46.

Butler C, Darrah J (2001) Effects of neurodevelopmental treatment (NDT) for cerebral palsy: an AACPDM evidence report. *Dev Med Child Neurol* 43: 778–790.

Campbell FA, Ramey CT (1995) Cognitive and school outcomes for high-risk African American students at middle adolescence: positive effects of early intervention. *Am Educ Res J* 32: 743–772.

Campbell FA, Pungello EP, Miller-Johnson S, Burchinal M, Ramey CT (2001) The development of cognitive and academic abilities: growth curves from an early childhood educational experiment. *Dev Psychol* 37: 231–242.

Catts HW, Fey ME, Tornblin JB, Zhang X (2002) A longitudinal investigation of reading outcomes in children with language impairments. *J Speech Lang Hear Res* 45: 1142–1157.

Cohen NJ, Menna R, Vallance DD, Barwick MA, Irn N, Horodezky NB (1998a) Language, social cognitive processing, and behavioral characteristics of psychiatrically disturbed children with previously identified and unsuspected language impairments. *J Child Psychol Psychiatry* 39: 853–864.

Cohen NJ, Barwick MA, Horodezky NB, Vallance DD, Irn N (1998b) Language, achievement, and cognitive processing in psychiatrically disturbed children with previously identified and unsuspected language impairments. *J Child Psychol Psychiatry* 39: 865–877.

Cohen NJ, Vallance DD, Barwick M, Irn N, Menna R, Horodezky NB (2000) The interface between ADHD and language impairment: an examination of language, achievement, and cognitive processing. *J Child Psychol Psychiatry* 41: 353–362.

Connolly B, Morgan S, Russell FF, Richardson B (1980) Early intervention with Down syndrome children: follow-up report. *Phys Ther* 60: 1405–1408.

Connolly BH, Morgan SB, Russell FF, Fulliton WL (1993) A longitudinal study of children with Down syndrome who experienced early intervention programming. *Phys Ther* 73: 170–179.

Dumont-Mathieu T, Fein D (2005) Screening for autism in young children: the Modified Checklist for Autism in Toddlers (M-CHAT) and other measures. *Ment Retard Dev Disabil Res Rev* 11: 253–262.

Dunst CJ, Snyder S, Mankinen M (1988) Efficacy of early intervention. In: Wang MC, Reynolds MC, Walberg HJ (eds) *Handbook of Special Education.* Oxford: Pergamon Press, pp 259–294.

Dunst CJ, Trivette CM, Jodry W (1997) Influences of social support on children with disabilities and their families. In: Guralnick MJ, Bennett FC (eds) *The Effectiveness of Early Intervention.* Baltimore: Paul H. Brookes, pp 499–522.

El Mallah MK, Chakravarthy U, Hart PM. (2000) Amblyopia: is visual loss permanent? *Br J Ophthalmol* 84: 952–956.

European Agency for Development in Special Needs Education (2005) *Early Childhood Intervention: Analysis of Situationsin Europe.* European Agency for Development in Special Needs Education.

Felsenfeld S, Broen PA, McGue M (1994) A 28-year follow-up of adults with a history of moderate phonological disorder: educational and occupational results. *J Speech Hear Res* 37: 1341–1353.

Francis K (2005) Autism interventions: a critical update. *Dev Med Child Neurol* 47: 493–499.

Gibson D, Harris A (1988) Aggregated early intervention effects for Down's syndrome persons: patterning and longevity of benefits. *J Ment Defic Res* 32: 1–17.

Gordon AM, Charles J, Wolf SL (2006) Efficacy of constraint-induced movement therapy on involved upper-extremity use in children with hemiplegic cerebral palsy is not age-dependent. *Pediatrics* 117: e363–373.

Guralnick MJ (1997) Second-generation research. In: Guralnick MJ, Bennett FC (eds) *The Effectiveness of Early Intervention.* Baltimore: Paul H. Brookes, pp 3–20.

Hawkins JD, Kosterman R, Catalano RF, Hill KG, Abbott RD (2005) Promoting positive adult functioning through social development intervention in childhood: long-term effects from the Seattle Social Development Project. *Arch Pediatr Adolesc Med* 159: 25–31.

Infant Health and Development Program (1990) Enhancing the outcomes of low-birth weight, premature infants: a multisite, randomized trial. *JAMA* 263: 3035–3042.

Johnston MV, Nishimura A, Harum K, Pekar J, Blue ME (2001) Sculpting the developing brain. *Adv Pediatr* 48: 1–38.

Law J (2004) The implications of different approaches to evaluating intervention: evidence from the study of language delay/disorder. *Folia Phoniatr Logop* 56: 199–219.

Law J, Garrett Z, Nye C (2003) Speech and language therapy interventions for children with primary speech and language delay or disorder. *Cochrane Database Syst Rev* 3: CD004110.

Lazar I, Darlington RD (1979) *Lasting effects after preschool.* US Department of Health, Education, and Welfare, DHEW Publication No. (OHDS) 79-30179.

Liepert J, Bauder H, Wolfgang HR, Miltner WH, Taub E, Weiller C (2000) Treatment-induced cortical reorganization after stroke in humans. *Stroke* 31: 1210–1216.

Lynch RG (2005) *Exceptional Returns: Economic, Fiscal and Social Benefits of Investment in Early Childhood Development.* Economic Policy Institute.

Mahoney G, Filer J (1996) How responsive is early intervention to the priorities and needs of families? *Topics in Early Childhood Special Education* 16: 437–457.

Mahoney G, Robinson C, Fewell RR (2001) The effects of early motor intervention on children with Down syndrome or cerebral palsy: a field-based study. *J Dev Behav Pediatr* 22: 153–162.

Martin SL, Ramey CT, Ramey S (1990) The prevention of intellectual impairment in children of impoverished families: findings of a randomized trial of educational day care. *Am J Public Health* 80: 844–847.

McAllister CL, Wilson PC, Green BL, Baldwin JL (2005) 'Come and take a walk': listening to Early Head Start parents on school-readiness as a matter of child, family, and community health. *Am J Public Health* 95: 617–625.

McCormick MC, Brooks-Gunn J, Buka SJ, Goldman J, Yu J, Salganik M, et al. (2006) Early intervention in low birth weight premature infants: results at 18 years of age for the infant health and development program. *Pediatrics* 117: 771–780.

Mendola JD, Conner IP, Roy A, Chan ST, Schwartz TL, Odom JV, et al. (2005) Voxel-based analysis of MRI detects abnormal visual cortex in children and adults with amblyopia. *Hum Brain Mapp* 25: 222–236.

Msall ME (2005) Measuring functional skills in preschool children at risk for neurodevelopmental disabilities. *Ment Retard Dev Disabil Res Rev* 11: 263–273.

Moeller MP (2000) Early intervention and language development in children who are deaf and hard of hearing. *Pediatrics* 106: E43.

Murphy KM, Duffy KR, Jones DG (2004) Experience-dependent changes in NMDAR1 expression in the visual cortex of an animal model for amblyopia. *Vis Neurosci* 21: 653–670.

Nelson HD, Nygren P, Walker M, Panoscha R (2006) Screening for speech and language delay in preschool children: systematic evidence review for the US Preventive Services Task Force. *Pediatrics* 117: e298–319.

Odding E, Roebroeck ME, Stam HJ (2006) The epidemiology of cerebral palsy: incidence, impairments and risk factors. *Disabil Rehabil* 28: 183–191.

Office of Special Education Programs (2005) *D.A.S. Report of infants and toddlers receiving early intervention services in accordance with Part C,* US Department of Education.

Olds D (2006) Progress in improving the development of low birth weight newborns. *Pediatrics* 117: 940–941.

Palfrey JS, Hauser-Cram P, Bronson MB, Warfield ME, Sirin S, Chan E (2005) The Brookline Early Education Project: a 25-year follow-up study of a family-centered early health and development intervention. *Pediatrics* 116: 144–152.

Palmer FB, Shapiro BK, Wachtel RC, Allen MC, Hiller JE, Harrymn SE, et al. (1988) The effects of physical therapy on cerebral palsy: a controlled trial in infants with spastic diplegia. *N Engl J Med* 318: 803–808.

Palmer FB, Shapiro BK, Allen MC, Mosher BS, Bilker SA, Harryman SE, et al. (1990) Infant stimulation curriculum for infants with cerebral palsy: effects on infant temperament, parent–infant interaction, and home environment. *Pediatrics* 85: 411–415.

Parry TS (1992) The effectiveness of early intervention: a critical review. *J Paediatr Child Health* 28: 343–346.

Petterson B, Leonard H, Bourke J, Sanders R, Chalmers R, Jacoby P, et al. (2005) IDEA (Intellectual Disability Exploring Answers): a population-based database for intellectual disability in Western Australia. *Ann Hum Biol* 32: 237–243.

Post RM, Weiss SR (1997) Emergent properties of neural systems: how focal molecular neurobiological alterations can affect behavior. *Dev Psychopathol* 9: 907–929.

Ramey CT, Ramey SL (1994) Which children benefit the most from early intervention? *Pediatrics* 94: 1064–1066.

Ramey SL, Ramey CT (1999) Early experience and early intervention for children 'at risk' for developmental delay and mental retardation. *Ment Retard Dev Disabil Res Rev* 5: 1–10.

Resnick MB, Armstrong S, Carter RL (1988) Developmental intervention program for high-risk premature infants: effects on development and parent–infant interactions. *J Dev Behav Pediatr* 9: 73–78.

Reynolds AJ, Temple JA, Robertson DL, Mann EA (2001) Long-term effects of an early childhood intervention on educational achievement and juvenile arrest: a 15-year follow-up of low-income children in public schools. *JAMA* 285: 2339–2346.

Rice C, Baio J, Van Naarden Braun K, Doernberg N (2007) Prevalence of autism spectrum disorders: autism and developmental disabilities monitoring network, 14 sites, United States, 2002, *MMWR Surveill Summ* 56: 12–28.

Rutter M (2005) Incidence of autism spectrum disorders: changes over time and their meaning. *Acta Paediatr* 94: 2–15.

Schweinhart LJ, Weikart DB (1980) *Young Children Grown Up: The Effects of the Perry Preschool Program on Youths Through Age 15.* Ypsilanti, Michigan: High/Scope Educational Research Foundation.

Schweinhart LJ, Weikart DB (1993) Success by empowerment: The High/Scope Perry Preschool Study through age 27. *Young Child* 49: 54–58.

Schweinhart LJ, et al. (1993) *Significant Benefits: The High/Scope Perry Preschool Study Through Age 27.* Ypsilanti, Michigan: High/Scope Press.

Schweinhart LJ et al. (2005) *Lifetime Effects: The High/Scope Perry Preschool Study Through Age 40.* Ypsilanti, Michigan. High/Scope Educational Research Foundation.

Shonkoff JP, Hauser-Cram P (1987) Early intervention for disabled infants and their families: a quantitative analysis. *Pediatrics* 80: 650–658.

Spiker D, Hopmann MR (1997) The effectiveness of early intervention for children with down syndrome. In: Guralnick ML (ed) *The Effectiveness of Early Intervention.* Baltimore: Paul H. Brookes, pp 271–305.

Taub E, Ramey SL, DeLuca S, Echols K (2004) Efficacy of constraint-induced movement therapy for children withcerebral palsy with asymmetric motor impairment. *Pediatrics* 113: 305–312.

US Department of Health and Human Services (1985) The impact of Head Start on children, families, and communities: Head Start Synthesis Project. Washington, DC: CSR, Inc. 105-81-C-026.

Vallance DD, Im N, Cohen NJ (1999) Discourse deficits associated with psychiatric disorders and with language impairments in children. *J Child Psychol Psychiatry* 40: 693–704.

Weiss AH, Kelly JP (2004) Spatial-frequency-dependent changes in cortical activation before and after patching in amblyopic children. *Invest Ophthalmol Vis Sci* 45: 3531–3537.

Westinghouse Learning Corporation (1969) *The Impact of Head Start: An Evaluation of Head Start on Children's Cognitive and Affective Development.* Executive Summary, Ohio University report to the Office of Economic Opportunity, Washington, DC: Clearinghouse for Federal Scientific and Technical Information (ED 036321).

Wong AM, Burkhalter A, Tychsen L (2005) Suppression of metabolic activity caused by infantile strabismus and strabismic amblyopia in striate visual cortex of macaque monkeys. *J AAPOS* 9: 37–47.

Yoshinaga-Itano C, Sedley AL, Coulter DK, Meh AL (1998) Language of early- and later-identified children with hearing loss. *Pediatrics* 102: 1161–1171.

22

SERVICE UTILIZATION AND HEALTH PROMOTION OF CHILDREN WITH NEURODEVELOPMENTAL DISABILITIES

Barbara Mazer and Annette Majnemer

QUALITY OF HEALTH SERVICES

According to the Academy for Health Services Research and Policy, health services research refers to the scientific investigation of the relationship between social factors, financial systems, organizational structures and processes, health technologies and personal behaviors with access to health care services, the quality and cost of care, and ultimately with health and well-being. The provision of health care services can be studied at various levels, ranging from individuals, families, organizations and institutions, to whole communities and specific populations (Freburger and Konrad 2002).

Quality of care is defined as the degree to which the health services that are provided:

1 Increase the likelihood of the desired health outcomes
2 Are consistent with current professional knowledge (Hammermeister et al. 1995, Seid et al. 2000)
3 Conform to the best available scientific information and generally accepted clinical principles and practices (Eldar 2000)

Ensuring quality of care is increasingly becoming an important aspect of the planning of services. In fact, professional and institutional accrediting bodies focus much attention on ensuring that the services individuals receive maintain a high level of quality (Wilkerson 2000).

Evaluating the quality of the care provided within a health care environment requires both direct and indirect evidence that the best strategy was selected and skillfully implemented (Donabedian 1992). Optimal care refers to the opportunity to obtain the required care, whether the care is appropriate and well provided, if it is delivered humanely and is consistent with patient preferences, and that the best possible outcomes are achieved (Seid et al. 2000). Quality of care can be judged according to how well the care provided conforms to a set of standards or expectations. These standards may relate to scientific evidence, personal values of the patients and their families, or society's social values (Donabedian 1990). Donabedian (1988) proposed a model that describes three types of evidence to evaluate the quality of care. This basic model is a simplification of the complex reality of health service delivery. In fact, it is difficult to clearly distinguish these three categories, as there are overlapping relationships between them. The different components of evidence that can be used to evaluate quality of care are outlined below.

1 *Structure:* includes the physical and organizational properties of the settings in which care is provided. It includes the physical facilities and equipment available, organizational properties, clinician:patient ratio, manpower available, credentials, qualifications and experience of the health care professionals offering services, as well as the type, frequency, and intensity of the programs offered (Hammermeister et al. 1995, Eldar 2000). Structure ultimately reflects the potential capacity of a service to provide adequate quality.

2 *Process:* comprises the activities of the treating professionals in the management of their patients. In the treatment of children with disabilities, providing services appropriate to an individual's level of impairment and disability may serve as criteria for quality of care. The process of care also encompasses the appropriate selection and inclusion of patients and the procedures instituted during admission, intake, assessment, and follow-up. Information for evaluating process may be abstracted from medical records. For parents of children receiving rehabilitation services, process elements, such as the provision of respectful and supportive care and co-ordination of care, were associated with overall satisfaction with services provided (King et al. 2001).

3 *Outcome:* relates to the results of care, specifically to the changes in health status (recovery, morbidity, mortality) that occur following intervention. Relevant outcomes for children with neurodevelopmental disabilities include level of function, school or work involvement, physical, emotional and social skills, as well as participation in leisure activities (Eldar 2000). The importance of outcome in evaluating the quality of care provided is dependent upon the strength of the causal relationship between process variables and outcome as well as between structure and outcome. Another important consideration is that these relationships may be modified by factors other than health care (Donabedian 1992), such as individual patient characteristics, clinical status, level of function, delay to rehabilitation, motivation, appropriateness of admission, and specific barriers to recovery (Eldar 2000). In fact, a particular outcome may be poor, but the care provided may have been the care most likely to do the most good.

A review examining the association between the process variables and outcome of care reported inconsistent results. Specifically, linkages between process and outcome have been positive when evaluating at the patient level, but not when

TABLE 22.1
Attributes of quality of care

Attribute	Description
Efficacy	What services achieve under the most favorable circumstances
Effectiveness	What services achieve under ordinary situations
Efficiency	Cost at which a given improvement is attained
Optimality	Balance of cost with the effect on health care
Acceptability	Modification of care to conform to the wishes, expectations, and values of patients and their families
Legitimacy	Acceptability to the ethical principles, values, norms, laws of the community and society at large
Equity	Fair distribution of health care among the members of a population

assessing at the overall hospital, community, or population level. Outcomes can be inefficient measures of quality because of the duration of time that often lapses between the provision of care and the ascertainment of outcome, and because of the difficulty in adequately adjusting for severity of illness, co-morbid conditions, and other patient risk factors (Hammermeister et al. 1995). Outcome reflects the contribution of all those involved in providing care and is intrinsic to the definition of quality of care, but it is not a direct measure of quality itself. In general, when evaluating care, it is often unclear what processes and structures would need to be changed in order to improve outcomes (Hammermeister et al. 1995). According to some (Donabedian 1990, 1993, Schiff and Rucker 2001), there are seven attributes that are necessary to judge overall quality of care. These are presented in Table 22.1.

Evaluating quality of care requires an examination of service provision from many different perspectives, ranging from the organizational properties of the health system to the direct services offered at the level of the individual patient. While the relationships between these various levels are not well understood and may in fact not be robust, each aspect of service provision is important to consider in order to direct efforts at improving deficits in each of the elements.

SERVICES FOR CHILDREN WITH DEVELOPMENTAL DISABILITIES

While there has been much discussion of the quality of health care services in general, the assessment of pediatric services requires attention to specific factors associated with pediatric care. Children are in continual transition, developing in many domains, and dependent on others for care and decision-making. In addition, children with special needs (i.e. those with neurodevelopmental disabilities) often receive care at multiple sites, including the health care system, the educational system, social services, as well as in the community and at home, resulting in potential co-ordination difficulties and challenges (American Academy of Pediatrics 1999, Seid et al. 2000). Services must address the many changing and interrelated needs of children and their families, as well as community members such as teachers (King et al. 2002). Collaboration is required to provide effective co-ordination of care and, ultimately, to optimize outcomes for children with special health care needs (American Academy of Pediatrics 1999). Children with disabilities have common requirements, including co-ordination of services, family support, technical assistance, communication between providers, and access to a team where care is co-ordinated and monitored on an ongoing basis (Kaplan 1999).

The Medical Expenditure Panel Survey in the United States recently examined the use of health care services and expenditure patterns by families of children with disabilities. These children had more than twice the number of physician visits and five times the number of non-physician professional visits compared to children without disabilities, indicating the great need for a wide range of health and rehabilitation services. Expenditures also were greatly increased. Children with disabilities (i.e. 7.3% of the population) accounted for 22.7% of total health care expenditures. The burden of out-of-pocket expenses was highly skewed, favoring a small subgroup of children with disabilities, indicating that the financial burden of childhood disability in the United States is unevenly distributed (Newacheck et al. 2004).

Rehabilitation services are an important long term component of the services provided to children with neurodevelopmental disabilities. An interdisciplinary collaborative team approach is used, with children and their families as active participants. The Life Needs Model of Service Delivery (King et al. 2002) suggests that services must place importance on four areas of child and family functioning:

1 Long-term outcomes such as social and community participation and quality of life
2 Spheres of life including personal, interpersonal, and external interactions
3 Commonly identified needs including the development of foundational skills and applied skill sets (i.e. life skills), providing support and information
4 Transitions and age-specific groups such as birth, infancy entry into elementary school, entrance to secondary school, and the beginning of adulthood

Quality should also include an evaluation of the effectiveness of teamwork, the extent to which children and families have been given the competence to participate in the care of their child, and the continuity of care (Eldar 2000). Table 22.2 describes the specific criteria that may be used to judge the quality of rehabilitation services (Larner 1997).

The focus of pediatric rehabilitation has been evolving from the assessment and treatment of conditions at the biomedical or organ (i.e. impairment) level, to a broader, more holistic approach, with greater emphasis on improving children's

TABLE 22.2
Criteria to judge quality of rehabilitation services

Criteria	Description
Competence	Meeting the clearly stated objectives, including the routine review of individual patients, monitoring of progress and performance, and the measurement of client satisfaction
Respect	Adapting clinical protocols to meet the psychologic and spiritual needs of individual children and their families
Choice	Making decisions regarding the planning of rehabilitation together with children and their families
Accessibility	Ensuring the physical access to and eligibility for services
Responsiveness	Adapting services offered through review of needs and resources

functional abilities as well as their overall participation in the community (King et al. 2002). Health and social service providers are increasingly interested in enhancing individual satisfaction, providing family-centered services, and recognizing strengths (i.e. an ecologic perspective) rather than problems (i.e. an individualistic perspective) of the child and family (King et al. 2002). The child's health and well-being and the involvement of the family are of increasingly greater interest. When evaluating quality of care and the association between process and outcome, it is important to consider whether specific treatment effects are carried over into everyday life skills and roles (Helders et al. 2003). Also, an individual and/or family-centered approach is favored, involving a partnership between family members and the interdisciplinary team of professionals in the planning of intervention (Allen et al. 1997). This collaborative approach ensures that families are included in decision-making regarding program planning, service delivery and the evaluation of the outcome of therapy (Allen et al. 1997, Rosenbaum et al. 1998). This approach is essential in achieving meaningful functional goals (Hanna and Rodger 2002). While the important factors associated with the provision of high quality services have been well defined, there are many families who report that they are not receiving the full range of services that their child requires.

BARRIERS TO RECEIVING SERVICES
WAITING TIMES
Time delays before receiving rehabilitation services may be influenced by organizational and consumer-specific factors. A study investigating the waiting times experienced by families referred for pediatric rehabilitation services in Montreal, Canada, found that of those referred for services, more than 50% had not received occupational therapy services and 36% had not started physical therapy 6 months after initial referral. Younger children received physical therapy services earlier, while

English-speaking families were more likely to receive occupational therapy services than French-speaking families. Interestingly, those families with shorter waiting times reported feeling more empowered in the care of their children when compared with families who had longer waiting times (Feldman et al. 2002). Parents of children newly diagnosed with developmental delay were surveyed regarding the rehabilitation services received within 6 months of diagnosis (Majnemer et al. 2002). Of the 129 participants, 23% reported receiving no services, 30% one service, and 47% two or more services. The majority of those receiving services were not yet being treated in a rehabilitation center, but were most likely to be followed in an acute care hospital (occupational therapy, 73%; physical therapy, 80%; speech therapy, 52%) or in private clinics.

In summary, while many children require and are referred for rehabilitation services, long waiting times and lack of resources in rehabilitation centers and in the community have led to the over-utilization of services in acute care institutions and to many young children not receiving needed services many months after diagnosis. Thus, the potential promise and benefits of early intervention may not be completely realized.

UNMET NEEDS FOR SERVICES

Families of children with disabilities require a range of services from a number of different professional disciplines and often experience difficulties receiving relevant and necessary care. A survey of parents of young children with severe physical impairments found that only 55% had a professional who helped them access and co-ordinate the input they received from different services (Sloper and Turner 1992). They reported an average of six unmet needs; the most important was related to receiving information.

Findings from the Participation and Activity Limitation Survey in Canada determined that 15.5% of all families with children with disabilities report an unmet health care need, primarily the absence of speech therapy and other health care services. Over 50% of unmet needs were a result of long waiting lists. Other reasons included lack of insurance coverage, cost, and the service not being available locally (Allen et al. 1997). Over 15% of American children with a limitation in activity brought about by a chronic illness experience one or more unmet health care needs, compared to an overall rate of 7% for all children surveyed in the National Health Interview Survey (Newacheck et al. 2000). Older children, those who are poor and uninsured, without a usual source of health care, living in the south or west of the United States, or living in a non-metropolitan area were the factors associated with an increased likelihood of having an unmet health care need. The Disability Supplement to the US National Health Interview Survey also reported disparities in the use of therapeutic and supportive services among school-age children (Benedict 2006). This study found that a higher level of household education, greater family income, having public insurance, and living in a family with more than four family members were associated with an increased rate in the child's use of therapeutic services provided in either rehabilitation or community settings. These factors were not predictive of services obtained within the school setting.

The impact of having unmet medical needs has been explored with different childhood disability groups. Parents of children with developmental delay, evaluated by a multidisciplinary team, were contacted 4 months after referral to determine which services were being received. Parents were successful in obtaining only 39% of social services, 71% of medical services, and 71% of educational and rehabilitation services. A proportion of families did not pursue the recommended service, with financial reasons being the primary barrier to receiving services (Roizen et al. 1996). Families of children who sustained a head injury also report unmet medical, rehabilitation, and social service needs, specifically for mental health intervention and counseling, information and referral, cognitive therapy, and respite services. In fact, those with the least severe injuries had the highest number of perceived unmet needs (Greenspan and Mackenzie 2000). Families with the highest number of unmet needs were likely to have experienced a high degree of strain from life events and to have children with mental retardation and physical impairments, and fathers were more likely to be unemployed (Sloper and Turner 1992). A sample of 81 parents of children with motor or multiple disabilities in the Netherlands also stated a need for more information from health professionals, and this unmet need was associated with an increase in familial feelings of social isolation (Hendriks et al. 2000).

Parents and health care providers may differ in their perception of the care provided to children with disabling conditions. Parents (n = 753) of adolescents with disabilities and health care providers (n = 141) completed questionnaires assessing the providers' level of involvement in the planning of the transition between childhood and adulthood. Health care providers rated themselves significantly higher than the parents did in their level of responsibility in assisting with the transition activities. Parents suggested that the service providers can be more helpful to families during these years by providing comprehensive co-ordinated care with a central person co-ordinating the health care plan and communicating with other involved professionals and agencies (Geenen et al. 2003). These findings underscore the importance for providers of services to understand the specific needs of those they are servicing and to develop strategies to address their concerns and resource requirements and enhance information transfer.

SATISFACTION WITH SERVICES
Individual (child and family) satisfaction with services is a consequence of the whole experience of care. It refers to the overall reaction to the structure, process,

and outcome of health care, with the interpersonal process being the most important aspect (Donabedian 1988). Patient satisfaction was operationally defined by
an interdisciplinary rehabilitation services committee to include access to care, the
physical environment, the human aspect of care, clinical features of the services,
and outcome (Davis and Hobbs 1989).

Several studies have focused on the relationship between practitioners and families of children with special health care needs and its association with satisfaction
with services. Overall, parent satisfaction is strongly associated with the personal
aspects of care, particularly communication between parent and providers (Keith
1998). A large cross-sectional survey of families in Ontario, Canada, evaluated
the factors related to parents' perception of family-centered service delivery and
satisfaction with services (Law et al. 2003). Results suggested that the factors
associated with greater parent satisfaction with services included the family-
centered service culture at the center or organization and having fewer locations
where different services were obtained. For mothers of young children receiving
services, there was an inverse relationship between their perception of family-
centered behaviors and parenting stress (O'Neil et al. 2001). In a study designed
to determine whether interventions based on the Family-Centered Functional
Therapy model improve task performance, three tasks were selected by parents
as being the most important goals for their child. Results indicated improved
performance in tasks for which intervention was provided as well as improved
parent satisfaction with their children's performance in those tasks (Lammi and
Law 2003). In fact, a review of patient satisfaction research found that higher
satisfaction was associated with patient compliance and improved outcomes, and
that reported levels of satisfaction were particularly high overall for rehabilitation
(Keith 1998).

King et al. (2001) explored the elements of service delivery that underlie
parents' satisfaction with pediatric rehabilitation services for their children. Parents
of 645 children with special needs treated in Ontario pediatric rehabilitation centers completed the Measure of Processes of Care Questionnaire (MPOC-56) and
the Client Satisfaction Questionnaire (CSQ). The 130 parents who were highly
satisfied were compared with the 101 relatively dissatisfied parents on 16 elements
of satisfaction and 16 elements of dissatisfaction. While the groups did not differ
on comments about the process of care, the relatively dissatisfied parents commented
more frequently about elements related to structure of care than did the satisfied
parents. Structural elements of service (e.g. access to services) are thus important
determinants of dissatisfaction. Interestingly, parents made few remarks about the
outcome of care for their child or family.

Families of adolescents (n = 49) and young adults (n = 39) with cerebral palsy
were questioned regarding their satisfaction with the services they had experienced
in the areas of health, education, recreation, employment, housing, and transportation

(Darrah et al. 2002). Factors contributing to dissatisfaction relate to the bureau-cratic structure of the systems as well as the attitudes of service providers. Specific-ally, four themes were identified:

1 Caring and supportive service providers positively influence the care experience
2 Fatigue from constantly having to 'work the system' and demand the provision of services leads to frustration
3 Poor parent–professional communication experiences, such as the use of sophis-ticated terminology or ignoring adolescents during conversations, relate to dissatisfaction with services
4 A lack of understanding of the needs and abilities of their child, including the discomfort associated with perceived and encountered societal attitudes

PARTICIPATION AND HEALTH PROMOTION FOR CHILDREN WITH DEVELOPMENTAL DISABILITIES
PARTICIPATION
Participation is of increasing importance for those providing health care and rehabilitation services (Law 2002). The World Health Organization's International Classification of Functioning, Disability and Health (WHO ICF) defines participa-tion as a person's involvement in life situations and includes, for example, areas of personal maintenance, mobility, social relationships, communication, education, leisure, spirituality, and domestic and community life (World Health Organization 2001, Majnemer and Limperopoulos 2002). For children, participation is the con-text in which they learn and develop skills, perform tasks and activities, develop friendships, and achieve personal satisfaction, and is therefore crucial for physical and psychologic health and well-being (Law 2002). Clinicians providing services to children must help select opportunities for participation that are congruent with each child's needs and desires for involvement. Intervention should focus on supporting children's mastery of tasks that are meaningful to them in order to encour-age successful participation (Goldstein et al. 2004). It has become clear that t' 's approach to treatment is preferable and more beneficial to the child than the direct treatment of organ-based impairments, as the assumed automatic carry-over of the effects of the treatment of impairments (e.g. increasing attention span, improving co-ordination) to actual improvement in functional tasks and enhanced participa-tion has not yet been demonstrated (Helders et al. 2003).

Children with disabilities are at increased risk for lower levels of participation (King et al. 2003) and the frequency and diversity of participation in community activities decreases throughout childhood (Brown and Gordon 1987). Several studies have examined the type and amount of participation experienced by chil-dren with disabilities as well as the factors that are associated with diminished participation. The daily activities of children and youth with (n = 239) and without (n = 519) disabilities were compared using personal diaries to ascertain activity patterns. Those with disabilities reported a reduction in the variety of their activities and were more likely to engage in activities requiring a slower pace. They spent more time in dependent activities, quiet recreation, and in personal care, and less time in social engagement and active recreation, household tasks, and activities away from home. While there was no association between daily activities and sex, race, number of children in the family, income, parent education, number of parents in the home, mother's work status, and access to a vehicle, only age was directly associated with activity patterns. With increasing age, the non-disabled children became more engaged in educational activities, whereas the children with disabilities spent more time watching television (Brown and Gordon 1987). Children with physical disabilities participated in more informal activities rather than formal activities and report participating in a mean of 12 recreational, 10 active, 9 social, 9 skill-based, and 10 self-improvement activities, as measured by the Children's Assessment of Participation and Enjoyment (CAPE) (Law et al. 2006a). Females were more likely to participate in social and skill-based activities, while males participated in more active physical activities. In another study, children with learning disabilities were also found to be less involved in academic activities. They spent more time participating in solitary activities at home compared to a control group of similar aged children, and their parents played a more important role in their free time. However, this group of young adolescents, with and without learning disabilities, did not differ in the amount of time spent watching television, reading books, playing games, spending time with friends, and participating in sport activities and hobbies (Margalit 1984).

The factors associated with participation in activities are complex and multi-factorial. It is important for clinicians and policy-makers to have a clear understanding of the factors that influence participation in order to design appropriate and effective programs to enable children to explore their full functional potential (Law et al. 2004). A conceptual model was developed identifying the environmental, family, and child factors thought to influence participation in recreation and leisure activities for children with physical disabilites. The primary environmental factors associated with participation include supportive physical and institutional environments, presence of supportive relationships for the child and for the parents. Family factors thought to enhance children's participation include the absence of a financial or time constraint on the family, supportive demographic factors such as parent education, employment, and income, a supportive home environment, and the preference to engage in recreation together as a family. Child factors include self-perception of athletic and scholastic competence, abilities in the areas of physical, cognitive, communication, emotional, behavioral, and social functioning, and the child's preferences for activity (King et al. 2003).

Law et al. (2004) recruited 427 children with neurologic and musculoskeletal disorders, 6 years of age and older, to determine whether participation differed with diagnosis. Children were assessed using the CAPE to determine their level of participation in a variety of activities. While the specific diagnostic group to which a child belonged was not a significant factor affecting participation scores, age, sex, and level of physical function as well as family participation in social and recreational activities, family values related to intellectual and cultural activities and the child's preferences for activity (Law et al. 2006b) were associated with participation in recreational and social activities. It is therefore important that when planning and implementing programs for children with special needs, the focus is not on specific diagnoses (Law et al. 2004). Also, the variety of activities was lower for families with low incomes, a single-parent structure, and low educational level (Law et al. 2006a). Other personal and environmental factors, such as skill or functional ability, age, sex, and activity preferences, are better determinants of the actual level of involvement in activity. Functional performance in everyday skills are more predictive of a child's ability to fully participate in school activities than level of impairment (Mancini et al. 2000).

Physical Activity

This is known to be an important aspect of participation, having both physical and psychosocial health benefits. A theoretical model describing how physical activity programs can be implemented to effect psychologic change explains the relationship among the components of a physical activity program, self-concept (i.e. perceived physical competence, social acceptance, general self-worth), and the performance of adaptive behaviors in individuals with disabilities. The model highlights the importance of competition and sport for individuals with neurodevelopmental disabilities (Weiss et al. 2003). In-depth interviews were used to examine the perceptions of 11 girls, 10–16 years of age, with physical disabilities regarding physical recreation pursuits. Results generated three general themes:

1 The personal meaning of physical activity, such as freedom, equalization with non-disabled peers, and opportunities for recreation
2 Ownership of disability, including perceptions of normalcy and body image
3 Access to role models (Bedini and Anderson 2005)

The results of a consensus conference aimed at identifying research priorities for physical activity and health among people with disabilities indicated that a greater emphasis must be placed on determining the risks and benefits of physical exercise (Cooper et al. 1999). Participation in physical activity, particularly for children with disabilities, can provide both physical and psychologic benefits.

HEALTH PROMOTION

There is an increasing focus on the promotion of health and healthy behaviors in children and adolescents by health care professionals, policy-makers, and educators. It is therefore equally critical that clinicians servicing children with special needs address these issues with the patients and their families. However, there is little evidence in the literature to help guide clinicians regarding selecting the most appropriate and effective approaches to promote healthy behaviors in children with disabling conditions.

Health promotion, health maintenance measures, and prevention strategies are not only necessary, but critical to the successful rehabilitation and integration of individuals with disabilities. The Healthy People 2010 initiative in the United States emphasizes improving the health of children and adults with disabilities. This represents a clear shift in focus from treating impairments and particular deficits to maintaining overall wellness and health, removing barriers, and restoring function and integration through accommodation of specific needs (Ayyangar 2002). Children's health may be affected by their disability and clinicians should pay particular attention to possible associated conditions. Health promotion is often a neglected area of practice. Health promotion issues should be discussed, including growth and development, immunizations, sleep patterns, continence, safety and injury prevention, and fitness. In addition, there is also a need to implement measures to prevent secondary health complications, such as contractures, spinal problems, fractures, and pressure ulcers. Other external factors potentially negatively affecting healthy behaviors include access to technology, psychosocial development and support, and environmental access and integration opportunities (Ayyangar 2002).

Maintaining and improving the physical fitness of children and adolescents with a disability or chronic disease will help ensure that they reach adulthood with an optimal level of physical function (Helders et al. 2003). A review of studies examining the level of physical fitness in persons with cerebral palsy suggested that these individuals must maintain higher levels of physical fitness than the general population in order to offset the expected decline in function that occurs with the natural aging process. These studies found that strength training helped improve the ability to complete more physically demanding tasks and maintain higher levels of physical independence (Rimmer 2001). Physical therapists are increasingly including exercise programs as part of their interventions for children with cerebral palsy. A review of research related to aquatic exercise reported that the buoyancy of water may provide children with movement disorders the opportunity to exercise with more freedom than on land. Also, aquatic exercise offers reduced levels of joint loading and less impact on unstable joints leading to less orthopedic difficulties (Kelly and Darrah 2005).

When examining the psychosocial aspects of adolescents with physical disabilities, a number of critical risk factors to which health promotion efforts should be directed were identified. These include lower levels of peer integration, dependence on adult relationships, low educational aspirations, and a poor knowledge of sexuality (Stevens et al. 1996). The recommendations for physical activity for the general population do not take into account the specific needs of those with mobility problems and may not be appropriate. Also, the available fitness equipment should be carefully examined to determine whether it is indeed accessible and safe with respect to each child's functional mobility, secondary conditions, and specific limb involvement. Fitness instructors in schools and in private gyms are not necessarily aware of the approaches required to adapt fitness programs for this population (Rimmer 2001) and it is imperative that trained health care professionals have input into fitness programs provided to children with physically disabling conditions.

CONCLUSIONS AND FUTURE DIRECTIONS
The evaluation of the quality of health services provided to children with developmental disabilities is complex and includes attention to many different levels of service delivery. Often, these children and their families must access and receive specialized interventions at a variety of locations and from many different service professionals. The literature indicates that many have difficulty receiving the full range of services they need. The factors associated with these problems can assist clinicians and policy-makers in improving access and quality of services. With the increased awareness of the importance of participation in leisure and recreational activities and the promotion of healthy behaviors, attention must now be paid to the specific resource needs of children with disabling conditions and the environmental factors that limit community integration and participation.

Further research to help guide and inform health policy and to enhance service delivery for children with developmental disabilities should focus on the processes that can improve access and co-ordination of services, with the ultimate goal of optimizing the health and well-being of these children and their families. Furthermore, health promotion strategies need to be developed in children and youth with disabilities, in order to develop autonomy, social participation, and life satisfaction.

REFERENCES
Allen KD, Wilczynski SM, Evans JE (1997) Pediatric rehabilitation: defining a field, a focus, and a future. *Int J Rehabil Health* 3: 25–40.
American Academy of Pediatrics (1999) Care coordination: integrating health and related systems of care for children with special health care needs (RE9902). *Pediatrics* 104: 978–981.
Ayyangar R (2002) Health maintenance and management in childhood disability. *Rehabil Clin North Am* 13: 793–821.
Bedini LA, Anderson DM (2005) I'm nice, I'm smart, I like karate: girls with physical disabilities' perceptions of physical recreation. *Ther Recreation J* 39: 114–130.
Benedict RE (2006) Disparities in use of and unmet need for therapeutic and supportive services among school-age children with functional limitations: a comparison across settings. *Health Serv Res* 41: 103–124.

Brown M, Gordon WA (1987) Impact of impairment on activity patterns of children. *Arch Phys Med Rehabil* 68: 828–832.

Cooper RA, Quatrano LA, Axelson PW, Harlan W, Stineman M, Franklin B, et al. (1999) Research on physical activity and health among people with disabilities: a consensus statement. *J Rehabil Res Dev* 36: 142–154.

Darrah J, Magil-Evans J, Adkins R (2002) How well are we doing? Families of adolescents or young adults with cerebral palsy share their perceptions of service delivery. *Disabil Rehabil* 24: 542–549.

Davis D, Hobbs G (1989) Measuring outpatient satisfaction with rehabilitation services. *Qual Rev Bull* June: 192–197.

Donabedian A (1988) The quality of care: how can it be assessed? *JAMA* 260: 1743–1748.

Donabedian A (1990) The seven pillars of quality. *Arch Path Lab Med* 114: 1115–1118.

Donabedian A (1992) The role of outcomes in quality assessment and assurance. *Qual Rev Bull* 1: 247–251.

Donabedian A (1993) Quality in health care: whose responsibility is it? *Am J Med Qual* 8: 32–36.

Eldar R (2000) A conceptual proposal for the study of the quality of rehabilitation care. *Disabil Rehabil* 22: 163–169.

Feldman DE, Champagne F, Korner-Bitensky N, Meshefedjian G (2002) Waiting time for rehabilitation services for children with physical disabilities. *Child Care Health Dev* 28: 351–358.

Freburger JK, Konrad TR (2002) The use of federal and state databases to conduct health services research related to physical and occupational therapy. *Arch Phys Med Rehabil* 83: 837–845.

Geenen SJ, Powers LE, Sells W (2003) Understanding the role of health care providers during the transition of adolescents with disabilities and special health care needs. *J Adolesc Health* 32: 225–233.

Goldstein DN, Cohn E, Coster W (2004) Enhancing participation for children with disabilities: application of the ICF enablement framework to pediatric physical therapist practice. *Pediatr Phys Ther* 16: 114–120.

Greenspan AI, Mackenzie EJ (2000) Use and need for post-acute services following paediatric head injury. *Brain Inj* 4: 417–429.

Hammermeister KE, Shroyer AL, ASethi GK, Grover FL (1995) Why it is important to demonstrate linkages between outcomes of care and processes and structures of care. *Med Care* 33: OS5–OS16.

Hanna K, Rodger S (2002) Towards family-centred practice in paediatric occupational therapy: a review of the literature on parent–therapist collaboration. *Aust Occup Ther J* 49: 14–24.

Helders PJ, Engelbert RH, Custers JW, Gorter JW, Takken T, van der Net J (2003) Creating and being created: the changing panorama of pediatric rehabilitation. *Pediatr Rehabil* 6: 5–12.

Hendriks AHC, De Moor JMH, Oud JHL, Franken WM (2000) Service needs of parents with motor or multiply disabled children in Dutch therapeutic toddler classes. *Clin Rehabil* 14: 506–517.

Kaplan LC (1999) Community-based disability services in the USA: a paediatric perspective. *Lancet* 354: 761–762.

Keith RA (1998) Patient satisfaction and rehabilitation services. *Arch Phys Med Rehabil* 79: 1122–1128.

Kelly M, Darrah J (2005) Aquatic exercise for children with cerebral palsy. *Dev Med Child Neurol* 47: 838–842.

King G, Cathers T, King S, Rosenbaum P (2001) Major elements of parents' satisfaction and dissatisfaction with pediatric rehabilitation services. *Child Health Care* 30: 111–134.

King G, Tucker MA, Baldwin P, Lowry K, LaPorta J, Martens L (2002) A life needs model of pediatric service delivery: services to support community participation and quality of life for children and youth with disabilities. *Phys Occup Ther Pediatr* 22: 53–77.

King G, Law M, King S, Rosenbaum P, Kertoy MK, Young NL (2003) A conceptual model of the factors affecting the recreation and leisure participation of children with disabilities. *Phys Occup Ther Pediatr* 23: 63–90.

Lammi BM, Law M (2003) The effects of family-centered functional therapy on the occupational performance of children with cerebral palsy. *Can J Occup Ther* 70: 285–297.

Larner S (1997) Quality rehabilitation: oasis or mirage? *Int J Health Care Qual* 10: 192–196.

Law M (2002) Enhancing participation. *Phys Occup Ther Pediatr* 22: 1–3.

Law M, Hanna S, King G, Hurley P, King S, Kertoy M, et al. (2003) Factors affecting family-centered service delivery for children with disabilities. *Child Care Health Dev* 29: 357–366.

Law M, Finkelman S, Hurley P, Rosenbaum P, King S, King G, et al. (2004) Participation of children with physical disabilities: relationships with diagnosis, physical function, and demographic variables. *Scand J Occup Ther* 11: 156–162.

Law M, King G, King S, Kertoy M, Hurley P, Rosenbaum P, et al. (2006a) Patterns of participation in recreational and leisure activities among children with complex physical disabilities. *Dev Med Child Neurol* 48: 337–342.

Law M, King G, King S, Kertoy M, Hurley P, Rosenbaum P, et al. (2006b) *Patterns and predictors of recreational and leisure participation for children with physical disabilities.* CanChild Centre for Childhood Disability Research.

Majnemer A, Limperopoulos C (2002) Importance of outcome determination in pediatric rehabilitation. *Dev Med Child Neurol* 44: 773–777.

Majnemer A, Shevell MI, Rosenbaum P, Abrahamowicz M (2002) Early rehabilitation service utilization patterns in young children with developmental delays. *Child Care Health Dev* 28: 29–37.

Mancini MC, Coster WJ, Trombly CA, Herren TC (2000) Predicting elementary school participation in children with disabilities. *Arch Phys Med Rehabil* 81: 339–347.

Margalit M (1984) Leisure activities of learning disabled children as a reflection of their passive life style and prolonged dependency. *Child Psychiatry Hum Dev* 15: 133–141.

Newacheck PW, Hughes DC, Hung Y, Wong S, Stoddard JJ (2000) The unmet health needs of America's children. *Pediatrics* 105: 989–997.

Newacheck PW, Inkelas M, Kim SE (2004) Health services use and health care expenditures for children with disabilities. *Pediatrics* 114: 79–85.

O'Neil ME, Palisano RJ, Westcott SL (2001) Relationship of therapists' attitudes, children's motor ability, and parenting stress to mothers' perceptions of therapists' behaviors during early intervention. *Phys Ther* 81: 1412–1424.

Rimmer JH (2001) Physical fitness levels of persons with cerebral palsy. *Dev Med Child Neurol* 43: 208–212.

Roizen NJ, Shalowitz MU, Komie KA, Martinez S, Miller LA, Davis S (1996) Acquisition of services recommended by a multidisciplinary medical diagnostic team for children under three years of age evaluated for developmental delays. *Dev Behav Pediatr* 17: 399–404.

Rosenbaum P, King S, Law M, King G, Evans J (1998) Family-centered services: a conceptual framework and research review. *Phys Occup Ther Pediatr* 18: 1–20.

Schiff GD, Rucker TD (2001) Beyond structure-process-outcome: Donabedian's seven pillars and eleven buttresses of quality. *Jt Comm J Qual Improve* 27: 169–174.

Seid M, Varni JW, Kurtin PS (2000) Measuring quality of care for vulnerable children: challenges and conceptualization of a pediatric outcome measure of quality. *Am J Med Qual* 15: 182–188.

Sloper P, Turner S (1992) Service needs of families of children with severe physical disability. *Child Care Health Dev* 18: 259–282.

Stevens SE, Steele CA, Jutai JW, Kalnins IV, Bortolussi JA, Biggar WD (1996) Adolescents with physical disabilities: some psychosocial aspects of health. *J Adolesc Health* 19: 157–164.

Weiss J, Diamond T, Demark J, Lovald B (2003) Involvement in Special Olympics and its relations to self-concept and actual competency in participants with developmental disabilities. *Res Dev Disabil* 24: 281–305.

Wilkerson DL (2000) Rehabilitation outcomes and accreditation. *J Rehabil Outcome Meas* 4: 42–48.

World Health Organization (2001) *International Classification of Functioning, Disability and Health (ICF)*. Geneva: World Health Organization.

23

CO-MORBID CONDITIONS IN NEURODEVELOPMENTAL DISABILITIES

Elysa J Marco

Developmental delay has a myriad of etiologies and consequently a variety and intensity of possible symptoms. Furthermore, the medical and behavioral difficulties that arise, either as a result, or in tandem with, the primary disorder, may often be far more disabling to the child and family than the primary cognitive, language, social, or motor disabilities. These co-morbidities of neurodevelopmental disabilities have tremendous impact on the overall well-being of the individual, family, and at times the broader social community. This impact has been magnified in the past decade as the prevalence of childhood disability and associated life expectancies have both increased dramatically. Familiarity with the behavioral and medical co-morbidities of developmental delay is crucial to comprehensive care as early identification of these co-morbidities and treatment can significantly improve an individual's quality of life and their ability to function harmoniously and participate more extensively in their surroundings.

In this chapter, the first section looks at symptoms or disorders that are broadly classified as psychiatric and behavioral, including challenging behavior, depression, anxiety, and psychosis. In clinical practice, it is clear that many behavioral disturbances will span traditional psychiatric syndromes making a parsimonious *Diagnostic and Statistical Manual of Mental Disorders, Fourth Edition Revised* (DSM-IVR) precise diagnosis difficult and treatment planning confusing. This challenge is further complicated by communication barriers and atypical features frequently found in this particular clinical population. The pragmatic clinical approach to these disorders is generally symptom-based or one-dimensional rather than categorical or syndromal, targeting the aggressive behavior rather than a conduct disorder. For more in-depth coverage of this topic, the interested reader is referred to Bouras (1999). The second section of this chapter addresses frequently encountered medical conditions such as epilepsy, sleep disorders, orthopedic disorders, and gastrointestinal compromise.

BEHAVIORAL AND PSYCHIATRIC DISORDERS
CHALLENGING BEHAVIOR
Challenging behavior is the most frequent reason for psychiatric referral and residential placement of individuals with developmental delay (Day 1985). While specific behaviors such as self-injury have become almost synonymous with specific rare

genetic and metabolic disorders such as Lesch–Nyhan, Rett, and Cornelia de Lange syndromes, these behaviors are also commonly seen in individuals with developmental disabilities with more frequent etiologies, including fragile X, traumatic brain injury, and severe hypoxic ischemic injury. Challenging behaviors are clearly multifactorial and consequently a multidisciplinary approach to their evaluation and effective treatment is crucial.

Definition

Emerson and Bromley (1995) defined challenging behavior as culturally abnormal behavior of such an intensity, frequency, or duration that the physical safety of the person or others in close proximity is likely to be placed in serious jeopardy, or behavior which is likely to seriously limit use of, or result in, the person being denied access to ordinary community facilities. Specifically, the behaviors often encountered are self-injurious, aggressive, destructive, impulsive, tantrum-like, verbally or physically abusive, and sexually explicit or inappropriate. The DSM-IVR conditions that are most closely aligned with these behaviors are conduct disorder and antisocial personality disorder; however, they can also be key aspects of obsessive-compulsive disorder, attention-deficit–hyperactivity disorder, autism spectrum disorders, or bipolar disorder.

Clinical features

While the clinical features of challenging behavior will vary with etiology and age, some attempts have been made to detail the incidence of particular types of challenging behaviors. Challenging behaviors are reported to reach a peak during adolescence and early adulthood, tapering off after 35 years of age (Day 1985, Oliver et al. 1987, Borthwick-Duffy 1994). Males tend to exhibit more aggressive behaviors, while females tend to show more self-injurious behaviors. Furthermore, the intensity of challenging behaviors appears to be inversely correlated with IQ (Borthwick-Duffy 1994). Stereotypic or repetitive self-injury has been shown to be a major source of ongoing stress for family and caregivers and these behaviors are believed to be the cause of institutionalization rather than a by-product of placement (Bromley and Emerson 1995).

In both fragile X and fetal alcohol syndrome, the behaviors that can be most disruptive tend to be those related to poor self-regulation and impulse control manifested as decreased attention, hyperactivity, stereotypies, and disruptive behaviors both at home and at school (Roebuck et al. 1999, Mattson and Riley 2000). In Rett syndrome, one sees the classic 'hand wringing,' while those afflicted with Lesch–Nyhan have hand and lip biting. The most common forms of aggression found in a mixed population of individuals with cognitive impairment were destruction of property and assault with head, teeth, fingers, hands and legs (Harris 1993, Emerson 2001). The use of weapons is infrequent. The self-injury topographies most commonly found in individuals with intellectual disabilities based on a total population survey in England were skin picking, self-biting, head punching/slapping, and head-to-object banging. Self-cutting with tools was only found in 2% of the sample (Oliver et al. 1987).

Prevalence and incidence
The prevalence of challenging behaviors varies tremendously depending on the definition of these behaviors, the ascertainment methodology used (i.e. surveys versus direct observation), and the actual population sampled. The two largest studies in England and California show rates of 7% and 14%, respectively; however, more inclusive studies have found rates up to 67% (Campbell and Malone 1991, Kiernan and Qureshi 1993, Borthwick-Duffy 1994). Most individuals displayed more than one type of challenging behavior and those who showed more severe behaviors tended to require a higher level of assistance with activities of daily living (Emerson 2001). There is also evidence to suggest that the severity of challenging behaviors is detrimental to the economic and psychiatric health of the mothers of these individuals above and beyond the impact of the intellectual impairment (Emerson and Bromley 1995).

Etiology and pathophysiology
Challenging behaviors are likely the manifestations of a complex interplay of genetic factors, endogenous neurotransmitters, physical discomfort, psychologic frustration, conditioned responses, and social disorder. Animal studies have consistently shown that structural lesions of the anterior hypothalamus lead to offensive aggressive behavior. Further studies have shown that the selective destruction of some D1 pathways, with the resultant hypersensitivity in the residual D1 receptors, may have a role in self-injurious behavior. It is unclear whether the dopamine system is acting alone or whether the challenging behaviors result from an interplay between the dopamine and serotonin systems. Non-human primate studies suggest that a deficit in serotonin activity correlates with impulsive and aggressive behaviors and that manipulation of the serotonin 5-HT receptor and serotonin transporter may affect the level of aggression (De Almeida et al. 2005). A more common and potentially reversible cause for self-injury and aggression are medical illnesses that cause pain such as migraine headaches, sinus infection, or gastrointestinal reflux. Poor sleep has also been found to be associated with increased irritability and aggressive behavior. In some cases, self-injurious behavior can be attributed to an obsessive-compulsive disorder and may be allieviated by treatment with serotonin agonists (King 1993). Furthermore, aggression may also be a manifestation of clinical depression which is ameliorated when this psychiatric condition is appropriately treated. Tantrums and aggression are also likely to be used as a means of

communication for individuals with language deficits. Operant conditioning or reinforcing responses from caregivers, may actually serve to habituate and reinforce these deleterious behaviors. Replacing these behaviors with more effective communication and removing the reinforcing behaviors has been shown to lead to amelioration of challenging behaviors (Lowry and Sovner 1992). Finally, some of the risk factors for challenging behaviors are common to children with and without developmental disabilities. For example, family factors such as an instability of home and family, parental adjustment issues, inadequate housing, and poverty are found to be correlated with challenging behaviors and conduct disorder (Rutter 1985).

Diagnosis

Evaluation of challenging behaviors usually requires a multidisciplinary team, ideally comprising from a medical perspective, a developmental pediatrician or pediatric neurologist, a child psychiatrist, and a behavioral psychologist. The medical evaluation should focus on the identification of possible reversible illnesses such as intercurrent or chronic infections (i.e. sinusitis or scabies), allergies, medication side effects, dental caries, headache, seizures, metabolic derangements, or dermatologic conditions. A genetic evaluation, when indicated by history and physical examination, may identify disorders commonly associated with developmental delay and challenging behaviors such as fragile X, Prader–Willi, Rubenstein–Taybi and Lesch–Nyhan syndromes. The psychiatric evaluation will help identify possible symptoms of depression, mania, anxiety, psychosis, or obsessional thoughts. The use of a symptom scale such as the Developmental Behavioral Checklist may be warranted. A behavioral formulation through observation and a direct rating based approach to define the behavior topography and possible drivers are essential to the treatment plan.

Treatment and management

Treatment should begin with the medical treatment of infection, metabolic derangement, and pain. In addition, co-morbid psychiatric conditions must be addressed. In targeting challenging behaviors, first line interventions are behavioral, with neurochemical treatments used to augment a well-constructed behavioral plan. The behavioral treatment paradigm implemented should seek to build competency through enabling activities, effect a modification of the environment to avoid overstimulation, crowding and unpredictability, together with the teaching of skills to replace maladaptive behaviors with more productive mechanisms of communication such as sign language and picture communication strategies. The plan must be reassessed and modified frequently with caregivers who are an integral part of the treatment planning team.

Neurochemical treatments must be used with caution in this population as individuals with neurologic impairment are often more sensitive to medication side effects. The best approach is to 'start low and go slow.' Choosing the best medication is still unfortunately a process of trial and error, with a subset of neuro-active medications. The process begins with identification of the target symptom and using a symptom rating scale to follow the specific response of the intervention. Ongoing monitoring of side effects such as lethargy, sleep dysregulation, extrapyramidal movement disorders, and additional cognitive impairment is important as is laboratory assessment of electrolytes, blood sugar levels, liver function tests, electrolytes, prolactin as indicated for specific medications.

The major categories of medications used in challenging behaviors modulate dopamine, serotonin, and opiate availability (Table 23.1). Based on the hypothesis of dopamine receptor hypersensitivity, dopamine antagonists such as clozapine (Clozaril), risperidone (Risperdal) and more recently aripiprazole (Abilify) have been used to target aggression and self-mutilation. Well-designed studies are limited for these medications with a single placebo-controlled cross-over study of Risperdal showing qualified success. Meanwhile the side effect profile of these medications, including tardive dyskinesia, sedation, weight gain, and seizure exacerbation, must be taken into account. Furthermore, close laboratory follow-up is required for many of the narcoleptics.

TABLE 23.1
Psychotropics for behavioral management

	Dopamine receptor activity	Serotonin receptor activity	Adrenergic receptor activity	Regimen
Risperidone (Risperdal)	Yes	Yes	Yes	0.25–0.5mg/day Increasing 0.25–0.5mg weekly
Olanzapine (Zyprexa)	Yes	Yes	Yes	2.5–5mg/day Increasing by 2.5–5mg weekly to max 20mg/day
Quetiapine (Seroquel)	Yes	Yes	Yes	12.5–25mg/day Increasing by 12.5–25mg/day weekly
Haloperidol (Haldol)	Yes	No	No	0.5mg/day Increasing by 0.5mg/day weekly
Pimozide (Orap)	Yes	No	No	0.5mg/day Increasing by 0.5mg/day weekly to max 10mg/day
Clonidine (Catapres)	No	No	Yes	0.05–0.10mg/day Increasing by 0.05–0.1mg/day weekly

Individual titration of all of the above essential, balancing therapeutic benefits and side effects (i.e. sedation, cognitive blunting, movement disorders).

The second neurotransmitter of interest is serotonin, primarily based on its observed efficacy in aggression, self-injurious behavior, and obsessive behaviors. In addition, patients with Cornelia de Lange syndrome have been shown to have low serotonin levels. Unfortunately, psychopharmacologic trials for challenging behaviors in general have a small number of patients, and lack controls and long-term follow-up, so study conclusions must be interpreted with caution. The serotonin reuptake inhibitors (SSRIs) are the most widely prescribed serotonergic therapeutic agents based on their relatively safe side effect profile. Paroxetine and sertraline have been shown to be efficacious for behavioral disorders in patients with developmental disabilities. In an effort to develop a more selective drug, the 5-HT1 agonists, such as eltoprazine, have been explored. Although showing initial promise in animal studies and individuals with high initial aggressive behavior, development has been halted because of high rates of medication-induced psychosis in early clinical trials.

Opiate blockers and beta-blockers have also been explored for treating self-injurious behaviors (Willemsen-Swinkels et al. 1995), but these studies include few subjects and are unblinded. There is some suggestion that naltrexone may be more effective in the early stages of self-injurious behaviors. The observed beneficial effect of beta-blockers may be a result of increased levels of concomitant medications through hepatic inhibition. The treatment of challenging behaviors is clinically problematic because of incomplete understanding of the underlying biology as well as apparently complex environmental influences. The most important lesson is to first define the challenging behavior, identify its occurrence and context, craft a flexible but specific behavioral plan, and then consider medications to augment targeting the specific behaviors.

AXIS I DISORDERS
Individuals with neurodevelopmental disabilities are several times more likely to present with a psychiatric disorder. Until relatively recently, mental retardation and mental illness were not clearly differentiated, either diagnostically or therapeutically (Scheerenberger 1987). It is exceedingly common for depression in this population to go undiagnosed for many years. According to Rutter's population study on the Isle of Wight, 50% of children with mental retardation had a psychiatric disorder (Rutter et al. 1976). The scarcity of child psychiatrists trained to meet this need and the difficulty of psychiatric diagnosis particularly in minimally verbal individuals makes treatment of these conditions especially challenging. Furthermore, most of the psychiatric treatment studies have specifically excluded patients with mental retardation so that data on treatment efficacy remains limited. However, the extremely high prevalence and the high impact on quality of life makes screening and treatment of psychiatric co-morbidities in patients with neurodevelopmental disabilities crucial.

Definition

The scope of psychiatric co-morbidity in neurodevelopmental disability in the literature ranges from maladaptive behaviors, which have been addressed in the preceding section, to Axis I diagnoses which include, but are not limited to, schizophrenia, mood disorders, and anxiety disorders. While individuals with developmental disabilities can develop the full spectrum of psychopathologic disorders, the phenomenology of the disorder becomes more difficult to recognize with declining IQ and verbal capabilities. Some researchers have approached these disturbances based on behavior domains (disruptive, self-absorbed, language disturbance, anxiety, social relating, and antisocial) rather than attempt a specific DSM-IVR or International Classification of Diseases (ICD) diagnosis (Tonge et al. 1996). In addition, a comprehensive mental health evaluation is time consuming, which has led to the development of several tools for relatively rapid screening and diagnosis of common conditions in this population.

Many scales have been developed. Some are checklists and others are based on direct interviewing. They all have limitations but can greatly facilitate the identification of specific psychiatric concerns. In the adult population with mental retardation, there are six instruments for assessing psychiatric symptoms: the Psychopathology Instrument for Mentally Retarded Adults (PIMRA), the Diagnostic Assessment Schedule for the Severely Handicapped (DASH-II), the Reiss Screen for Maladaptive Behavior (RSMB), the Psychiatric Assessment Schedule for Adults with Developmental Disabilities Checklist (PAS-ADD Checklist), the Aberrant Behavior Checklist (ABC), and, most recently, the Developmental Behavior Checklist for Adults (DBC-A) (Mohr et al. 2005). For children, the most commonly used scales include the Developmental Behavior Checklist for Pediatrics (DBC-P) (Clarke et al. 2003), the Children's Depression Inventory (Meins 1993), and the parents' version of the Anxiety Disorders Interview Schedule.

Clinical features

Expression of psychiatric disorders is similar to that found in the general population for patients with mild disability; however, more severe neurodevelopmental disabilities render the ICD-10 and DSM-IVR criteria less applicable. Major depression requiring observations of irritability, psychomotor agitation, increased behavior problems, loss of adaptive behavior, and decreased sleep is common. Psychosis, which is manifested by delusions, hallucination, and change in mood, may also be established based on direct observation. The behaviors to watch for include shouting at unseen people, social withdrawal, blunted affect, and suspiciousness. This diagnosis is generally not made in individuals less than 7 years old or in those with an IQ <45. Anxiety disorders, defined in the DSM-IVR, are clinically significant, unpleasant emotions that have the quality of fear, dread, and alarm. Anxiety disorders often manifest in crying or tantrums experienced with transitions or exposure to novel environments.

Prevalence and incidence

The reported prevalence of major psychiatric disorders in those with neurodevelopmental disabilities varies dramatically depending on the diagnostic methodology, population source, and the diagnosis under study. An adult outpatient sample found 9% of patients affected with depression or dysthymia. In general, rates of depression are felt to mirror that found in the general population; however, higher rates are reported in patients with Down syndrome than mixed groups with developmental delay. This is thought to be related to co-incidence of dementia. Furthermore, depression is compounded by stressful life events, which often afflict this population, such as separation from a long-time caregiver, school demands, or traumatic events. The rates of schizophrenia are reported to be 2–6% in samples of patients with mixed etiologies and documented severity of mental retardation, compared to 1% in the general population (Bouras 1999). Anxiety has been found in up to 23% of children with developmental disability using the anxiety subscale of the DBC questionnaire (Tonge et al. 1996). This is considerably higher than the 2–5% prevalence of anxiety in typically developing children.

Diagnosis

In assessing psychiatric symptoms, developmental age and cognitive abilities must be taken into consideration. For example, separation anxiety, self-talk, concrete play, and fleeting attention are expected in late infancy through preschool. Therefore, a team approach combines detailed neuropsychologic evaluation, family assessment, direct symptom assessment, behavioral questionnaires, a medical history, and physical examination.

Medical evaluation may yield either related co-morbidities or specific causes of psychiatric symptoms. For example, deafness can lead to language delay, social withdrawal, and aggressive behavior, while epilepsy is known to produce hallucinations which can overtly mimic psychosis. Clearly, these pathologies require an altogether different evaluation and treatment plan from depression and psychosis. An evaluation to rule out organic causes of Axis I psychiatric conditions includes a complete medical history with emphasis on perinatal history, development, review of systems and family history, plus a detailed general and neurologic examination. This history will inform subsequent diagnostic procedures including laboratory evaluations, genetic evaluation, imaging studies, and electrophysiologic studies.

Treatment and management

The mainstays of treatment for anxiety, mood disorders, and psychosis are a combination of behavioral techniques with psychopharmacology. For anxiety, higher functioning patients have been shown to benefit from progressive relaxation strategies. In all cases, the environment must be reviewed with the goal of minimizing possible triggers. Some powerful examples of effective environmental changes

TABLE 23.2
Targeting behaviors with psychopharmacology

Behavioral target	Category of medication	Specific medication
Aggression	Atypical antipsychotics	Aripiprazole Olanzapine Quetiapine Risperidone Ziprasidone
	Mood stabilizers	Carbamazepine Lithium Valproic acid Oxcarbazepine Gabapentin Tiagabine Lamotrigine
	Beta-blockers	Propranolol Nadolol
	Antidepressants	SSRIs: Citalopram Escitalopram Fluoxetine Fluvoxamine Paroxetine Sertraline Others: Atomoxetine Bupropion Clomipramine Imipramine Mirtazapine Trazodone Venlafaxine
Self-injurious	Atypical antipsychotics Antidepressants Opiate antagonist	 Low-dose SSRIs Naltrexone
Impulsive	Atypical antipsychotics Mood stabilizers Antidepressants Stimulants	 Methylphenidate Amphetamine
Stereotypic/ritual	Antidepressants Atypical antipsychotics	SSRI

SSRI, selective serotonin reuptake inhibitor.

include reducing caregiver variation, decreasing novel stimuli, and preparation for transitions with visual cues and ample allotted time to effect transition. After a full medical evaluation, persistent symptoms of anxiety, psychosis, and mood symptoms may need to be addressed with medication.

A detailed discussion of psychopharmaceuticals is beyond the scope of this chapter as psychiatric treatment requires careful diagnosis, an in-depth familiarity of medication side effects and interactions, together with ongoing monitoring of benefits, adverse reactions, and, in some cases, laboratory follow-up. A thorough review on pharmacology in patients with dual diagnosis of psychiatric disorders and developmental delay was recently carried out by Antochi et al. (2003). Table 23.2 provides a summary of behavioral targets and possible beneficial psychoactive agents. Whenever possible, we urge the simplification of medications such that a single medication may target several co-morbidities. It is sometimes the case that an anticonvulsant such as carbamazepine or valproic acid can be used to treat both emotional lability and a seizure disorder, or an antidepressant can be used to ameliorate pain as well as insomnia.

MEDICAL CONDITIONS
SPELLS, SEIZURES, AND EPILEPSY
Seizure disorders are both a potential cause and effect of neurodevelopmental disability. It is estimated that up to 40% of individuals with mental retardation or cerebral palsy have epilepsy (Aicardi 1994). Down syndrome, Angelman syndrome, and many other known genetic disorders place individuals at much higher risk for epilepsy. Similarly, acquired etiologies of developmental delay such as hypoxic ischemic injury, periventricular hemorrhage/venous infarction, and neonatal meningitis can also greatly increase an individual's risk for a dual diagnosis. In addition, there is ongoing concern that recurrent and especially prolonged seizures can lead to lasting cortical injury and disability. The long-term effect of seizures on cognition and behavior remains an area of great interest, controversy, and research efforts.

Definition
There are many types of 'spells' or paroxysmal events and all can be found in children with developmental delay. The first question is whether the 'spell' is a seizure or not. The term 'seizure' is generally used to denote abnormal paroxysmal behavior which is the result of excessive hypersynchronic discharges of cortical and/or subcortical neurons. Observation and careful questioning can often answer this question, but ultimately an electroencephalogram (EEG) or even prolonged video telemetry may be necessary to differentiate the many possible etiologies of 'spells' (including syncope). The etiologies of these spells can include, but are not limited to, syncope, self-stimulation, gastroesophageal reflux, cardiovascular compromise, migraine equivalents, stereotypies, tics, and epileptic seizures (Table 23.3).

TABLE 23.3
Spells other than seizures in the neurodevelopmentally disabled population

Non-epileptiform paroxysmal events

Cardiovascular	Syncope
	Cardiac arrhythmia-related spells
	Tetralogy spells
Gastrointestinal	Gastroesophageal reflux/Sandifer syndrome
	Rumination
Neurologic	Benign sleep myoclonus
	Cerebrovascular events
	Dystonia
	Elevated intracranial pressure
	Migraine: classic, hemiplegic, and ocular variants
	Paroxysmal dyskinesias
	Periodic paralysis
	Startle response
	Sucking
	Tics/Tourette syndrome
	Torticollis
	Tremor
Psychiatric/behavioral	Hallucinations
	Head banging
	Head nodding
	Masturbation
	Panic attacks
	Pseudoseizures
	Rage
Respiratory	Apnea
	Breath holding
	Hyperventilation
Sleep disorders	Cataplexy
	Narcolepsy
	Nightmares
	Sleep terrors
	Sleep walking

In the case of a seizure, the next question is whether the event is caused by an inherently hyperexcitable or injured brain tissue (i.e. epilepsy) or if the seizure is secondary to a transient reversible condition such as an infection or a metabolic abnormality. As children and adults with cognitive impairment are often unable to provide verbal descriptions of any subjective symptomatology (i.e. auras, psychiatric changes), pain and mental status changes are more difficult to infer and assess objectively, care providers must have a higher suspicion for treatable causes such as intercurrent infection, hydrocephalus, possible electrolyte derangements, or intoxication. Patients with recurrent non-provoked seizures are said to have epilepsy. Often, patients with developmental delay and epilepsy syndromes will have more than one type of seizure. Identifying the specific seizure type and choosing medication accordingly will contribute to successful management.

Clinical features

Generally, epilepsy in patients with developmental delay begins in childhood and often persists into adolescence and adulthood. The most common seizure type in this group is a generalized seizure which may be primary or more typically secondary in origin. However, children often have multiple seizure types, including simple and complex partial seizures, myoclonic seizures, absence seizure (frequently atypical in its features), infantile spasms, and atonic seizures. One common epilepsy syndrome that co-occurs with mental retardation is Lennox–Gastaut syndrome, which consists of a triad of minor motor seizures (tonic seizures, atonic seizures, atypical absence seizures), with or without associated generalized tonic–clonic seizures, cognitive disability, and a low frequency (often 2–3Hz) alpha-wave EEG abnormality. Tuberous sclerosis is known to often be present in those with infantile spasms, while electrographic status epilepticus during slow-wave sleep with global delay and dysmorphic features should prompt a detailed genetic evaluation for Angelman syndrome. These particular seizure syndromes often respond to certain anticonvulsants so it is important to take both the underlying etiology and the actual seizure type into consideration when deciding treatment options.

Parents will often report an increased seizure frequency upon falling asleep or awakening. This is likely a result of hypnogogic/hypnosomnic hypersynchrony which occurs in early Stage 1 sleep. In addition, patients with epilepsy often have a dramatic increase in their seizure frequency in the setting of intercurrent illness and are at higher risk for status epilepticus or prolonged seizures during these events. In general, patients with an underlying neurologic abnormality are at substantially higher risk for clusters of seizures, status epilepticus, seizure recurrence after a first seizure, and manifesting an ultimately medically refractory epilepsy (Goulden et al. 1991, Camfield et al. 1993, Berg and Shinnar 1994). Furthermore, mental retardation has been found to increase the risk for sudden unexplained death in epilepsy (Walczak et al. 2001).

Prevalence and incidence

In general, the prevalence of epilepsy appears to increase with increased severity of developmental delay, mental retardation, and intellectual disability. Goulden et al. (1991) prospectively studied a cohort of 221 children with mental retardation in Aberdeen, Scotland. They reported an overall prevalence of 15% by the age of 22 years while the coincidence of mental retardation and cerebral palsy increased the prevalence of epilepsy to 38%. Severe mental retardation further increased this prevalence to 59% (Goulden et al. 1991). Furthermore, the risk of epilepsy increases with multiple disabilities and specific genetic syndromes. One familial study of patients with tuberous sclerosis found a 62% incidence of 'fits' (Webb et al. 1991). In Angelman syndrome, seizures of various types are reported in 90% of patients (Clayton-Smith and Pembrey 1992). The co-occurrence of epilepsy in this population can have dire consequences, with mortality rates doubling in the presence of epilepsy (McKee and Bodfish 2000).

Diagnosis
The most important part of accurately diagnosing 'spells' is the history. It is often necessary to gather history from multiple sources as the affected individual may be too young or disabled to give adequate or accurate information. In group home situations, caregivers often change and the primary caregiver may not accompany the affected individual to office visits. A phone call to an actual eye witness of these spells can often clarify the history and 'spell' frequency, thus greatly enhancing chances for successful diagnosis and treatment planning. A video recording of the spells can be a tremendous help.

Additional work-up includes a physical examination, EEG, neuroimaging, and relevant laboratory evaluations. The medical examination aims to identify possible focality that will guide the interpretation of historical, EEG, and imaging studies. It may be necessary to conduct extended video telemetry to determine the origins of particular spells if they are occurring frequently enough. Obtaining an EEG may be more difficult in this population because of the frequent need for sedation. It is helpful to choose a sedative with a known minimal impact on the actual EEG tracing such as chloral hydrate, but the need for sedation can be greatly reduced by creating a comfortable environment. An ultrasound in infants and CT scans in older individuals may be warranted in the acute setting of new onset seizures to rule out hemorrhage, ischemia, and hydrocephalus. In general, magnetic resonance imaging (MRI) is often necessary because it aids in the diagnosis of subtle cortical malformations or the extent of an acquired CNS injury. The relevant laboratory evaluation needs to reflect the differential determined by the seizure type and presentation, patient's age, and family history. This may reflect the possibility of a metabolic disorder, a persistent electrolyte or endocrine abnormality, or the influence of a suspected genetic etiology.

Treatment and management
Any good treatment plan begins with establishing the goals of treatment with the patient and caregivers. Treatment goals often start with improved seizure control

but equally important is improving the quality of life, decreasing attached social stigma, eliminating or minimizing side effects, physical injury or death, and enhancing the affected individual's desired activity or participation in the broader community (de Silva et al. 1996). A medication that eradicates seizures but results in excessive somnolence is clearly not an option. It should be anticipated that this group of patients may be more sensitive to side effects. Often, side effects and efficacy will need to be monitored using non-verbal cues, laboratory values, and observed seizures. Keeping a calendar of 'spells' is always helpful.

The choice of anticonvulsant can be daunting. As a rule, the newer anticonvulsants with broad-spectrum coverage, minimal interactions, simple regimens, and cross-over behavioral benefits such as lamotrigine (Lamictal) and topiramate (Topamax) may be preferred to the traditional first line approach of anticonvulsants utilized in non-disabled populations (Rutecki and Gidal 2002), (Singh and White-Scott 2002). Additionally, the actual route of administration can be crucial as orally fed children may require a liquid, dissolvable, or sprinkle formulation (Smith et al. 2004). Frequent reassessment of benefits and side effects of medical intervention implemented is the mainstay of a successful treatment plan.

The ketogenic diet and surgery (i.e. lesional and non-lesional) are also important treatment options for some seizure disorders. The ketogenic diet, which markedly restricts carbohydrate intake, was found in a multicenter study to reduce seizures by >50% in almost half of the children with medically refractory seizures at 12 months. It is not recommended for children with metabolic disorders or impaired immune systems. Vagal nerve stimulators, a recent therapeutic modality, can result in a 34–90% seizure reduction depending on length of follow-up (Hosain et al. 2000). For patients with epilepsy caused by discrete structural lesions (i.e. tuberous sclerosis), surgical resection can greatly reduce – and in some cases eliminate – overall seizure burden. Aggressive management of intercurrent sleep disorders can also decrease seizure frequency and intensity. Figure 23.1 provides a simplified approach to seizure control from a medical perspective.

HEARING/VISION IMPAIRMENT

Children with neurodevelopmental disabilities are at higher risk for vision and auditory impairments. These conditions, which can be congenital or acquired, can dramatically impair a child's ability to learn as well as adequately interact and participate in their environment. Unfortunately, because of their other disabilities, these deficits often remain undiagnosed and untreated (MMWR 1997). Clearly, identification of these sensory impairments and early appropriate intervention can improve developmental outcome. Vigilant vision and hearing screening for early detection, correction, and amplification is essential in this population of children (Yoshinaga-Itano 2003).

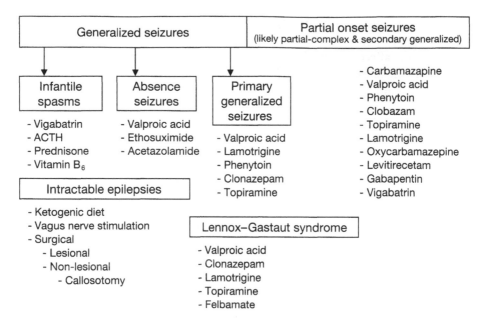

Figure 23.1 A suggested simplified approach to anticonvulsant management. ACTH, adenocorticotropic hormone.

Definition

Hearing loss can result from abnormalities all along the auditory pathway, including craniofacial dysgenesis, middle ear obstruction, inner ear dysfunction, and third cranial nerve, brainstem (pons/midbrain), or cortical injury. The Metropolitan Atlanta Developmental Disabilities Surveillance Program defines hearing impairment as a bilateral pure tone hearing loss at frequencies of 500–2000Hz averaging 40 decibels (dB) or more unaided in the better ear as indicated by the results of formal audiologic testing (MMWR 1997). Current recommendations from the American Academy of Pediatrics (AAP) include universal newborn screening which will help detect some, but not all, of these auditory deficits. However, the nature of the hearing loss (e.g. conductive, sensorineural, mixed, retrocochlear, or central) as well as the timing, temporal evolution, severity, and laterality of the deficit will help determine the location of injury and target treatment efforts. Failure to detect hearing loss magnifies pre-existing challenges in patients with developmental impairment. This may additionally contribute to lifelong deficits in speech and language acquisition, poor academic performance, personal–social maladjustment, and emotional difficulties (Cunningham and Cox 2003).

Vision loss can result from dysgenesis, injury, or degeneration along the visual pathway. Disease processes often affect a particular point along the pathway. Retinal lacunae can make a clinician consider the diagnosis of Aicardi syndrome in the right context (i.e. female infant with infantile spasms). Congenital and early onset cataracts will elicit an entirely different differential diagnosis. Acquired intrauterine infections, such as cytomegalovirus (CMV), may cause both retinal and cortical injury and should prompt through evaluation for infection. Thus, detection of the specific type of sensory deficit may help to establish the underlying etiology of the neurodevelopmental disorder.

Clinical features

Clinically, the vocalizations of deaf children are the same as hearing children up to mid-infancy. As children move towards monosyllabic and polysyllabic babble, qualitative and quantitative differences in vocalizations can often be appreciated between deaf and hearing children (Berg 1996). Parents and caregivers have been found to be sensitive to these differences in speech production as well as the child's diminished response to verbal engagement. In fact, medical diagnosis of hearing loss can lag behind parental suspicion by up to 5 months with an additional 3–4 months for intervention and amplification devices (Harrison and Roush 1996).

Ascertaining vision loss can also be a challenge in the context of the young child with a neurodevelopmental disability. An investigation for vision loss is often prompted by observations that clinically suspected children or adults will bring objects, or the television, close for inspection. However, other behaviors are similarly concerning and should prompt further evaluation. Head turning for visual fixation can be an indicator of strabismus, nystagmus, or hemianopia. Parents of children with severe developmental disabilities may report eye poking as a form of self-stimulation. This behavior can be encountered in the context of primary retinal disease such as Leber congenital amaurosis or acquired retinal infectious disorders such as CMV infection. It is hypothesized that this orbital pressure generates pleasing visual self-stimulation (Berg 1996). Individuals with retinal disease or optic nerve injury are also noted to look above or askew at objects of interest to obtain a sharper visual focus. Staring at bright lights often occurs with retrogeniculate or cortical visual impairment.

Prevalence and incidence

Significant hearing loss is present in 1–6/1000 newborn infants; however, some congenital hearing loss may not be apparent until later in childhood. Hearing loss can also be acquired during childhood. Sensorineural hearing loss was reported in 29% of children with at least one other developmental disability (MMWR 1997). Almost half of this group of children went undiagnosed until after 3 years of age. Vision impairment has been found in 13–25% of children with global developmental delay. Institutionalized adults have a 10-fold higher incidence of vision impairment. In addittion, these rates do not reflect the recent increased survival of infants with birth weight less than 1000g, who are at particular enhanced risk for hearing loss, visual loss, and developmental delay. An added complication is that individuals with intellectual impairments have more difficulty tolerating and completing behavioral audiometric and standardized visual testing.

Pathophysiology

Disorders of the auditory and visual systems can occur because of direct injury to the involved structures or from secondary degeneration from decreased or abnormal input during a critical developmental window (Zhang et al. 2002). Fetal alcohol syndrome (FAS) provides an interesting model of acquired toxic injury during fetal development which results in four possible types of hearing impairment: (1) sensorineural hearing loss, (2) conductive hearing loss from serous otitis media, (3) central hearing loss from injury to the auditory cortex (transverse gyri of Hershel), and (4) slow auditory processing. The convergence of craniofacial and ocular anomalies in this disorder is thought to reflect primary injury to the first and second brachial arches which share a similar fetal epoch of vulnerability to toxic injury (Church and Kaltenbach 1997). It is likely that the first two components of FAS hearing impairments additionally create the preconditions for the second two deficits. Sensorineural and conduction hearing loss may lead to deprivation and deafferentiation of the auditory cortex. This impoverished afferent input is believed to cause abnormal auditory cortex mapping and disruption of higher order auditory connectivity. It is also important to note that while unilateral hearing loss, as seen in chronic middle ear effusions, may have less of an effect on language learning, binaural hearing is important for accurately localizing sounds in space as well as optimal speech perception within a noisy background. Similarly, direct injury to the orbit, retina, or optic nerve has direct and indirect consequences on vision that are more pronounced when they occur in the setting of a non-intact or immature brain.

Diagnosis

Periodic standardized objective hearing and vision screening or assessment is important for all children with neurodevelopmental disabilities. There are several tests currently used for hearing assessment, each with benefits and limitations. Evoked otoacoustic emission in the newborn infant tests the cochlear stimuli response. It allows independent ear testing; however, it does not assess cranial nerve, brainstem, or cortical processing. Auditory brainstem response measures the brainstem, not cortical, response to broad-band repetitive click responses presented at frequencies greater than 1000Hz in each ear. This test does not require subjective participation; however, some children are resistant to the earphones used for testing. In addition, the results are pass or fail. Visual reinforced audiometry detects observable behavioral response to speech sounds to frequency-specific stimuli but misses unilateral deficits. Finally, conventional audiometry tests speech and frequency-specific stimuli by requiring the individual to raise the ipsilateral hand when the sound is appreciated. While this test is generally attempted for children 4 years of age and older, it requires understanding and participation that may be beyond the capability of some individuals regardless of their chronologic age.

When deficits are detected, further inquiry is indicated. On physical evaluation, the examination should include ophthalmoscope, pneumatic otoscopy, and tympanometry, but equally important is a careful eye and craniofacial and cutaneous evaluation to consider possible stigmata of chromosomal disorders, neurofibromatosis, and other indicators of abnormal fetal development. In cases of hearing and vision loss, dedicated MRI to focus on the area of interest is clearly the modality of choice. Computed tomography (CT) and ultrasound assessment should be considered in the event of acute symptom onset or progressive macrocephaly; however, they will often, and perhaps routinely, miss subtle disorders of migration. In addition, urine should be examined for muchopolysaccharides as children less than 18 months may not yet exhibit the dysmorphic features associated with Hunter-Hurler disease. CMV can be detected in urine for the first 3 weeks of life if a TORCH (toxoplasmosis, other agents, rubella, CMV, herpes simplex) infection is suspected and thyroid function should always be screened if not performed routinely in the newborn infant. The type of hearing and vision impairment documented will clearly direct further genetic, infectious, and exposure evaluation. A referral to a pediatric ophthalmologist or otolaryngologist is strongly recommended.

Treatment and management
Early identification has repeatedly been shown to reduce communication disability associated with hearing impairment (Mauk et al. 1991). The mainstays of treatment are amplification devices and in some cases cochlear implants. Behavioral treatment for hearing and vision loss is equally important. Furthermore, surgical correction of severe strabismus and cataracts is crucial to maintaining conjugate vision and cortical input bilaterally during the cortical developmental window. Eye glasses and contact lenses are increasingly comfortable and therefore more tolerated. Often, the earlier glasses are introduced, the easier child compliance will be.

SLEEP DISORDERS
Definition
Sleep disorders are often split into dyssomnias and parasomnias, which is reflected in the International Classification of Sleep Disorders–Revised 10. Dyssomnias are primary sleep disorders that result from intrinsic, extrinsic, and circadian rhythm disorders. They can interfere with initiation or maintaining sleep. Obstructive sleep apnea, narcolepsy, and involuntary limb movements are common intrinsic factors, while an inappropriate sleep environment and parenting factors largely contribute

to extrinsic factors. Circadian rhythm disorders refer to the disorganization of sleep phases or sleep–wake timing. Parasomnias are episodic behavioral disorders that occur during sleep and may lead to inappropriate waking. They are commonly divided by sleep phase occurrence. Head banging generally occurs upon the transition from the sleep to wake state, while sleep walking (somnambulism) and night terrors typically occur during Stage IV sleep. Nightmares are generally found during REM sleep. Enuresis and bruxism can occur at any time (Stores 1999, Didden and Sigafoos 2001, Didden et al. 2002).

Clinical features
The consequences of sleep disorders are far reaching and can be severe, both for the individual and the family unit. These manifestations include daytime sleepiness, challenging behavior, additional psychomotor retardation, headaches, and increased seizure activity (Quine 1991, Koh et al. 2000, Symons et al. 2000, Lindblom et al. 2001). A recent review of the literature shows that sleep disordered breathing can have adverse effects on cognition (i.e. lower IQ), behavior (i.e. attention-deficit–hyperactivity disorder [ADHD]), and an enhanced seizure frequency with a negative impact on already developmentally delayed children (Bass et al. 2004). Even in healthy populations, sleep disturbances are shown to produce memory, attention, and visuospatial impairment. For the most part, these deficits are thought to be reversible. Mood and behavior, like cognition, is similarly affected by poor quality and reduced quantity of sleep. Depressed mood and irritability are already exacerbated by impoverished sleep.

The signs of poor sleep may be different for children and individuals with neurodevelopmental disability. Instead of reduced activity, inattention and hyperactivity may be seen. Parents may note increased aggression, bedtime tantrums, and frequent night time wandering. Furthermore, parasomnias (night terrors and sleep walking) can be frightening or embarrassing, affecting the individual as well as the family unit. There is even some suggestion that the physiologic stress response from these disorders can lead to impaired growth and immune function. Clinically, it is important to ascertain whether the problem is with shortened sleep duration, disruption of sleep, snoring, or atypical sleep timing (i.e. daytime sleeping) as this will help target effective intervention.

Prevalence and incidence
The prevalence of sleep disturbance in neurodevelopmental disability ranges from 13 to 86%. This huge range is a reflection of the type and severity of illness, the varied criteria for diagnosing a sleep disorder, variety of measurement tools and strategies, and wide range of home environments. For example, in children with severe mental retardation cared for at home, the rates for a broadly defined and

observable sleep difficulty were 77–86%. When the definition of sleep disorder is more restricted, the occurrence of at least one sleep problem is around 16% (Didden et al. 2002). This same study correlated sleep problems with the severity of intellectual disability, medication use, epilepsy, a younger age at time of assessment, and the co-occurrence of cerebral palsy. An increased occurrence of aggression, noncompliance, and hyperactivity was shown in affected individuals.

A Finnish adult sample found similar risk factors such as poorly controlled severe locomotor disability, blindness, and active epilepsy for fragmented and abnormal sleep distribution (Lindblom et al. 2001). While the finding of an increased sleep disturbance in the blind is quite reproducible, there has been some disagreement regarding the role of IQ and age in sleep disruption (Piazza et al. 1996, Espie et al. 1998, Didden et al. 2002). It was highlighted in a study of children with Down syndrome that some of the behaviors that are found most commonly (i.e. difficulty settling, night waking, and sleeping with parents) have a strong behavioral component. These behaviors may result, in part, from maternal stress, marital discord, and issues relating to the diagnosis and co-morbidities of illness. It is also interesting to note that these same behaviors are reported in up to 20% of typically developing toddlers (Richdale 2000).

While it is believed that there is an increased prevalence of sleep disorders in those with neurodevelopmental disability, there are some specific syndromes with enhanced frequency. For example, individuals with Prader–Willi syndrome are well characterized as having daytime somnolence, snoring, and restlessness. Although there are some conflicting data, these difficulties may result from both an obstructive sleep apnea as well as a sleep onset REM disorder (Vela-Bueno et al. 1984, O'Donoghue et al. 2005). The obstructive sleep apnea is thought to result from the obesity frequently seen in this syndrome which is secondary to unrestrained hyperplasia; however, patients with Down syndrome are also found to have increased sleep apnea which is not always associated with individual obesity.

Sleep apnea, including obstructive and central etiologies, is the most common sleep disorder. These disorders can lead to compromise of central respiratory regulation, the neural control of respiratory muscles, and hypotonic nasopharyngeal airways. It is important to note that children can present with less sleep fragmentation and oxygen desaturations than adults with this disorder. Angelman syndrome, which, like Prader–Willi syndrome, results from a disruption at 15q11 which reflects the differential effects of imprinting, has a high incidence of disordered sleep. Patients with Angelman syndrome are frequently found electrographically to have 2–3 cycles/second spike and slow wave complexes during sleep with decreased overall REM time (Clarke and Marston 2000, Miano et al 2004). Unfortunately, such slow wave sleep abnormalities are often treatment resistant. Although epilepsy is associated with sleep dysregulation, it is unclear whether the relationship is the result of actual nocturnal seizures or the use of anticonvulsant medications. However, treating sleep apnea has been shown to improve overall seizure control.

Diagnosis
An evaluation for sleep disorders is indicated for all individuals with neurodevelopmental disabilities. This evaluation should begin with observation by the parents or caregivers, focused on possible difficulty with initiation or maintenance of sleep. In addition, increased challenging behaviors focused on naps or bedtime should prompt a more thorough evaluation. Snoring or other breathing difficulties during sleep are strongly suggestive of obstructive sleep apnea and merit a sleep study and medical evaluation of the oropharynx. In some cases, difficulty with sleep can indicate discomfort related to severe gastroesophageal reflux, and an upper gastrointestinal series or pH probe can be helpful. Behavioral assessments for triggers and reinforcers are essential to address the frequent behavioral aspects of sleep problems which often form a core and possibly intractable component of these disorders.

Treatment and management
The treatment and management of sleep disorders varies depending on the underlying etiology. Psychiatric and medical conditions such as depression, obstructive sleep apnea, and gastroesophageal reflux must be identified and treated. For problems with sleep initiation that are likely to be behavioral in origin (e.g. bedtime tantrums), there are several approaches that have been shown to be helpful but require a firm plan and consistent enactment. Withholding parental attention, extinction, gradual distancing, and a regular sleep–wake schedule are some approaches recommended by behavioral therapists (Didden et al. 1998). The behavioral triggers, such as the fear of a dark bedroom, must be identified and used for the formulation of a treatment approach. It is also important for individuals to create a restful sleep environment devoid of nocturnal distractions.

For sleep difficulties related to disrupted circadian cycles, it is helpful to synchronize the endogenous circadian cycle with the individual's daily schedule. Exposure to bright light upon awakening to synchronize circadian rhythm and limiting daytime sleeping can also reset the internal chronobiologic clock. Limiting daily caffeine intake (i.e. soft drinks), particularly evening imbibing, may be helpful and regular exercise has also been reported to improve overall sleep. Melatonin, a hormone released by the pineal gland, serves to regulate our circadian pacemaker. Exogenous treatment with melatonin may be beneficial in decreasing time to sleep onset but has shown no benefits in fragmented sleep patterns or early morning awakening. Long-term safety of this hormone is unknown and there are some reports of increased seizure frequency.

GASTROINTESTINAL FEEDING AND REFLUX

Individuals with neurodevelopmental disabilities often have difficulties with nutritional intake, food motility, and growth (Canadian Pediatric Society 1994). Oromotor inco-ordination, dysphagia, gastroesophageal reflux, diarrhea, and constipation are frequent observations from the newborn period through to adulthood. These difficulties can be transient, chronic, or progressive and can lead to discomfort, failure to thrive, ulceration of the gastrointestinal lining, and bowel obstruction if not adequately evaluated and treated. Feeding issues can also lead to serious discord in the home with 'the inability to manage mealtimes was (is) a common reason for taking a child out of a home and placing him or her in an institution' (Perske et al. 1986).

Definition

Problems with food intake may be related to decreased tone and poor motor planning. While some gastrointestinal difficulty is 'normal' during infant development, it becomes pathologic when it causes distress or leads to health complications such as recurrent pneumonia, painful esophagitis, dehydration, and poor growth (failure to thrive). Dysphagia, or difficulty with swallowing, is manifest by repeated choking during feeding. Gastroesophageal reflux, which reflects the retrograde movement of stomach contents into the esophagus, will generally occur following every feed. The more forceful vomiting is thought to arise from active spasms of the pylorus muscle. The definitions of constipation and diarrhea can be difficult as the consistency of stool will change dramatically based on age and type of food ingested. Constipation is defined as the passage of fewer than three stools per week or a history of painful large hard stools, while diarrhea is defined as a sudden increase in loose stools, generally more than three watery stools per day.

Clinical features

Difficulties with nutrition and gastrointestinal motility can mimic other medical conditions as well as lead to secondary medical problems. Nutritionally, discomfort from feeding can lead to a reduced poor appetite, poor compliance with feeding, and inadequate weight gain. Furthermore, children who have been fed with a feeding tube may develop oral aversion and texture intolerance if oral stimulation is not continued in some way. Dysphagia and gastroesophageal reflux (GER) have also been correlated with food refusal (Field et al. 2003). The most obvious signs of dysphagia and GER are spitting up and vomiting. However, clinicians must also be aware of apnea, stridor, wheezing, chronic cough, aspiration pneumonia, throat and chest pain as alternative manifestations of this disorder. In an infant, GER can also manifest as Sandifer syndrome, which appears as a triad of head tilt, back arching, and repeated jerking associated with swallowing. This can be easily confused with an epileptic seizure. Overall, gastrointestinal disorders can contribute to decreased energy, immune function, and functional status (Kuhn and Matson 2004).

Indeed, in cases requiring enteral feeding, there has been reported improvement not only with growth but also with improvements in spasticity and affect (Sanders et al. 1990). At the other extreme, overeating and obesity, as can be seen with Prader–Willi syndrome, can lead to serious morbidity in this population.

Prevalence and incidence

The prevalence of gastrointestinal disorders and nutritional deficits is unknown and will vary depending on the etiology of neurodevelopmental disability. Using parental interviews and direct assessments of children with cerebral palsy, 60% were found to have intercurrent feeding problems, 43% of the children assessed were undernourished, and 9% showed evidence of overnutrition (Dahl et al. 1996). Conversely, in a sample of children referred for feeding evaluations and treatment, 64% were identified to have neurodevelopmental disabilities (Field et al. 2003). Severe disability and younger age were significant risk factors for poor nutritional status.

In the Oxford Feeding Study, children with neurodevelopmental disability and reported feeding problems were queried regarding the nature of feeding problems as well as the predictors for those difficulties. In this selected group, 89% of children with neurodevelopmental disabilities were found to require help with feeding, 56% exhibited choking, but, surprisingly, 64% of these children had not been formally assessed for feeding or nutritional needs (Sullivan et al. 2000). Furthermore, significant familial caregiving time and stress surrounded these significant feeding issues (Johnson and Deitz 1985).

The etiology of malnutrition in this population is certainly mulitfactorial, including an alteration in hormonal control, mechanical difficulty with chewing, swallowing, and digesting, as well as gastrointestinal discomfort caused by the use of a variety of medications and GER. It is encouraging, however, that improved nutrition has yielded observable developmental benefits (Sanders et al. 1990).

Diagnosis

A detailed nutrition and feeding history must be carried out for all children with neurodevelopmental disabilities. This should include time and duration of feeding, types and quantity of food/drinks taken, difficulties encountered, as well as reports of protracted constipation or diarrhea. The physical examination should focus on axial muscle tone and posture of the head. In addition, craniofacial abnormalities that affect feeding, such as cleft palate or relative macroglossia, will need to be identified for treatment planning.

If there is concern regarding oropharyngeal incoordination, aspiration, or reflux, observed feeding with video fluoroscopy is warranted to assess feeding safety. Upper gastrointestinal endoscopy may be necessary for assessing structural barriers and possible mucosal breakdown and ulceration from the mouth to the small intestine. Radiologic evaluations with swallowed barium are typically less effective than direct endoscopy. The 'criterion standard' for diagnosing GER is the 24-hour pH probe. In this test, a small flexible catheter with a pH sensitive tip is passed through the nose into the esophagus. This sensor can then record each event of acid reflux, which is especially helpful when correlated with directly observable behavioral events in largely non-verbal and non-communicative individuals. A wireless capsule device to monitor pH in the esophagus has recently been introduced. It has the benefit of being less conspicuous; however, it remains expensive and is less consistent in obtaining recordings. Finally, to assess motility one can perform esophageal motility testing using a pressure-sensitive catheter in the esophagus in addition to gastric emptying studies. Laboratory evaluations are seldom useful in the diagnosis of GER; however, investigation for food allergies is warranted when specific intolerances are evident as suggested by a listing of particular food related symptomatology.

Treatment and management
It is important to realize that individuals with neurodevelopmental disabilities will have special nutritional and gastrointestinal needs. For example, some individuals may take less exercise, while others may have substantially more physical demands from typical activities of daily living and/or frequent intractable seizures. Some may have motility and GER disorders, whereas others have oral aversion. A well-developed plan must consider appetite, specific nutritional needs, behavioral and medical barriers to oral feeding, and motility. Appetite can be affected in both directions by various medications. Consequently, stimulants and medications that cause gastrointestinal upset should be given after meals or replaced if a medication with a more tolerable gastrointestinal profile and similar neurologic effectiveness is available.

The issue of oral feeding versus direct enteric feeding is at times controversial. The indications for nasogatric or percutaneous enterostomy include recurrent aspiration and continued malnutrition despite aggressive oral feeding strategies with nutritionally enriched foods. Caregivers report that enteric feeding can improve quality of life for the affected individual and his or her family. For the patient, these benefits include less coughing, choking, vomiting, and respiratory infection. For the caregivers, the benefits include an ease of medication administration and more time to devote to other needs of their children and families. Unfortunately, enteric feeding without ongoing oral feeding programs can lead to impaired eating strategies and oral aversion. Oral programs stress appropriate upright head, neck, and body positioning during feeding and altering the texture of administered foods. Creative strategies to overcome tongue thrusting and rooting, a variety of food textures and tastes, a relaxed feeding environment, and adaptive feeding equipment can make all the difference for eventual success in this important domain.

Similarly, GER can be approached with behavioral, medical, or surgical approaches. Affected individuals should avoid trigger foods such as citrus or acidic foods and juices, avoid large meals, and wait 3 hours (where practical) after a meal before lying down. Antacids can be tried after meals and before bedtime, but often an H_2-blocker or a proton pump inhibitor will be necessary to control reflux symptoms. Promotility agents can be helpful in conjunction with an acid-suppressing medication. There are also surgical procedures to limit the retrograde flow of stomach contents (i.e. Nissen fundoplication). Constipation can be treated with a high fiber diet and increased fluid intake. Food allergies can be identified and avoided. Typically, the approach to intervention in gastrointestinal disorder requires input from a gastrointestinal specialist, occupational therapist, physiotherapist, or, if necessary, a general surgeon.

CONCLUSION

The early recognition and treatment of NDD co-morbidities is crucial to the daily well being of affected individuals. Patients should be routinely screened for psychiatric and medical disorders, including vigilant hearing and vision assessments. Most importantly, the primary care givers need to be firmly integrated into treatment assessment and planning as they are often called to speak for the patient and implement the plan of care.

REFERENCES

Aicardi J (1994) Syndromic classification in the management of childhood epilepsy. *Child Neurol* 9: 14–18.

Antochi R, Stavrakaki C, Emery PC (2003) Psychopharmacological treatments in persons with dual diagnosis of psychiatric disorders and developmental disabilities. *Postgrad Med J* 79: 139–146.

Bass JL, Corwin M, Gozal D, Moore C, Nishida H, Parker S, et al. (2004) The effect of chronic or intermittent hypoxia on cognition in childhood: a review of the evidence. *Pediatrics* 114: 805–816.

Berg AT, Shinnar S (1994) Relapse following discontinuation of antiepileptic drugs: a meta-analysis. *Neurology* 44: 601–608.

Berg BO (1996) *Principles of Child Neurology*. New York: McGraw-Hill Health Professions Divis .

Borthwick-Duffy SA (1994) Epidemiology and prevalence of psychopathology in people with mental retardation. *J Consult Clin Psychol* 62: 17–27.

Bouras N (1999) *Psychiatric and Behavioural Disorders in Developmental Disabilities and Mental Retardation*. Cambridge, UK; New York, NY: Cambridge University Press.

Bromley J, Emerson E (1995) Beliefs and emotional reactions of care staff working with people with challenging behaviour. *J Intellect Disabil Res* 39: 341–352.

Camfield C, Camfield P, Gordon K, Smith B, Dooley J (1993) Outcome of childhood epilepsy: a population-based study with a simple predictive scoring system for those treated with medication. *J Pediatr* 122: 861–868.

Campbell M, Malone RP (1991) Mental retardation and psychiatric disorders. *Hosp Community Psychiatry,* 42: 374–379.

Canadian Pediatric Society (1994) Undernutrition in children with a neurodevelopmental disability. Nutrition Committee, Canadian Paediatric Society. *Can Med Assoc J* 151: 753–759.

Church MW, Kaltenbach JA (1997) Hearing, speech, language, and vestibular disorders in the fetal alcohol syndrome: a literature review. *Alcohol Clin Exp Res* 21: 495–512.

Clarke AR, Tonge BJ, Einfeld SL, Mackinnon A (2003) Assessment of change with the Developmental Behaviour Checklist. *J Intellect Disabil Res* 47: 210–212.

Clarke DJ, Marston G (2000) Problem behaviors associated with 15q-Angelman syndrome. *Am J Ment Retard* 105: 25–31.

Clayton-Smith J, Pembrey ME (1992) Angelman syndrome. *J Med Genet* 29: 412–415.

Cunningham M, Cox EO (2003) Hearing assessment in infants and children: recommendations beyond neonatal screening. *Pediatrics* 111: 436–440.

Dahl M, Thommessen M, Rasmussen M, Selberg T (1996) Feeding and nutritional characteristics in children with moderate or severe cerebral palsy. *Acta Paediatr* 85: 697–701.

Day K (1985) Psychiatric disorder in the middle-aged and elderly mentally handicapped. *Br J Psychiatry* 147: 660–667.

De Almeida RMM, Ferrari PF, Parmigiani S, Miczek KA (2005) Escalated aggressive behavior: Dopamine, serotonin and GABA. *European Journal of Pharmacology* 182: 116–127.

de Silva M, MacArdle B, McGowan M, Hughes E, Stewart J, Neville BG, et al. (1996) Randomized comparative monotherapy trial of phenobarbitone, phenytoin, carbamazepine, or sodium valproate for newly diagnosed childhood epilepsy. *Lancet* 347: 709–713.

Didden R, Curfs LM, Sikkema SP, de Moor J (1998) Functional assessment and treatment of sleeping problems with developmentally disabled children: six case studies. *J Behav Ther Exp Psychiatry* 29: 85–97.

Didden R, Korzilius H, van Aperto B, van Overloop C, de Vries M (2002) Sleep problems and daytime problem behaviours in children with intellectual disability. *J Intellect Disabil Res* 46: 537–547.

Didden R, Sigafoos J (2001) A review of the nature and treatment of sleep disorders in individuals with developmental disabilities. *Res Dev Disabil* 22: 255–272.

Emerson E, Bromley J (1995) The form and function of challenging behaviours. *J Intellect Disabil Res* 39: 388–398.

Emerson E, Kiernan C, Alborz A, Reeves D, Mason H, Swarbrick R, Mason L, Hatton, C. (2001) The prevalence of challenging behaviors: a total population study. *Research in Developmental Disabilities,* 22: 77–93.

Espie CA, Paul A, McFie J, Amos P, Hamilton D, McColl JH, et al. (1998) Sleep studies of adults with severe or profound mental retardation and epilepsy. *Am J Ment Retard* 103: 47–59.

Field D, Garland M, Williams K (2003) Correlates of specific childhood feeding problems. *J Paediatr Child Health* 39: 299–304.

Goulden KJ, Shinnar S, Koller H, Katx M, Richardson SA (1991) Epilepsy in children with mental retardation: a cohort study. *Epilepsia* 32: 690–697.

Harris P (1993) The nature and extent of aggressive behaviour amongst people with learning difficulties (mental handicap) in a single health district. *J Intellect Disabil Res* 37: 221–242.

Harrison M, Roush J (1996) Age of suspicion, identification, and intervention for infants and young children with hearing loss: a national study. *Ear Hear* 17: 55–62.

Hosain S, Nikalov B, Harden C, Li M, Fraser R, Labar D (2000) Vagus nerve stimulation treatment for Lennox–Gastaut syndrome. *J Child Neurol* 15: 509–512.

Johnson CB, Deitz JC (1985) Time use of mothers with preschool children: a pilot study. *Am J Occup Ther* 39: 578–583.

Kiernan C, Qureshi H (1993). Challenging behaviour. In C. Kiernan (Ed.). Research to Practice? Implications of Research on the Challenging Behaviour of People with Learning Disabilities. Kidderminster: British Institute of Learning Disabilities.

King BH (1993) Self-injury by people with mental retardation: a compulsive behavior hypothesis. *Am J Ment Retard,* 98: 93–112.

Koh S, Ward SL, Lin M, Chen LS (2000) Sleep apnea treatment improves seizure control in children with neurodevelopmental disorders. *Pediatr Neurol* 22: 36–39.

Kuhn DE, Matson JL (2004) Assessment of feeding and mealtime behavior problems in persons with mental retardation. *Behav Modif* 28: 638–648.

MMWR (1997) Serious hearing impairment among children aged 3–10 years: Atlanta, Georgia, 1991–1993. *Morb Mortal Wkly Rep* 46: 1073–1076.

Lindblom N, Heiskala H, Kaski M, Nevanlinna A, Iivanainen M, Laakso ML (2001) Neurological impairments and sleep–wake behaviour among the mentally retarded. *J Sleep Res* 10: 309–318.

Lowry MA, Sovner R (1992) Severe behaviour problems associated with rapid cycling bipolar disorder in two adults with profound mental retardation. *J Intellect Disabil Res* 36: 269–281.

Mattson SN, Riley EP (2000) Parent ratings of behavior in children with heavy prenatal alcohol exposure and IQ-matched controls. *Alcohol Clin Exp Res,* 24: 226–231.

Mauk GW, White KR, Mortensen LB, Behrens TR (1991) The effectiveness of screening programs based on high-risk characteristics in early identification of hearing impairment. *Ear Hear* 12: 312–319.

McKee JR, Bodfish JW (2000) Sudden unexpected death in epilepsy in adults with mental retardation. *Am J Ment Retard* 105: 229–235.

Meins W (1993) Assessment of depression in mentally retarded adults: reliability and validity of the Children's Depression Inventory (CDI). *Res Dev Disabil* 14: 299–312.

Miano S, Bruni O, Leuzzi V, Elia M, Verrillo E, Ferri R (2004) Sleep polygraphy in Angelman syndrome. *Clin Neurophysiol* 115: 938–945.

Mohr C, Tonge BJ, Einfeld SL (2005) The development of a new measure for the assessment of psychopathology in adults with intellectual disability. *J Intellect Disabil Res* 49: 469–480.

O'Donoghue FJ, Camfferman D, Kennedy JD, Martin AJ, Couper T, Lack LD, et al. (2005) Sleep-disordered breathing in Prader–Willi syndrome and its association with neurobehavioral abnormalities. *J Pediatr* 147: 823–829.

Oliver C, Murphy GH, Corbett JA (1987) Self-injurious behaviour in people with mental handicap: a total population study. *J Ment Defic Res* 31: 147–162.

Perske R, Clifton A, et al. (1986) *Mealtimes for Persons with Severe Handicaps.* Baltimore; London: Brookes Publishing.

Piazza CC, Fisher W, Kahng SW (1996) Sleep patterns in children and young adults with mental retardation and severe behavior disorders. *Dev Med Child Neurol* 38: 335–344.

Quine L (1991) Sleep problems in children with mental handicap. *J Ment Defic Res* 35: 269–290.

Richdale A, Francis A, Gavidia-Payne S et al (2000). Stress, behaviour, and sleep problems in children with an intellectual disability. *J Intellect Dev Dis* 25: 147–161.

Roebuck TM, Mattson SN, Riley EP (1999) Behavioral and psychosocial profiles of alcohol-exposed children. *Alcohol Clin Exp Res,* 23: 1070–1076.

Rutecki PA, Gidal BE (2002) Antiepileptic drug treatment in the developmentally disabled: treatment considerations with the newer antiepileptic drugs. *Epilepsy Behav* 3: 24–31.

Rutter M (1985) Family and school influences on cognitive development. *J Child Psychol Psychiatry* 26: 683–704.

Rutter M, Tizard J, Yule W, Graham P, Whitmore K (1976) Research report: Isle of Wight Studies, 1964–1974. *Psychol Med* 6: 313–332.

Sanders KD, Cox K, Cannon R, Blanchard D, Pitcher J, Papathakis P, et al. (1990) Growth response to enteral feeding by children with cerebral palsy. *JPEN* 14: 23–26.

Scheerenberger RC (1987) *A History of Mental Retardation: A Quarter Century of Promise.* Baltimore: PH Brookes.

Singh BK, White-Scott S (2002) Role of topiramate in adults with intractable epilepsy, mental retardation, and developmental disabilities. *Seizure* 11: 47–50.

Smith MC, Centorrino F, Welge JA, Collins MA (2004) Clinical comparison of extended-release divalproex versus delayed-release divalproex: pooled data analyses from nine trials. *Epilepsy Behav* 5: 746–751.

Stores G (1999) Children's sleep disorders: modern approaches, developmental effects, and children at special risk. *Dev Med Child Neurol* 41: 568–573.

Sullivan PB, Lambert B, Rose M, Ford-Adams M, Johnson A, Griffiths P (2000) Prevalence and severity of feeding and nutritional problems in children with neurological impairment: Oxford Feeding Study. *Dev Med Child Neurol* 42: 674–680.

Symons FJ, Davis ML, Thompson T (2000) Self-injurious behavior and sleep disturbance in adults with developmental disabilities. *Res Dev Disabil* 21: 115–123.

Tonge BJ, Einfeld SL, Krupinski J, Mackenzie A, McLaughlin M, Florio T, et al. (1996) The use of factor analysis for ascertaining patterns of psychopathology in children with intellectual disability. *J Intellect Disabil Res* 40: 198–207.

Vela-Bueno A, Kales A, Soldatos CR, Dobladez-Blanco B, Campos-Castello J, Espino-Hurtado P, et al. (1984) Sleep in the Prader–Willi syndrome: clinical and polygraphic findings. *Arch Neurol* 41: 294–296.

Walczak TS, Leppik IE, D'Amelio M, Rarick J, So E, Ahman P, et al. (2001) Incidence and risk factors in sudden unexpected death in epilepsy: a prospective cohort study. *Neurology* 56: 519–525.

Webb DW, Fryer AE, Osborne JP (1991) On the incidence of fits and mental retardation in tuberous sclerosis. *J Med Genet* 28: 395–397.

Willemsen-Swinkels SH, Buitelaar JK, Weijnen FG, van Engeland H (1995) Placebo-controlled acute dosage naltrexone study in young autistic children. *Psychiatry Res* 58: 203–215.

Yoshinaga-Itano C (2003) Early intervention after universal neonatal hearing screening: impact on outcomes. *Ment Retard Dev Disabil Res Rev* 9: 252–266.

Zhang LI, Bao S, Merzenich MM (2002) Disruption of primary auditory cortex by synchronous auditory inputs during a critical period. *Proc Natl Acad Sci U S A* 99: 2309–2314.

24

OUTCOMES IN CHILDREN WITH DEVELOPMENTAL DISABILITIES

Annette Majnemer and Catherine Limperopoulos

IMPORTANCE OF OUTCOME DETERMINATION

An outcome can be considered as the end result of a process such as a treatment or service, or the effect(s) of a disease process over time. Outcome determination involves tracking a defined group of individuals longitudinally and characterizing their status at key points in their individual trajectories (Majnemer and Limperopoulos 2002). Outcome measures are tools used to document the characteristics or attributes of interest. These measures may be used serially to objectively document changes that occur as the individual matures, so as to determine the impact of a health condition on an individual and/or the effects of particular treatments or programs. Measures selected must be reliable (i.e. consistency of measurement) and valid (i.e. accuracy in measuring the construct of interest) (Kenny et al. 1991, Law et al. 1999).

Outcomes are important to determine for a variety of reasons. There is a need for greater accountability in a health care system that is facing increasing financial constraints (Stanger and Oresic 2003). New medical and rehabilitation treatment options need to demonstrate their effectiveness in order to be considered an essential, integral, and mandated part of high quality services. A greater emphasis on evidence-based practice further emphasizes the requirement for objective evidence to justify the need for particular services or resources to enhance outcomes as applied to children and youth with developmental disabilities.

Rehabilitation services focus on the enabling–disabling process, and as such are directed at outcomes holistically from pathology to disability and the environmental context (Seelman 2000). Indeed, there is a shift in attention from impairments or deficits to function in spite of actual deficits and from child to family and community. Furthermore, there is an increasing interest in the intrinsic and extrinsic factors that shape developmental progress. Therefore, outcome measures used in clinical practice or research need to cover the spectrum of individual and family health and functioning to reflect this broader focus (Whyte 1998, Helders et al. 2003). Concomitant with this broader focus has been the emergence of many new assessment tools appropriate for children with disabilities.

A variety of 'stakeholders' benefit from outcomes data (Majnemer and Limperopoulos 2002). *Consumers* of our services (i.e. children and especially their families) want objective quantitative evidence of improvements following interventions. Use of standardized outcome measures provides empirical evidence to families of the changes that have occurred with treatment in the domain(s) of interest (Helders et al. 2003, Stanger and Oresic 2003). Outcomes data in the literature on target populations of interest also enable clinicians to counsel families more effectively with respect to realistic expectations for their child's future development. Children and families are increasingly implicated in setting goals and establishing priorities for interventions (i.e. family centered care). Therefore, measures such as the Canadian Occupational Performance Measure allow families to identify areas of greatest personal concern (Law et al. 1999, Manns & Darrah 2006).

Service providers use outcome measures to ascertain the extent to which they are meeting their selected goals of treatment. This promotes a more reflective practice approach, providing necessary feedback to adjust on an ongoing basis intervention strategies to achieve individualized goals (Majnemer and Limperopoulos 2002). Clinicians need to be more accountable, demonstrating to third party payers the benefits of their services. Therefore measures used should be multidimensional so as to capture all possible areas of improvement (Vivier et al. 1994).

Administrators and managers are preoccupied with measuring the impact of health care services so as to justify resource needs (Helders et al. 2003). In addition to measuring outcomes relating to a child's performance and functioning, there is increasing interest in measuring structure and process elements of service delivery itself such as access to care and service utilization, as they can impact on the quality of services and patient satisfaction (Vivier et al. 1994).

Researchers rely on the use of psychometrically sound outcome measures to quantify independent and dependent variables of interest in research studies relating to mechanisms that underlie disability, its natural history, possible predictor variables, and the assessment of treatment efficacy or effectiveness (Kenny et al. 1991, Johnston et al. 2006).

ADVANCES IN OUTCOME RESEARCH
A BROADER FRAMEWORK FOR OUTCOME DETERMINATION
There is an increasing appreciation by clinicians and researchers that a more comprehensive approach to the evaluation of children with disabilities is needed, so that strengths and limitations in all relevant domains may be considered. Recently, the World Health Organization (WHO) endorsed a new classification scheme of health and functioning that provides a broader conceptual framework in which to consider outcomes. The International Classification of Functioning, Disability and Health (ICF) includes components of body structures and functions (structural, psychologic, and physiologic impairments at the organ system level), activity limitations in everyday tasks, and restrictions in participation in various life roles. In addition, contextual factors, whether personal or environmental, that can act

as obstacles or facilitators to functioning and health are also considered in this approach (WHO 2001).

This ICF framework has greatly facilitated a broader approach to outcome determination, as health and functioning is inherently and increasingly recognized as multidimensional, and therefore a comprehensive view of the child is necessary to fully appreciate the impact of a particular health condition (Vivier et al. 1994, Majnemer 2006). For example, when evaluating a 7-year-old child with global developmental delay, it would be important to determine areas of difficulty across developmental domains (i.e. impairments in body function), as well as the impact of any delays on functioning in everyday age-appropriate activities (i.e. personal care, mobility, communication, and socialization skills) and any restrictions in participating fully in all life habits (i.e. at school, in recreational activities, social relationships, domestic chores). In addition, it would be essential to evaluate the primary factors within this child (e.g. motivation, personal preferences) or in his/her environment (e.g. family functioning, resources in the community) that can enhance or limit functioning, as these factors are potentially modifiable.

Traditionally, outcome research in populations with or at risk for developmental disability has focused on mortality and morbidities, such as cognitive impairment (IQ), visual or hearing loss, and objectively documented neurologic abnormalities. High-risk groups were typically compared with a normative sample, and risk factors identified were primarily biomedical in nature, such as gestational age or evidence of a brain lesion. In the past, it was assumed by clinicians that by improving or 'normalizing' one component (e.g. motor impairments such as muscle tone and strength), this would causally and linearly translate into improvements in other components (e.g. increased independence and better quality of life). It is increasingly recognized that without measuring the outcomes that are expected to improve directly or indirectly with treatment, we cannot make the simplistic assumption that these areas will indeed progress (Helders et al. 2003).

Contemporary studies that embrace a more holistic view of the child with a disability apply a wider range of outcome measures that capture a child's functioning more comprehensively (Vivier et al. 1994, Majnemer and Mazer 2004). Recent studies in the literature now focus more on functional limitations and participation in life roles such as maintaining relationships, participating in all school-related tasks, and involvement in community life and recreational activities. There is an apparent greater interest in aspects of the environment that can optimize activity and participation or limit functioning. This includes the physical environment, such as access to services, transport, and adaptations available, the social environment, which includes emotional support by peers and family, and the attitudinal environment, comprises of the level of encouragement and inclusiveness experienced from all individuals within the broader community (Colver 2005). Studies examining determinants of outcomes have also considered a wider range of intrinsic and extrinsic predictor variables, in recognition of the dynamic interplay between an individual's genetic blueprint, possible anatomic anomalies, impairments and activity limitations, and personal and environmental contextual factors (Majnemer and Mazer 2004, Manns and Darrah 2006). This social model of disability and the wide endorsement of the ICF by the clinical and research community have been key facilitators to adoption of a broader view of outcomes and their determinants (Stanger and Oresic 2003, Colver 2005).

COMPLEXITY OF STUDY DESIGNS

In the past, outcome studies were often cross-sectional, involving convenience samples of children, with a primary focus on the first 5 years of life. Increasingly, there are longitudinal cohort studies that follow a well-defined population with or at risk for developmental disability over infancy, childhood, and adolescence, with outcome assessments at key transition points in a child's development (Johnson 1991). There is a growing interest in the risk and resilience factors that can modify (either positively or negatively) a child's developmental trajectory, as this knowledge can guide therapeutic strategies as well as health and social policy to optimize eventual outcomes. For example, family-centered care approaches in rehabilitation have evolved in part because of a greater appreciation of child and family factors that can positively modify outcomes. As a result, identifying a child's activity preferences and a family's priorities for goal-setting, providing active family supports, and addressing resource needs are viewed as important elements of rehabilitation service delivery (Majnemer and Mazer 2004). There is a greater attention in the design of outcome studies to ensure that the subjects recruited are representative of real clinical populations of interest. Furthermore, evaluations are more routinely conducted in a blinded fashion by expert evaluators who are unaware of the specific hypotheses of the study or the medical history of the subjects so as to minimize potential evaluator bias (Kenny et al. 1991, Johnston et al. 2006). Efforts are also directed at minimizing attrition, a further potential source of bias. Finally, there is greater consideration paid to the use of reliable and valid outcome measures (Majnemer and Mazer 2004, Johnston et al. 2006).

This added rigor to study design ensures that policy-makers and health administrators are better informed with respect to the possible resource needs of children and youth with disabilities. Greater understanding of the evolution and progression of outcomes through the lifespan assists clinicians in providing appropriate anticipatory guidance to families. What is increasingly appreciated is that environmental facilitators (i.e. supportive environments) and individual adaptability, in the context of a static medical situation, can enhance the life quality of youth and their family, thus providing mechanisms and strategies to improve these outcomes.

STATISTICAL APPROACHES

Outcomes studies are shifting from descriptive accounts of the proportion of children with delays in particular domains to complex depictions of a range of outcomes with the key intrinsic and extrinsic factors identified that can provide points of intervention to modify outcomes. Theoretical frameworks such as the ICF are applied to statistical approaches and conceptual models are being developed that capture the variables that, either directly or indirectly, collectively influence the outcomes of interests. Increasing statistical and methodologic sophistication is being applied to outcome research (Johnson 1991, Johnston et al. 2006). Efforts to increase sample size are made with multicentre studies to provide adequate statistical power to ask more complex research questions applied to heterogeneous, more representative samples. For observational outcome studies, there is now greater theoretical consideration given to adjustments for possible recognized confounding effects (Greene and Ernhart 1991). Complex statistical approaches such as structural equation modeling are being used to determine the influence, through direct or indirect pathways, of child, family, and environmental factors that collectively modify or influence the outcomes of interest. As a result, statisticians are more actively involved in the research teams that are investigating these complex issues.

In summary, outcome studies embrace a new paradigm of disability as a holistic dynamic interaction between the individual and the environment (Seelman 2000) and, as such, influence strongly the approaches to measurement. Families are ultimately interested in their child's well-being and competency in everyday life skills, not the characteristics of disability (Colver 2005). Traditionally, outcome measures have focused on describing impairments and functional limitations (what they 'can't do'). In order to evaluate the effectiveness of our health and social services, a more holistic perspective of health is needed (Fuhrer 2000). Recently, the concept of health has expanded to invariably include psychosocial elements (i.e. a focus on well-being) in addition to traditional biomedical aspects (i.e. a disease focus). Greater methodologic sophistication and statistical rigor have further enhanced the ability to carefully address complex research questions with regards to the outcomes of children and youth with disabilities.

OUTCOMES IN CHILDREN WITH DEVELOPMENTAL DELAY

Developmental disabilities comprise a heterogeneous group of related chronic disorders of early onset that collectively share a fundamental disturbance in the acquisition of cognitive, motor, language, and/or social skills that result in a substantial and ongoing impact on a child's individual developmental trajectory (Petersen et al. 1998, Shevell et al. 2005a). Essentially, these disorders are considered 'clinical symptom complexes' that lack an objective marker for validation (Shevell 1998). Developmental disabilities currently represent a large proportion of childhood disorders commonly seen in clinical practice. The WHO estimates that worldwide

15–20% of children have disabilities, with global developmental delay and developmental language impairment representing the two most common subtypes of early childhood neurodevelopmental disability encountered in clinical practice (Peterson et al. 1998).

Outcome research in children with developmental delays has focused primarily on biologically 'at risk' children (e.g. neonatal intensive care survivors), or children with an established risk or diagnosis (e.g. Down syndrome, Rett syndrome, cerebral palsy). Conversely, research in children with developmental delay has largely focused on clinical investigations to determine etiological yield and on the development of identification approaches and practice parameters for these disorders (Shevell et al. 2001, 2003, Whelen et al. 2003, Tsai et al. 2005, McDonald et al. 2006, Rydz et al. 2006, Srour et al. 2006). Very few studies have examined outcomes in children with developmental delay in the absence of a known etiologic diagnosis or established risk. The remainder of this chapter focuses on a selective review of outcomes in children diagnosed with global developmental delay and developmental language impairment.

GLOBAL DEVELOPMENTAL DELAY

Global developmental delay constitutes the most common subtype of childhood developmental disability (Petersen et al. 1998). Global developmental delay may be operationally defined as a significant delay (i.e. scores 1.5–2.0 standard deviations below the mean on norm-referenced age-appropriate assessments) in two or more domains including gross/fine motor, cognitive, speech/language, personal/social, or daily living activities (Shevell 1998). Despite the reported high prevalence of global developmental delay, there is a remarkable paucity of studies delineating the outcomes of this population of interest. Consequently, this glaring lack of outcome data has resulted in a limited ability to prognosticate, effectively counsel families, and target early intervention services (Shevell et al. 2005b).

Nevertheless, available evidence from retrospective studies would suggest that older children with mental retardation were initially labeled as globally delayed and that early developmental difficulties do indeed correlate with later academic problems (Silva et al. 1983, Montgomery 1988, Shapiro et al. 1990). For example, early developmental delays have been shown to precede school-aged deficits in handwriting (Sandler et al. 1992), while early perceptual motor difficulties have been documented to precede poor performance on early academic mathematic concepts (Feder and Kerr 1996). Similarly, early motor and cognitive delays have been associated with significant reading difficulties at school age (Shapiro et al. 1990).

A recent prospective study of a relatively large cohort of children with a preschool diagnosis of global developmental delay provided converging evidence for persistent significant difficulties at school age from both a developmental and functional perspective (Shevell et al. 2005a). Poor motor performance was associated with an identified etiology for a child's global developmental delay. Interestingly, the degree of initial delay predicted later functional disabilities, but *not* eventual developmental outcome. Maternal employment and paternal post-secondary education were associated with higher functional communication and socialization skills, suggesting that children in families with a higher socioeconomic status are better able to adapt to their impairments and these parent more effectively advocate for and access needed resources (Shevell et al. 2005a, 2005b).

In summary, a diagnosis of global developmental delay in preschool children has high prognostic validity with regard to persisting global developmental and functional disabilities at school age. Longer term follow-up studies are needed to better delineate early and later predictors of outcome in this group of children.

DEVELOPMENTAL LANGUAGE IMPAIRMENT

Developmental language impairment (DLI) is a common childhood developmental disability with an estimated prevalence of 7.5% (range 5–15%) (Silva 1980, Tomblin et al. 1997, Law et al. 2001, 2003) that is characterized by a primary impairment in language (expressive or receptive language) in a child with normal hearing, cognitive and social function (Nass and Koch 1992). Although the term DLI is increasingly used to characterize this group of children, DLI has also been known as developmental language disorder, specific language impairment, and developmental dysphasia (Silva 1980). For the purposes of this review, DLI will be used to summarize the outcome of this group of children. Importantly, children with a language impairment that is secondary to a neurologic or autism spectrum disorder or global developmental disability or hearing impairment would not fall into the specific diagnostic category or context of DLI.

Typically, children with DLI are diagnosed by health care providers at preschool age (Shevell et al. 2005c). However, delayed acquisition of language milestones is the first indication of language impairment and can be identified at an earlier age. The importance of identifying and distinguishing transient from persistent language delay at an early age has received considerable attention from clinicians. Longitudinal reports have found that more than 40% of 2-year-old toddlers diagnosed with an early language delay have persisting language difficulties at preschool age (3–4 years of age). However, while a high proportion of toddlers do appear to catch up in language development, they may often remain below norms for typically developing children or age-matched controls (Thal and Katich 1996, Paul 2000, Rescorla et al. 2000).

For many children, delayed language development often persists throughout childhood, and interferes with everyday communication and academic attainment (Bishop et al. 2003). Controversy exists regarding the accuracy of prediction of DLI in children diagnosed with a language delay early in life (i.e. 2 years). Some studies have shown that the accuracy of prediction is relatively poor for discriminating persistent versus transient difficulties (Bishop et al. 2003), while others suggest that the vulnerability of early language delay persists at school age (Miniscalco et al. 2005, 2006) and that the observed recovery by school entry may be 'illusionary' (Rescorla et al. 2000, Snowling et al. 2001, Rescorla 2002, 2003, Dale et al. 2003). Overall, diagnostic accuracy appears to improve with increasing age at the time of diagnosis and longer term follow-up of these children.

DLI is operationally defined as a primary impairment in language in a child with otherwise normal cognitive function. However, a review of the literature indicates that 16–89% of children with DLI identified at *preschool age* not only experience ongoing language impairment, but also have more wide-ranging difficulties in development (Webster et al. 2005). Specifically, cognitive impairment is frequently documented in children with DLI at *school age*. Furthermore, DLI is associated with academic and social difficulties that can persist into adulthood (Silva et al. 1983, Aram et al. 1984). Apraxia, sensorimotor, and oromotor difficulties have also been documented on neurologic examination in school-age children with DLI (Mandelbaum et al. 2006). Moreover, several studies have demonstrated that impaired gross and fine motor function is an important and prevalent (range 51–90%) probable co-morbidity associated with DLI in school-aged children (Robinson 1991, Owen et al. 1997, Preis et al. 1997, Rintala et al. 1998, Hill 2001, Bishop 2001, Webster et al. 2005, Mandelbaum et al. 2006). These data strongly suggest that cognitive and motor impairments in preschool children with apparently 'isolated' language impairments are underdiagnosed, or alternatively the possibility of an evolving profile of a more global developmental impairment evident over time has been suggested (Webster et al. 2004).

Evidence from both cross-sectional and prospective longitudinal studies of children with DLI has also demonstrated a heightened risk for psychiatric disorders, particularly attention-deficit–hyperactivity disorder (ADHD) (Beitchman et al. 1996, Snowling et al. 2006). It is important to note that attentional disorders are often underappreciated and inadequately addressed in this population because they are overshadowed by the more evident and troubling neurodevelopmental disorder (Ewen and Shapiro 2005). Broadly speaking, the psychosocial outcomes in *adolescence* of children with a preschool history of DLI are favorable unless the language impairment persists into the school years. Severity and persistence of DLI diagnosed in preschool and low non-verbal IQ children are associated with an increased incidence of attention and social difficulties in adolescence. In a recent longitudinal study, adolescents with attention problems had a profile of specific expressive language difficulties, whereas those with social difficulties had receptive and expressive language difficulties. The presence of both attention and social difficulties was associated with a lower IQ and with more globally apparent language difficulties (Snowling et al. 2006).

Although several studies have examined the longitudinal trajectory of childhood DLI and adult outcomes, methodologic limitations including heterogeneous samples, varied inclusion and exclusion criteria, as well as retrospective or cross-sectional study designs have limited their clinical applicability and utility. Nonetheless, available reports have documented that DLI, once diagnosed, tends to persist into later childhood (Johnson et al. 1999, Conti-Ramsden et al. 2001) and adolescence (Aram et al. 1984, Tomblin et al. 1997, Stothard et al. 1998). Deficits in literacy development and later academic attainment have been shown to become apparent over time and have been identified as important consequences of an early diagnosis of DLI (Stothard et al. 1998, Mawhood et al. 2000, Conti-Ramsden et al. 2001). In a recent study, receptive DLI was associated with significant deficits in a theory of mind, verbal short-term memory, and phonologic processing. In addition to cognitive and memory deficits, substantial social adaptation difficulties and an increased risk of psychiatric disorders have also been reported in *adult* life (Clegg et al. 2005). However, little is known about the impact of DLI on adolescent and adults.

In summary, a diagnosis of DLI is often associated with ongoing language impairment, in addition to far-reaching developmental consequences that extend well beyond the language domain and beyond childhood. Further studies are needed to better delineate possible early predictors of persistent versus transient DLI, as well as other co-morbidities.

CONCLUSIONS AND FUTURE DIRECTIONS

Studies to date strongly support the importance of systematic and programmatic developmental surveillance at key intervals in the lifespan in order to monitor developmental progress to identify, perhaps in an active anticipatory way, ongoing difficulties that will lead to target interventions and resource needs for children continuing to struggle. Ongoing studies delineating the outcomes of children with global development delay and DLI will require the systematic use of operationally defined study populations to ensure that results are clinically applicable. Furthermore, greater focus needs to be placed on evaluating the multiple domains in a child's health and well-being, as well as the relationship between the child's impairments and his/her activity limitations, in order to target services that minimize barriers to school and community participation.

Although there is an increasing number of high quality developmental outcome studies, strong evidence of the broad range of outcomes for children with GDD and DLI is still lacking (Johnston et al. 2006). Future prospective cohort studies should use a broader framework for outcome determination in well-defined clinical populations evaluated intermittently at key transition points in child, adolescent, and adult development. These cohort studies should be scientifically rigorous using large sample sizes, complex statistical approaches, blinded evaluation, reliable and valid outcome measures, and efforts to minimize ongoing study attrition. In particular, examination of potential intrinsic and extrinsic risk factors that may positively or negatively influence outcomes need to be identified so as to rationally guide service delivery and health policy planning.

REFERENCES

Aram DM, Ekelman BL, Nation JE (1984) Preschoolers with language disorders: 10 years later. *J Speech Hear Res* 27: 232–244.

Beitchman JH, Brownlie EB, Inglis A, Wild J, Ferguson B (1996) Seven-year follow up of speech/language impaired and control children: psychiatric outcome. *J Child Psychol Psychiatry* 37: 961–970.

Bishop DM (2001) Motor immaturity and specific language impairment: evidence from a common genetic basis. *Am J Med Genet* 114: 56–63.

Bishop DV, Price TS, Dale PS, Plomin R (2003) Outcomes of early language delay: II. Etiology of transient and persistent language difficulties. *J Speech Lang Hear Res* 46: 561–575.

Clegg J, Hollis C, Mahwood L, Rutter M (2005) Developmental language disorders: a follow-up in later adult life. Cognitive, language and psychosocial outcomes. *J Child Psychol Psychiatry* 46: 128–149.

Colver A (2005) A shared framework and language for childhood disability. *Dev Med Child Neurol* 47: 780–784.

Conti-Ramsden G, Botting N, Simkin Z, Knox E (2001) Follow-up of children attending infant language units: outcomes at 11 years of age. *Int J Lang Commun Disord* 36: 207–220.

Dale PS, Price TS, Plomin R (2003) Outcomes of early language delay: I. Predicting persistent and transient language difficulties at 3 and 4 years. *J Speech Lang Hear Res* 46: 544–560.

Ewen JB, Shapiro BK (2005) Disorders of attention or learning in neurodevelopmental disorders. *Semin Pediatr Neurol* 12: 229–241.

Feder K, Kerr R (1996) Aspects of motor performance and pre-academic learning. *Can J Occup Ther* 63: 293–303.

Fuhrer MJ (2000) Subjectifying quality of life as a medical rehabilitation outcome: review. *Disabil Rehabil* 22: 481–489.

Greene T, Ernhart CB (1991) Adjustment for cofactors in pediatric research. *Dev Behav Pediatr* 12: 378–386.

Helders PJM, Engelbert RHH, Custers JWH, Gorter JW, Takken T, Van Der Net J (2003) Creating and being created: the changing panorama of paediatric rehabilitation. *Pediatr Rehabil* 6: 5–12.

Hill EL (2001) Non-specific nature of specific langue impairments: a review of the literature with regard to concomitant motor impairments. *Int J Lang Commun Disord* 36: 149–171.

Johnson SB (1991) Methodological considerations in pediatric behavioural research: measurement. *Dev Behav Pediatr* 12: 361–369.

Johnson CJ, Beitchman JH, Young A, Escobar M, Atkinson L, Wilson B, et al. (1999) Fourteen-year follow-up of children with and without speech/language impairments: speech/language stability and outcomes. *J Speech Lang Hear Res* 42: 744–760.

Johnston MV, Sherer M, Whyte J (2006) Applying evidence standards to rehabilitation research. *Am J Phys Med Rehabil* 85: 292–309.

Kenny TJ, Holden EW, Santilli L (1991) The meaning of measures: pitfalls in behavioural and developmental research. *Dev Behav Pediatr* 12: 355–360.

Law J, Boyle J, Harris F, Harkness A, Nye C (2001) Prevalence and natural history of primary speech and language delay: findings from a systematic review of the literature. *Int J Commun Disord* 35: 165–188.

Law J, Garrett Z, Nye C (2003) Speech and language therapy interventions for children with primary speech and language delay or disorder (Review). *Cochrane Database Syst Rev* CD004110.

Law M, King G, Russell D, MacKinnon E, Hurley P, Murphy C (1999) Measuring outcomes in children's rehabilitation: a decision protocol. *Arch Phys Med Rehabil* 80: 629–636.

Majnemer A (2006) Assessment tools for cerebral palsy: new directions. *Future Neurol* 1: 755–763.

Majnemer A, Limperopoulos C (2002) Importance of outcome determination in pediatric rehabilitation. *Dev Med Child Neurol* 44: 773–777.

Majnemer A, Mazer B (2004) New directions in the outcome evaluation of children with cerebral palsy. *Semin Pediatr Neurol* 11: 11–17.

Mandelbaum DE, Stevens M, Rosenberg E, Wiznitzer M (2006) Sensorimotor performance in school-age children with autism, developmental language disorder, or low IQ. *Dev Med Child Neurol* 48: 33–39.

Manns PJ, Darrah J (2006) Linking research and clinical practice in physical therapy: strategies for integration. *Physiotherapy* 92: 88–94.

Mawhood L, Howlin P, Rutter M (2000) Autism and developmental receptive language disorder: a comparative follow up in early adult life: I. Cognitive and language outcomes. *J Child Psychol Psychiatry* 41: 547–559.

McDonald L, Rennie A, Tolmie J, Galloway P, McWilliam R (2006) Investigation of global developmental delay. *Arch Dis Child Fetal Neonatal Edn* 91: 701–705.

Miniscalco C, Nygren G, Hagberg B, Kadesjö B, Gillberg C (2006) Neuropsychiatric and neurodevelopmental outcome of children at age 6 and 7 years who screened positive for language problems at 30 months. *Dev Med Child Neurol* 48: 361–366.

Miniscalco C, Westerlund M, Lohmander A (2005) Language skills at age 6 years in Swedish children screened for language delay at $2^1/2$ years of age. *Acta Paediatrica* 94: 1798–1806.

Montgomery TR (1988) Clinical aspects of mental retardation: the chief complaint. *Clin Pediatr* 27: 529–531.

Nass RD, Koch D (1992) Disorders of higher cognitive cortical function in preschoolers. In: David R (ed) *Neurology for the Clinician.* Norwalk, Connecticut: Appleton & Lange, pp 493–514.

Owen SE, McKinlay IA (1997) Motor difficulties in children with developmental disorders of speech and language. *Child Care Health Dev* 23: 315–325.

Paul R (2000) Predicting outcomes of early expressive language delay: ethical implications. In: Bishop DVM, Leonard LB (eds) *Speech and Language Impairments in Children: Causes, Characteristics, Intervention and Outcome.* Philadelphia: Psychology Press, pp 195–209.

Petersen MC, Kube DA, Palmer FB (1998) Classification of developmental delays. *Semin Pediatr Neurol* 5: 2–14.

Preis S, Schittler P, Lenard HG (1997) Motor performance and handedness in children with developmental language disorder. *Neuropediatrics* 28: 324–327.

Rescorla L (2002) Language and reading outcomes to age 9 in late-talking toddlers. *J Speech Lang Hear Res* 45: 360–361.

Rescorla L (2003) Do late-talking toddlers turn out to have reading difficulties a decade later? *Ann Dyslexia* 50: 87–102.

Rescorla L, Dayosgaard K, Singh L (2000) Late-talking toddlers: MLU and IPSyn outcomes at 3;0 and 4;0. *J Child Lang* 27: 293–311.

Rintala P, Pienimaki K, Ahonen T, Cantell M, Kooistar L (1998) The effects of a pyschomotor training programme on motor skill development in children with developmental language disorders. *Human Move Sci* 17: 721–731.

Robinson RJ (1991) Causes and associations of severe and persistent specific speech and language disorders in children. *Dev Med Child Neurol* 33: 943–962.

Rydz D, Srour M, Oskoui M, Marget N, Shiller M, Birnbaum R, et al. (2006) Screening for developmental delay in the setting of a community pediatric clinic: a prospective assessment of parent-report questionnaires. *Pediatrics* 118: 1178–1186.

Sandler AD, Watson TE, Footo M (1992) Neurodevelopmental study of writing disorders in middle childhood. *Dev Behav Pediatr* 13: 17–23.

Seelman KD (2000) Rehabilitation science. *Technol Disabil* 12: 77–83.

Shapiro BK, Palmer FB, Antell S, Bilker S, Ross A, Capute AJ (1990) Precursors of reading delay: neurodevelopmental milestones. *Pediatrics* 85: 416–420.

Shevell M, Ashwal S, Donley D, Flint J, Gingold M, Hirtz D, et al. (2003) Quality Standards Subcommittee of the American Academy of Neurology, Practice Committee of the Child Neurology Society. Practice parameter: evaluation of the child with global developmental delay: report of the Quality Standards Subcommittee of the American Academy of Neurology and The Practice Committee of the Child Neurology Society. *Neurology* 60: 367–380.

Shevell M, Majnemer A, Platt RW, Webster R, Birnbaum R (2005a) Developmental and functional outcomes at school age of preschool children with global developmental delay. *J Child Neurol* 20: 648–653.

Shevell M, Majnemer A, Platt RW, Webster R, Birnbaum R (2005b) Developmental and functional outcomes in children with global developmental delay or developmental language impairment. *Dev Med Child Neurol* 47: 678–683.

Shevell MI (1998) The evaluation of the child with a global developmental delay. *Semin Pediatr Neurol* 5: 21–26.

Shevell MI, Majnemer A, Rosenbaum P, Abrahamowicz M (2001) Etiologic determination of childhood developmental delay. *Brain Dev* 23: 228–235.

Shevell MI, Majnemer A, Webster RI, Platt RW, Birnbaum R (2005c) Outcomes at school age of preschool children with developmental language impairment. *Pediatr Neurol* 32: 264–269.

Silva PA (1980) The prevalence, stability and significance of developmental language delay in preschool children. *Dev Med Child Neurol* 22: 768–777.

Silva PA, McGee R, Williams SM (1983) Developmental language delay from three to seven years and its significance for low intelligence and reading difficulties at age seven. *Dev Med Child Neurol* 25: 783–793.

Snowling M, Adams C, Bisohp DVM, Stothard SE (2001) Educational attainments of school leavers with a preschool history of speech-language impairments. *Int J Lang Commun Disord* 36: 173–183.

Snowling MJ, Bishop DV, Stothard SE, Chipchase B, Kaplan C (2006) Psychosocial outcomes at 15 years of children with a preschool history of speech-language impairment. *J Child Psychol Psychiatry* 47: 759–765.

Srour M, Mazer, B, Shevell MI (2006) Analysis of clinical features predicting etiologic yield in the assessment of global developmental delay. *Pediatrics* 118: 139–145.

Stanger M, Oresic S (2003) Rehabilitation approaches for children with cerebral palsy: overview. *J Child Neurol* 18: S79–S88.

Stothard SE, Snowling MJ, Bishop DVM, Chipchase BB, Kaplan CA (1998) Language-impaired preschoolers: a follow-up into adolescence. *J Speech Lang Res* 41: 407–418.

Thal DJ, Katich J (1996) Predicaments in early identification of specific language impairment: does the early bird always catch the worm? In Cole KN, Dale PS, Thal DJ (eds) *Assessment of Communication and Language.* Baltimore, Maryland: Paul H Brookes, pp 1–28.

Tomblin JB, Records NL, Buckwater P, Smith E, O'Brien M (1997) Prevalence of specific language impairment in kindergarten children. *J Speech Lang Hear Res* 40: 1245–1260.

Tsai JT, Kuo HT, Chou IC, Tsai MY, Tsai CH (2005) A clinical analysis of children with developmental delay. *Acta Paediatr Taiwan* 46: 192–195.

Vivier PM, Bernier JA, Starfield B (1994) Current approaches to measuring health outcomes in pediatric research. *Curr Opin Pediatr* 6: 530–537.

Webster RI, Majnemer A, Platt RW, Shevell MI (2004) The predictive value of a preschool diagnosis of developmental language impairment. *Neurology* 63: 2327–2331.

Webster RI, Majnemer A, Platt RW, Shevell MI (2005) Motor function at school age in children with a preschool diagnosis of developmental language impairment. *J Pediatr* 146: 80–85.

Whelen M, Crawford T, Comi A, Freeman JM, Kossoff EH, Singer H, et al. (2003) Practice parameter: evaluation of the child with global developmental delay (comments). *Neurology* 61: 1315–1316.

Whyte J (1998) Enabling America: a report from the Institute of Medicine on Rehabilitation Science and Engineering. *Arch Phys Med Rehabil* 79: 1477–1480.

World Health Organization (2001) *International Classification of Functioning, Disability and Health.* Geneva: WHO (www.who.int/classification/icf).

INDEX